EVIDENCE-BASED
PRACTICE

ACROSS THE HEALTH PROFESSIONS

FOURTH
EDITION

EVIDENCE-BASED PRACTICE

ACROSS THE HEALTH PROFESSIONS

TAMMY **HOFFMANN**

SALLY **BENNETT**

CHRIS **DEL MAR**

ELSEVIER

ELSEVIER

Elsevier Australia. ACN 001 002 357
(a division of Reed International Books Australia Pty Ltd)
Tower 1, 475 Victoria Avenue, Chatswood, NSW 2067

ISBN: 978-0-7295-4443-6

Notice

Practitioners and researchers must always rely on their own experience and knowledge in evaluating and using any information, methods, compounds or experiments described herein. Because of rapid advances in the medical sciences, in particular, independent verification of diagnoses and drug dosages should be made. To the fullest extent of the law, no responsibility is assumed by Elsevier, authors, editors or contributors for any injury and/or damage to persons or property as a matter of products liability, negligence or otherwise, or from any use or operation of any methods, products, instructions, or ideas contained in the material herein.

National Library of Australia Cataloguing-in-Publication Data

A catalogue record for this book is available from the National Library of Australia

---

Senior Content Strategist: Natalie Hunt and Dorothy Chiu
Content Project Manager: Kritika Kaushik
Copy edited by Robyn Flemming
Proofread by Tim Learner
Cover design by Gopalakrishnan Venkatraman
Index by SPi Global

Typeset by GW Tech

Printed in China by 1010 Printing International Ltd.

Last digit is the print number: 9 8 7 6 5 4 3 2 1

Dedication

Tammy and Sally dedicate this edition to Professor Chris Del Mar, who passed away shortly before it was published. Chris was renowned locally, nationally and internationally for his superior skills in, and commitment to, teaching evidence-based practice. He was a passionate advocate for evidence, clinical research, patient-centredness, and questioning assumptions in health care. Chris leaves an enormous legacy in his various fields of research. One indelible legacy is the immeasurable contribution that he made towards training and inspiring thousands of students and clinicians to provide evidence-based care. This book has influenced our lives in ways that we never could have imagined, and we are deeply privileged to have been able to learn from and partner with him.

From Tammy: to the most wonderful husband I could have ever wished for. Thank you for every moment. I will be forever grateful to this book for bringing us together. You are so very dearly missed.

FOREWORD

The COVID-19 pandemic highlighted the critical importance of research evidence to inform clinical practice and policy worldwide. Never before have we seen such a pressing demand for evidence from the public, clinicians and policy makers. Unfortunately, alongside the COVID-19 pandemic, we also experienced a massive, global misinformation pandemic. The impact of misinformation is substantial—eroding public trust and causing deaths and increased morbidity worldwide. This impact was particularly harsh for those with compounding vulnerabilities. In turn, the misinformation pandemic shone light on the need for all decision makers to seek and appraise evidence. But how is this done?

This fourth edition of *Evidence-Based Practice Across the Health Professions*, edited by Professors Tammy Hoffmann, Sally Bennett and Chris Del Mar, is well-timed to meet this need! This book provides the foundations of evidence-based practice from asking questions, through to seeking, appraising and using evidence in decision making. Particularly helpful are the tips on embedding evidence into routine clinical care, which targets individual clinicians and organisations. At the individual clinician level there is much needed discussion of shared decision making and the book provides practical approaches to incorporating this into clinical care. Some of the commonly reported barriers to evidence-based practice are identified and strategies for overcoming these provided.

Optimising research evidence use in decision making must happen at all levels within the health care system and include the public, clinicians, patients, managers and policy makers. Without this focus, research will be wasted and its impact on patients and the health care (and public health) system will not be realised. We have an ethical and moral imperative to avoid research waste and to use high-quality evidence in health decision making. The latest edition of this book provides the way forward.

Finally, this work is a wonderful legacy of the amazing Professor Del Mar. His commitment to evidence-based practice in his own practice and teaching, while also advancing its methods, served as an exemplar for all of us. This book ensures that his legacy and impact on patients and clinicians continues into the future.

Sharon E Straus, CM, MD, MSc, FRCPC, CAHS, FRSC
Professor, Department of Medicine
University of Toronto

AUTHORS

Tammy Hoffmann OAM, BOccThy (Hons 1), PhD, FOTARA, FAHMS

Professor of Clinical Epidemiology, Institute for Evidence-Based Healthcare, Faculty of Health Sciences and Medicine, Bond University, Gold Coast, Australia

Tammy has been teaching and researching about evidence-based practice and shared decision making for over 20 years and has an international reputation in her various areas of research. Her research spans many aspects of shared decision making, evidence-based practice, informed health decisions, improving the reporting and uptake of effective interventions, reporting guidelines, knowledge translation, minimising waste in research and the teaching of evidence-based practice.

Sally Bennett BOccThy (Hons), PhD, FOTARA

Professor in Occupational Therapy, School of Health and Rehabilitation Sciences, The University of Queensland, Brisbane, Australia

Sally has extensive experience in teaching and research about evidence-based practice and knowledge translation. Her research interests are about building capacity for knowledge translation and translating knowledge for care of people living with dementia. She was one of the leaders of the internationally recognised OTseeker database that provided evidence relevant to occupational therapy. She has been actively involved at the professional level both nationally and internationally, including having been associate editor on a number of occupational therapy journals.

Chris Del Mar AM, BSc, MA, MB BChir, MD, FRACGP, FAFPHM, FAHMS

Professor of Public Health and academic General Practitioner, Institute for Evidence-Based Healthcare, Faculty of Health Sciences and Medicine, Bond University, Gold Coast, Australia

Chris worked as a full-time general practitioner for many years before becoming Professor of General Practice at the University of Queensland. He was invited to become the Dean of a new Health Sciences and Medicine Faculty and to develop a new medical program at Bond University. He was also Pro-Vice Chancellor (Research) at Bond University. After overseeing the graduation of the first cohort of medical students, he stepped back from those roles so that he could return his focus to research and teaching and was Professor of Public Health until 2022. Chris's international reputation is in the management of acute respiratory infections (for 20 years, he was the coordinating editor of the Cochrane Acute Respiratory Infections Group); general practice research; evidence-based medicine and systematic reviews; and randomised controlled trials, in both clinical medicine and health services research.

CONTRIBUTORS

Bridget Abell BAppSc (HMS-Exercise Science), MSc, PhD
Implementation Scientist and Early Career Health Services Researcher, Australian Centre for Health Services Innovation, Queensland University of Technology (QUT), Brisbane, Australia

Loai Albarqouni MD, MSc, PhD
Assistant Professor, Institute for Evidence-Based Healthcare, Faculty of Health Sciences and Medicine, Bond University, Gold Coast, Australia

Mina Bahkit BMedSurg, MA, PhD
Research Fellow, Institute for Evidence-Based Healthcare, Faculty of Health Sciences and Medicine, Bond University, Gold Coast, Australia

Lauren Ball BAppSc, Grad Cert (Higher Ed), Grad Dip Health Economics and Health Policy, M Nutrition & Dietetics (Honours), PhD
Professor of Community Health and Wellbeing, The University of Queensland, Brisbane, Australia

John Bennett BMedSc, MBBS, BA (Hons), PhD, FRACGP, FACHI
General Practitioner, UQ Healthcare, The University of Queensland, Brisbane, Australia

Fiona Bogossian RN, RM, DipAppSci (NEd), BAppSci, MPH, PhD, FACM
Professor, Practice Education in Health, Academic Lead USC Clinical School, University of the Sunshine Coast, Sunshine Coast, Australia

Malcolm Boyle ADipBus, ADipHSc (Amb Off), MICA Cert, BInfoTech, MClinEpi, PhD
Associate Professor and Academic Lead in Paramedicine Education, School of Medicine and Dentistry, Griffith University, Gold Coast, Australia

Mary Bushell BPharm (Hons), AACPA, GCTLHE, AFACP, MPS, PhD
Clinical Assistant Professor, Discipline of Pharmacy, School of Health Sciences, Faculty of Health, University of Canberra, Canberra, Australia

Ryan Causby B Podiatry, M Podiatry, PhD
Program Director Podiatry, Allied Health and Human Performance Unit, University of South Australia, Adelaide, Australia

Justin Clark BA
Senior Research Information Specialist, Institute for Evidence-Based Healthcare, Faculty of Health Sciences and Medicine, Bond University, Gold Coast, Australia

Jeff Coombes BEd (Hons), BAppSc, MEd, PhD
Professor, School of Human Movement and Nutrition Sciences, The University of Queensland, Brisbane, Australia

Scott Devenish MaVEdT, BNur, Dip Para Sc, RN, RPara (Aus), FACP, FHEA, PhD
Associate Professor in Paramedicine and Head of Discipline, School of Nursing, Midwifery and Paramedicine, Faculty of Health, Australian Catholic University, Brisbane, Australia

Fiona Dobson BAppSc (Physiotherapy), Postgraduate Diploma (Health Research Methods), PhD
Associate Professor, Department of Physiotherapy, Melbourne School of Health Sciences, The University of Melbourne, Melbourne, Australia

Jenny Doust BEcons, BMBS, Grad Dip Clin Epi, FRACGP, PhD
Clinical Professor Research Fellow, Australian Women and Girls' Health Research (AWaGHR) Centre, School of Public Health, Faculty of Medicine, The University of Queensland, Brisbane, Australia

Carolyn Ee MBBS, FRACGP, BAppSci (Chinese Med), MMed, GradCert Med Acup, PhD
Senior Research Fellow, NICM Health Research Institute, Western Sydney University, Penrith, Australia

Roma Forbes BHSc (Physiotherapy), MHSc (Hons), Grad Cert (HigherEd), PhD
Senior Lecturer in Physiotherapy, School of Health and Rehabilitation Sciences, The University of Queensland, Brisbane, Australia

Elizabeth Gibson BOccThy, PhD
Senior Research Fellow, Institute for Evidence-Based Healthcare, Faculty of Health Sciences and Medicine, Bond University, Gold Coast, Australia

Paul Glasziou AO, MBBS, FRACGP, MRCGP, FAHMS, PhD
Professor of Evidence-Based Medicine and Director of the Institute for Evidence-Based Healthcare, Bond University, Gold Coast, Australia

Ian Graham FCAHS, FNYAM, FRSC, PhD

Distinguished Professor, Senior Scientist, Centre for Practice-Changing Research, Ottawa Hospital Research Institute, Ottawa, Canada

Romi Haas BPhysio (Hons), MPH, PhD

Research Fellow, Department of Epidemiology and Preventive Medicine, School of Public Health and Preventive Medicine, Monash University; and Monash-Cabrini Department of Musculoskeletal Health and Clinical Epidemiology, Cabrini Health, Melbourne, Australia

Karin Hannes MSc Edu, MSc Med, PhD

Professor in Transdisciplinary Studies, Creative Research Methodology and Meta-Synthesis at Research Group SoMeTHin'K (Social, Methodological and Theoretical Innovation / Kreative), Faculty of Social Sciences, University of Leuven, Leuven, Belgium

Joanna Harnett MHSc, BHSc (Complementary Medicines), Grad Cert Educational Studies (HigherEd), PhD

Senior Lecturer, School of Pharmacy, The University of Sydney, Sydney, Australia

Joy Higgs AM, BSc, MHPEd, PhD, PFHEA

Emeritus Professor in Higher Education, Charles Sturt University, Sydney, Australia

Kylie Hill BSc (Physiotherapy), PhD

Associate Professor, Curtin School of Allied Health, Faculty of Health Sciences, Curtin University, Perth, Australia

Isabelle Jalbert OD, MPH, PhD

Associate Professor, School of Optometry and Vision Science, Faculty of Medicine and Health, The University of New South Wales, Sydney, Australia

Jacqueline Jauncey-Cooke RN, MN, Grad Dip Crit Care, Grad Cert Health Prof Educ, PhD

Senior Lecturer, School of Nursing, Midwifery and Social Work, The University of Queensland, Brisbane, Australia

Sohil Khan MPharm (Clin Pharm), MBA, PhD

Faculty of Pharmacotherapeutics and Evidence Based Practice, School of Pharmacy and Medical Sciences, Griffith University, Gold Coast, Australia

Nerida Klupp BAppScPod (Hons), PhD

Senior Lecturer, School of Health Sciences, Western Sydney University, Penrith, Australia

Karl Landorf Dip App Sc, Grad Cert Clin Instr, Grad Dip Ed, PhD

Professor of Podiatry, Associate Dean, Research and Industry Engagement, School of Allied Health and La Trobe Sport and Exercise Medicine Research Centre, La Trobe University, Melbourne, Australia

David Long Adv Dip Paramed Sc (Amb), BEd (Hab), BHlthSc (Pre-Hosp Care), GCertAcadPrac, PhD

Senior Lecturer (Paramedicine), School of Health and Medical Sciences, University of Southern Queensland, Ipswich, Australia

Amary Mey BPharm (Hons), PhD

Lecturer, School of Pharmacy and Medical Sciences, Griffith University, Gold Coast, Australia

Zachary Munn Grad Dip (Health Sciences), B Med Radiation (Nuclear Medicine), PhD

Director of Evidence-based Healthcare Research, JBI, Faculty of Health and Medical Sciences, The University of Adelaide, Adelaide, Australia

Natalie Munro BAppSc (Speech Pathology) (Hons I), Grad Cert (HigherEd), CPSP, SFHEA, PhD

Associate Professor, Faculty of Medicine and Health, The University of Sydney, Sydney, Australia

Shannon Munteanu BPod (Hons), PhD

Professor of Podiatry, Discipline of Podiatry, School of Allied Health, Human Services and Sport, La Trobe University, Melbourne, Australia

Denise O'Connor BAppScOT (Hons), PhD

Associate Professor (Research), School of Public Health and Preventive Medicine, Monash University, Melbourne, Australia

Rebecca Packer BSpPath (Hons), GCHEd, PhD

Lecturer in Speech Pathology, School of Health and Rehabilitation Sciences, The University of Queensland, Brisbane, Australia

Matthew Page BBSc (Hons), PhD

Senior Research Fellow, Deputy Head of the Methods in Evidence Synthesis Unit, School of Public Health and Preventive Medicine, Monash University, Melbourne, Australia

Toby Pavey BSc, MSc, PhD

Associate Professor in Physical Activity, Sedentary Behaviour and Health, School of Exercise and Nutrition Sciences, Queensland University of Technology, Brisbane, Australia

John Pierce BSpPath, Postgraduate Diploma (Health Research Methodology), PhD
Postdoctoral Research Fellow, Centre of Research Excellence in Aphasia Recovery and Rehabilitation, School of Allied Heath, Human Services and Sport, La Trobe University, Melbourne, Australia

Emma Power BAppSc (Speech Path, Hons 1), PhD
Associate Professor, Speech Pathology, Graduate School of Health, University of Technology Sydney, Sydney, Australia

Claire Rickard BN, RN, GradDip (CriticalCare), FAHMS, FACN, PhD
Professor of Infection Prevention and Vascular Access, Metro North Health and School of Nursing, Midwifery and Social Work, The University of Queensland, Brisbane, Australia

Sharon Sanders BSc (Pod), MPH, PhD
Assistant Professor, Institute for Evidence-Based Healthcare, Faculty of Health Sciences and Medicine, Bond University, Gold Coast, Australia

Katrina Schmid BAppSc (Opt) (Hons), Grad Cert (Ocular Therapeutics), Therapeutically Endorsed Optometrist, Grad Cert (HigherEd), SFHEA, AFHEA (Indigenous), PhD
Associate Professor, School of Optometry and Vision Science, Faculty of Health, Queensland University of Technology, Brisbane, Australia

Michal Schneider BSc, Grad Dip Ed, M Rep Sc, Grad Cert Health Prof Edu, PhD
Professor, Department of Medical Imaging and Radiation Sciences, Monash University, Melbourne, Australia

Ian Scott FRACP, MHA, MEd
Professor and Director of Internal Medicine and Clinical Epidemiology, Princess Alexandra Hospital, Brisbane, Australia and Faculty of Medicine, The University of Queensland, Brisbane, Australia

Nichola Shelton BA (Hons), MA, GDip, MSLP, CPSP
PhD candidate, Faculty of Medicine and Health, The University of Sydney, Sydney, Australia

Rachel Thompson BPsySci (Hons), PhD
Senior Lecturer, School of Health Sciences, Faculty of Medicine and Health, The University of Sydney, Sydney, Australia

Leigh Tooth BOccThy (Hons), PhD
Associate Professor, Principal Research Fellow and Deputy Director of the Australian Longitudinal Study on Women's Health, School of Public Health, The University of Queensland, Brisbane, Australia

Adrian Traeger MPhty, BSc (Hons I), PhD
Research Fellow, School of Public Health, The University of Sydney, Sydney, Australia

Merrill Turpin BOccThy, Grad Dip Counsel, PhD
Senior Lecturer, School of Health and Rehabilitation Sciences, The University of Queensland, Brisbane, Australia

Adam P Vogel BA, MSc (SpPth), PhD
Professor, Head of Speech Pathology, School of Health Sciences, The University of Melbourne, Melbourne, Australia; and Redenlab Inc., Australia

Cynthia Wensley RN, MHSc, PGDip Health Systems Management, BA Social Sciences (Nursing), PhD
Lecturer, Faculty of Medical and Health Sciences, Nursing, University of Auckland, New Zealand

Shelley Wilkinson BSc (Hons) (Psyc), Grad Dip Nut & Diet, PhD
Associate Professor, School of Human Movement and Nutrition Sciences, Faculty of Health and Behavioural Sciences, The University of Queensland, Brisbane, Australia

Kylie Williams BPharm, Grad Dip Hosp Pharm, PhD
Professor and Head, Discipline of Pharmacy, University of Technology Sydney, Sydney, Australia

Caroline Wright BSc (Hons), MSc, DCR Therapy, PGCE, PhD
Associate Professor, Department of Medical Imaging and Radiation Sciences, Monash University, Melbourne, Australia

Joshua R Zadro BAppSc (Phty) (Hons 1), PhD
Research Fellow, Institute for Musculoskeletal Health, Sydney School of Public Health, Faculty of Medicine and Health, The University of Sydney, Sydney, Australia

Leanne Bisset MPhty (Manipulative), MPhty (Sports), BPhty, PhD
Griffith University, Gold Coast, Queensland, Australia

Melissa Carey BN, MN, MAP (HCR)
University of Southern Queensland, Queensland, Australia

Anne Cusick MA (Psych), MA (Interdisc Stud), Grad Dip Beh Sc, Grad Cert Bus Admin, BAppSc (OT), Dip AICD, PhD
Professor, Faculty of Medicine and Health, The University of Sydney, Sydney, New South Wales, Australia; Adjunct Professor, College of Health & Human Sciences, Charles Darwin University, Casuarina, Northern Territory, Australia; Emeritus Professor, Western Sydney University, Campbelltown, New South Wales, Australia

Thanya Pathirana MPH, MBBS, PhD
Senior Lecturer in Medical Education, Associate Lead in Doctor and Health in the Community theme, MD program, School of Medicine and Dentistry, Griffith University, Sunshine Coast, Queensland, Australia

Cynthia Wensley MHSc, BA, RN, PhD
School of Nursing, Faculty of Medical and Health Sciences, The University of Auckland, Auckland, New Zealand

PREFACE

Each time we work on a new edition of this book, there are various methodological developments and new resources and literature to incorporate. The field of evidence-based practice continues to mature and, gratifyingly, it is becoming expected and commonplace in more health settings, disciplines and curricula. The COVID-19 pandemic accentuated the importance of being able to rapidly generate, appraise and disseminate quality evidence for decision making (at individual, health system and global policy levels).

An interdisciplinary approach is best in evidence-based practice and health care, and we are delighted that there are now 16 disciplines represented in the book. We are very appreciative of the 56 contributors to this edition, who are national or international experts in their fields and readily prepared the chapters and worked examples for this edition. Thank you for partnering with us to help teach the skills of evidence-based practice and further its uptake.

Since the book's previous edition, the three of us have had numerous interactions with the health system as patients and family for very serious and minor health conditions. In some of these encounters, we have experienced evidence-based *and* patient-centred care. What a difference it has made when this has occurred. We urge all health professionals, and soon-to-be health professionals, who use this book to learn skills in evidence-based practice to not underestimate the impact that *your* interaction can have on a patient and their family. Providing advice and care that is based on the best available evidence, and carefully considering the way in which you discuss the options with your patient and involve them in the decision making, are powerful strategies that are at your disposal. We hope that you can use this book to learn or refine these skills so that your patients receive the best care possible.

Tammy Hoffmann, Sally Bennett, Chris Del Mar

ACKNOWLEDGMENTS

Thank you to the reviewers who provided useful suggestions. We are particularly grateful to our colleagues, especially Dr Libby Gibson, Dr Sharon Sanders and Dr Romi Haas, who willingly stepped in to assist with finalising content for this edition when its timely completion was threatened.

The publisher would like to remember Professor Chris Del Mar who passed away shortly before the publication of this text. Alongside his extensive contribution to the field of evidence-based practice, Chris's invaluable work on all editions of this text is greatly acknowledged with much thanks.

CONTENTS

Introduction to Evidence-Based Practice

Tammy Hoffmann, Sally Bennett and Chris Del Mar

LEARNING OBJECTIVES

After reading this chapter, you should be able to:
- Explain what is meant by the term 'evidence-based practice'
- Understand the origins of evidence-based practice
- Explain why evidence-based practice is important
- Describe the scope of evidence-based health care
- List and briefly explain each of the five steps that make up the evidence-based practice process

WHAT IS EVIDENCE-BASED PRACTICE?

There is a famous definition by Professor David Sackett and some of his colleagues that declares evidence-based medicine to be explicit and conscientious attempts to find the best available research evidence to assist health professionals to make the best decisions for their patients.[1] This definition was originally given with respect to evidence-based *medicine*. However, its use has extended beyond the medical profession to all health professions and services, where the phrase 'evidence-based *practice*' is used, often with the same original definition. The definition may sound rather ambiguous, so in the first section of this chapter we will pick its elements apart so that you can fully appreciate what is meant by the term 'evidence-based practice'. As we do, we will come across various concepts that are important in understanding evidence-based practice and we will indicate which chapters of the book explore these concepts in more depth.

Evidence-based practice is a problem-based approach where research evidence is used to assist in clinical decision making. To make informed clinical decisions, we need to integrate lots of pieces of information. As health professionals, we are typically very good at seeking information from our patients and their families, and from the settings in which we work; however, traditionally, we have not been as aware of the information that we can gain from research. When Sackett and his colleagues refer to 'evidence', they clarify it by specifying that they mean 'evidence from research', which refers to information or data that comes from research studies. So, although we need information from many sources (including from patients), evidence-based practice shows how evidence from research can also play a role in informing clinical decisions.

In this chapter, you will learn that as part of the process of evidence-based practice, you turn your clinical information need into a question, search for evidence from research, assess the quality of the evidence that you find, and then decide if and how to use that evidence to help answer your question.

What is different about evidence from research?

It is worth pausing for a moment to consider how evidence from research can enhance our clinical decision making and how this type of information differs from other types of science-based information that you may already be familiar with, such as information that comes from testing theories and the background information that forms part of our clinical knowledge. Knowledge of subjects such as anatomy, pathology, psychology and social structures is essential to our work and has been refined over many years through research. Our science-based training gives us models on which to base the clinical management of our patients. Understanding the mechanisms of illnesses and conditions is also important; for example, we could never have made sense of heart failure or diabetes without understanding the basic mechanisms of these illnesses. Yet, focusing *only* on the mechanisms of illness, and hence of treatments, can be misleading. Evidence-based practice encourages us to

TABLE 1.1   Examples of how focusing only on the mechanisms of illness can be misleading

Previous recommendation (based on a mechanism approach)	Rationale based on a mechanism approach	The empirical research that showed it was wrong
Put babies onto their fronts when they go to sleep	If they should vomit in their sleep, they might swallow the vomit into their lungs and develop pneumonia (Dr Spock in the 1950s)[2]	Observational data have shown that babies are more likely to die of sudden infant death syndrome (SIDS) if they lie on their fronts, rather than on their backs, when sleeping.[3]
Bed rest after a heart attack (myocardial infarct)	The heart needs resting after an insult in which some of the heart muscle dies	Randomised controlled trials showed that bed rest makes thromboembolism (a dangerous condition in which a clot blocks the flow of blood through a blood vessel) much more likely.[4]
Covering skin wounds after removal of skin cancer	To prevent bacteria gaining access and therefore causing infection	A randomised controlled trial showed that leaving skin wounds open does not increase the infection rate.[5]

concentrate instead on research that has tested the information (such as a hypothesis about the effectiveness of a treatment) directly. Table 1.1 gives some clinical examples to illustrate how the two approaches differ.

Each element in the definition of evidence-based practice is important

Returning to exploring the elements of the definition of evidence-based practice, the definition very deliberately states that attempts to find evidence should be 'explicit' and 'conscientious'. There is a good reason for this. Prior to the advent of evidence-based practice, the way in which many health professionals accessed research was somewhat haphazard, and their understanding of how to accurately interpret research results was often superficial. In other words, we may not have been making the best use of research to inform our clinical decision making. For example, simply using whatever evidence from research that you happen to obtain from reading the few journals that you subscribe to will not sufficiently meet your clinical information needs or keep you up to date with new research.[6] Hence, the definition of evidence-based practice encourages us to be 'explicit' and 'conscientious' in our attempts at locating the 'best available evidence from research'.

This understanding leads us to explore what is meant by the term 'best available evidence from research'. There is not one research study design that is most suited to providing the type of information that we seek from research studies. As you will learn in Chapter 2, the 'best type' of study design depends on the type of question that is being

asked. It is important to understand the main types of study designs and to be clear about what each study design can and cannot help you with. That is, what type of useful information can they provide, and what are their pros and cons? Part of the skill of evidence-based practice is being able to locate the type of study design that is best suited to providing the most appropriate type of information for a particular clinical decision. Further, as we explain in more detail later in this chapter, some studies are not designed or conducted very well, and this reduces the confidence we have in their conclusions. So, as well as looking for the best type of research study, we also need to attempt to find the best-quality research that is available.

The beginning of the definition of evidence-based medicine according to Sackett and colleagues (1996), introduced at the start of this chapter, is well known and often quoted. However, the section that follows it is also important. It reads:

The practice of evidence-based medicine means integrating individual clinical expertise with the best available external clinical evidence from systematic research. By individual clinical expertise we mean the proficiency and judgement that individual clinicians acquire through clinical experiences and clinical practice. Increased expertise is reflected in many ways, but especially in more effective and efficient diagnosis and in the more thoughtful identification and compassionate use of individual patients' predicaments, rights, and preferences in making clinical decisions about their care.[1]

This definition makes it clear that evidence-based practice also requires clinical expertise, which includes thoughtfulness and consideration of the patient and their preferences and situations, as well as knowledge of effectiveness and efficiency. The importance of exploring patient preferences for healthcare options, and strategies for incorporating these into the decision-making process, are addressed in Chapter 14, and the concept of clinical expertise is covered in more depth in Chapter 15.

A simple definition of evidence-based practice

Over time, the definition of evidence-based practice has been expanded and refined. One of the current most frequently used and widely known definitions of evidence-based practice acknowledges that it involves the integration of the best research evidence with clinical expertise and the patient's values and circumstances.[7] It also requires the health professional to consider characteristics of the local and broader practice context. This is illustrated in Figure 1.1. As you read this book, keep this definition in mind. Evidence-based practice is *not* just about using research evidence, as some critics

of it may suggest. It is also about valuing and using the education, skills and experience that you have as a health professional. Furthermore, and just as importantly, it is about considering the patient's preferences and values when making a decision, as well as considering characteristics of the practice context (for example, the resources available, policies, and socio-cultural and geographical factors). This requires judgment and artistry, as well as science and logic. The *process* that health professionals use to integrate all of this information is *clinical (or professional) reasoning* (which is discussed in more detail in Chapter 15). When you take these four elements and combine them in a way that enables you to make decisions about the care of a patient, then you are engaging in evidence-based practice.

A note about the language we use throughout the book: we use the word 'patient' but acknowledge that different words ('client' or 'consumer') are used in different disciplines. Similarly, some disciplines use the phrase 'evidence-informed practice'. We have chosen to use 'evidence-based practice' throughout this book, as it is more widely used, but the intentions are the same.

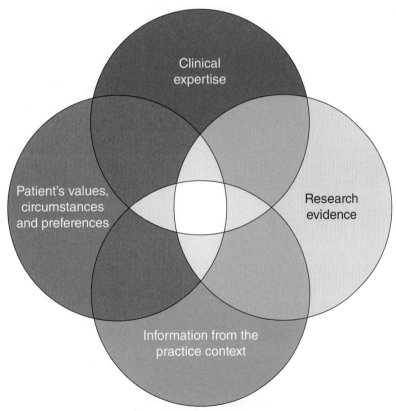

Fig 1.1 Evidence-based practice involves using clinical reasoning to integrate information from four sources: research evidence; clinical expertise; the patient's values, preferences and circumstances; and the practice context.

Where did evidence-based practice come from?

Evidence-based practice came from a new medical school that started in the 1970s at McMaster University in Canada. The new medical program was unusual in several respects. For example, it was very short (only three years). This meant its teachers realised that the notion of teaching medical students everything they needed to know was clearly impossible. All the teachers could hope for was to teach students how to find for themselves what they needed to know. How could they do that? The answer was the birth of evidence-based medicine, and hence evidence-based practice.

What happened before evidence-based practice?

This is a good question, and one that patients often ask whenever we explain to them what evidence-based practice is all about. We often relied on 'experience'; on the expertise of colleagues who were older and 'better'; and on what we were taught as students. Each of these sources of information can be flawed and there are data to show this.[8] Experience is very subject to flaws of bias. We overemphasise the mistakes of the recent past and underestimate the rare mistakes. What we were taught as students is often woefully out of date,[9,10] and health knowledge changes rapidly (with estimates that 20% of core knowledge, in medicine at least, changes in one year because of changes in evidence).[11] The health professions are often conservative, and so relying on colleagues who are older and more experienced (so-called eminence-based practice[12]) risks providing us with information that is out of date, biased and, quite simply, wrong.

This is not to say that clinical experience is not important. It is so important that it is a key feature in the definition of evidence-based practice. Clinical experience (discussed further in Chapter 15) is knowledge that is generated from practical experience and involves thoughtfulness and compassion as well as knowledge about the practices and activities that are specific to a discipline. However, rather than simply relying on clinical experience alone for decision making, we need to use our clinical experience *together* with other types of information. To help us make sense of all the information that we have—from research, from clinical settings, from our patients and from clinical experience—we use clinical reasoning processes.

Is evidence-based practice the same as randomised controlled trials?

No. Randomised controlled trials are one study design. As you will see in Chapter 4, they are the cornerstone of research investigating whether *interventions* (treatments) work. However, questions about the effectiveness of interventions are not the only type of clinical question. For example, health professionals also need good information about questions of: *aetiology* (what causes disease or makes it more likely); *frequency* (how common it is); *diagnosis* (how we know if the patient has the disease or condition of interest); *prognosis* (what happens to the condition over time); and what *patients' experiences and concerns* are in particular situations. This book focuses primarily on how to answer four main types of questions—concerning the effects of interventions, diagnosis, prognosis, and patients' experiences and concerns—as these questions are relevant to a range of health professionals and are commonly asked by them. Each question type requires a different type of research design to address it. Other research designs include *case-control studies*, *cross-sectional studies* and *cohort studies*, and various types of *qualitative research* designs. There are many others. They can all be examples of the best evidence for some research questions. This topic is explored in more depth in Chapter 2.

Is evidence-based practice the same as just following 'guidelines'?

No. Just as there are different types of research study designs, there are also now many ways in which evidence from primary research studies is synthesised, such as into systematic reviews (which are explained in detail in Chapter 12) and clinical practice guidelines (explained in Chapter 13). As you will see in Chapter 13, clinical guidelines are just one route to getting the best available evidence into clinical practice and, unfortunately, some guidelines are *not* evidence-based (for example, they may contain recommendations that are derived from expert opinion).

Is evidence-based practice the same as practice-based evidence?

No. The idea of 'practice-based evidence' recognises that there is sometimes the need to systematically collect data about local clinical practices and experiences that are commonly used but may not have been formally researched. In some settings, health professionals are encouraged to systematically gather data about real-time outcomes from patients and/or to access outcome data that has been routinely collected and collated in that specific setting. Such data can help to identify the impact of local practice(s) on the setting's patients and can be considered alongside information obtained from formal research; as such, it can complement evidence-based practice.

Can anyone practise evidence-based practice?

Yes. With the right training, practice and experience, any of us can learn how to do evidence-based practice competently. You do not have to be an expert in anything. Having access to the internet and databases (such as PubMed and the Cochrane Library) is important. And, particularly as you are learning how to do this, it is useful to have some trustworthy colleagues to check your more surprising findings.

In recent years, a set of core competencies in evidence-based practice have been developed.[13] These competencies are grouped into the key steps in the evidence-based practice process that is explained later in this chapter. This book covers most of these core competencies. For some competencies, just reading and knowing about them is sufficient, while others (such as critical appraisal and shared decision making) require practice to develop the skill.

Do health professionals have time for an activity such as evidence-based practice?

While there can be various barriers to doing evidence-based practice, there are also enablers to it. You, as an individual, and your workplace should make every effort to overcome these barriers. Some of these barriers and enablers are described in Chapter 17. Evidence-based practice is not an optional activity for health professionals. It should be the standard way that health care is practised, and you have a responsibility as a health professional to ensure that the care you are providing is evidence-based. It is no longer an emerging concept and is now expected, as reflected by its embodiment in the curriculum, registration competencies and accreditation standards for nearly all health professions. Try not to view evidence-based practice as an 'add on' and something else you need to find time to fit into your day. Instead, strive to find ways to integrate evidence-based decision making into your everyday practice and carefully choose which continuing professional development activities you engage in. As you will see in Chapter 2, a lot of the learning activities that health professionals traditionally used (such as simply reading a journal as a new issue catches your eye or attending a conference or in-service) are not helpful at enabling evidence-based practice—although there are ways that some of these activities (such as journal clubs) can be performed so that they form part of evidence-based practice (as described in Chapter 17).

WHY IS EVIDENCE-BASED PRACTICE IMPORTANT?

Evidence-based practice's greatest importance lies in its goal to help both health professionals and patients make an evidence-informed decision about what might be the best decision for *that* patient at *that* point in time. Without this, optimal patient outcomes and care are unlikely to be attained. There are many other important benefits. Patients are increasingly bringing information about their health conditions to their clinician, and we need to be able to assess the accuracy of this information, determine the suitability of the intervention for them and work with them to decide if this intervention is an appropriate and effective option for them.

Evidence-based practice promotes an attitude of inquiry in health professionals and gets us thinking about questions such as: Why am I doing this in this way? Is there evidence that can guide me to do this in a more effective way? Evidence-based practice has an important role in facilitating our professional accountability. By definition, we are *professionals* whose job is to provide health care to people who need it (hence the term 'health professionals'). As part of providing a professional service, it is our responsibility, whenever possible, to ensure that our practice is informed by the best available evidence. When we integrate the best available evidence with information from our clinical knowledge, patients and practice context, the reasoning behind our clinical decisions becomes more apparent and this serves to reinforce both our professional accountability and our claim of being a health professional.

Evidence-based practice also has an important role to play in ensuring that health resources are used wisely and that relevant evidence is considered when decisions are made about funding health services. There are finite resources available to provide health care to people. Accordingly, we need to be responsible in our use of healthcare resources. For example, if there is good-quality evidence that a particular intervention is harmful or not effective and will not produce clinically meaningful improvement in our patients, we should not waste precious resources providing this intervention—even if it has been provided for years. This is not to say, however, that if no research exists that clearly supports what we do, then the interventions that we provide should not be funded. As discussed later in this book, absence of evidence and evidence of ineffectiveness (or evidence of harm) are quite different things.

During the COVID-19 pandemic, the importance of rapidly generating, appraising and disseminating quality evidence for decision making (at individual, health system and global policy levels) took centre stage. We saw the harm (such as through the use of ineffective or harmful treatments) that arose when policies and clinical decisions were not based on evidence, but instead on anecdotes, expert opinion, research that did not use the ideal study type for the question being asked (such as observational studies instead of randomised trials for questions about intervention effectiveness) or poor-quality studies.[14] We also saw the power of coordinated international randomised trials that provided convincing evidence about the effectiveness of various treatments. And on a scale not previously seen, we saw the challenges of researchers and clinicians trying to keep up with and to synthesise the tsunami of COVID-19 research.[15]

SCOPE OF EVIDENCE-BASED HEALTH CARE

As mentioned earlier, evidence-based practice is a concept that emerged out of evidence-based medicine. Although this book will concentrate largely on the use of evidence-based practice in clinical settings, evidence-based concepts now permeate all of health care (and beyond). That is why you will hear, from time to time, terms such as 'evidence-based purchasing' (where purchasers are informed by research to make purchases of health- and social-care services and resources that are useful and safe), 'evidence-based policy' (where policy makers integrate research evidence into the formation of policy documents and decisions to address the needs of the population) or 'evidence-based management' (where managers integrate research findings into a range of management tasks). Evidence-based practice has had a significant impact in more than just the clinical domain and its influence can be seen in many of the major health systems and government health policies across the world. In fact, if you are interested, you might like to do a quick internet search that will show that 'evidence-based' principles are now being applied in social care, criminology, education, conservation, engineering, sport and many other disciplines. Although its focus is only on randomised controlled trials, the book *Randomistas* is a fascinating read about their application and attempts at evidence-based decision making in health, public policy, education and other fields.[16]

COMMON CRITICISMS OF EVIDENCE-BASED PRACTICE

Once you start reading widely in this area, you will notice that there are some criticisms of evidence-based practice.[17–20] Sometimes this is from a lack of knowledge or from misinformation and is easily rebutted. Others have developed very thoughtful concerns about unintended negative consequences from the adoption of evidence-based practice. Some of these criticisms are summarised in Table 1.2, along

TABLE 1.2 Some criticisms of evidence-based practice, and some responses

Criticisms	Responses
Relies too heavily on quantitative research.	Qualitative research is very important in helping us to understand more about how individuals and communities perceive and manage their health and make decisions related to health service usage. Appreciation of the value of qualitative research to evidence-based practice is growing. This is partially reflected in the growth of mixed-methods research papers (that use a combination of qualitative and quantitative approaches) in both primary studies and systematic reviews.
Limitations of relying on research to provide the evidence upon which to base practice, particularly in areas where there is limited research available.	While we acknowledge that there is little research and/or inconsistencies in evidence for some clinical questions, evidence-based practice emphasises using the best research evidence available. The other components of evidence-based practice (clinical experience and reasoning, patient preferences) must be relied on even more where there is a lack of evidence or uncertainty between the various options.
The amount of evidence available is overwhelming.	This is more of a problem for some disciplines and topics than others. There certainly are areas where there is much research, overlap and a huge amount of synthesised evidence (such as systematic reviews and guidelines, which sometimes are conflicting). For areas such as this, being an efficient searcher of evidence, being guided by the pyramid of evidence-based information (see Chapter 3) and having critical appraisal skills (even for synthesised evidence) are very important.
Contemporary large, randomised trials over-focus on achieving small gains in health.	Proper practice of evidence-based practice should include careful consideration of the size of the effect (both benefits and harms). Hence, clinical significance from the patient's perspective, not just statistical significance (see Chapters 2 and 4), should be considered, as well as that the trials measured outcomes that matter to the patient.
Clinicians (particularly inexperienced ones) may slavishly follow 'the evidence' (and associated rules and algorithms) without considering patient factors (including preferences and multimorbidity).	Proper practice of evidence-based practice is not about following rules. Clinical judgment and reasoning are crucial to it and should include careful consideration of the patient's 'whole-person' best interests and their preferences. This is sometimes called 'individualising evidence decisions'. In Chapter 14, you will learn about how shared decision making is a crucial component of evidence-based practice.

with some responses. While the debate can sometimes become very academic and nuanced, it can be useful to ask yourself, 'If not evidence-based practice, then what is the alternative?' While evidence-based practice is not without its flaws and challenges, it is the best process we currently have and is superior to clinical decision making that is guided by expert opinion, claims from industry (such as pharmaceutical or device companies) or clinical anecdotes.

THE PROCESS OF EVIDENCE-BASED PRACTICE

Rather than just being a vague concept that is difficult to incorporate into everyday clinical practice, the process of evidence-based practice is actually quite structured. It can be viewed as a number of steps that health professionals need to perform when an information need (that can be answered by research evidence) arises:[7]

1. Convert your information needs into an answerable clinical question.
2. Find the best evidence to answer your clinical question.
3. Critically appraise the evidence for its validity (risk of bias), impact and applicability.
4. Integrate the evidence with clinical expertise; the patient's values, preferences and circumstances; and information from the practice context.
5. Evaluate the effectiveness and efficiency with which steps 1–4 were carried out, and think about ways to improve your performance of them next time.

Some people may prefer to remember these steps as the five As:[21]

- **Ask a question.**
- **Access the information.**
- **Appraise the articles found.**
- **Apply the information.**
- **Audit.**

It has been wisely suggested that even prior to beginning the first step of asking a question, health professionals should undertake Step 0, which is recognising our uncertainties.[22] This can include acknowledging that we often have basic uncertainties about common tests and treatments. Uncertainty is an inherent part of health care. And it often makes health professionals uncomfortable. Acknowledging the uncertainties is important. It is also important to recognise the uncertainties in evidence for a clinical question and to incorporate this into your discussions with patients. This issue is covered in other chapters of this book.

Regardless of which list you prefer to use to remember the process of evidence-based practice, the basic steps are the same and they are explained in more detail below.

Step 1: Convert your information needs into an answerable clinical question

The process of evidence-based practice begins with the recognition that you, as a health professional, have a clinical information need. Some types of clinical information needs can be answered with the assistance of research evidence. Chapter 2 describes the different types of clinical information needs and which of these research evidence can help to answer. An important step in the evidence-based practice process is turning this information need into an answerable clinical question. There are some easy ways to do this, which are demonstrated in Chapter 2.

You may have a question about the following:

- **Intervention** (that is, treatment)—for example, in adults with rheumatoid arthritis, is education about joint protection techniques effective in reducing hand pain and improving function?
- **Diagnosis**—for example, in adults admitted to a chest pain unit, which elements of serial diagnostic testing are the most sensitive and specific predictors of cardiac involvement?
- **Prognosis**—for example, in people undergoing total knee replacement for osteoarthritis, what improvement in walking ability is expected after six weeks?
- **Patients' experiences and concerns**—for example, what does the lived experience of older adults transitioning to residential aged care facilities mean for their ability to integrate and find a sense of identity?

The type of question will determine the type of research that you need to look for to answer your question. This process is explained further in Chapter 2.

Step 2: Find the best evidence to answer your clinical question

Once you have structured your clinical question appropriately and know what type of question you are asking and, therefore, what sort of research you need to look for, the next step is to find the research evidence to answer your question. It is important that you are aware of the many online evidence-based resources and which of these will be most appropriate for you to use to search for the evidence to answer your question. Being able to *efficiently* search online evidence-based resources is a crucial skill for anyone engaged in evidence-based practice. Chapter 3 contains information about the key online evidence-based resources and how to efficiently search for evidence.

Step 3: Critically appraise the evidence for its validity (risk of bias), impact and applicability

Upon finding the evidence, you will need to critically appraise it. That is, you need to examine the evidence closely to determine whether it is worthy of being used to inform your clinical practice.

Why do I need to critically appraise the evidence? Surely all published research is good quality?

Unfortunately, it is not. A number of studies suggest that much published research is of poor quality, poorly reported or wrong.[23–29] Sadly, much clinical research is not useful, as it is often not sufficiently pragmatic, or it is not built upon information gained from systematic reviews of existing research, or is not patient-centred (that is, it does not reflect patients' top priorities or use outcomes that are meaningful to them), or is not sufficiently transparent or feasible.[24] These deficiencies lead to waste in research.[25–28] How is it that poor-quality research can pass through peer review? Unfortunately, peer review is a flawed process, with peer reviewers sometimes no more informed about appropriate study design, analysis and reporting than the researchers who conducted the studies; as a result, flawed studies are published.[30–33]

There is now a growing awareness, by researchers, peer reviewers and journal editors, of the importance of strong study design (thanks, in part, to the proliferation of evidence-based practice). As you will see in various chapters throughout the book, guides have been developed for how certain types of studies should be reported. (For example, in Chapter 4, you will learn about the CONSORT statement for randomised controlled trials.) A list of the reporting guidelines for various study types is available at the website of the EQUATOR Network (www.equator-network.org). A growing number of journals now require authors of studies to follow these guides closely if they wish their article to be considered for publication. All of this is good news for us (as health professionals using evidence to inform our clinical decisions), as it has the potential to make it easier to appraise and interpret research reports.

Because of this, before you can use the results of a research study to assist you in making a clinical decision, you need to determine whether the study methods are sound enough to provide you with potentially useful information or, alternatively, whether the methods are so flawed that they might potentially provide misleading results. Studies that are poorly designed may produce results that are distorted by bias (and often more than one type of bias). Some of the common types of bias are introduced in Chapter 2. The main types of bias that are relevant to each of the question types are explained in detail in the corresponding chapter that discusses how to appraise the evidence for each question type.

What is involved in critically appraising evidence?

There are three main aspects of the evidence (that is, each study) that you need to appraise (in the following order):

1. **Internal validity (or risk of bias).** This refers to whether the evidence is trustworthy. That is, can you believe the results of the study? You evaluate the validity of the study by determining whether the study was carried out in a way that was methodologically sound. In this step, we are concerned with the study's *internal validity*—this is explained more fully in Chapter 2. This term can be interchanged with 'risk of bias', and our focus is on appraising the extent to which the design and conduct of a study are likely to have minimised its bias. In qualitative research, the concept of internal validity is not used; as Chapter 10 explains, the concepts of trustworthiness and credibility of a study are used instead.

2. **Impact.** If you decide that the validity of the study is sufficient that you can believe the results, you then need to look closely at those results. The main thing you need to determine is the impact (that is, the clinical importance) of the evidence. For example, in a study that compared the effectiveness of a new intervention with an existing intervention, did the new intervention have a *large enough effect* on the clinical outcome(s) of interest that you would consider altering your practice and using the new intervention with your patient?

3. **Applicability.** If you have decided that the validity of the study is adequate and that the results are clinically important, the final step in critical appraisal is to evaluate whether you can apply the results of the study to your patient. Essentially, you need to assess whether your patient is so different from the participants in the study that you cannot apply the results of the study to that individual. This step is concerned with assessing the *external validity* (or the 'generalisability' or 'applicability') of the study, as explained more fully in Chapter 2. In qualitative research, the concept of transferability may be used, rather than generalisability, and this is discussed in Chapter 10.

Many of the chapters of this book (Chapters 4–12) are devoted to helping you learn how to critically appraise various types of evidence. There are plenty of appraisal checklists that you can use to help you to critically appraise the evidence. Many of the checklists are freely available on the internet. Most of them contain more-or-less the same key items. The checklists that we have used in this book as a general guide for the appraisal of quantitative research are mostly based on those that were developed by the UK National Health Service Public Health Resource Unit as part of the Critical Appraisal Skills Programme (CASP). In turn, these checklists were largely derived from the well-known *Journal of the American Medical Association (JAMA)* Users' Guides.[34] The CASP checklists are freely available at www.casp-uk.net. For the appraisal of qualitative research, we have used the Qualitative Assessment and Review Instrument (QARI), which was developed by the Joanna Briggs Institute and can be accessed through https://jbi.global. The CASP checklist for appraising qualitative studies has also been described, and the two approaches are compared in Chapter 10.

Each of the CASP checklists begins by asking a screening question about whether the study addressed a clearly focused question (such as in terms of the population, intervention and outcomes studied). This question is to help you not waste your time proceeding to appraise the validity, impact and applicability of a study that is going to be of too poor quality for you to use in clinical decision making. In the worked examples in Chapters 5, 7, 9 and 11, you will notice that this screening question is not included in the examples. This is because, prior to appraising their chosen article, the authors of each of the worked examples had already conducted a screening process to decide which article was the best available evidence to use to answer their clinical question; as part of this, they also checked that it addressed a clearly focused question. When you are critically appraising research articles, keep in mind that no research is perfect and that it is important not to be overly critical of research articles. An article just needs to be *good enough* to assist you to make a clinical decision.

Ideally, the evidence for all clinical questions would already be pre-appraised and synthesised in a resource such as a guideline. Unfortunately, this is not yet the situation for many, many clinical questions and far less so for health professions other than medicine. The reality is that there will be times when you will need to use primary studies as the best available evidence to answer your clinical question. And you will need the skills to critically appraise these studies. Skills in critical appraisal need to go beyond just knowing how to assess risk of bias. Knowing how to interpret other aspects such as the quality and certainty of a body of evidence, magnitude of an effect and the applicability of evidence are also important. We follow this broader approach to critical appraisal skills throughout this book.

Step 4: Integrate the evidence with clinical expertise; the patient's values, preferences and circumstances; and information from the practice context

The fourth step in the evidence-based practice process involves integrating the findings from the critical appraisal step with your clinical expertise; your patient's values, preferences and circumstances; and the practice (clinical) context. As discussed earlier in this chapter and

illustrated in Figure 1.1, these four elements form the definition of evidence-based practice. 'Clinical expertise' refers to a health professional's accumulated experience, education and disciplinary and clinical skills. As evidence-based practice is a problem-solving approach that initially stems from a patient's needs, any clinical decision that is made in relation to that individual should involve consideration of the unique needs, values, preferences, concerns and experiences that each patient brings to the situation. Evidence alone is never sufficient to guide clinical decisions. Many decisions are preference-sensitive and what is the 'best choice' for one person will not be the best choice for another, even though the clinical question may be the same. Many of the chapters of this book discuss the need for and process of integrating research evidence with clinical expertise and the patient's preferences, with appropriate consideration also given to the practice context. When thinking about the practice context, it is not only the local context that should be considered (such as the nature of the setting, resources available, roles of various disciplines, local service delivery priorities and policies) but sometimes also the impact of the broader context in which the care is being delivered (such as relevant state or federal policies, funding mechanisms and socio-cultural and geographical factors).

Step 5: Evaluate the effectiveness and efficiency with which steps 1–4 were carried out, and think about ways to improve your performance of them next time

As evidence-based practice is a process intended for health professionals to incorporate into their routine clinical practice, it is important that you learn to do it as efficiently as possible so that it does not become a time-consuming or onerous task. Asking yourself self-reflection questions after you have completed the previous four steps of the evidence-based practice process can be a useful way to identify which steps you are doing well and areas where you could improve. Box 1.1 contains some examples of self-reflection questions that you could ask when evaluating how well you performed steps 1–4 of the evidence-based practice process.

HOW THIS BOOK IS STRUCTURED

The process of evidence-based practice that was just described is used as the main structure for this book. In addition to the key steps in the process, there are other topics that health professionals who wish to do evidence-based practice should know about. Hence, these topics

---

BOX 1.1   Examples of self-reflection questions when evaluating your performance of steps 1–4 of the evidence-based practice process

- Am I asking well-formulated clinical questions? (See Chapter 2.)
- Am I aware of the best sources of evidence for the different types of clinical questions? (See Chapter 3.)
- Am I searching the databases efficiently? (See Chapter 3.)
- Am I using the hierarchy of evidence for each type of clinical question as my guide for the type of evidence that I should be searching for? (See Chapter 2.)
- Where possible, am I searching for and using information that is higher up in the pyramid of levels of organisation of evidence (e.g. synthesised summaries, systematically derived recommendations, systematic reviews)? (See Chapter 3.)
- Am I integrating the 'findings' from critically appraising relevant studies into my clinical practice? (See Chapters 4–12.)
- Can I clearly explain what the options are and what the evidence means to my patients and collaborate with them in shared decision making where appropriate? (See Chapter 14.)
- Am I proactively monitoring for newly emerging evidence in my field of practice?[35] (See Chapter 3.)

(such as sharing decisions with patients and how to implement evidence into practice) also have their own chapters in the book.

Chapter 1: Introduction to evidence-based practice

Addresses some of the background information about evidence-based practice, such as what it is, why it was developed, why it is important, and the five key steps that underlie the process of evidence-based practice.

Chapter 2: Information needs, asking questions, and some basics of research studies

Provides details about clinical information needs, how to convert them into an answerable question, and how the type of research that you look for differs according to the type of question that you are asking.

Contains some of the background statistical information that you need to understand before being able to critically appraise research evidence.

Chapter 3: Finding the evidence

Contains information about how to undertake the second step of the evidence-based practice process: searching for evidence to answer your clinical question.

Chapter 4: Evidence about effects of interventions

Explains what to do when you have a clinical question about the effects of an intervention, with a focus on how to perform the third and fourth steps of the evidence-based practice process.

Provides details about how to assess the risk of bias of the evidence, understand the results and use the evidence to inform practice.

Chapter 5: Questions about the effects of interventions: examples of appraisals from different health professions

As the steps of evidence-based practice become easier with practice, this chapter provides you with multiple worked examples of questions about interventions so that you can see, step-by-step, for various clinical scenarios how questions are formulated and evidence is found, appraised and applied. In keeping with the multidisciplinary nature of this book, examples from a range of health professions are provided.

Chapter 6: Evidence about diagnosis

Uses the same structure as Chapter 4, but the content is focused on how to appraise the evidence when your clinical question is about diagnosis (or assessment).

Chapter 7: Questions about diagnosis: examples of appraisals from different health professions

Contains multiple worked examples of questions about diagnosis from a range of health professions that commonly have diagnostic or assessment informational needs.

Chapter 8: Evidence about prognosis

Follows the same structure as Chapters 4 and 6, but the content is focused on how to appraise evidence when your clinical question is about prognosis.

Chapter 9: Questions about prognosis: examples of appraisals from different health professions

Contains multiple worked examples of questions about prognosis from a range of health professions that commonly consider prognostic issues.

Chapter 10: Understanding evidence from qualitative research

Provides details about how to appraise the evidence when your question is about patients' experiences and concerns and you are using qualitative research to answer the question.

Chapter 11: Understanding evidence from qualitative research: examples of assessment of quality (critical appraisal) from different health professions

Contains multiple worked examples of questions about patients' experiences and concerns from a range of health professions.

Chapter 12: Appraising and interpreting systematic reviews

Explains how to appraise and make sense of systematic reviews and meta-analyses, which are a very important research study type in evidence-based practice.

Chapter 13: Clinical practice guidelines

Explains what clinical practice guidelines are, why they can be a useful tool in evidence-based practice, how they are developed, where to find them, and how to assess their quality before deciding whether to use them in clinical practice.

Chapter 14: Shared decision making

Explains the importance of and skills needed to collaborate with patients in the decision-making process, clearly explain

evidence to them and integrate their preferences—a crucial final step of evidence-based practice.

Chapter 15: Clinical reasoning and evidence-based practice

Addresses the role of clinical reasoning in decision making and explains the process by which health professionals integrate information from many different sources.

Chapter 16: Implementing evidence and closing research–practice gaps

Acknowledges that after finding and appraising the evidence, patient outcomes will only be altered if the evidence is then implemented into clinical practice.

Describes the process for doing this, along with some of the barriers that may be encountered during the process and strategies for overcoming them.

Chapter 17: Embedding evidence-based practice into routine clinical care

Acknowledges that while individual health professionals will always be key in advancing evidence-based practice, an organisational environment that recognises the value of, and encourages, evidence-based practice is also important.

Describes why organisations should promote evidence-based practice, characteristics of organisations that do this, and specific strategies organisations can use to support evidence-based practice.

SUMMARY

- Evidence-based practice is a problem-based approach where research evidence is used to inform clinical decision making. It involves the integration of the best available research evidence with clinical expertise; our patient's values, preferences and circumstances; and consideration of the clinical (practice) context.
- Evidence-based practice is important because it aims to improve patient outcomes, it is what our patients expect, and it can help to assure that the care provided is appropriate and aligned with a patient's values. It also has a role in facilitating professional accountability and guiding decisions about the funding and resourcing of health services.
- Evidence-based practice has extended to all areas of health care and is also used in areas such as policy formulation and implementation, purchasing and management.

- There are five main steps (5 As) in the evidence-based practice process: (1) asking a question (Ask); (2) searching for evidence to answer it (Access); (3) critically appraising the evidence (Appraise); (4) integrating the evidence with your clinical expertise, information from the practice context, and the patient's values, preferences and circumstances (Apply); and (5) evaluating how well you performed steps 1–4 and how you can improve your performance the next time you do this (Audit).
- Much research evidence is not of sufficient quality for you to confidently use it to inform clinical decision making. Therefore, you need to critically appraise it as part of deciding whether to use it. The three main aspects of the evidence that you need to critically appraise are its: (1) validity/risk of bias (can you trust it?); (2) impact (are the results clinically important?); and (3) applicability (can you apply it to your patient?).

REFERENCES

1. Sackett D, Rosenberg W, Gray J, et al. Evidence based medicine: what it is and what it isn't: it's about integrating individual clinical expertise and the best external evidence. BMJ 1996;312:71–2.
2. Spock B. Baby and child care. London: The Bodley Head; 1958.
3. Gilbert R, Salanti G, Harden M, et al. Infant sleeping position and the sudden infant death syndrome: systematic review of observational studies and historical review of recommendations from 1940 to 2002. Int J Epidemiol 2005;34:874–87.
4. Allen C, Glasziou P, Del Mar C. Bed rest: a potentially harmful treatment needing more careful evaluation. Lancet 1999;354:1229–33.
5. Heal C, Buettner P, Raasch B, et al. Can sutures get wet? Prospective randomised controlled trial of wound management in general practice. BMJ 2006;332:1053–6.
6. Hoffmann T, Erueti C, Thorning S, et al. The scatter of research: a cross-sectional comparison of randomised trials and systematic reviews across specialties. BMJ 2012;344:e3223.
7. Straus S, Glasziou P, Richardson W, et al. Evidence-based medicine: how to practice and teach EBM. 5th ed. Edinburgh: Elsevier Churchill Livingstone; 2018.
8. Oxman A, Guyatt G. The science of reviewing research. Ann NY Acad Sci 1993;703:125–33, discussion 133–4.
9. Sibley J, Sackett D, Neufeld V, et al. A randomized trial of continuing medical education. N Engl J Med 1982;306:511–5.
10. Ramsey P, Carline J, Inui T, et al. Changes over time in the knowledge base of practising internists. JAMA 1991;266:1103–7.
11. Alper, B. How much does practice-guiding medical knowledge change in one year? 2012; https://www.semanticscholar.org/paper/How-Much-Does-Practice-Guiding-Medical-Knowledge-in-Alper/d431658fb5b9ae20bf4b6cce2c4fdbef7da86a07.
12. Isaacs D, Fitzgerald D. Seven alternatives to evidence based medicine. BMJ 1999;319:1618.
13. Albarquoni L, Hoffmann T, Straus S, et al. Core competencies in evidence-based practice for health professionals: consensus statement based on a systematic review and Delphi survey. JAMA Netw Open 2018;1(2):e180281.
14. Glasziou P, Sanders S, Hoffmann T. Waste in Covid-19 research. BMJ 2020;369:m1847. doi:10.1136/bmj.m1847.
15. Pearson H. How COVID broke the evidence pipeline. The pandemic stress-tested the way the world produces evidence—and revealed all the flaws. Nature 2021;593:182–5. doi: https://doi.org/10.1038/d41586-021-01246-x.
16. Leigh A. Randomistas: how radical researchers changed our world. Carlton, Vic: La Trobe University Press; 2018.
17. Greenhalgh T, Howick J, Maskrey N. Evidence based medicine: a movement in crisis? BMJ 2014;348:g3725.
18. Greenhalgh T, Snow R, Ryan S, et al. Six 'biases' against patients and carers in evidence-based medicine. BMC Med 2015;13:1–11.
19. Ioannidis J. Evidence-based medicine has been hijacked: a report to David Sackett. J Clin Epidemiol 2016;73:82–6.
20. Straus S, McAlister F. Evidence-based medicine: a commentary on common criticisms. Can Med Assoc J 2000;163:837–41.
21. Jackson R, Ameratunga S, Broad J, et al. The GATE frame: critical appraisal with pictures. ACP J Club 2006;144:2.
22. Glasziou P. Six proposals for EBM's future. Evidence based medicine (EBM) toolkit. BMJ Publishing Group Limited; 2021. https://bestpractice.bmj.com/info/toolkit/discuss-ebm/six-proposals-for-ebms-future/.
23. Ioannidis J. Why most published research findings are false. PLoS Med 2005;2(8):e124.
24. Ioannidis J. Why most clinical research is not useful. PLoS Med 2016;13(6):e1002049.
25. Ioannidis J, Greenland S, Hlatky M, et al. Increasing value and reducing waste in research design, conduct, and analysis. Lancet 2014;383(9912):166–75.
26. Glasziou P, Altman D, Bossuyt P, et al. Reducing waste from incomplete or unusable reports of biomedical research. Lancet 2014;383(9913):267–76.
27. Chan A, Song F, Vickers A, et al. Increasing value and reducing waste: addressing inaccessible research. Lancet 2014;383(9913):257–66.
28. Macleod M, Michie S, Roberts I, et al. Biomedical research: increasing value, reducing waste. Lancet 2014;383(9912):101–4.
29. Turner L, Shamseer L, Altman D, et al. Consolidated standards of reporting trials (CONSORT) and the completeness of reporting of randomised controlled trials (RCTs) published in medical journals. Cochrane Database Syst Rev 2012;(11):MR000030.
30. Patel J. Why training and specialization is needed for peer review: a case study of peer review for randomized controlled trials. BMC Med 2014;12:128.
31. Smith R. Peer review: a flawed process at the heart of science and journals. J R Soc Med 2006;99:178–82.
32. Stahel P, Moore EE. Peer review for biomedical publications: we can improve the system. BMC Med 2014;12(1):179.
33. Chauvin A, Ravaud P, Baron G, et al. The most important tasks for peer reviewers evaluating a randomized controlled trial are not congruent with the tasks most often requested by journal editors. BMC Med 2015;13:158.
34. Guyatt G, Rennie D. Users' guides to the medical literature. JAMA 1993;270:2096–7.
35. Keister D, Tilson J. Proactively monitoring for newly emerging evidence: the lost step in EBP? Evid Based Med 2008;13:69.

Information Needs, Asking Questions, and Some Basics of Research Studies

Chris Del Mar, Tammy Hoffmann and Paul Glasziou

This chapter provides background information that you need to know in order to understand the details of the evidence-based practice process presented in the following chapters. The combination of topics is eclectic but no less important. First, we describe the types of clinical information needs that health professionals commonly have and discuss some of the methods they use to obtain information to answer those needs. In Chapter 1, we saw how the first step in the process of evidence-based practice is converting an information need into an answerable, well-structured question. This chapter explains how to do this. We then explain the importance of matching the type of question asked with the most appropriate study design. As part of this, we introduce and explain the concept of 'hierarchies of evidence' for each type of question. In the last sections of this chapter, we explain some concepts that are fundamental to the critical appraisal of research evidence, which is the third step in the evidence-based practice process. These concepts include internal validity, chance, bias, confounding, statistical significance, clinical significance and power.

CLINICAL INFORMATION NEEDS

Health professionals need information all the time to help them assess patients, make decisions, reassure patients, formulate treatment, make practical arrangements, and so on. Some of the necessary questions can be usefully answered from existing research, and some cannot. Table 2.1 provides examples of some of the obvious types of questions that can or cannot be answered by research. This book helps you to learn how to deal with information needs that can be answered, at least to some extent, by research. Along the way, we will also discuss the types of information that come from patients and those that come from clinical experience. When we consider this information together—from research, patients and experience—we are working within an evidence-based practice framework.

DEALING EFFECTIVELY WITH INFORMATION NEEDS

Having established that health professionals have many information needs, this section explains how you can deal

TABLE 2.1 Clinical information needs—examples of questions that can, and questions that cannot, be answered by evidence-based practice

	Information		Examples
These questions typically *cannot* be answered by research	Local	Background information	Is this patient eligible for treatment subsidy?
			What are the regulations for the use of a type of treatment?
			Who can be referred to this service?
			What are the opening hours of the hospital outpatients' administration?
			Is there an organisation that runs a chronic disease self-management program in this community?
			What is a Colles fracture?
These questions *can* usually be informed by research	General	Aetiology/frequency	Is this risk factor associated with that disease?
			How many people with those symptoms have this disease?
		Prognosis	What happens to this illness without treatment?
		Diagnosis	If I elicit this sign among people with these symptoms, how many have that disease?
			If this test is negative, how sure can I be that the patient does *not* have the disease?
		Treatment/intervention	How much improvement can I expect from this intervention?
			How much harm is likely from the intervention?
			Is this intervention more effective than that intervention?
		Patients' experiences and concerns	What is the experience of patients concerning their condition or intervention?
			What is happening here, and why is it happening?

effectively with these needs. A simple overview of one way of doing this is as follows:

- Recognise when we have a question.
- Record the question—do not lose that moment!
- Attempt to find the answer.
- Record the answer so that it can be re-used later.
- Stop and reflect on what you have been looking up and dealing with. Is it helping you to answer your question?

The size of the problem

The clinical literature is big. Just *how* big is staggering. Thousands of new studies are published every week. For example, on average, about 75 randomised controlled trials and 11 systematic reviews (this is where primary studies have been systematically located, appraised and synthesised) are published each day.[1] That is about one trial published every 19 minutes! And randomised controlled trials are only a small proportion (less than 5%) of the research that is indexed in PubMed, which, as you will see in Chapter 3, is just one of several databases available for you to search to find evidence. This means that the accumulated literature is a massive haystack to search for that needle of information you need. The information might mean the difference between effective or ineffective (or even harmful) care for your patient. One of the purposes of this book, then, is to help you find evidence needles in research haystacks.

Noting down your clinical question

It is important that we keep track of the questions we ask. It is all too easy to lose track of them and the opportunity evaporates. If you cannot remember what you wanted to know when in the midst of managing a patient, the chances are you will never go back to answering that question.

How should we do this? One way is to keep a notebook with you in which to write them down. Date and scribble. A more modern way, of course, is to make notes electronically, using a smartphone, tablet or computer (if simultaneously making patient records). Some health professionals tell the patient what they are doing:

> 'I'm just making a note of this to myself to look it up when I have a moment. Next time I see you, I'll be able to let you know if we need to discuss changing anything.'

Or:

> 'Let's get online and look that up right now, because I want to make sure that we're using the latest research when we make decisions about your ...'

(This second strategy feels risky until you have had a lot of practice with the first!)

In Chapter 1, we discussed the general process of looking up, appraising and applying the evidence that we find. Remember also to keep track of the information that you have found (in other words, write it down!), and how you evaluated and applied it. In the end, the information you find might convince you to change (hopefully, improve) your clinical practice. The way it does this is often uncoupled

from the processes you undertook, so it takes some time to realise what led you to make the changes—often systematic—to the way you do things. Chapter 17 has more information about good ways of doing this. Sometimes the research information just reassures us, the health professional, that we are on the right track, but this is important also.

DIFFERENT WAYS OF OBTAINING INFORMATION: PUSH OR PULL? JUST-IN-CASE OR JUST-IN-TIME?

Push: 'just-in-case' information

In advertising jargon, the term 'push' means that the information is sent out, or broadcast. This is the traditional means of disseminating information and is how journals work. After research has been undertaken, it is either sent directly to you, or is pre-digested in some way (perhaps as an editorial, review article, systematic review or guideline). 'Just-in-case' information is made available when it is generated, or when it is thought health professionals, such as you, ought to hear about it.

Figure 2.1 shows some examples of information that can be *pushed*. Others (not shown) include conferences, professional newsletters, textbooks, social media, and informal chats with colleagues and people from other professional groups.

Although there are many ways in which a piece of research can reach you as a health professional, it is actually more complicated: what is picked up for review, systematic review and so on is determined by several factors, including which journals the primary data were first published in, how relevant readers think the research is and how well it fits into the policy being formulated or already in existence. There are, in fact, different sorts of information that we might want to access, as explained in Chapter 3 (see Figure 3.1).

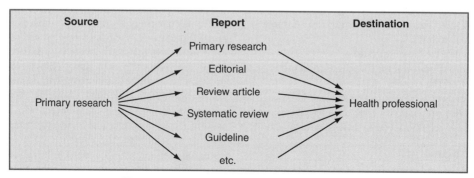

Fig 2.1 Ways in which research data get to you

All of these methods rely on the information arriving at your place of work (or home, post box, email inbox, online blog, etc.). But it has to be managed before it is put into practice. How does this happen? The different stages are described in Table 2.2.

This is not an easy process—how do we get to read just the best articles from among the thousands available? We can often feel overloaded by this, but a famous quote says: '*It's not information overload. It's filter failure.*'[2] There are a number of different filtering processes. It is important to minimise any distortion of the information they might create.

One solution is to sign up for alerts from one of the specialist databases and federated search engines that contain articles which have been carefully critically appraised. We describe this type of resource in more depth in Chapter 3. Another filtering option is journal scanning—often provided by clinical services (such as hospital libraries). However, most of these are insufficient for health professionals to rely on as a method for keeping up to date. This is partly due to the problem of research scatter, where articles that might be relevant (even systematic reviews of primary research papers) can be published in any of hundreds of specialty and general journals.[3] 'Scatter' also means, of course, that the traditional means of keeping up to date by personal journal subscriptions (even supplemented by scanning several specialty journals) is insufficient. Another problem is the lack of any filter for quality

---

TABLE 2.2 The processes involved in using just-in-case information in clinical practice

Task		Explanation
Read the title Read the abstract		Decide whether something is worth reading at all.
Read the full paper		We have obviously not tossed this paper aside (that means we have turned the page).
Decide whether it is ...	**(a)** relevant	A lot of research is not aimed at health professionals who are looking for better information to manage their patients. Much of it is researcher-to-researcher information. Just some of it is information that we think might be useful, either now or in the future when this might become part of everyday practice.
	(b) believable	Methodologically sound. That means the information is not biased to the extent that we cannot believe the result. This is explained further later in this chapter and in Chapters 4–12.
Check whether the technique is available		Many research reports do not spell out the intervention, diagnostic procedure or other management in enough detail to put it into practice—even if we believe the research!
Store the paper so we can recall it when the right patient comes along		Different health professionals do this in different ways: • tear out the paper and file it • meticulously make out reference cards • store a copy electronically (through a reference manager) • just try to remember it. Most health professionals do the last. But then forget!
Ensure that we have the necessary resources to incorporate the research into our practice		There may be prerequisites, such as availability of resources and skills to carry it out, or perhaps some policy needs to be instituted before this can happen.
Discuss with the patient		... how the benefits and harms of *this* management compare with the alternative options. This is explained in Chapter 14.

and relevance offered by journal scanning services. Happily for health professionals, however, there is an alternative to 'just-in-case' information.

Pull: 'just-in-time' information

'Pull' is advertising jargon for information that potential customers look for (rather than simply waiting for it to be *pushed* to them). This is information that the health professional seeks in relation to a specific question arising from their clinical work, and so this gives it certain characteristics. This process is illustrated in Table 2.3 using the five As that were introduced in Chapter 1 as a way of simply describing the steps in the evidence-based practice process.

If this looks familiar to you, it is not surprising—it is the essential core of evidence-based practice. How feasible is it to incorporate this way of finding information 'just-in-time'? Again, there are several steps, which are not easy—they all need mastering and practice (as with almost everything in clinical care). For example, asking questions can initially be difficult. It requires health professionals to be open to not knowing everything, which can be difficult for some—and particularly for disciplines where, traditionally, the health professional is expected to 'know the best thing to do'. Luckily, nowadays, most people welcome the honesty that goes with questioning the management you are proposing. It shows how we health professionals are taking extra and meticulous care.

How often do we ask questions? Is this something that we can realistically aspire to? Many health professionals are worried that they do not ask enough questions. You can relax, because you probably do. A review of primary care literature showed that doctors and nurses had a lot of information needs.[4] A systematic review that examined the frequency with which clinical questions are raised, pursued and successfully answered by health professionals (including doctors, medical residents, nurses, dentists and care managers) found that the mean frequency of questions

raised was 0.57 (95% confidence interval [CI] 0.38 to 0.77) per patient.[5] (We explain confidence intervals later in this chapter.) This was much higher than clinicians' own estimates. Although clinicians frequently raised questions in daily practice and were effective at finding answers approximately 80% of the time, they only looked for answers about half of the time.

A Spanish study found that doctors had a good chance (nearly 100%) of finding an answer if it took less than 2 minutes, but were much less likely to do so (<40%) if it took 30 minutes.[6] In an analysis of logs of patient interactions by general practitioner (GP) trainees, most (61%) of the searching for answers was done during consultations, and the searches took an average of 4 minutes.[7] Despite advances in electronic access, health professionals typically do not effectively search for answers to clinical questions,[8] often preferring to ask colleagues,[5,8] even though there is evidence from a randomised trial that getting information this way (that is, just-in-time) improves clinical decision making.[9]

Often, in the hurly-burly of daily clinical practice, we are not able to look up questions immediately, which is why it is important (as mentioned earlier) to write them down. This then forms a questions logbook, which can be either paper-based or electronic.

HOW TO CONVERT YOUR INFORMATION NEEDS INTO AN ANSWERABLE CLINICAL QUESTION

We will now look at how you can take a clinical question and convert it into an answerable clinical question that you can then effectively search for answers to. Remember from Chapter 1 that forming an answerable clinical question is the first step in the evidence-based practice process. Asking a good question is central to successful evidence-based practice. Converting our clinical question into an

---

TABLE 2.3   Processes involved in *just-in-time* information: The five As

Task	Explanation
Ask a question: re-format the question into an answerable one	This ensures relevance—by definition!
Access the information: searching	Decide whether to look now (in front of the patient) or later. Searching is a special skill, which is described in Chapter 3.
Appraise the papers found	We talk about this (in fact, we talk about this a lot!) in Chapters 4–12.
Apply the information	This means using the information with the patient who is in front of you.
Audit	Check whether the evidence-based practice processes that you are engaged in are working well.

'answerable question' is necessary because it prevents the health professional from forgetting any of the important components of the clinical question. Typically, there are four components,[10] which can be easily remembered using the PICO mnemonic:

Patient or **P**roblem (or **P**opulation or **P**erson)
Intervention (or diagnostic test or prognostic factor or issue)
Comparison
Outcome(s).

A few questions are only POs—Population and Outcome. For example, '*What is the chance that an elderly person who falls (P) will have a second fall within 12 months (O)?*' But most questions have three or four PICO elements. We will now address each component in turn.

Patient or problem (or population or person)

This component makes sure that you are clear *who* the question relates to. It may include information about the patient, their primary problem or disease, or coexisting conditions—for example, '*In children with autism ...*' Sometimes we specify the sex and age of a patient if that is going to be relevant to the diagnosis, prognosis or intervention—for example, '*In elderly women who have osteoporosis ...*' In qualitative research, you may also want to specify whose perspective is being considered.

Intervention (or diagnostic test or prognostic factor or issue)

The term 'intervention' is used here in a broad sense. It may refer to the intervention (that is, treatment) that you wish to use with your patient—for example, '*In people who have had a stroke, is home-based rehabilitation as effective as hospital-based rehabilitation in improving ability to perform self-care activities?*' In this case, home-based rehabilitation is an intervention that we are interested in. If you have a diagnostic question, this component of the question may refer to the diagnostic test that you are considering using with your patients—for example, '*Is the "Mini-Cog" examination as accurate as the "Mini-Mental State Examination" in detecting the presence of cognitive impairment in older community-living people?*' In this example, the Mini-Cog is the diagnostic test that we are interested in (the 'I'). A question about prognosis may specify a particular factor or issue that might influence the prognosis of your patient—for example, in the question '*What is the likelihood of hip fracture in women who have a family history of hip fracture?*', the family history of hip fracture is the particular factor that we are interested in. If you want to understand more about patients' perspectives, you may want to focus on a particular issue. For example, in the question '*In adolescents who are being treated with chemotherapy, what are their experiences and perceptions of hospital environments?*', the issue of interest is adolescent perceptions of hospital environments.

Comparison

Your questions may not always include this component, but it is useful to consider whether there is a comparison and, if so, what it is. It is mainly questions about the effects of intervention (and sometimes diagnosis) that use this component. Adding a comparison element to your question enables you to compare the intervention component of your question with another when you wish to know if one intervention is more effective than the other—which might consist of 'doing nothing'. In the example we used above, '*In people who have had a stroke, is home-based rehabilitation as effective as hospital-based rehabilitation in improving ability to perform self-care activities?*', the comparison is with hospital-based rehabilitation. Often, the comparison that you are interested in is the 'usual' (standard) care. Question types that usually do not have this component include: PO prognosis questions (for example, '*How long before a runner with an ankle sprain can return to training?*') and qualitative questions (for example, '*In adolescents who are being treated with chemotherapy, what are their experiences and perceptions of hospital environments?*').

Outcome(s)

Thinking about this element of the question forces you to think very specifically about what it is you want to have been measured. Just asking 'What is better?' begs that the word 'better' be defined (into something like 'less pain', 'greater function' or 'fewer admissions'—with the units of measure declared). In some outcomes, you may also need to specify whether you are interested in increasing the outcome (such as the score on a functional assessment or chance of recovery) or decreasing it (such as the reduction of pain or the risk of relapse, for example). In the stroke question example above, the outcome of interest was an improvement in the ability to perform self-care activities. As you will see in Chapter 14, when we explore shared decision making, it is important to involve your patient in choosing the goals of intervention that are most important to them. This means that patients' preferences often guide the outcome component of your question, and this is the basis of *patient-centred care*.[11] In other words, make sure you are choosing outcomes that are important to your patient, and not just to you!

The exact way that you structure your clinical question will vary, depending on the type of question. This is explained more in the relevant chapter—Chapter 4 for questions about the effects of intervention, Chapter 6 for diagnostic questions, Chapter 8 for prognostic questions and Chapter 10 for qualitative questions.

NOW THAT THE QUESTION HAS BEEN FORMULATED, WHAT TYPES OF INFORMATION SHOULD BE LOOKED FOR?

Not all types of information are equally useful—some are much more useful than others. Useful pieces of information are those that are more *relevant*, or more *believable*, than others.

Relevant information

The main problem when searching is that there is so much information. This means that what you use might be distorted by having found something that *nearly* answers your question, but not quite. It is all too easy to be distracted by interesting-looking (but, sadly, not directly relevant) information. So, when you have found a candidate article from your search, check its PICO against your original PICO to see how well it matches. This will help to ensure that you are thinking about the relevance of each of the components of your question.

Believable information: validity

When the results of research are not true, they are said to be *invalid*. Some information *appears* to answer your question, but either does not or, worse, cannot. Much published research is unhelpful to health professionals. There are several reasons why results may not be valid:

- The research study (even if attempting to answer your question) used a design that cannot answer the question. This is often because the **wrong study type** was used. There are many different study designs, and the right one must be used to answer the question at hand. Using the wrong study design risks not being able to glean a direct answer or distorting the information with so much bias that the results cannot be relied on as true.
- The research (even though it does attempt to answer your question) had some **flaws in its conduct** that leave it vulnerable to bias, leaving too much uncertainty to answer the question confidently. For example, the research may have failed in a large number of different ways so that we are unsure that the apparent 'result' is true.
- There were not enough numbers of participants or 'events'. ('Events' are things of clinical importance that happen—such as deaths, hospital admissions, or falls or recoveries. They can be good or bad things.) When this occurs, it is called **insufficient statistical power**.

We will now look in detail at these reasons why results may be invalid.

WHAT ARE THE DIFFERENT STUDY TYPES?

First, we need to understand some of the different study types that exist. They are briefly illustrated in Figure 2.2 and explained in Table 2.4.

There are some important things to notice about the study types listed in Table 2.4:

1. Only one study type is particularly good at addressing intervention questions—*randomised controlled trials*. Even better is a pooled analysis of several randomised controlled trials, something called a *meta-analysis* (a type of *systematic review* where the results from individual studies are combined). Systematic reviews and meta-analyses are discussed in detail in Chapter 12.

2. A sub-group of randomised controlled trials is the *n-of-1 trial*, described in Table 2.4. This study type may represent the best evidence for an individual patient, because it is undertaken in the same individual that the results will be applied to.

3. The other study types are either *observational studies* or *qualitative research studies*. They are not the best at answering questions about the effect of interventions (you will see in Chapter 4 why a randomised controlled trial is the best primary study type for answering intervention questions), but they can be good at answering *other* types of questions, including questions about prognosis, diagnosis, frequency, aetiology and experiences.

4. Different questions require different study designs; this is explained more fully in the next section. Although randomised controlled trials can sometimes answer questions about prognosis (for example), by examining just the control group (who did not receive any intervention) of a randomised controlled trial, this method can be inefficient.

This means that there is no *single* 'hierarchy of evidence' (a rank order of study types from 'good' to 'bad'), as is sometimes claimed. However, hierarchies of evidence do exist for each question type (except for questions about experiences, which are best answered by qualitative research, as explained in Chapter 10).

Figure 2.2 illustrates the various types of questions that can arise from a particular clinical scenario (patients with stroke) and how different quantitative study types are most appropriate to answer each of these question types. Starting on the left before the disease has become manifest, you might ask '*What risk factors lead to stroke?*' (for example, hypertension, diabetes and so on). There are two principal study types that can be used to answer these questions: a cohort study or a case-control study, both of which have pros and cons (see Table 2.4).

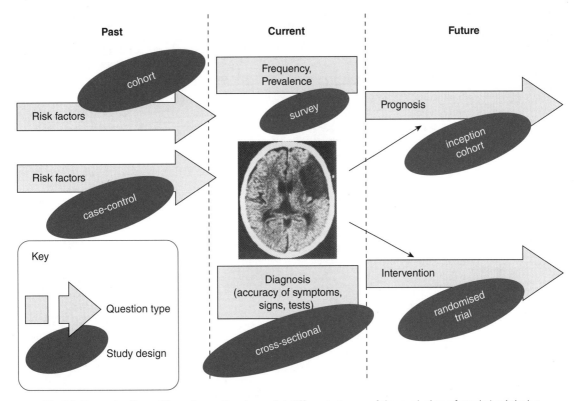

Fig 2.2 Example: How different question types (at different stages of the evolution of stroke) might be posed and the study types that might answer them. CT scan reproduced with permission from Crawford MH et al. Cardiology, 3rd ed. Mosby; 2010, Figure 11.1A.

TABLE 2.4   Some of the main study types that you need to know about for evidence-based practice

Study type	How it works	The types of questions that it is good at answering
Randomised controlled trial	This is an experiment. Participants are randomised into two (or more) different groups and each group receives a different intervention. At the end of the trial, the effects of the different interventions are measured.	Questions about interventions, such as: • *Is the intervention effective?* • *Is one intervention more effective than another?*
n-of-1 randomised trial	This is a sub-group of a randomised controlled trial and is conducted on just *one* participant. Different time periods are randomised, and the participant receives one treatment in one time period and a different treatment in another (a procedure that can be repeated several times). The average differences in clinical outcomes between the two time periods are compared.	Intervention questions—particularly those that address stable illnesses (such as chronic ones that cannot be 'cured'), so that the intervention can be tested over time.

Continued

TABLE 2.4 **Some of the main study types that you need to know about for evidence-based practice—cont'd**

Study type	How it works	The types of questions that it is good at answering
Cohort	This is an observational study. It is a type of longitudinal study where participants are followed over time. Participants with specific characteristics are identified as a 'cohort', differences between them are measured and they are followed over time. Finally, differences in outcome are observed and related to the initial differences.	Several questions: • Risks—*what risk factors predict disease?* • Aetiology—*what factors cause these outcomes?* • Prognosis—*what happens with this disease over time? What is the natural history of this condition?* • Diagnosis—*if the test is positive, what happens to the patient?*
Case-control	Observational study. Participants (i.e. 'cases') who have experienced an outcome already (such as developing a disease) are identified. They are then 'matched' with other participants who are similar (i.e. 'controls')—except they do *not* have the outcome (e.g. the disease being studied). Differences in risk factors between the two groups of participants are then analysed.	Several questions: • Risks—*what risk factors predict disease?* • Prognosis—*what happens with this disease over time?* • Diagnosis—*does this new test perform as well as the old 'gold standard'?* Intervention, particularly for rare events such as harms (which occur too infrequently in many randomised trials).
Cross-sectional	These studies sample a population at a particular point in time and measure them to see who has the outcome. Often, associations between risk factors and a certain outcome are analysed. Or comparisons are made between an established test ('gold standard') and a new candidate test.	Observational questions: • Frequency—*how common is the outcome (disease, risk factor, etc.)?* • Aetiology—*what risk factors are associated with these outcomes?* • Diagnosis—*does the new test perform as well as the 'gold standard'?*
Qualitative	There are many different qualitative research designs, but they usually make use of one or more of the following methods of data collection: • Interviews (asking people) • Focus groups (a representative group of people who will provide a wide spectrum of information) • Participant observation (the researcher joins the group to understand what is going on, or observes from a distance)	Observational questions: • *Why do people ...?* • *What are the possible reasons for ...?* • *How do people feel about ...?*
Case-series	Descriptions of a series of patients (i.e. 'cases') who are exposed to the factor (such as an intervention or an outcome of interest) that is being studied. They usually do not provide definitive evidence, but more usually are 'hypothesis-generating' (meaning that they give rise to questions that need one of the higher level of study designs to answer). There is no control group involved.	*Should we research this question?* (which might be about intervention, prognosis, diagnosis, etc.)

Or you might ask about the prevalence of stroke—for example, 'How common is a history of stroke in nursing home residents who are older than 70 years?' For this question, a simple cross-sectional survey would be the best way of providing the answer and the type of study you should look for. A similar cross-sectional study design may be best for answering diagnosis questions (although sometimes a cohort design is necessary). For example, 'Which depression screening instrument is as good at diagnosing post-stroke depression as the "gold standard" assessment of depression?' Another method for testing diagnostic alternatives is a cohort study, especially when there is no gold standard and the patient outcome ('Did the patient become clinically depressed?') has to be the gold standard instead.

The right-hand side of the figure shows the two types of questions that often occur when looking to the future: (1) prognosis questions (what will happen questions— such as 'How likely is it that a stroke patient with expressive aphasia will experience full recovery of their speech?'), which are best answered by an inception cohort study (see Table 2.4); and (2) intervention questions (such as 'Is mirror therapy effective at improving upper limb function in people who have had a stroke?'), which are best answered by a randomised controlled trial.

HIERARCHIES OF EVIDENCE FOR EACH QUESTION TYPE

Hierarchies of evidence help you decide what study type is likely to provide the most robust (that is, most free of bias) evidence, and therefore what you should look for first. There are different hierarchies for each question type, when using quantitative research. If there are no relevant studies of the type that are at the top of the hierarchy (for example, systematic reviews of randomised controlled trials for an intervention question), proceed to search for the type of study next down the hierarchy (for example, randomised controlled trials). This method ensures that you select from the best available evidence. The higher up the hierarchy it appears, the more likely it is that a study can minimise the impact of bias on its results. We can also think of the hierarchy as representing a continuum of certainty (with higher levels of certainty at the top of the hierarchy). Consider, for example, the hierarchy of evidence for intervention questions—the continuum of certainty represents how certain we are that the effects found in the study are actually due to the intervention and not to something else. This introduces two very important concepts in evidence-based practice, bias and confounding, which are explained in the next section of this chapter.

There are several published hierarchies of evidence that have been assembled by different organisations. Although these are generally similar, they have subtle differences. However, most 'hierarchies' are slowly being replaced by the Grading of Recommendations, Assessment, Development and Evaluation (GRADE) approach, which is explained in Chapter 13. The GRADE approach implicitly uses a hierarchy, but always begins with a systematic review of the most appropriate study design for the type of question, such as randomised trials for questions about intervention effectiveness.

The hierarchies of evidence for various types of questions shown in Table 2.5 are a simplified version of the hierarchies that have been developed by the Centre for Evidence-Based Medicine at the University of Oxford to show the sequence you would look for when searching for evidence. (Chapter 3 gives more details on searching.) Once you have found the best available type of evidence, you would need to consider its quality, size and precision of the results, and so on, to decide whether and how to use it in decision making. We explain the appraisal process for individual studies and systematic reviews in Chapters 4–12. As you will see in Chapter 13, many clinical practice guidelines now use the GRADE approach for assessing the quality of evidence.

Most of the study types included in Table 2.5 have been explained already in this chapter. The intricate details of the main study types are explained in the relevant chapter that deals with how to appraise evidence for each of the question types. Here we briefly consider study types additional to those in Table 2.5 and not already explained elsewhere in this chapter. Figure 2.3 shows how you can identify the main study type by asking some simple questions about assignment of exposure and use of a comparison group.

- A **non-randomised experimental trial** is essentially the same as a randomised controlled study except that there is no randomisation (hence it is lower down the hierarchy, as this opens it up to several kinds of bias). Participants are allocated to either an intervention or a control group by a process that is not random, and the outcomes from each group are compared.
- The basic premise of a **case-control study** was explained in Table 2.4.
- **Interrupted time series studies** also attempt to test interventions. Trends in an outcome are measured at several points of time before, and then after, the intervention occurs. The analysis compares the before and after outcomes. A stronger (meaning less vulnerable to bias) variant of this design is to compare the differences in before and after values with a control group of participants who did not receive the same intervention.

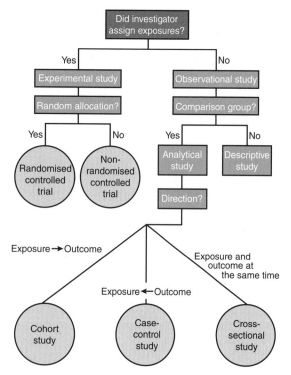

Fig 2.3 Algorithm for classification of types of clinical research
Based on Grimes DA, Schulz KF. An overview of clinical research: the lay of the land. Reprinted with permission from Elsevier (The Lancet, 2002, Vol. 359, pp. 57–61).

- In a **historical control study**, the key word is 'historical', as the control group does not participate in the study at the same time as the intervention group. There are two main forms that this type of study can take. Data about outcomes are prospectively collected for a group of participants who received the intervention of interest. These data are compared with either:
  - data about outcomes from a group of people who were treated at the same institution before the intervention of interest was introduced—this group is, in a sense, considered to be a control group who received standard care; or
  - data about outcomes from a group of people who received the control (or an alternative) intervention, but the data come from a previously published document.
- A **two or more single arm study** gathers the data from two or more studies and compares the outcomes of a single series of participants (in each study) who received the intervention of interest.
- In a **diagnostic (test) accuracy study**, the outcomes from the test that is being evaluated (known as the 'index test') are compared with outcomes from a *reference standard test* to see how much agreement there is between the two tests. The outcomes are measured in people who are suspected of having the condition of interest. A reference standard test (often called the 'gold standard' test) is the test considered to be the best available method for establishing the presence or absence of the target condition of interest.

TABLE 2.5   Hierarchies of evidence: steps in the process of searching for the best evidence for different types of questions

Question	Step 1 (Level 1*)	Step 2[†] (Level 2*)	Step 3[†] (Level 3*)	Step 4[†] (Level 4*)
Does this intervention help? (Intervention benefits and harms)	Systematic review of randomised controlled trials	Randomised controlled trial	Non-randomised controlled cohort/ follow-up study[§]	Case-series, case-control studies or historically controlled study
What might happen if we do not add an intervention? Or **What might happen over time?** (Prognosis)[‡]	Systematic review of inception cohort studies	Inception cohort study	Cohort study or control arm of a randomised controlled trial	Case-series or case-control studies, or poor-quality prognostic cohort study
Is this diagnostic or monitoring test accurate? (Diagnosis)	Systematic review of cross-sectional studies (of test accuracy) with consistently applied reference standard and blinding (and among consecutive persons)	Individual cross-sectional study (of test accuracy) with consistently applied reference standard and blinding (and among consecutive persons)	Non-consecutive studies, or studies without consistently applied reference standards	Case-control studies, or poor-quality or non-independent reference standard

TABLE 2.5   Hierarchies of evidence: steps in the process of searching for the best evidence for different types of questions—cont'd

Question	Step 1 (Level 1*)	Step 2[†] (Level 2*)	Step 3[†] (Level 3*)	Step 4[†] (Level 4*)
Is this (early detection) test worthwhile? (Screening)	Systematic review of randomised trials	Randomised trial	Non-randomised controlled cohort/ follow-up study	Case-series, case-control or historically controlled study
How common is the problem?	Local and current random sample surveys (or censuses)	Systematic review of surveys that allow matching to local circumstances	Local non-random sample	Case-series

*Level may be graded down on the basis of study quality, imprecision, indirectness (e.g. study PICO does not match your PICO well), because of inconsistency between studies or because the absolute effect size is very small; Level may be graded up if there is a large or very large effect size. See GRADE details in Chapter 13 for more detailed explanations.

[†]As always, a systematic review is generally better than an individual study.

[‡]Questions might be about what happens without intervention (i.e. the natural history of the condition) or what might happen with intervention.

[§]For questions about common harms, there needs to be sufficient numbers to rule out a common harm. For long-term harms, the duration of follow-up must be sufficient.

Adapted from the 'The Oxford 2011 Levels of Evidence' table. OCEBM Levels of Evidence Working Group. The Oxford 2011 Levels of Evidence. Oxford Centre for Evidence-Based Medicine. http://www.cebm.net.

- The basic idea of a **cohort study** was explained in Table 2.4, but there are two broad types of cohort studies that can be conducted that sit at different levels in the hierarchy of evidence for prognostic questions. The reasons for this are explained in Chapter 8, but for now we will just explain the main difference between them.
  - In a **prospective cohort study**, groups of participants are identified as a 'cohort' (based on whether they have or have not been exposed to a certain intervention or situation) and then followed prospectively over time to see what happens to them.
  - In a **retrospective cohort study**, the cohorts are defined from a previous point in time and the information is collected (for example, from past records) about the outcome(s) of interest. Participants are not followed up in the future to see what happens to them, as happens in a prospective cohort study.

Hierarchy of evidence for questions about experiences and concerns

Questions about experiences and concerns (usually of patients or members of the public, but they can also be of health professionals) are answered using qualitative evidence. The various qualitative research methodologies are explained in depth in Chapter 10. There is currently no universally agreed-upon hierarchy of evidence for study types that seek to answer questions about patients' experiences and concerns.

INTERNAL VALIDITY: WHAT ARE *BIAS* AND *CONFOUNDING*?

Internal validity and external validity

As we saw in Chapter 1 when the process of evidence-based practice was explained, when reading a research study you need to know whether you can believe its results. In this section, we will cover some of the key points that need to be considered when using *quantitative* research. Understanding the results from *qualitative* research will be addressed in Chapter 10. First, we need to explain briefly what external validity is, so that you do not confuse it with internal validity. *External validity* refers to the generalisability of the results of a study. That is, to what extent can we apply the results of the study to people other than the participants of the study? *Internal validity* refers to whether the evidence is trustworthy. That is, are the conclusions of a particular study true ('valid'), or could the result be explained by something else? There are three common alternative explanations that must be considered for the association or effect that is found in a study: (1) chance, (2) bias, and (3) confounding. Let us look at each of these in turn.

Chance

One possible explanation for a study's results—a difference between two groups, say—could be that the differences are due to random variation in the data. This means that any differences occurred just by chance alone. As we explain later in this chapter, determining whether findings are due to chance is what *statistical analysis* helps us decide. Random variation is smaller when the sample size (that is, the number of participants or, more properly, the number of *events*) of the study is greater. We discuss this in more detail later in the chapter.

Bias

Bias can be likened to the characteristic of lawn bowls that enables the bowl to roll in a curve. Although this is useful in the game of lawn bowls, 'not running true' (that is, not moving in a straight line) is a problem in study design: we use the term 'bias' for any effect that prevents the study conclusions from running true. Whereas chance is caused by *random* variation, bias is caused by *systematic* variation. Bias is a systematic error in the way that participants are selected for a study, outcomes are measured or data are analysed, each of which can lead to inaccurate results.

Biases can operate in either direction—to underestimate or overestimate an effect reported in a study. For example, consider a randomised controlled trial of the effectiveness of a new intervention for back pain. Imagine that the participants allocated to the new intervention had more severe symptoms (that is, had more back pain) at the start of the trial than those allocated to the control group. Any differences at the end of the study might be the result of that initial difference rather than the effect of the new intervention. This bias is called 'allocation bias'—a bias introduced by how participants were allocated to the two groups rather than by any differences attributable to the new intervention. It is an apparent, rather than a real, effect.

There are dozens of other kinds of bias, and we need to be able to look for and recognise them. Table 2.6 briefly describes some of the common kinds of bias that can occur. Some are relevant to non-randomised studies and some to randomised studies. Chapter 4 discusses the biases that can occur in randomised controlled trials in more detail.

The Centre for Evidence-Based Medicine at the University of Oxford has created a Catalogue of Bias (https://catalogofbias.org/), which describes over 50 types of bias that

TABLE 2.6   Some common kinds of bias

Type	How it operates	How study design can prevent it	What to look for when critically appraising an article
Selection or sampling bias	Systematic differences between those who are selected for study and those who are not selected. This means that the results of the study may not be generalisable to the population from which the sample is drawn.	Good sampling ensures that the people who are participating are representative of the population you want to generalise to.	Check how the sampling was done. Look for any data that compare this sample with the population's characteristics.
Allocation bias	In experimental studies, 'allocation bias' or 'selection bias' can refer to intervention and control groups being systematically different.	Randomisation attempts to evenly distribute both known and unknown confounders. Assess differences between groups at baseline. Statistically control for differences in analysis.	Check the article for a comparison of the groups before an intervention to see if they look sufficiently similar (also known as 'baseline similarity').
Maturation bias	The effect might be due to changes that have occurred naturally over time, not because of any intervention.	Use a control group and random allocation to intervention or control group.	Check to see if a control group and random allocation were used.

TABLE 2.6 Some common kinds of bias—cont'd

Type	How it operates	How study design can prevent it	What to look for when critically appraising an article
Attrition bias	Participants who withdraw from studies may differ systematically from those who remain. Alternatively, there may be more participants lost from one group in the study than from the other group.	Minimise loss to follow-up.	Be concerned about articles with a loss to follow-up of >15%.
		Analyse the results by intention-to-treat.	Check whether results were analysed by intention-to-treat.
Measurement bias in experimental studies	Errors in measuring exposure or outcome can lead to differential accuracy of information between groups. In other words, if the way that data are measured differs systematically between groups, this introduces bias. In experimental studies, this can be due to bias in the expectations of study participants, health professionals or researchers.	'Blinding' participants, health professionals or researchers will reduce this bias. Blinding is discussed further in Chapter 4.	Look to see if the study used methods to reduce the participants', health professionals' and/or researchers' awareness of a participant's group allocation (blinding).
Placebo effect	An improvement in the participants' condition may occur because they expect or believe that the intervention they are receiving will cause an improvement.	Have a control group of participants that receive approximately the same intervention (i.e. raise no different expectations). 'Blinding' participants, health professionals or researchers will reduce this bias.	Check whether there is a suitable control group and look to see whether the study used methods to reduce the participants', health professionals' and/or researchers' awareness of a participant's group allocation (blinding).
Hawthorne effect	Participants may experience changes because of the attention that they are receiving from being a part of the research process.	Have a control group that is studied in the same way (except for the intervention)—i.e. a randomised controlled trial.	Check whether there is a suitable control group to control for attention and whether the randomised controlled trial is designed properly.

affect health evidence. But there is no need to worry—you are not required to know them all! It may help to consider that all the biases fundamentally fall into two types: *selection bias* or *measurement bias*. For a single sample, such as a survey, this would be (a) bias in the selection of participants, and (b) bias in the 'measurement' of the participants selected. In studies that compare two groups, such as in a controlled trial, the selection bias becomes allocation bias (that is, there is some difference in the selection of

participants into the two groups); and the measurement bias becomes 'differential' measurement bias (that is, there is some difference in the way the exposure or outcomes were measured which creates a spurious difference between the groups). You might like to try applying this classification of bias—selection or measurement—to the biases listed in Table 2.6.

Assessing whether bias has occurred in a study is the focus of the first step (*Is the evidence valid?*) in the three-step critical appraisal process that was described in Chapter 1. Being able to assess whether the evidence is valid is a fundamental skill for evidence-based practice. So, we give it a lot of attention in this book, primarily in Chapters 4, 6, 8, 10 and 12.

Confounding

'Confound' comes from the Latin *confundere* [*com-* (together) + *fundere* (to pour)], meaning to confuse. Imagine adding red paint to a tin of pure white paint: the white becomes tainted in a way that they can never be separated. So it is with confounding factors. The factor of interest becomes irreducibly confused with the confounding factor (the 'confounder'). Confounders do not cause error in *measurement*; rather, they involve error in the *interpretation* of what may be an accurate measurement.

There are ways to minimise confounders. For intervention research ('does it work?' questions), the easiest way of doing this is to randomly allocate participants to groups—which is why the randomised controlled trial is the prime study design for these types of questions (Table 2.4). The intention is to distribute any confounders randomly—and hence evenly—between the intervention and the control groups. Randomisation will ensure that the sample is large enough (see below). In other study designs, a list of possible confounders is drawn up and either accounted for in the analysis (by stratification or statistical adjustment—such as 'regression analysis'—methods) or restricted to sub-groups. This is the method employed for observational studies (since there is no other option).

The problem with adjusting for confounders is that some confounders are *unknown*—factors that we either cannot measure or do not even know about. For example, participants' level of motivation to participate fully in an intervention (consider one that required people to perform certain exercises daily) is very difficult to measure accurately and could be a potential unknown confounder for a study that was examining the effectiveness of this intervention. Randomisation is the key, because the act of randomisation distributes all confounders, both known and unknown, fairly. A problem remains, though: what about the chance of an unequal distribution of confounders between groups? The answer to that is to do with two things: statistics, and the numbers in the study.

STATISTICAL SIGNIFICANCE, CLINICAL SIGNIFICANCE AND POWER

Statistical significance

We saw above that a randomised controlled trial could be biased because of a chance uneven distribution of confounders across the groups. The chance of this happening is reduced if the number of participants in the trial is increased. (As the numbers increase, the chance of unevenness decreases.) The chance of unevenness never decreases to zero, though, regardless of how large the trial is. In other words, there is always a chance of bias from confounders, so we have to tolerate some uncertainty. As the trial size (meaning the number of participants) increases, we become more confident that confounders will be minimised. The question is: how large should the trial be? The answer comes from statistics, which is the science of dealing with and quantifying this uncertainty. There are two main ways of deciding whether a difference in the summaries of two groups of participants is due to chance or to a real difference between them.

The *p* value

The *p* here is short for *probability*. This test is based on one of the cornerstones of scientific philosophy: that we cannot ever attempt to prove anything; rather, we can only attempt to *dis*prove it.[12] This means that we have to invert the question from the 'proving' form:

> 'Are the measurements between the two groups different enough to assume that it is because of some factor other than chance?'

to the 'disproving' form:

> 'Are the measurements between the two groups similar enough to assume that it is because of chance alone?'

If we can show that the latter statement is unlikely, then we can say that there must be some *other* factor responsible for the difference. In other words, the *p* value is estimated to establish 'how likely it is that the difference is because of chance alone'. Statisticians estimate a value of *p* that will be somewhere between 1.0 (absolutely sure that the difference is because of chance alone) and 0.0 (absolutely sure that the difference is *not* because of chance alone). Traditionally, we set the arbitrary value of *p* as <0.05, at which point we assume that chance was so unlikely that we can rule it out as the cause of the difference. A value of 0.05 ($\frac{5}{100}$) is the same as 5%, or 1:20. What we mean when we use this cut-off point for the *p* value is: 'We would have to repeat the study an average of 20 times for the result to happen once by chance alone.' When a study produces a result where the *p* value is <0.05, that result is considered to be '*statistically significant*'.

Confidence intervals

Confidence intervals take a different approach, and instead estimate what range of values the true value lies within.

True value refers to the population value, not just the estimate of a value that has come from the sample of one study (such as an estimate of how effective an intervention is, which is explained in more detail in Chapter 4). The range of values is called the *confidence interval* and is most commonly set at the same arbitrary level as *p* values (0.95, or 20:1), which is also called the '95% confidence interval'. Another way to think of the value is graphically, as shown in Figure 2.4.

The figure shows the range of possible values for an estimated measurement for two different studies, A and B. In each figure, the two vertical lines indicate the two limits (or boundaries) of the confidence interval. The values in between these lines indicate the range of values within which we are 95% certain (or confident, hence the term 'confidence intervals') that the true value is likely to lie. The probability that the true value lies outside of this confidence interval is 0.05 (or 5%), with half of this value

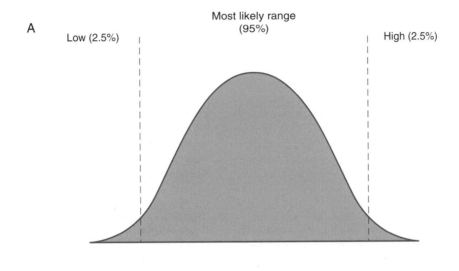

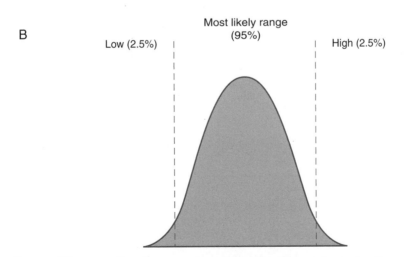

Fig 2.4 For two different studies, the range of possible values for an estimated measurement (with the 95% confidence interval) is shown. In the study represented by figure B, the 95% confidence interval is smaller (narrower) than the one in figure A. A smaller confidence interval can occur when the sample size of a study is larger.

(2.5%) lying in each tail of the curve. The most likely value is central and, in most cases, the distribution of possible values forms a normal distribution (that is, a bell-shaped curve). The spread of values will form a different shape according to different influences on the 95% confidence interval. For example, in the study that is represented by Figure 2.4B, the sample size is larger. This has the effect of narrowing the 95% confidence interval because the normal curve is more peaked. The same effect is achieved by samples that yield greater uniformity of the participants (that is, decreased variance of the sample). This is summarised in Table 2.7.

Confidence intervals are an important concept to understand in evidence-based practice as they help you with the second step (*What is the impact of the evidence?*) of the three-step critical appraisal process described in Chapter 1. The role that confidence intervals play in helping you to determine the impact of the evidence is explained in more detail in Chapter 4. Despite their usefulness and calls for studies to report effect size and confidence intervals rather than just isolated *p* values, in many articles this does not occur,[13] so we will also explain how to calculate confidence intervals where appropriate.

Clinical versus statistical significance

There is one more essential consideration: how big a difference is worthwhile? Once we have established a difference that is unlikely to be attributable to chance (that is, it is statistically significant), how can we decide whether the difference is important? *Clinical significance* is defined as just that: the minimum difference that would be important to patients. (Because of this, some people use the term 'clinical importance', rather than 'clinical significance', to refer to this concept.)

We cannot use statistics to measure clinical significance, because it is a judgment: we have to decide what difference would be important. This means choosing some difference based on what you (or your patients) judge is clinically important. For example, consider an intervention study where the outcome being measured was pain, using a visual analogue scale (a straight line with one end meaning 'no pain' and the other end meaning 'the most pain imaginable'). If the intervention had the effect of reducing participants' pain (on average) by 4 points on a 10-point visual analogue scale (where 1 = 'no pain' and 10 = 'the most pain imaginable'), we would probably judge a difference of this size to be clinically significant, while we probably would not consider a reduction of 0.5 to be clinically significant. Chapter 4 discusses in further detail the various approaches that can be used to help determine clinical significance.

It should now be clear that there are four main categories into which the results of a study can fall. As visualised in Figure 2.5, a result may be:

1. **Statistically significant *and* clinically significant.** This is the type of result that is clear: there is a real and meaningful difference that can potentially inform our clinical practice and you can proceed to the third step in the three-step critical appraisal process—deciding whether the evidence can be applied to your patient.
2. **Not statistically significant but possibly clinically significant.** When this is the case, you will need to find— or wait for—more research to clarify, as you cannot even be sure that the result was not due to chance.
3. **Statistically significant but not *clinically* significant.** This is common, unfortunately. It means that the difference is not large enough to be important even though it is a 'real', not-by-chance, difference.
4. **Not statistically significant and not clinically significant.** When this is the case, you cannot even be sure that the result was not due to chance, but in any case, the effect is unlikely to be clinically significant.

Outcome measures—what do we need to know about them?

The issue of clinical significance raises another matter that is important when it comes to appraising articles: you need

TABLE 2.7 Effect of sample size and variance on a study's confidence interval	
Factor	**Effect on the confidence interval**
Sample size (the number of participants in the study)	The confidence interval narrows as the sample size increases—there is more certainty about the effect estimate. This is one of the reasons why it is important that studies have an adequate sample size. The importance of a smaller (narrower) confidence interval is explained in Chapter 4.
Variance (the amount of 'noise' or differences in values between participants in the sample)	The confidence interval widens as the variance increases— there is less certainty about the effect estimate.

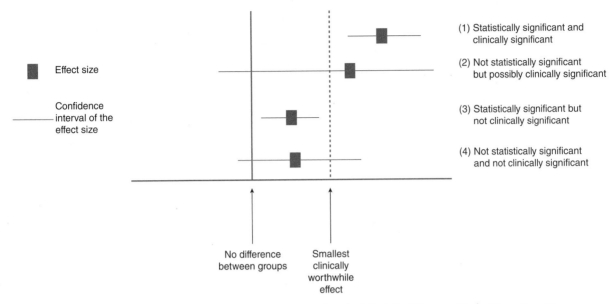

Fig 2.5 Interpreting confidence intervals for statistical and clinical significance. Adapted from Berry G. Statistical significance and confidence intervals. Med J Aust 1986;144(12):618–19.

to know about the outcome measure that a study used, as this helps you to make a judgment about clinical significance. In our pain study example, if the visual analogue scale that was used to measure pain was a 0–100 scale, then we would probably no longer consider a reduction in pain of 4 points (on a 100-point scale) to be clinically significant (even though on a 10-point scale, we decided that it was). If you are lucky, the study that you are reading will include the scale range of the continuous outcome measures used in the study somewhere in the article (usually in the methods section or in a results table). If it does not, then you will need to find this information out for yourself. If it is an outcome measure that you are familiar with, great! If not, perhaps searching for it on the internet (Google can be useful in this instance) may help you to find out more about it.

In addition to knowing about the actual measures used in a study to measure the outcomes, it is important that you consider whether the outcomes themselves are relevant, useful and important to your patient. For example, consider a patient who has had a stroke and now has difficulty using his arm to perform functional activities such as eating and getting dressed. The patient's goal is to return to doing these activities independently. You are considering using a physical rehabilitation technique with him to improve his ability to carry out these activities, primarily by working on the quality of the movement in his affected arm. Let us suppose that when evaluating the evidence for

the effectiveness of this intervention, there are two studies that you can use to inform your practice. (For the sake of simplicity, we will assume that they both have a similar level of internal validity.) The outcomes measured in one study (study A) are arm function and the ability to perform self-care activities, whereas the outcome measured in the other study (study B) is quality of arm movement. In this (very simplified!) example, if you choose study A to inform your clinical practice you will be able to communicate the results of the study to the patient and explain to them the estimated effect that the intervention may have on their ability to perform these activities. Remember that this is what your patient primarily wants to know. Although study B may provide you with information that is useful to you as a health professional, the effect that the intervention may have on the quality of arm movement may be of less interest to your patient than knowing how it may improve the function of their arm. Considering whether the outcomes measured are useful to your patient is one way of considering how *patient-centred* the study is. Chapter 14 explains patient-centred care and the importance of encouraging patients' involvement in decisions about their health care.

Putting it all together: thinking about power

As we mentioned earlier, we can have results that are statistically significant but not clinically significant. But statistical significance can be made more likely by increasing the size of the sample (or reducing the 'noise'—more properly called 'variance'). If a study is large enough, its results will become statistically significant even though the differences are not important clinically—which is why we call on clinical significance to decide what is worthwhile. This means we can decide on the minimum size a study's sample has to be to give a definitive answer. This is important because it helps us decide what would be wasteful. (Above the minimum is wasteful of research resources.)

When we estimate the minimum, this is called a 'power calculation'. A study has enough *power* (meaning that there is a large enough sample) if a statistically significant difference is found. In other words, the power of a study is the degree to which we are certain that, if we conclude that a difference does *not* exist, that it in fact does *not* exist. The accepted level of power is generally set at the arbitrary level of 80% (or 0.80).

What happens if the minimum sample size is not reached? Such a study is called 'underpowered', meaning that if a difference is found that is not significant, either there really *is* no effect (that is, any difference can be attributed to chance), or there is a real difference but it was not detected because the sample was too small. If the authors or readers incorrectly conclude that a difference does not exist, this is called a 'type-2 error'. Because of the risk of this type of error occurring, when evaluating a study you need to decide whether it had adequate power (that is, a large enough sample size). One way to determine this is to check an article to see if the researchers did a power calculation. Researchers do a power analysis prior to conducting the study because it enables them to estimate how many participants they will need to recruit to be reasonably sure (to a given level of uncertainty) that they will detect an important difference if it really exists. You can then check if they actually did recruit at least as many participants as they estimated would be needed.

Can a study be too large? Surprisingly, the answer is 'yes'. If a research study is unnecessarily large, then effort and money have been wasted. A more subtle reason is that a difference that is statistically significant can be found, but the difference may be so small that we judge its significance not to be meaningful. This can mean having a situation that we discussed earlier in this chapter, where a difference is *statistically* significant but *clinically* not significant.

SUMMARY

- Questions about frequency, diagnosis, prognosis, the effects of interventions and people's experiences are among the types of clinical questions that can usually be answered using evidence-based practice.
- Converting your information needs into answerable clinical questions is the first step in the evidence-based practice process. A well-structured question can be achieved by using the PICO (Patient/Problem, Intervention, Comparison, Outcome[s]) format.
- Systematic reviews, randomised controlled trials, cohort studies, cross-sectional studies, case-control studies and qualitative research designs are some of the common study types that are used in evidence-based practice.
- For each type of question, there is a different hierarchy of evidence. The higher up the hierarchy that a study is, the more likely it is that the study can minimise the impact of bias on its results. You should use the hierarchy of evidence that is appropriate to your question to guide your search for and selection of quantitative evidence to answer your question. Qualitative research is considered differently, and this is discussed in Chapter 10.
- For all question types, a systematic review of the individual study type that is at the top of the hierarchy is what you should search for first. What type of study this is differs for each question type. For example, for intervention questions it is a randomised controlled trial; for prognostic questions, it is a prospective inception cohort study; and for diagnostic studies, it is a cross-sectional study of test accuracy that involved an independent, blinded comparison with a valid reference standard, among consecutive persons.
- Being able to recognise whether bias and/or confounding have occurred in a study is a crucial part of the critical appraisal process, as it enables you to determine the internal validity of the evidence. There are many types of bias and you need to be able to recognise them. 'Internal validity' refers to how much we can trust the results of a quantitative study and is influenced by how chance, bias and/or confounding operated in a study.
- If the result of a study is statistically significant, it means that we are reasonably sure that the result (such as a difference in outcomes between two groups in a study) did not occur because of chance. Statistical significance can be indicated by *p* values or confidence intervals. In evidence-based practice, confidence intervals are much more useful than *p* values. If a result is statistically significant, you then need to consider if it is also clinically significant—that is, is the result important enough that you will use it in your clinical practice? Clinical significance is typically best determined by judgment and, ideally, in conjunction with your patient.

REFERENCES

1. Bastian H, Glasziou P, Chalmers I. Seventy-five trials and eleven systematic reviews a day: how will we ever keep up? PLOS Med 2010;7:e1000326.

2. Shirky C. It's not information overload. It's filter failure. Web 2.0 Expo, New York; 2008.

3. Hoffmann T, Erueti C, Thorning S, et al. The scatter of research: a cross-sectional comparison of randomised trials and systematic reviews across specialties. BMJ 2012; 344:e3223.

4. Clarke MA, Belden JL, Koopman RJ, et al. Information needs and information-seeking behaviour analysis of primary care physicians and nurses: a literature review. Health Info Libr J 2013;30:178–90.

5. Del Fiol G, Workman TE, Gorman PN. Clinical questions raised by clinicians at the point of care: a systematic review. JAMA Intern Med 2014;174:710–18.

6. Gonzalez-Gonzalez A, Dawes M, Sanchez-Mateos J, et al. Information needs and information-seeking behavior of primary care physicians. Ann Fam Med 2007;5:345–52.

7. Kortekaas MF, Bartelink M-LEL, Boelman L, et al. General practice trainees' information searching strategies for clinical queries encountered in daily practice. Fam Prac 2015;32:533–7.

8. Coumou H, Meijman F. How do primary care physicians seek answers to clinical questions? A literature review. JAMA 2006;94:55–60.

9. McGowan J, Hogg W, Campbell C, et al. Just-in-time information improved decision-making in primary care: a randomized controlled trial. PLOS ONE 2008;3:e3785.

10. Straus S, Richardson W, Glasziou P, et al. Evidence-based medicine: how to practice and teach EBM. 4th ed. Edinburgh: Churchill Livingstone; 2011.

11. Kitson A, Marshall A, Bassett K, et al. What are the core elements of patient-centred care? A narrative review and synthesis of the literature from health policy, medicine and nursing. J Adv Nurs 2013;69:4–15.

12. Hacking I. An introduction to probability and inductive logic. New York: Cambridge University Press; 2001.

13. Chavalarias D, Wallach J, Li A, et al. Evolution of reporting p values in the biomedical literature, 1990–2015. JAMA 2016;315:1141–8.

Finding the Evidence

Justin Clark

LEARNING OBJECTIVES

After reading this chapter, you should be able to:
- Describe the principles of efficient searching
- Understand how to navigate your way around literature services
- Understand how each of the major evidence-based resources fits into evidence-based practice

- Identify discipline-specific evidence-based resources
- Know which databases are likely to supply an answer when searching for evidence for each type of question (that is, intervention, diagnosis, prognosis and qualitative)
- Know how to search for evidence for each type of question

Finding current best evidence relevant to your clinical question can pose a challenge when implementing evidence-based practice. The internet has improved access to information but has also caused an information explosion. This makes finding the current best evidence challenging. Resources compete to claim that they are 'evidence-based' but often do little to authenticate such claims. You can probably relate to some or all of the following obstacles when attempting to answer a clinical question:
- the challenge of knowing which sources to use and when
- the excessive amount of time required to find information
- difficulty in sorting high-quality information from low-quality information
- failure of the selected resource to provide an answer.[1,2]

Using a systematic approach to search for the best evidence can help you to harness the way the literature is organised to your advantage. This chapter will show you how you can do this. Starting from the basics of searching, we will outline a helpful way to navigate evidence-based information services. We will consider how evidence is processed and presented. Within each category of this model, we will describe the types of evidence that are included. We will then map these to the resources that can be used to find each particular type of evidence. We will

emphasise resources with the strongest evidence base, as these have the most potential to inform your clinical practice. These are typically the resources that are easier and faster to use. We will finish with some examples of clinical questions and how you might search for evidence to answer them.

THE BASICS OF SEARCHING

Effective searching for evidence starts from the following principles:
1. Carefully define your clinical question.
2. Choose your key search terms.
3. Broaden your search if necessary, with synonyms, truncation and/or wildcards.
4. Use Boolean operators.

Carefully define your clinical question

If you have already constructed a well-formulated clinical question using the PICO format that was explained in Chapter 2, you are well placed to start defining the components of your search strategy.

Choose your key search terms

Structuring your clinical question using the PICO format simplifies the process of choosing key search terms.

Normally, you start searching with the 'P' (patients [or population]) and 'I' (intervention) terms. For example, if your question is '*In people with chronic low back pain, is spinal manipulation more effective than light massage in reducing pain and functional disability?*' you would start your search with the phrases "chronic low back pain" ('P' terms) and "spinal manipulation" ('I' terms). If this produces too many results, add your 'O' (Outcome) terms—in this example, it would be "pain" and "function" ('O' terms). If you still have too many results, you could add "light massage" (the 'C'—comparator—term) to the search.

Broaden your search if necessary

Using only a single term or phrase for each of your search terms means you may miss relevant articles or return no relevant articles at all. The terms that an author chooses to use when writing the title and abstract of their article may not be the same as the terms you use when searching for it. To improve your chances of finding relevant results, you should broaden your search, particularly if your initial search yields no relevant articles. Here are some ways of doing this:

- Consider using **synonyms and related terms**. For example, when searching for articles on patients with "rheumatoid arthritis" you can broaden your search by adding the terms "RA" and "rheumatologic disease". Resources that list synonyms and related terms for many diseases and conditions may prove useful (such as the National Library of Medicine MeSH database: https://www.ncbi.nlm.nih.gov/mesh/). It is also common to find a few examples of the type of study you are looking for. Then look at the words used by the authors in the title and abstract, or at the subject headings, and note any useful alternative terms.
- Widen your search using **truncation** and **wildcards**.
  - Truncation involves entering the first part of a keyword followed by a symbol (usually an asterisk symbol[*]). The system then identifies any variant spellings or word endings from the occurrence of the symbol onwards. For example, "disease*" would retrieve records with the word *disease*, as well as the words *diseases*, *diseased*, etc. However, truncating a word too much can result in irrelevant words—in this case, truncating at *dis** would retrieve *disaster*.
  - A wildcard differs from truncation in replacing a single character, rather than a word ending. You usually enter a wildcard character (such as "?") within, or at the end of, a keyword to substitute for only one character. Wildcards are particularly useful when

searching for some plural forms, such as "wom?n", which would retrieve records with the words *woman* and *women*. Wildcards are also useful in searching for variations in spelling—for example, orthopedic/orthopaedic and pediatric/paediatric. Searching with the term "orthop?edic" will find articles that use *orthopaedic* as well as *orthopedic*.

- Truncation symbols and wildcard characters are usually specific to each database or database provider. Most databases use an asterisk (*); however, some use other characters such as a colon (:) or a dollar sign ($). Their use also varies between databases—for example, PubMed supports only end-character truncation (not single wildcard characters within words).

Use Boolean operators

Once you have chosen the terms or phrases to include in your search, you should consider how you are going to combine these terms using the Boolean logical operators AND/OR.

- Use the Boolean AND operator when you want *all* of the search terms to be present in each article that is retrieved. For example, when searching using 'P' terms and 'I' terms, you combine these terms using the Boolean AND operator to retrieve articles with *both* your patient/population of interest *and* the intervention of interest. Using the back pain example from earlier in the chapter, the search combination would be "(chronic low back pain) AND (spinal manipulation)".
- You use the Boolean OR operator when you want *any* of the specified search terms to be present in the articles. Typically, you combine synonyms using the Boolean OR operator—for example, "rheumatoid arthritis OR RA OR rheumatologic disease"—thus broadening your search. This search retrieves articles that use either 'rheumatoid arthritis' *or* 'RA' *or* 'rheumatologic disease'.

Be aware that although most databases use AND and OR when combining terms, the command language (for example, paragraph names, symbols and punctuation) is specific to each database. You should translate commands from the command language of one database to those of another when you search using another interface. Consult each database's Help function, seek advice from an information specialist or librarian, or use an automatic translator (such as the Polyglot Search Translator:[3] https://sr-accelerator.com/#/polyglot).

BASICS OF SEARCHING: AN EXAMPLE

To illustrate these basics of searching further, we will work through a step-by-step example.

Step 1: Identify the components of your question in PICO format

P **Patient population**	I **Intervention (therapy, diagnostic test, prognostic factor)**	C **Comparison**	O **Outcomes**
Work-related neck muscle pain	Strength training of the painful muscle	General fitness training	Pain relief

Step 2: Compose your clinical question

Patients with work-related neck muscle pain	Patients
Strength training of the painful muscle	Intervention
General fitness training without direct involvement of the painful muscle	Comparison
Greater pain relief	Outcomes

Step 3: Construct the final clinical question

For patients with work-related neck muscle pain, does strength training of the painful muscle versus general fitness training without direct involvement of the painful muscle result in greater pain relief?

Clinical scenario

You are a rehabilitation consultant who has recently seen a number of individuals with work-related neck muscle pain, especially pain from the descending part of the trapezius muscle. You know that physical exercise is generally recommended, but you do not know which type of training is more effective in relieving muscle pain—strength training of the painful muscle, or general fitness training without direct involvement of the painful muscle.

Step 4: Record keywords and phrases

Keyword 1:	**Keyword 2:**	**Keyword 3:**	**Keyword 4:**
Neck muscle pain	Muscular strength training	General fitness	Pain relief

Step 5: Identify synonyms and variant words

Keyword 1:	**Keyword 2:**	**Keyword 3:**	**Keyword 4:**
Neck strain	Strength training	Exercise	Pain
Neck strains	Muscle strengthening		
Neck strain injury			
Neck strain injuries			
Neck sprain			
Neck sprains			
Stiff neck			
Trapezius muscle pain			

Step 6: Use truncation and wildcards where appropriate and Boolean operators to combine terms

(Neck muscle pain OR Neck strain* OR Neck strain injur* OR Neck sprain* OR Stiff neck OR Trapezius muscle pain) AND (Strength training OR Muscle strengthening) AND (General fitness OR Exercise) AND (Pain*)

Note: The truncation symbol used in this example is for conducting a search in PubMed.

Step 7: Decide which online resource(s) to search

The online resource that you decide to search in will depend on the type of question you are asking (for example, an intervention, diagnostic, prognostic or qualitative question). As explained in Chapter 2, for each type of question there is a hierarchy of evidence. This hierarchy should be used to guide your search so that you know what type of study design you are hoping to find. The type of study design you are looking for will, in turn, influence which online resource(s) you should search in. For example, if your clinical question is a prognostic one related to rehabilitation, then you will be looking for a cohort study (or a systematic review of cohort studies). Therefore, there is no point in searching resources such as PEDro, as it does not contain cohort studies. The best resource for you to start your search in would probably be PubMed, using the *Clinical Queries* feature, or the Rehabilitation subset of ACCESSSS 2.0 (see later in this chapter). All of these resources, and many others, are described in the following section and in the examples at the end of this chapter.

HOW TO NAVIGATE EVIDENCE-BASED INFORMATION SERVICES

In this chapter, we use a five-layer pyramid to navigate the various evidence-based information services.[4] This five-layer model (see Figure 3.1), known as the Evidence-Based HealthCare (EBHC) 5.0 pyramid, offers a structured and efficient way to navigate information sources. **As you are seeking the current best evidence, begin your search as high up the pyramid as possible. The higher you are in the pyramid, the more work has been done for you in collecting, sifting and synthesising the evidence base and the information should be more useful for guiding clinical decision making.** As the synthesis and evaluation has already been done by others, using evidence from the higher layers saves you time and effort. It also helps you to identify and apply the best-quality available evidence. Starting at the top and working down, the layers are:

- **Systems:** integrated decision support services—evidence from lower levels of the pyramid integrated with individual patient records.
- **Synthesised summaries for clinical reference:** overviews of management options for diseases or conditions arranged by clinical topics—for example, evidence-based texts (also known as 'point-of-care information tools') such as UpToDate, DynaMed Plus or BMJ Best Practice.
- **Systematically derived recommendations (Guidelines):** this might be a synthesis of multiple guidelines or single guidelines.

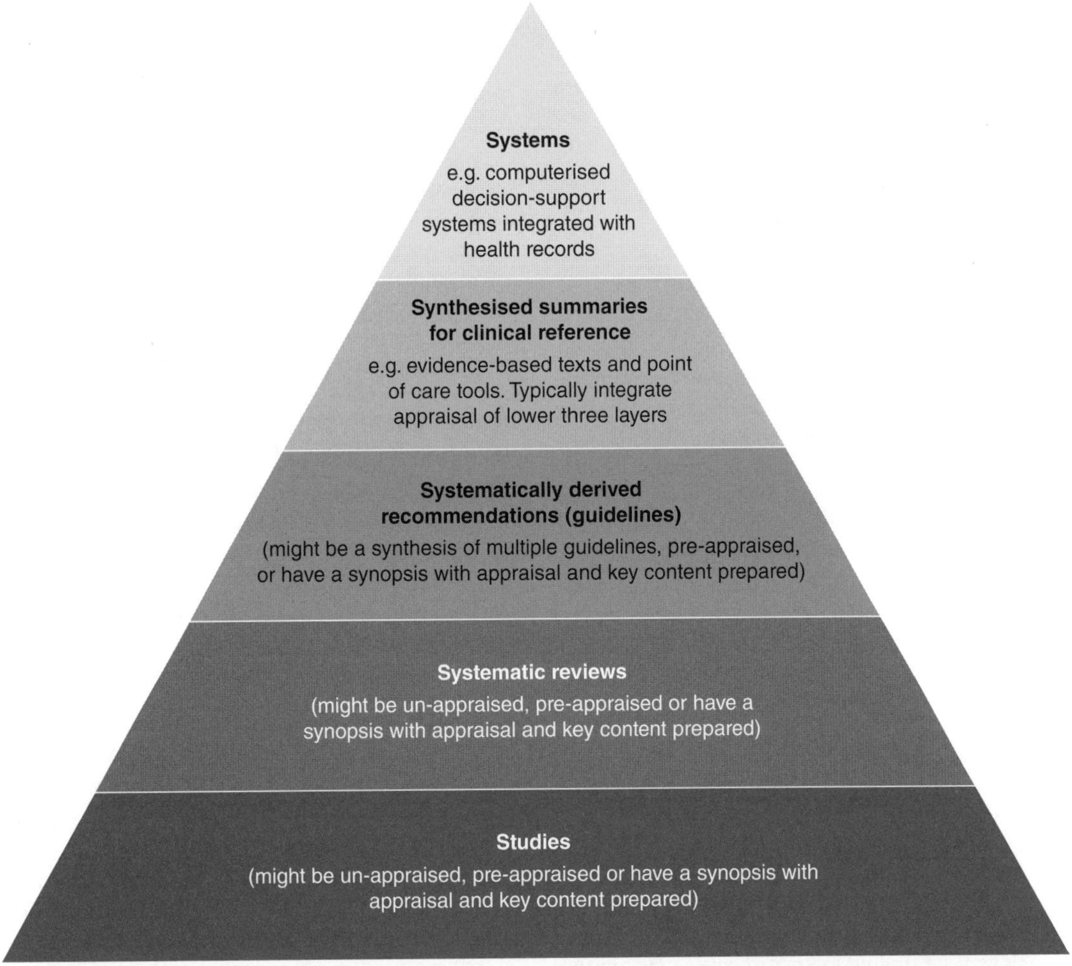

Systems
e.g. computerised decision-support systems integrated with health records

Synthesised summaries for clinical reference
e.g. evidence-based texts and point of care tools. Typically integrate appraisal of lower three layers

Systematically derived recommendations (guidelines)
(might be a synthesis of multiple guidelines, pre-appraised, or have a synopsis with appraisal and key content prepared)

Systematic reviews
(might be un-appraised, pre-appraised or have a synopsis with appraisal and key content prepared)

Studies
(might be un-appraised, pre-appraised or have a synopsis with appraisal and key content prepared)

Fig 3.1 The Evidence-Based HealthCare (EBHC) 5.0 pyramid showing the organisation of evidence from healthcare research
Adapted with permission from Alper BS, Haynes RB. EBHC pyramid 5.0 for accessing preappraised evidence and guidance. BMJ Evid Based Med 2016;21:123–5.

- **Systematic reviews:** systematic reviews (the evidence across several studies on the same topic) of the literature.
- **Studies:** single studies published in journals.

Where you start within the pyramid depends largely on the question that you are asking and the resources available to you. As explained in Chapter 2, be guided by the hierarchy of evidence for the type of question that you are asking. Additionally, you will find that most content available at the higher layers of the pyramid is aimed at the medical profession. Most evidence for other health professions is located within the lower layers (as guidelines, systematic reviews and individual studies).

Within the bottom three layers, content from some resources will be critically appraised. This might be in the form of pre-appraised (or filtered) studies or reviews or a synopsis of them (where an appraisal and extraction of key content has been done). However, for information from many resources in the lower layers, users of the evidence must appraise the quality of the evidence presented to ensure that the methods used to generate this evidence were sound. Detailed information about how to critically appraise evidence, once you have found it, is presented later in this book. Each layer of the pyramid is now discussed further, starting at the top of the pyramid, where the most highly synthesised evidence is found.

Systems—first layer (top) of the pyramid

Systems are found at the top of the pyramid. A system is an integrated clinical decision support service designed to improve clinical decision making. Such a system may be integrated into an electronic patient health record system or hospital clinical information system. Alternatively, the system may allow for entry of patient-specific characteristics, such as age, gender and allergy history. These computerised decision support systems link patient characteristics with the current evidence-based guidelines for care. The system generates patient-specific recommendations (for example, lower the dose of insulin because of hypoglycaemic events, or schedule a blood test because it is due next month). A key component of a clinical decision support service that differentiates it from other types of evidence-based information services is that it integrates the evidence with patient-specific variables. Systematic reviews of the effects of computerised clinical decision support systems show that some systems may improve health professionals' performance or prevent morbidity but are unlikely to have an effect on mortality.[5] However, systems that integrate the evidence base with patient-specific details are still uncommon; therefore, most health professionals will be unable to start their search for the current best evidence at this layer.

Synthesised summaries for clinical reference—second top layer of the pyramid

Summaries are information resources that provide regularly updated evidence, usually arranged by clinical topic. They may resemble traditional textbook chapters in form and content but differ in the frequency of their update and usually in the quality thresholds for the evidence they cite. Summaries provide guidance and/or recommendations for patient management and often provide links to other aspects of the disease or condition. These are typically available on subscription, but your workplace, particularly if an academic or healthcare institution, may have an institutional subscription.

- **BMJ Best Practice** (https://bestpractice.bmj.com/info/) combines the latest research evidence, guidelines and expert opinion regarding symptom evaluation, test ordering and treatment, with links provided to supporting evidence.
- **UpToDate** (https://www.uptodate.com) is a comprehensive electronic textbook that is organised into topic outlines for each medical specialty (for example, primary care, internal medicine, cardiovascular medicine, endocrinology and diabetes). *UpToDate* provides specific recommendations (guidelines), and the primary references. Most, but not all, of these recommendations include an assessment of the quality of the evidence.
- **DynaMed Plus** (https://www.dynamed.com/) is a clinical reference tool for use at the point of care (for example, at the bedside or in the clinic). It offers clinically organised summaries for thousands of topics. The source offers recommendations for practice supported by accompanying evidence.

Systematically derived recommendations (Guidelines)—third layer of the pyramid

Evidence-based clinical guidelines are located within this layer of the pyramid. (Chapter 13 discusses guidelines in detail, including where to search for them.) An example of a resource for locating them is **EBM Guidelines** (https://www.ebm-guidelines.com/dtk/ebmg/home)—a frequently updated collection of about 1,000 concise primary care practice guidelines and about 4,000 evidence summaries.

Systematic reviews—fourth layer of the pyramid

Systematic reviews provide syntheses of the highest quality evidence for a specific clinical question. How to appraise systematic reviews is explained in Chapter 12. Systematic reviews can be found in the following resources:

- **Cochrane Database of Systematic Reviews** (www.thecochranelibrary.com) is part of the Cochrane Library and is made up of outputs from numerous topic-based review groups who concentrate and synthesise the evidence in specific healthcare areas. For example, the

Cochrane Musculoskeletal Group focuses on synthesising the evidence from randomised controlled trials of interventions related to the prevention and treatment of musculoskeletal disorders.

This database originally focused on healthcare interventions; however, the scope has broadened to include reviews on diagnostic test accuracy, prognosis and qualitative evidence syntheses. For now, the Cochrane Library is a subscription-based resource available by institutional subscription in many academic or hospital environments. However, residents in many low- or middle-income countries can access the Cochrane Library for free, while in other countries (such as Australia) the government purchases a national subscription. Cochrane has committed to full open access publishing by 2025. Cochrane systematic reviews are indexed in several large biomedical databases such as MEDLINE.

The Cochrane Database of Systematic Reviews has numerous search functions, such as Quick Search, Advanced Search and MeSH search. (See Box 3.1 for an explanation of MeSH.) As the Cochrane Library is such an important evidence-based practice resource, you should learn how to search it efficiently. We recommend that you read the free, easy-to-read Cochrane Library Reference Guide (https://www.cochranelibrary.com/help/how-to-use).

Some Cochrane reviews are updated regularly, and superseded versions of a review are archived on the Cochrane Library website under an 'Other versions' tab.

- **Campbell Collaboration** (https://www.campbellcollaboration.org/) conducts and maintains systematic reviews in a broad range of social science topics, including the fields of ageing, disability, education, nutrition, and knowledge translation and implementation.

BOX 3.1   What are index terms and textwords?

Index terms

- Index terms are 'look up words' that point you to the best terms to use for searching. They are designed to overcome the problem of different authors using different terms to describe the same concept. Typically 10–20 index terms are assigned to each article by indexing staff using a database-specific thesaurus. Unfortunately, database producers have no incentive to coordinate the terms they use and different databases use different index terms. For example, MEDLINE uses MeSH (Medical Subject Headings), CINAHL uses CINAHL subject headings and EMBASE uses Emtree.
- Index terms are organised hierarchically, using a tree structure, with broader terms higher up the 'tree'. This structure allows you to make your search broader conceptually by moving up the tree or narrower by moving down the tree to a more specific term. For example, the MeSH tree structure for 'stroke' includes the following:

Nervous System Diseases
    Central Nervous System Diseases
        Brain Diseases
            Cerebrovascular Disorders
                Stroke
                    Brain Infarction
                        Hemorrhagic stroke
                        Ischemic stroke

- New topics, or those where little research has appeared, may not have been assigned corresponding index terms. This is often the case for many interventions that are used by allied health professionals. When this occurs, you need to search using textwords. Using textwords has the benefit of identifying studies that contain the exact term that you are looking for. However, if the author of a study has used a different label for the same intervention, you will miss this relevant article.
- How do you know which MeSH terms to choose? You can search the MeSH browser on the National Library of Medicine website (https://www.ncbi.nlm.nih.gov/mesh); commercial versions of MEDLINE allow you to choose to map your search automatically to relevant MeSH; or you can look at relevant articles to examine which MeSH are assigned to those articles.

Textwords

You can also search using textwords. These are free-text words that are found in the title and abstract of the article and therefore are the words used by the authors of articles. The limitation of this method is that the authors may have used a different term (for example, 'cerebrovascular accident') from the search term that you are using (for example, 'stroke'). Although you are both describing the same thing, you may not retrieve their article in your search. The obvious way to overcome this is to use the relevant index term as well as textwords. However, if there is no corresponding index term, you can use a wide range of synonyms and related terms (combining them with the Boolean operator OR) and truncation and wildcard symbols to help to broaden your search.

- **Epistemonikos** (www.epistemonikos.org) is a collaborative, multilingual database of research evidence and knowledge translation products developed and maintained by systematically searching electronic databases and other sources for relevant systematic reviews. It aims to bring together all the systematic reviews answering the same PICO question. A unique feature is that it links together systematic reviews and primary studies, so that a searcher can move between reviews and their included studies in an evidence matrix. For this reason, Epistemonikos does not claim to be a comprehensive database of health research. It only includes primary studies that have been included in a systematic review.
- **L·OVE: Living OVerview of Evidence** (https://iloveevidence.com/) combines artificial intelligence algorithms and a wide network of experts to organise and categorise the collection of around 300,000 systematic reviews from the Epistemonikos database. This allows easy browsing of health systematic reviews by topic, condition or problem using the PICO format. It enables the saving of questions so you will be notified when new evidence emerges.

- **Various biomedical databases**—details of many systematic reviews may be retrieved from large electronic biomedical databases such as MEDLINE and EMBASE. MEDLINE is available free of charge through PubMed. Both databases are offered through various providers on a subscription basis. The sheer volume of articles that these large databases contain, together with the fact that they also contain many other types of articles that are not useful for answering clinical questions, makes it challenging to identify systematic reviews. To overcome the challenge of retrieving systematic reviews, these databases have search filters (usually as an 'article type' or 'publication type') that narrow down the results to only systematic reviews.
- **Discipline-specific databases** that contain systematic reviews or index systematic reviews are shown in Table 3.1.
- Various discipline journals (such as **Evidence-Based Nursing**: https://ebn.bmj.com/ and the **Journal of Physiotherapy**: https://www.journals.elsevier.com/journal-of-physiotherapy) critically appraise and publish a summary of new research (both systematic reviews and primary studies), along with an expert commentary.

TABLE 3.1 Discipline-specific databases for systematic reviews and primary studies

Database name	URL	Content coverage	Study types	Access
Health Evidence	www.healthevidence.org	Approximately 8,400 systematic reviews evaluating the effectiveness of **public health** interventions. Reviews are screened for relevance and critically appraised by two database staff and quality scores displayed.	Systematic reviews	Free
EvidenceAlerts and ACCESSSS 2.0	https://www.evidencealerts.com https://www.accessss.org/ Subsets relevant to Medicine (MD+), Nursing (N+), and Rehabilitation (R+) can be searched separately	These resources are described in the chapter in the 'Federated search engines' and 'Alerting services' sections.	Guidelines, primary studies and systematic reviews	Free (although within ACCESSSS, a personal or institutional subscription is needed to access the electronic textbook content)
PEDro— Physiotherapy Evidence Database	www.pedro.org.au	57,000 abstracts of studies of **physiotherapy interventions**. Most trials have been critically appraised.	Systematic reviews, randomised trials and clinical practice guidelines	Free

TABLE 3.1 **Discipline-specific databases for systematic reviews and primary studies—cont'd**

Database name	URL	Content coverage	Study types	Access
Diagnostic Test Accuracy database	https://dita.org.au/	A database that indexes diagnostic test accuracy studies relevant to physiotherapy.	Systematic reviews of diagnostic test accuracy and primary diagnostic test accuracy studies	Free
NeuroBITE	https://neurorehab-evidence.com/web/cms/content/home	About 5,000 abstracts of studies on cognitive, behavioural and other treatments for **psychological problems and issues following acquired brain impairment**. Studies have been critically appraised.	Systematic reviews, randomised trials, non-randomised controlled trials, case series and single-participant designs	Free
speechBITE (Speech Pathology Database for Best Interventions and Treatment Efficacy)	www.speechbite.com	About 5,000 abstracts of studies on **speech pathology interventions**. Randomised and non-randomised trials have been critically appraised.	Systematic reviews, randomised trials, non-randomised controlled trials, case series and single-participant designs	Free
PDQ Evidence	www.pdq-evidence.org	Evidence for informing decisions about **health systems**. It has direct connections between systematic reviews, broad syntheses of reviews and their included studies, making it easy for the searcher to derive a broad synthesis of the evidence and to find what they are looking for.	Systematic reviews and their included studies.	Free
Health Systems Evidence	www.healthsystems evidence.org	Evidence (syntheses) to support policy makers, stakeholders and researchers interested in how to **strengthen or reform health systems** and in implementation strategies to support change in health strategies.	Syntheses include evidence briefs for policy, overviews of systematic reviews, systematic reviews, systematic review protocols and registered titles. Economic evaluations, descriptions of health systems and reforms.	Free; creating a free account enables additional features

Studies—bottom layer of the pyramid

The top layers of the pyramid hold the potential to save you time and to offer information that is either quality assessed, accumulated from multiple sources, or both. When none of the upper layers provide an answer to your clinical question, you must look for individual studies. With millions of individual studies, it is challenging to find efficiently the evidence that you need to answer your clinical question. When selecting an individual article, be aware of your own values and beliefs, and of how your biases might influence which articles, from the many that are retrieved from a search, you choose to explore further. When searching for individual studies, where possible, start your search using databases that have screened many sources for you, that include only the most important clinical studies and that have pre-appraised the studies for you. Examples are shown in Table 3.1.

Cochrane central register of controlled trials

This registry is part of the Cochrane Library and is the largest electronic registry of randomised trials in existence. The Cochrane Central Register is available via a Cochrane Library subscription or is free to some low- or middle-income countries. It is a companion database to the Cochrane Database of Systematic Reviews described earlier. The references in this registry are sourced from large databases including MEDLINE and EMBASE, hand-searches of major healthcare journals across many health disciplines, and other sources managed by the Cochrane Collaboration review groups. It also incorporates the records of registered, ongoing, clinical trials from such places as the International Clinical Trials Registry Platform (ICTRP) (https://trialsearch.who.int/) and Clinicaltrials.gov (https://clinicaltrials.gov/).

If you cannot find an answer to your clinical question using one of the specialised databases listed in Table 3.1, your next step is to search one or more of the large electronic bibliographic databases. When searching these, it can help to combine terms identified by the database (index terms) with free text terms used by yourself, colleagues and study authors. These are explained in Box 3.1.

MEDLINE

MEDLINE currently has over 35 million citations. It is produced by the US National Library of Medicine and is available free of charge through PubMed (https://pubmed.ncbi.nlm.nih.gov/). In comparison with the smaller databases listed in Table 3.1, searching efficiently on MEDLINE requires very precise, targeted searches. It also includes many articles and subjects that are not helpful in evidence-based practice.

- In recognition of this, the **Clinical Queries screen in PubMed** (https://pubmed.ncbi.nlm.nih.gov/clinical/) offers a search window for specific clinical research areas. This search interface seeks to narrow down otherwise overwhelming search results by providing ready-to-use search filters. These search strategies identify terms most likely to be used in the titles, abstracts and indexing of primary study types appropriate for the clinical categories of **therapy, diagnosis, aetiology, prognosis** and **clinical prediction guides**. For example, when searching for an article about therapy, you can select from a drop-down menu a *Therapy* search filter that retrieves articles containing features commonly found within a randomised trial design.
- A similar facility for appropriate study types for **healthcare costs** and **healthcare quality** (and **qualitative topics**) can be accessed using the **Health Services Research (HSR) PubMed Queries** screen (www.nlm.nih.gov/nichsr/hedges/search.html).

When using the *Clinical Queries* interface, you simply:

1. Enter basic topic information (such as the keywords from your clinical question—try starting with the 'P' and 'I' keywords and then broaden or narrow your search as needed) and click on 'Search'.
2. Then select the type of question that you are searching for an answer to (in *Clinical Queries*, you can choose from therapy, prognosis, diagnosis, aetiology or clinical prediction guides).
3. Decide if you want to conduct a broad (sensitive) or narrow (specific) search:
   a. A **sensitive (broad) search** increases the likelihood of retrieving every possible relevant study, which in PubMed can often result in an unmanageable number of search results.
   b. You may wish to begin with a **specific (narrow) search**, which will minimise the number of irrelevant studies that are returned. If you get very few, or no, search results, you can then repeat the search and change the emphasis to sensitive (broad).

That is all you have to do. Everything else, such as narrowing down your results using a methodological search filter, is done for you. The first five results are presented, sorted by the most recent articles. To view the other results, click the 'See all results in PubMed' link. A useful feature of PubMed that you will see once you click on an article is that it automatically maps your words to any relevant MeSH terms (without you having to select them). A further feature is *Similar Articles*—a list of articles matched by the computer as relevant.

Figure 3.2 shows the search page of *Clinical Queries* and a basic search related to the clinical scenario described

PubMed Clinical Queries

This tool uses predefined filters to help you quickly refine PubMed searches on clinical or disease-specific topics. To use this tool, enter your search terms in the search bar and select filters before searching.

Note: The Systematic Reviews filter has moved; it is now an option under the 'Article Type' filter on the main PubMed search results page.

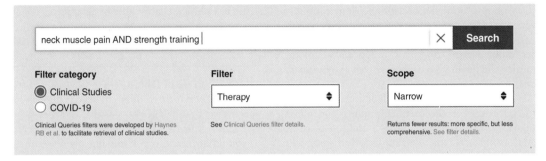

Results for Clinical Studies: Therapy/Narrow

5 of 91 results sorted by: Most Recent

See all results in PubMed (91)

Effect of Progressive Step Marching Exercise on Balance Ability in the Elderly: A Cluster Randomized Clinical Trial.
Sitthiracha P, et al. Int J Environ Res Public Health. 2021. PMID: 33803720 Free PMC article. Clinical Trial.

The Effect of Physical Exercise Training on Neck and Shoulder Muscle Function Among Military Helicopter Pilots and Crew: A Secondary Analysis of a Randomized Controlled Trial.
Murray M, et al. Front Public Health. 2020. PMID: 33330303 Free PMC article. Clinical Trial.

[Effect of *Fu's* subcutaneous needling on thickness and elasticity of affected muscles in shoulder neck pain based on ultrasonic elastography].
Zhang YH, et al. Zhongguo Zhen Jiu. 2020. PMID: 32959587 Clinical Trial. Chinese.

Motor control integrated into muscle strengthening exercises has more effects on scapular muscle activities and joint range of motion before initiation of radiotherapy in oral cancer survivors with neck dissection: A randomized controlled trial.
Chen YH, et al. PLoS One. 2020. PMID: 32760097 Free PMC article. Clinical Trial.

Fig 3.2 The *Clinical Queries* search page in PubMed
Reproduced courtesy of National Center for Biotechnology Information/US National Library of Medicine.

earlier in this chapter. You can check details of the search that *Clinical Queries* ran by going to the advanced search page (https://pubmed.ncbi.nlm.nih.gov/advanced/) by clicking the 'Advanced' button just under the search box. Then click the arrow in the 'Details' column. In the example shown in Figure 3.2, simply typing in *neck muscle pain AND strength training* was expanded by an automated term mapper on PubMed into the following actual query:

("neck muscles"[MeSH Terms] OR ("neck"[All Fields] AND "muscles"[All Fields]) OR "neck muscles"[All Fields] OR ("neck"[All Fields] AND "muscle"[All Fields]) OR "neck muscle"[All Fields]) AND ("pain"[MeSH Terms] OR "pain"[All Fields]) AND ("resistance training"[MeSH Terms] OR ("resistance"[All Fields] AND "training"[All Fields]) OR "resistance training"[All Fields] OR ("strength"[All Fields] AND "training"[All Fields]) OR "strength training"[All Fields]) AND ("randomized controlled trial"[Publication Type] OR ("randomized"[Title/Abstract] AND "controlled"[Title/Abstract] AND "trial"[Title/Abstract]))

Other large databases

- **EMBASE** is a large European database with over 24 million citations. EMBASE has similar coverage to

MEDLINE and provides greater coverage of European and non-English-language publications, conference proceedings and a broader coverage of topics concerned with pharmaceuticals, psychiatry, toxicology and alternative medicine. EMBASE is offered through various providers on a subscription basis. Your organisation may have an institutional subscription. Many commercial versions of EMBASE allow you to limit your search query by a *Clinical Queries* filter to retrieve individual studies about therapy, diagnosis, prognosis, aetiology, economics and qualitative studies, as well as systematic reviews.

- **CINAHL** (Cumulative Index to Nursing and Allied Health Literature) is the premier nursing and allied health database and contains over 3 million records. CINAHL is only available on a subscription basis. You can limit CINAHL content searches by *Clinical Queries* to retrieve individual studies about therapy, prognosis, aetiology and qualitative studies, as well as systematic reviews.
- **PsycINFO** is a comprehensive international bibliographic database of psychological literature and contains over 4 million records. As with the other large databases, multiple access routes are available and all require a subscription. Again, a *Clinical Queries* filter is offered by some database providers to limit retrieval to individual studies about therapy or to qualitative studies, as well as systematic reviews.

When searching large electronic databases, you should explore the Help function to learn tips on how to search each database efficiently. Features and interfaces of databases change over time and databases use different notation for specific search techniques, such as different symbols for truncation (for example, * or $) and the use of double quotation marks or parentheses for combining terms.

Some tips for locating qualitative research

Finding qualitative research can be more challenging. Unlike many quantitative study designs (such as a randomised trial), using study designs to identify relevant studies is not straightforward and there is no hierarchy of evidence. Using the term 'qualitative' on its own as a search term is not always useful, as sometimes qualitative research is indexed by the specific method used to collect data (for example, focus group or in-depth interview) and other times it is indexed according to the specific methodology used (for example, phenomenology or grounded theory). Table 3.2 shows empirically derived[6–9] search filters that you can use to identify qualitative studies in CINAHL, PubMed/MEDLINE, EMBASE and PsycINFO. As methodological search filters, they focus on the *methods of qualitative research* rather than the content. Combine these methodological search filters (words such as 'qualitative' or 'themes') with your content terms (keywords from your clinical question).

For example, to locate qualitative research about spinal cord injury in women, you could try the following search string in PubMed (tiab = 'title or abstract'):

> spinal cord injur* [tiab] AND (women[tiab] OR woman[tiab]) AND (qualitative[tiab] OR themes[tiab])

As you can see in Table 3.2, in most cases you are offered a choice between three different search filters—'sensitive', 'specific' or 'best balance of sensitive and specific':
- Use the 'sensitive' search filter for a broad search when you do not want to risk missing any relevant articles.
- Use the 'specific' search filter to narrow your search and find just a few relevant articles.
- Use the 'best balance' search filters when you want a good balance between sensitivity and specificity.

Federated search engines

One of the challenges with efficient searching is that you do not know at which level of the pyramid you will find the best results for your clinical question. When you face a clinical question where the best choice of evidence-based resource is not readily apparent for answering your particular clinical problem, using a 'federated search engine' provides a means to search many resources, with the retrieval of results organised according to the source of evidence. Although not specifically on the EBHC pyramid, the following are examples of evidence-based sources:
- **ACCESSSS** 2.0 (https://www.accessss.org/) is a free health-related meta-search engine that searches multiple databases with just one entry of your search term(s). ACCESSSS 2.0 is designed to find the best evidence-based answer to your clinical questions by simultaneously searching the leading evidence-driven medical publications and high-quality clinical literature. Research staff review over 120 top clinical journals for articles that are scientifically sound and potentially clinically relevant. A network of experienced health professionals then rate high-quality articles for relevance to their practice and newsworthiness. Over 35,000 articles are reviewed each year. By filtering the articles based on methodology, relevance and newsworthiness, there is over 90% 'noise reduction', which greatly assists health professionals and students to keep up to date with the best, most relevant research in their field. ACCESSSS also incorporates evidence-based textbooks (for example, DynaMed, Best Practice, EBM Guidelines), automated PubMed searches, with the search results

TABLE 3.2 Search filters for locating qualitative research in PubMed/MEDLINE, CINAHL, EMBASE and PsycINFO

Hedge	MEDLINE (PubMed)	MEDLINE (Ovid syntax)	CINAHL (EBSCO syntax)	EMBASE (Ovid syntax)	PsycINFO (Ovid syntax)
Sensitive (Broad)	(interview*[tiab] OR psychology[sh:noexp] OR health services administration[mh])	(interview*.tw. OR psychology. fs. OR exp Health Services Administration/)	((MH "study design+" not MM "study design+") or MH "attitude" or (MH "interviews+" not MM "interviews+"))	interview:.tw. OR qualitative. tw. OR exp health care organization/	experience:.mp. OR interview:. tw. OR qualitative:.tw.
Specific	(qualitative[tiab] OR themes[tiab])	(qualitative.tw. OR themes.tw.)	((MH "grounded theory" not MM "grounded theory") or (TI thematic analysis or AB thematic analysis or MW thematic analysis))	qualitative.tw. OR qualitative study.tw.	qualitative:.tw. OR themes.tw.
Best balance of sensitive and specific	Not available	Not available	((TI interview or AB interview) or (MH "audiore-cording" not MM "audiore-cording") or (TI qualitative stud* or AB qualitative stud*))	interview:.tw. OR exp health care organization/ OR experiences. tw.	experiences.tw. OR interview:. tw. OR qualitative.tw.

PubMed syntax: tiab = title or abstract; mh = MeSH heading; noexp = non-exploded; sh = subheading:noexp
Ovid syntax: colon (:) = truncation; exp = explosion; fs = floating subheading;.mp = multi-purpose (searches title, abstract, original title, name of substance word, subject heading word, keyword heading word, protocol supplementary concept word, rare disease supplementary concept word, unique identifier); tw = textword (searches title and abstract)
EBSCO syntax: + = explode; AB = abstract; MH = subject heading; MM = exact major subject heading; MW = subject heading word; TI = title

displayed hierarchically according to the EBHC pyramid. You can search a subset of it by choosing to search in Nursing+, MD+ or Rehab+ for articles relevant to nursing, medicine and rehabilitation, respectively.
- You can also register to receive alerts by selecting your disciplines and patient populations of interest. When an article meets your criteria, you will receive an email alert that there is a new, high-quality, relevant and newsworthy article available in your area of interest.

- **TRIP** (Turning Research Into Practice, https://www.tripdatabase.com/) searches multiple databases and other evidence-based resources with just one entry of your search term(s). TRIP groups the search results into systematic reviews, evidence-based synopses, clinical guidelines, key primary research, clinical questions and answers, and more. You can also subscribe to the premium version, TRIP Pro, which has more content, more functionality and no advertisements.

Alerting services

Although not on the EBHC pyramid specifically, you may also find that emails can be useful as a way to alert you to newly published studies. Unlike the resources outlined earlier in this chapter that require you to proactively search for the evidence, alerting services bring the research literature to you in the form of email alerts. This can be described as 'push' or 'just-in-case' information (see Chapter 2). Several alerting systems target individual health professionals. Examples include:

- **EvidenceAlerts** (and its subset databases) are described in Table 3.1. It has the same functionality and service as the journal screening component of ACCESSSS 2.0 that was described earlier (but does not incorporate the other resources, such as DynaMed that ACCESSSS does). It also offers a free service where users can tailor alerts for their own clinical discipline and set cut-offs for their clinical relevance and importance from newly published studies and systematic reviews from over 120 leading journals. Users can also use Evidence Alerts as a database for looking up studies and systematic reviews accumulated to date.
- **My NCBI** (www.ncbi.nlm.nih.gov/sites/myncbi) is an alerting service within PubMed that will email users with new citations in the clinical areas they have specified. Users set up a search that will automatically email them citations of newly published articles based on content (for example, asthma in adolescents). However, the newly published articles are not filtered by methodological rigour and you will need to critically appraise the articles when considering whether to use them in clinical practice.
- **Journals** may enable you to register to have the table of contents emailed to you as each new issue of the journal is published. You may wish to do this for journals that you frequently consult. Newly published articles are not filtered by methodological rigour, so you will need to critically appraise the articles that are sent to you.

Other resources

When you use a search engine such as Google, you are not searching a defined database but are searching the internet in general. A negative aspect of these search engines is that evidence-based information can be difficult to find. On the other hand, an internet search can be a quick way to track down a specific article and is useful for policy- or time-sensitive information such as listings of country-specific vaccination rules for travellers.

Google Scholar (https://scholar.google.com/) is a free academic search engine that searches the scholarly literature. From one site, you can search across many disciplines and sources such as peer-reviewed articles, theses, books, abstracts and articles that are from academic publishers, professional societies, preprint repositories, universities and other scholarly organisations. Google Scholar weights articles by likely relevance according to the full text of the article, the author, the publication in which it appears and how often the article is cited in other scholarly literature.

SEARCH EXAMPLES

This section demonstrates how resources we have previously described can be used to answer some of the different question types covered in this book. For these examples, and indeed for most searching activities, it is important to note that many routes (that is, different databases, different combinations of terms) can lead to the same evidence— your challenge is to make the searching as efficient and productive as possible.

Clinical question about the effects of intervention

You are a physiotherapist and currently have two patients who are pregnant and experiencing pelvic and back pain. You wonder:

> In pregnant women, is acupuncture more effective than standard treatment in relieving pregnancy-related pelvic and back pain?

Starting at the top of the pyramid, you confirm that there is nothing on the top three layers of the pyramid, as is often the case for allied health clinical questions. As your question relates to intervention effectiveness, you are ideally seeking a systematic review of randomised controlled trials. Therefore, your next step is to look for a systematic review (systematic review layer of the pyramid). To do this, you could search various resources, including PEDro, the Cochrane Database of Systematic Reviews, PubMed Clinical Queries or TRIP. As PEDro contains guidelines, systematic reviews and pre-appraised articles related to physiotherapy and indexes Cochrane reviews, you start there.

On the advanced search page, you type in the term 'pregnancy' in the *Abstract & Title* field and select 'acupuncture' in the *Therapy* field, 'pain' in the *Problem* field, and 'lumbar spine, sacro-iliac joint and pelvis' in the *Body Part* field. Note that in PEDro you do not need to type in Boolean operators; just tick the box at the bottom of the advanced search page indicating whether you want to Match all search terms (AND) or Match any search term (OR). Your search retrieves 21 records, and seven of these are systematic reviews—a number of which look relevant.[10]

Clinical question about diagnosis

You are an occupational therapist who works in a community health centre. Your team is designing an initial assessment form for newly referred patients, and they wish to include some screening questions that will provide useful information to various members of the team. You are interested in including a brief cognitive screening test, such as the Mini-Mental State Examination (MMSE), as part of this initial assessment. However, you are unsure how accurate this test is at predicting cognitive impairment in older people who live in the community. Your question is:

> Does the MMSE accurately detect the presence of cognitive impairment in older community-living people?

After confirming that there is nothing available within the top three layers of the pyramid, you proceed to the fourth layer of the pyramid. You conduct a search in the Cochrane Database of Systematic Reviews, and you retrieve one highly relevant review.[11]

The fact that this review is recently published takes away some of the need to search more extensively. However, if you had not found a review, or had only found an older review, you could try searching PubMed Clinical Queries (with 'diagnosis' selected as the category and a narrow search chosen). You could start with search terms such as:

> (MMSE OR Mini-Mental State Examination) AND (older OR elder* OR Aged) AND community

Clinical question about prognosis

As a recently graduated speech pathologist, you have just commenced working in a stroke rehabilitation unit. One of your patients is two months post-stroke with severe dysphagia (difficulty swallowing). His wife asks you how likely it is that his swallowing will get better in the next few months and that he will be able to return to eating a normal diet. Being new to clinical practice with little experience to guide your answer, you form the following clinical question:

> In adults with dysphagia following stroke, what is the likelihood of recovery within 6 months of the stroke?

You search using PubMed Clinical Queries (with prognosis selected as the clinical category and a narrow search chosen) with the terms:

> (dysphag* OR swallow*) AND (stroke OR CVA) and (recover*)

This search produces 83 results. From a quick glance at the titles, it appears that some of these are relevant to your question.[12,13]

SUMMARY

- Using the PICO format to structure your clinical question makes choosing key search terms easier.
- Combining search terms using the Boolean operators (AND, OR) helps to narrow or broaden your search as required, with wildcard and truncation symbols also proving useful.
- Organising your literature search using the EBHC pyramid is an effective and efficient way to find the best evidence.

- Where you start on the EBHC pyramid depends largely on the type of question you are asking and what resources are available to you.
- Although many evidence-based resources require a subscription, other excellent resources are readily available on the internet free of charge.
- Many clinical questions can be answered by searching online for the best evidence.

ACKNOWLEDGMENTS

The updated version of this chapter for this edition is based on Chapter 3 in the previous editions of this book, which were authored by Nancy Wilczynski, Ann McKibbon and Andrew Booth. Their valuable contribution to the content and structure of this chapter is gratefully acknowledged.

REFERENCES

1. Ely JW, Osheroff JA, Ebell MH, et al. Obstacles to answering doctors' questions about patient care with evidence: qualitative study. BMJ 2002;324(7339):710.
2. van der Keylen P, Tomandl J, Wollmann K, et al. The online health information needs of family physicians: systematic review of qualitative and quantitative studies. J Med Internet Res 2020;22(12):e18816.

3. Clark JM, Sanders S, Carter M, et al. Improving the translation of search strategies using the Polyglot Search Translator: a randomized controlled trial. J Med Libr Assoc 2020;108(2):195–207.

4. Alper BS, Haynes RB. EBHC pyramid 5.0 for accessing preappraised evidence and guidance. BMJ Evid Based Med 2016;21:123–5.

5. Moja L, Kwag KH, Lytras T, et al. Effectiveness of computerized decision support systems linked to electronic health records: a systematic review and meta-analysis. Am J Public Health 2014;104(12):e12–22.

6. Wong SS, Wilczynski NL, Haynes RB. Developing optimal search strategies for detecting clinically relevant qualitative studies in MEDLINE. Stud Health Technol Inform 2004;107(Pt 1):311–16.

7. Wilczynski NL, Marks S, Haynes RB. Search strategies for identifying qualitative studies in CINAHL. Qual Health Res 2007;17(5):705–10.

8. Walters LA, Wilczynski NL, Haynes RB. Developing optimal search strategies for retrieving clinically relevant qualitative studies in EMBASE. Qual Health Res 2006;16(1):162–8.

9. McKibbon KA, Wilczynski NL, Haynes RB. Developing optimal search strategies for retrieving qualitative studies in PsycINFO. Eval Health Prof 2006;29(4):440–54.

10. Yao X, Li C, Ge X, et al. Effect of acupuncture on pregnancy related low back pain and pelvic pain: a systematic review and meta-analysis. Int J Clin Exp Med 2017;10(4):5903–12.

11. Creavin ST, Wisniewski S, Noel-Storr AH, et al. Mini-Mental State Examination (MMSE) for the detection of dementia in clinically unevaluated people aged 65 and over in community and primary care populations. Cochrane Database Syst Rev 2016;(1):CD011145.

12. Kumar S, Doughty C, Doros G, et al. Recovery of swallowing after dysphagic stroke: an analysis of prognostic factors. J Stroke Cerebrovasc Dis 2014;23(1):56–62.

13. Maeshima S, Osawa A, Hayashi T, et al. Factors associated with prognosis of eating and swallowing disability after stroke: a study from a community-based stroke care system. J Stroke Cerebrovasc Dis 2013;22(7):926–30.e1.

Evidence about Effects of Interventions

Sally Bennett and Tammy Hoffmann

LEARNING OBJECTIVES

After reading this chapter, you should be able to:

- Understand more about study designs appropriate for answering questions about effects of interventions
- Generate a structured clinical question about an intervention for a clinical scenario
- Appraise the risk of bias (validity) of randomised controlled trials

- Understand how to interpret the results from randomised controlled trials and calculate additional results (such as confidence intervals) where possible
- Describe how evidence about the effects of intervention can be used to inform practice

This chapter focuses on research that can inform us about the effects of interventions. Let us first consider a clinical scenario that will be useful for illustrating the concepts that are the focus of this chapter.

◎ CLINICAL SCENARIO

You are working in a community health centre. During a regular team meeting, the general practitioner notes that there are a few people diagnosed with heart failure who are having difficulty with depression. The general practitioner has started them on anti-depressants but believes that psychological support such as cognitive behaviour therapy (CBT) may be effective. She suggests that those involved in providing psychosocial care for these people form a small group to look at the research regarding CBT for people with heart failure who also have depression. In your experience of working with people who have depression and heart failure, you are aware that many of them also have problems with anxiety. You are therefore particularly interested in finding evidence about the effectiveness of CBT programs that have looked at improving participants' anxiety as well as depression.

This clinical scenario raises several questions about the interventions that might be effective for reducing anxiety and depression among people with heart failure. Is cognitive behaviour therapy alone effective in reducing anxiety and depression in people with heart failure? Does CBT in addition to anti-depressants have a beneficial effect over and above the use of anti-depressants alone? If it is effective, how long does the effect last? Is CBT cost-effective for reducing anxiety and depression for people with heart failure?

As we saw in Chapter 1, clinical decisions are made by integrating information from the best available research evidence with information from our patients, the practice context and our clinical experience. Given that one of the most common information needs in clinical practice relates to questions about the effects of interventions, this chapter will begin by reviewing the role of the study design that is used to test intervention effects before explaining the process of finding and appraising research evidence about the effects of interventions.

STUDY DESIGNS THAT CAN BE USED FOR ANSWERING QUESTIONS ABOUT THE EFFECTS OF INTERVENTIONS

There are many different study designs that can provide information about the effects of interventions. Some are more convincing than others in terms of the degree of bias that might be in play given the methods used in the study. From Chapter 2, you will recall that *bias* is any systematic error in collecting and interpreting data. In Chapter 2, we also introduced the concept of *hierarchies of evidence*. The higher up the hierarchy that a study design is positioned, in the ideal world, the more likely it is that the study design can minimise the impact of bias on the results of the study. That is why randomised controlled trials (sitting second from the top of the hierarchy of evidence for questions about the effects of interventions) are so commonly recommended as the study design that best controls for bias when testing the effectiveness of interventions. Systematic reviews of randomised controlled trials are located above them (at the top of the hierarchy) because they can combine the results of multiple randomised controlled trials. Combining multiple trials can potentially provide an even clearer picture about the effectiveness of interventions provided they are undertaken rigorously. Systematic reviews are explained in more detail in Chapter 12.

One of the best methods for limiting bias in studies that test the effects of interventions is to have a control group.[1] A control group is a group of participants in the study who should be similar in as many ways as possible to the intervention group except that they do not receive the intervention being studied. Let us first have a look at studies that do not use control groups and identify some of the problems that can occur.

Studies that do not use control groups

Uncontrolled studies are studies where the researchers describe what happens when participants are provided with an intervention, but the intervention is not compared with other interventions. Examples of uncontrolled study designs are case reports, case series, and before and after studies. These study designs were explained in Chapter 2. The big problem with uncontrolled studies is that when participants are given an intervention and simply followed for a period of time with no comparison against another group, it is impossible to tell how much (if any) of the observed change is due to the effect of the intervention itself or is due to some other factor or explanation. There are some alternative explanations for effects seen in uncontrolled studies, and these need to be kept in mind if you use this type of study to guide your clinical decision making. Some of the forms of bias that commonly occur in uncontrolled studies are described below.

- **Volunteer bias.** People who volunteer to participate in a study are usually systematically different from those who do not volunteer. They tend to be more motivated and concerned about their health. If this is not controlled for, it is possible that the results can make the intervention appear more favourable (that is, more

effective) than it really is. This type of bias can be controlled for by randomly allocating participants, as we shall see later in this chapter.

- **Maturation.** A participant may change between the time of pre-test (that is, before the intervention is given) and post-test (after the intervention has finished) as a result of maturation. For example, consider that you wanted to measure the improvement in fine motor skills that children in grade 2 of school experienced as a result of a fine-motor-skill intervention program. If you test them again in grade 3, you will not know if the improvements that occurred in fine motor skills happened because of natural development (maturation) or because of the intervention.

- **Natural progression.** Many diseases and health conditions will naturally improve over time. Improvements that occur in participants may or may not be due to the intervention that was being studied. The participants may have improved on their own with time, not because of the intervention.

- **Regression to the mean.** This is a statistical trend that occurs in repeated non-random experiments, where participants' results tend to move progressively towards the mean of the behaviour/outcome that is being measured. This is due not to maturation or improvement over time, but to the statistical likelihood of someone with high scores not doing as well when a test is repeated or of someone with low scores being statistically likely to do better when the test is repeated. Suppose, for example, that you used a behavioural test to assess 200 children who had attention deficit hyperactivity disorder and scored their risk of having poor academic outcomes, and that you then provided the 30 children who had the poorest scores with an intensive behavioural regimen and medication. Even if the interventions were not effective, you would still expect to observe some improvement in the children's scores on the behavioural test when it is next given, due to regression to the mean. When outliers are repeatedly measured, subsequent values are less likely to be outliers (that is, they are expected to be closer to the mean value of the whole group). This always happens, and health professionals who do not expect this to occur often attribute any improvement that is observed to the intervention. The best way to deal with the problem of regression to the mean is to randomly allocate participants to either an experimental group or a control group. The regression to the mean effect can only be accounted for by using a control group (which will have the same regression to the mean if the randomisation succeeded and the two groups are similar). How to determine this is explained later in this chapter.

- **Placebo effect.** This is a well-known type of bias where an improvement in the participants' condition occurs because they expect or believe that the intervention they are receiving will cause an improvement (even though, in reality, the intervention may not be effective at all).
- **Hawthorne effect.** This is a type of bias that can occur when participants experience improvements not because of the intervention that is being studied, but because of the attention that participants are receiving from being a part of the research process.
- **Rosenthal effect.** This occurs when participants perform better because they are expected to and, in a sense, this expectation has a similar sort of effect as a self-fulfilling prophecy.

Controlled studies

It should now be clear that the best way to limit the influence of bias and extraneous factors on the results of a study is to have a control group that can be compared with the intervention group in the study. However, it is not as simple as just having a control group as part of the study. The way in which the control group is created can make an enormous difference to how well the study design actually controls for bias.

Non-randomised controlled studies

You will recall from the hierarchy of evidence about the effects of interventions (in Chapter 2) that case-control and cohort studies are located above uncontrolled study designs. This is because they make use of control groups. Cohort studies follow a cohort that has been exposed to a situation or intervention and have a comparison group of people who have not been exposed to the situation of interest (for example, they have not received any intervention). However, because cohort studies are observational studies, the allocation of participants to the intervention and control groups is not under the control of the researcher. It is not possible to tell whether the participants in the intervention and the control groups are similar in terms of all the important factors and, therefore, it is unclear to what extent the exposure (that is, the intervention) might be the reason for the outcome rather than some other factor.

We saw in Chapter 2 that a case-control study is one in which participants with a given disease (or health condition) in a given population (or a representative sample) are identified and are compared with a control group of participants who do not have that disease (or health condition). When a case-control study has been used to answer a question about the effect of an intervention, the 'cases' are participants who have been exposed to an intervention and

the 'controls' are participants who have not. As with cohort studies, because this is an observational study design, the researcher cannot control the assembly of the groups under study (that is, which participants go into which group). Although the controls that are assembled may be similar in many ways to the 'cases', it is unlikely that they will be similar with respect to both known and unknown confounders. Chapter 2 explained that confounders are factors that can become confused with the factor of interest (in this case, the intervention that is being studied) and obscure the true results.

In a non-randomised experimental study, the researchers can control the assembly of both experimental and control groups, but the groups are not assembled using random allocation. In non-randomised studies, participants may choose which group they want to be in, or they may be assigned to a group by the researchers. For example, in a non-randomised experimental study that is evaluating the effectiveness of a particular public health intervention (such as an intervention that encourages walking to work) in a community setting, a researcher may assign one town to the experimental condition and another town to the control condition. The difficulty with this approach is that the people in these towns may be systematically different from each other and so confounding factors, rather than the intervention that is being trialled, may be the reason for any difference that is found between the groups at the end of the study.

So, not only are control groups essential, but to make valid comparisons between groups, they must also be as similar as possible at the beginning of a study. This is so that we can say, with some certainty, that any differences found between groups at the end of the study are likely to be due to the factor under study (that is, the intervention) rather than because of bias or confounding. To maximise the similarity between groups at the start of a study, researchers need to control for both known and unknown variables that might influence the results. The best way to achieve this is through randomisation. Non-randomised studies are inherently biased in favour of the intervention that is being studied, which can lead researchers to reach the wrong conclusion about the effectiveness of the intervention.[2]

Randomised controlled trials

The key feature of randomised controlled trials is that the participants are randomly allocated to either an intervention (experimental) group or a control group. The outcome of interest is measured in participants in both groups before (known as pre-test) and again after (known as post-test) the intervention has been provided. Therefore, any changes that appear in the intervention group pre-test to

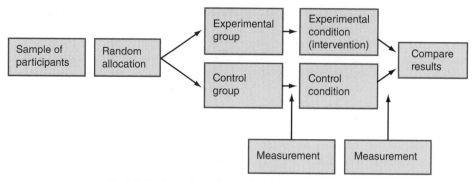

Fig 4.1 Basic design of a randomised controlled trial

post-test, but not in the control group, can reasonably be attributed to the intervention. Figure 4.1 shows the basic design of a randomised controlled trial.

You may notice that we keep referring to how randomised controlled trials can be used to evaluate the effectiveness of an intervention. It is worth noting that they can also be used to evaluate the efficacy of an intervention. *Efficacy* refers to interventions that are tested in ideal circumstances, such as where intervention protocols are very carefully supervised and participant selection is very particular. *Effectiveness* is an evaluation of an intervention in circumstances that are more like real life, such as where there is a broader range of participants included and a typical clinical level of intervention protocol supervision. In this sense, effectiveness trials are more pragmatic in nature (that is, they are accommodating of typical practices) than are efficacy trials.

There are a number of variations on the basic randomised controlled trial design that partly depend on the type or combination of control groups used. There are many variations on what the participants in a control group in a randomised controlled trial actually receive. For example, participants may receive no intervention of any kind (a 'no intervention' control), or they may receive a placebo, some form of social control or a comparison intervention. In some randomised controlled trials, there are more than two groups. For example, in one study there might be two intervention groups and one control group; or, in another study, there might be an intervention group, a placebo group and a 'no intervention' group. Randomised crossover studies are a type of randomised controlled trial in which all participants take part in both intervention and control groups, but in random order. For example, in a randomised crossover trial of a closed-loop device or a sensor-augmented pump (open loop) for insulin therapy, children with diabetes were assigned to receive one of the devices for a

72-hour inpatient period followed by a 6-week home phase. Participants crossed over to the other device after a 1-week washout period.[3] A difficulty with crossover trials is that there needs to be a credible wash-out period. That is, the effects of the intervention provided in the first phase must no longer be evident prior to commencing the second phase. In the example we used here, the effect of the first device must be cleared prior to the alternative device being provided.

As we have seen, the advantage of a randomised controlled trial is that any differences found between groups at the end of the study are likely to be due to the intervention rather than to extraneous factors. But the extent to which these differences can be attributed to the intervention is also dependent on some of the specific design features that were used in the trial, and these deserve close attention. The rest of this chapter will look at randomised controlled trials in more depth within the context of the clinical scenario that was presented at the beginning of this chapter. In this scenario, you are a health professional who is working in a small group at a community health centre and you are looking for research regarding the effectiveness of CBT for people with heart failure who also have anxiety and depression. To locate relevant research, you start by focusing on what it is that you specifically want to know about.

HOW TO STRUCTURE A QUESTION ABOUT THE EFFECT OF AN INTERVENTION

In Chapter 2, you learnt how to structure clinical questions using the PICO format: Patient/Problem/Population, Intervention/Issue, Comparison (if relevant) and Outcomes. In our depression and anxiety in heart failure clinical scenario, the *population* that we are interested in is people who have been diagnosed with heart failure and also have anxiety and depression. We know from our clinical experience and the literature that this sub-group of people with heart failure are at risk of poorer health outcomes.

The *intervention* that we think could make a difference is cognitive behaviour therapy. This is because you know that CBT has been shown to be effective with people with major depressive disorders, but who do not have heart failure. Are we interested in a *comparison* intervention? While we could compare the effectiveness of one type of intervention with another, for this scenario it is probably more useful to start by first thinking about whether the intervention is effective over and above usual care. To do this, we would need to compare the intervention to either a placebo (a concept we will discuss later) or to usual care.

There are several *outcomes* that we could consider important for people with heart failure who have depression and anxiety. The most obvious outcome of interest is a reduction in anxiety and depressive symptoms. However, we could also look for interventions that consider objective outcomes such as re-hospitalisation and even mortality. Another outcome (of a more subjective nature) that is likely to be important to people with heart failure is quality of life.

◎ CLINICAL SCENARIO (CONTINUED)

Structuring the question
While there are several questions about interventions that can be drawn from the scenario presented at the beginning of this chapter, you decide to form the following clinical question:

In people with heart failure who also have depression and anxiety, is CBT effective in reducing depression and anxiety compared with usual care?

HOW TO FIND EVIDENCE TO ANSWER QUESTIONS ABOUT THE EFFECTS OF AN INTERVENTION

Our clinical scenario question is one about the effectiveness of an intervention for reducing anxiety and depression. You can use the hierarchy of evidence for this type of question as your guide in deciding which type of study you are looking for and where to start searching. In this case, you are looking for a systematic review of randomised controlled trials. If there is no relevant systematic review, you should next look for a randomised controlled trial. If no relevant randomised trials are available, you would then

need to look for the next best available type of research, as indicated by the hierarchy of evidence for this question type shown in Chapter 2.

As we saw in Chapter 3, a useful source of systematic reviews of randomised controlled trials is the Cochrane Database of Systematic Reviews, so this would be a logical place to start searching. The Cochrane Library also contains the Cochrane Central Register of Controlled Trials, which includes a large collection of citations of randomised trials.

Once you have found a research article that you are interested in, it is important to critically appraise it. That is, you need to examine the research closely to determine whether and how it might inform your clinical practice. As we saw in Chapter 1, when critically appraising research, there are three main aspects to consider: (1) its risk of bias (that is, its internal validity); (2) its impact (the size and importance of any effect found); and (3) whether or how the evidence might be applicable to your patient or clinical practice.

◎ CLINICAL SCENARIO (CONTINUED)

Finding evidence to answer your question
You search the Cochrane Database of Systematic Reviews and find no reviews concerning cognitive behaviour therapy for anxiety and depression in people with heart failure. A search of PubMed found a number of reviews about the treatment of depression in people with heart failure, although they did not include methods important to systematic reviews such as appraisal of the risk of bias in individual studies or did not focus on cognitive behaviour therapy or on heart failure.

You therefore decide to look for randomised controlled trials in PubMed—Clinical Queries using the search string: depression AND heart failure AND cognitive behaviour therapy (using PubMed—Clinical Queries' narrow scope function). Your search finds some relevant randomised controlled trials and you choose the one that most closely matches your PICO. It is a randomised controlled trial that has investigated the effectiveness of CBT for depression and self-care in people with heart failure.[4] You obtain the full text of the article in order to critically appraise it, to determine whether the trial also measured anxiety as an outcome, and if it did, to examine the results of the trial and determine whether the findings may be applicable to your clinical scenario.

◎ CLINICAL SCENARIO (CONTINUED)

Structured abstract of our chosen article

Citation: Freedland K, Carney R, Rich M, et al. Cognitive behavior therapy for depression and self-care in heart failure patients: a randomized clinical trial. JAMA Intern Med 2015;175:1773–82.

Design: Randomised controlled trial.

Setting: Outpatients enrolled through a university medical centre in Missouri, United States.

Participants: 158 outpatients with heart failure diagnosed ≥3 months prior to screening for the study and also diagnosed with a current major depressive episode.

Intervention: The intervention followed standard CBT manuals, and a manual of CBT designed for people with heart disease. Treatment was individualised, based on a collaboratively determined problem list. A manual describing the treatment in detail is available as supplementary material. The intervention involved 6 months of weekly 1-hour sessions and was provided by experienced, trained therapists who also had weekly supervision. Intervention tapered off as a set of depression, heart failure self-care and CBT skills were met. Up to four 20- to 30-minute telephone calls were made as relapse prevention from 6 to 12 months following randomisation.

Comparator: Enhanced usual care, which consisted of a cardiac nurse reviewing educational materials on heart failure self-care at baseline, then by three 30-minute telephone calls 3 to 4 weeks following randomisation.

Outcomes: The primary outcome was severity of depressive symptoms measured by the Beck Depression Inventory-II (BDI-II) at 6 months and the Self-Care Maintenance and Confidence subscale of the Self-Care of Heart Failure Index. Authors stated that remission of depression was indicated by a score of 9 or less on the BDI-II. Secondary outcomes included: anxiety, other measures of depressive symptoms, health-related quality of life, social roles, fatigue and physical function. Of particular interest to this clinical scenario is that anxiety was measured using the Beck Anxiety Inventory.

Follow-up period: Follow-up measurement occurred at 3, 6, 9 and 12 months post-randomisation.

Main results: At 6 months, scores on the Beck Depression Inventory (BDI-II) were lower in the CBT group than in the usual care group (mean 12.8 [SD 10.6] versus mean 17.3 [SD 10.7]; $p = 0.008$), with higher remission rates in the CBT group compared with the usual care group (46% versus 19%; number needed to treat [NNT] = 3.76; 95% CI 3.62 to 3.90; $p < 0.001$). Anxiety was also lower in the CBT group compared with the usual care group, with a between group mean difference of −4.47 (CI −7.70 to −1.25; $p = 0.007$). These reductions in depressive symptoms and anxiety, and higher rates of remission from depression, were sustained at 9 and 12 months follow-up.

Conclusion: CBT can reduce depressive symptoms, increase its rate of remission and reduce symptoms of anxiety in people with heart failure.

IS THIS EVIDENCE LIKELY TO BE BIASED?

In this chapter, we will discuss six criteria that are commonly used for appraising the potential risk of bias in a randomised controlled trial. These six criteria are summarised in Box 4.1 and can be found in the *Users' guides to the medical literature*[5] and in many appraisal checklists such as the Critical Appraisal Skills Program (CASP) checklist and the PEDro scale.[6] A number of studies have demonstrated that estimates of treatment effects may be distorted in trials that do not adequately address these issues.[7–11] As you work through each of these criteria when appraising an article, it is important to consider the direction of the bias (that is, is it in favour of the intervention or the control group?) as well as its magnitude. As we pointed out in Chapter 1, all research has flaws. However, we do not just want to know what the flaws might be, but whether and how they might influence the results of a study.

BOX 4.1 Key questions to ask when appraising the risk of bias (validity) of a randomised controlled trial

1. Was the assignment of participants to groups randomised?
2. Was the allocation sequence concealed?
3. Were the groups similar at the baseline or start of the trial?
4. Were participants, health professionals and study personnel 'blind' to group allocation?
5. Were all participants who entered the trial properly accounted for at its conclusion, and how complete was follow-up?
6. Were participants analysed in the groups to which they were randomised using intention-to-treat analysis?

Was the assignment of participants to groups randomised?

Randomised controlled trials, by definition, randomise participants to either the experimental or the control condition. The basic principle of randomisation is that each participant has an equal chance of being assigned to any group, such that any difference between the groups at the beginning of the trial can be assumed to be due to chance. The main benefit of randomisation is related to the idea that, this way, both known and unknown participant characteristics should be evenly distributed between the intervention and control groups. Therefore, any differences between groups that are found at the end of the study are likely to be because of the intervention.[12]

Random allocation is best done using a random numbers table, which can be computer-generated. Sometimes it is done by tossing a coin or 'pulling a number out of a hat'. Additionally, there are different randomisation designs that can be used, and you should be aware of them. Researchers may choose to use some form of restriction, such as blocking or stratification, when allocating participants to groups in order to create a greater balance between the groups at baseline in known characteristics.[13] The different randomisation designs are summarised below.

- **Simple randomisation:** involves randomisation of individuals to the experimental or the control condition.
- **Cluster randomisation:** involves random allocation of intact *clusters* of individuals, rather than individuals (for example, randomisation of schools, towns, clinics or general practices).
- **Stratified randomisation:** in this design, participants are matched and randomly allocated to groups. This method ensures that potentially confounding factors such as age, gender or disease severity are balanced between groups. For example, in a trial that involves people who have had a stroke, participants might be stratified according to their initial stroke severity as belonging to a 'mild', 'moderate' or 'severe' stratum. This way, when randomisation to study groups occurs, researchers can ensure that, within each stratum, there are equal numbers of participants in the intervention and control groups.
- **Block randomisation:** in this design, participants who are similar are grouped into 'blocks' and are then assigned to the experimental or control conditions within each block. Block randomisation often uses stratification. An example of block randomisation can be seen in a randomised controlled study of the effectiveness of an educational intervention for health professionals to improve knowledge about acute stroke.[14] Groups of physicians, nurses and paramedics were recruited (64 in each group). Then, using block randomisation, 32 participants in each group were randomly assigned to either the intervention or waiting list control group. To ensure that there were comparable numbers within each group across the disciplines, block randomisation was used. By using block randomisation, selection bias due to differences across the disciplines was avoided.

◎ CLINICAL SCENARIO (CONTINUED)

Was the assignment of participants to groups randomised?

In the CBT trial for depression in heart failure, it is explicitly stated that participants were randomised and that the randomisation was carried out using permuted blocks of 2, 4 or 6 pairs stratified by anti-depressant use at baseline.

Was the allocation sequence concealed?

As we have seen, the major benefit of a randomised controlled trial over other study designs is the fact that participants are randomly allocated to the study groups. However, the benefits of randomisation can be undone if the allocation sequence is manipulated or interfered with in any way. As strange as this might seem, a health professional who wants their patient to receive the intervention being evaluated may swap their patient's group assignment so that their patient receives the intervention being studied. Similarly, if the person who recruits participants to a study knows which condition the participants are to be assigned to, this could influence their decision about whether to enrol them in the study. This is why assigning participants to study groups using alternation methods, such as every second person who comes into the clinic, or methods such as date of birth is problematic because the randomisation sequence is known to the people involved.[12]

Knowledge about which group a participant will be allocated to if they are recruited into a study can lead to the selective assignment of participants, and thus introduce bias into the trial. This knowledge can result in manipulation of either the sequence of groups that participants are to be allocated to or the sequence of participants to be enrolled. Either way, this is a problem. The problem can be dealt with by concealing the allocation sequence from the people who are responsible for enrolling patients into a trial, or from those who assign participants to groups, until the moment of assignment.[15] Allocation can be concealed by having the randomisation sequence administered by someone who is 'off-site' or at a location away from where people are being enrolled into the study. Another way to conceal allocation is by having the group allocation placed in sealed, opaque envelopes. Opaque envelopes are used so that the group allocation cannot be seen if the envelope is held up to the light! The envelope is not to be opened until the patient has been enrolled into the trial (and is therefore now a participant in the study).

Hopefully, the article that you are appraising will clearly state that allocation was concealed, or that it was done by an independent or off-site person, or that sealed opaque envelopes were used. Unfortunately, though, many studies do not give any indication about whether allocation was concealed,[16,17] so you are often left wondering about this, which is frustrating when you are trying to appraise a study. It is possible that some of these studies did use concealed allocation, but you cannot tell this from reading the article.

 CLINICAL SCENARIO (CONTINUED)

Concealed allocation
In the CBT trial for depression in heart failure, allocation was concealed. The article states that randomisation was done using sequentially numbered opaque envelopes (1 set per stratum) and opened by the study coordinator after the baseline evaluation.

Were the groups similar at the baseline or start of the trial?

One of the principal aims of randomisation is to ensure that the groups are similar at the start of the trial in all respects, except for whether or not they received the experimental condition (that is, the intervention of interest). However, the use of randomisation does not guarantee that the groups will have similar known baseline characteristics. This is particularly the case if there is a small sample size. Authors of a research article will usually provide data in the article about the baseline characteristics of both groups. This allows readers to make up their own minds as to whether the balance between important prognostic factors (variables that have the potential for influencing outcomes) is sufficient at the start of the trial. Consider, for example, a study about the effectiveness of acupuncture for reducing pain from migraines compared with sham acupuncture. If the participants who were allocated to the acupuncture group had less severe or less chronic pain at the start of the study than the participants who were allocated to the sham acupuncture group, any differences in pain levels that were seen at the end of the study might be the result of that initial difference and not of the acupuncture that was provided.

Differences between the groups that are present at baseline after randomisation have occurred due to chance. Therefore, it is not appropriate to use p values to assess whether these differences are statistically significant.[18] That is, rather than using the p value that is often reported in studies, it is important to examine these differences by comparing means or proportions visually. The extent to which you might be concerned about a baseline difference between the groups depends on how large a difference it is and whether it is a key prognostic variable, both of which require some clinical judgment. The stronger the relationship between the characteristic and the outcome of interest, the more the differences between groups will weaken the strength of any inference about efficacy.[5] For example, consider a study that is investigating the effectiveness of group therapy in improving communication for people who have chronic aphasia following stroke compared with usual care. Typically, such a study would measure and report a wide range of variables at baseline (that is, prior to the intervention), such as participants' age, gender, education level, place of residence, time since stroke, severity of aphasia, side of stroke, and so on. Some of these variables are more likely to influence communication outcomes than others. The key question to consider is: are any differences in key prognostic variables between the groups large enough that they may have influenced the outcome(s)? Hopefully, if differences are evident the researchers will have corrected for this in the data analysis process.

As a reader (and critical appraiser) of research articles, it is important that you are able to see data for key characteristics that may be of prognostic value in both groups. Many articles will present such data in a table, with the data for the intervention group presented in one column and the data for the control group in another. This enables you to easily compare how similar the groups are for these variables. As well as presenting baseline data about **key socio-demographic characteristics** (for example, age and gender), articles should *also* report data about important **measures of the severity of the condition** (if that is relevant to the study—most times it is) so that you can see whether the groups were also similar in this respect. For example, in a study that involves participants who have had a stroke, the article may present data about the initial stroke severity of participants, as this variable has the potential to influence how participants respond to an intervention. In most cases, socio-demographic variables alone are not sufficient to determine baseline similarity.

One other area of baseline data that articles should report is the **key outcome(s)** of the study (that is, the pre-test measurement(s)). To illustrate why this is important, let us consider the example presented earlier of people receiving group communication treatment for aphasia. Although such an article would typically provide information about socio-demographic variables and clinical variables (such as severity of aphasia, type of stroke and side of stroke), having information about participants' initial (that is, pre-test) scores on the communication outcome measure that the study used would be helpful for considering baseline similarity. This is because, logically, participants' pre-test scores on a communication measure are likely to be a key prognostic factor for the main outcome of the study, which is communication ability.

When appraising an article, if you do conclude that there are baseline differences between the groups that are likely to be big enough to be of concern, hopefully the researchers will have statistically adjusted for these in the analysis. If they have not, you will need to try to take this into account when interpreting the study.

◎ CLINICAL SCENARIO (CONTINUED)

Baseline similarity

In the CBT trial for depression in heart failure, the baseline characteristics shown in Tables 1 and 2 of the article are similar between the study groups (except for a slight difference between groups in racial status) and include most of the likely confounders. Notably, both groups had the same number of participants taking anti-depressants. The baseline scores of the outcome measures were also similar between the two groups. For example, the CBT group had a baseline BDI-II score of 30.7 and the usual care group a BDI-II score of 29.6 (from a possible score range of 0–63).

Were participants, health professionals and study personnel 'blind' to group allocation?

People involved with a trial, whether they be the participants, the treating health professionals or the study personnel, usually have a belief or expectation about what effect the experimental condition will or will not have. This conscious or unconscious expectation can influence their behaviour, which in turn can affect the results of the study. This is particularly problematic if they know which condition (experimental or control) the participant is receiving. Blinding (also known as 'masking') is a technique that is used to prevent participants, health professionals and study personnel from knowing which group the participant was assigned to so that they will not be influenced by that knowledge.[13]

In many studies, it is difficult to achieve blinding. Blinding means more than just keeping the name of the intervention hidden; the experimental and control conditions need to be indistinguishable. This is because even if they are not informed about the nature of the experimental or control conditions (which, for ethical reasons, they usually are) when they sign informed consent forms, participants can often work out which group they are in. Whereas pharmaceutical trials can use placebo medication to prevent participants and health professionals from knowing who has received the active intervention, blinding of participants and the health professionals who are providing the intervention is very difficult (and often impossible) in many non-pharmaceutical trials. We will now look a little more closely at why it is important to blind participants, health professionals and study personnel to group allocation.

A **participant's** knowledge of their treatment status (that is, if they know whether they are receiving the intervention that is being evaluated) may consciously or unconsciously influence their performance during the intervention or their reporting of outcomes. For example, if a participant was keen to receive the intervention that was being studied and they were instead randomised to the control group, they may be disappointed and their feelings about this might be reflected in their outcome assessments, particularly if the outcomes being measured are subjective in nature (for example, pain, quality of life or satisfaction). Conversely, if a participant knows or suspects that they are in the intervention group, they may be more positive about their outcomes (such as exaggerating the level of improvement they have experienced) when they report them, as they wish to be a 'polite patient' and are grateful for receiving the intervention.[19]

The **health professionals** who provide the intervention often have a view about the effectiveness of interventions, and this can influence the way they interact with the study participants and the way they deliver the intervention. This, in turn, can influence how committed they are to providing the intervention in a reliable and enthusiastic manner, affecting participants' compliance with the intervention and responses on outcome measures. For example, if a health professional believes strongly in the value of the intervention that is being studied, they may be very enthusiastic and diligent in their delivery of the intervention, which may in turn influence how participants respond to it. It is easy to see how a health professional's enthusiasm (or lack of it) could influence outcomes. Obviously, some interventions (such as medications) are not able to be influenced easily by the way in which they are provided, but for many other interventions (such as rehabilitation techniques provided by therapists) this can be an issue.

Study personnel who are responsible for measuring outcomes (the assessors) and who are aware of whether the participant is receiving the experimental or control condition may provide different interpretations of marginal findings or differential encouragement during performance tests, either of which can distort results. For example, if an assessor knows that a participant is in the intervention group, they might be a little more generous when scoring the participant's performance on a task than they would be if they thought the participant was in the control group. Studies should aim to use blinded assessors to prevent measurement bias from occurring. This can be done by ensuring that the assessor who measures the outcomes at baseline and at follow-up is unaware of the participant's group assignment. Sometimes this is referred to as the use of an *independent assessor*. The more objective the outcome that is being assessed, the less critical this issue becomes.[12] However, there are not many truly objective outcome measures, as even measures that appear to be reasonably objective (for example, measuring muscle strength manually or functional ability) have a subjective component and, as such, can be susceptible to measurement bias. Therefore, where it is at all possible, studies should try to ensure that the people who are assessing participants' outcomes are blinded. Estimates from a systematic review revealed that non-blinded assessors (for subjective measures) exaggerated the pooled effect size by 68%.[11] Ideally, studies should also check and report on the success of blinding assessors and, where this information is not provided, you may wish to reasonably speculate about whether or not the outcome assessor was actually blinded as claimed.

However, there is a common situation that occurs, particularly in many trials in which non-pharmaceutical interventions are being tested, that makes assessor blinding not possible to achieve. If the participant is aware of their group assignment, then the assessment cannot be considered to be blinded. For example, consider the outcome measure of pain that is assessed using a visual analogue scale. The participant has to complete the assessment themselves, due to the subjective nature of the symptom experience. In this situation, the participant is really the assessor and, if the participant is not blind to which study group they are in, then the assessor is also not blind to group allocation. Research articles often state that the outcome assessors were blind to group allocation. Most articles measure more than one outcome, and often a combination of objective and subjective outcome measures is used. So, while this statement may be true for objective outcomes, if the article involved outcomes that were assessed by participant self-report and the participants were not blinded, you cannot consider that these subjective outcomes were measured by a blinded assessor.

 CLINICAL SCENARIO (CONTINUED)

Blinding

In the CBT trial for depression in heart failure, it was not possible to blind participants to which group (CBT or usual care) they had been allocated to, nor to blind therapists to the group allocation. The primary outcome measure was the BDI-II depression score, and this was measured by participant self-report. As the primary outcome measure was measured by participant self-report and participants were not blinded, technically the measurement of the primary outcome measure was not done by a blinded assessor. However, participant self-report is an appropriate, and widely used and accepted, measure of collecting data about depression and anxiety and there is not really any other feasible method that enables this type of data to be collected in a blinded manner. However, the authors state that the outcome assessors were blinded to group assignments. Blinding is certainly possible to achieve for the objective measurements taken in this trial, such as the 6-minute walk test.

Were all participants who entered the trial properly accounted for at its conclusion, and how complete was follow-up?

In randomised trials, it is common to have missing data at follow-up. There are many reasons why data may be missing. For example, some questionnaires may not have been fully completed by participants, some participants may have decided to leave the study, or some participants may have moved house and cannot be located at the time of the follow-up assessment. How much of a problem this is for the study, with respect to the bias that is consequently introduced, depends on how many participants left the study and *why*.

It is therefore helpful to know whether all the participants who entered the trial were properly accounted for. In other words, we want to know what happened to them. Could the reason that they dropped out of the study have affected the results? This may be the case, for example, if they left the study because the intervention was making them worse or causing adverse side effects. If this was the case, this might make the intervention look more effective than it really was. Did they leave the study simply because they changed jobs and moved away, or was the reason that they dropped out related to the study or to their health? For example, it may not be possible to obtain data from participants at follow-up measurement points because they became unwell, or maybe because they improved and no longer wanted to participate. Hopefully, you can now see why it is important to know why there are missing data for some participants.

The more participants who are 'lost to follow-up', the more the trial may be at risk of bias because participants that leave the study are likely to have different prognoses from those who stay. It has been suggested that 'readers can decide for themselves when the loss to follow-up is excessive by assuming, in positive trials [that is, trials that showed that the intervention was effective], that all patients lost from the treatment group did badly, and all lost from the control group did well, and then recalculating the outcomes under these assumptions. If the conclusions of the trial do not change, then the loss to follow-up was not excessive. If the conclusions would change, the strength of inference is weakened (that is, less confidence can be placed in the study results).'[5]

When large numbers of participants leave a study, the potential for bias is enhanced. Various authors suggest that *if more than 15–20% of participants leave the study* (with no data available for them), then the results should be considered with much greater caution.[19,20] Therefore, you are looking for a study to have a minimum follow-up rate of at least 80–85%. To calculate the loss to follow-up, you divide the number of participants included in the analysis at the time point of interest (such as the 6-month follow-up) by the number of participants who were originally randomised into the study groups. This gives the percentage of participants who were followed up. Some articles will clearly report this, while in others it can be straightforward to find the necessary data that you need to calculate this, particularly if the article has provided a flow diagram (see Figure 4.2). It is highly recommended that trials do this, and this is explained more fully later in the chapter when the recommended reporting of a randomised trial is discussed. In other articles, this information can be obtained from the text, typically in the results section. In some articles, the only place to locate information about the number of participants who remain in the groups at a particular time point is from the column headers in a results table. And finally, in some articles, despite all of your best hunting efforts, there may be no information about the number of participants who were retained in the study. This may mean that there were no participants lost to follow-up (which is highly unlikely, as at least some participants are lost to follow-up in most studies) or the authors of the article did not report the loss of participants that occurred. Either way, as you cannot determine how complete the follow-up was, you should be suspicious of the study and consider the results to be potentially biased.

It is worth noting that where there is loss to follow-up in both the intervention and the control groups and the reasons for these losses are both *known* and *similar* between these groups, it is less likely that bias will be problematic.[21] When the reasons why participants leave the study are unknown, or when they are known to be different between the groups and potentially prognostically relevant, you should be more suspicious about the validity of the study. That is why it is important to consider the reasons for loss to follow-up and whether the number of participants lost to follow-up was approximately the same for both study groups, as well as the actual percentage of participants who were lost to follow-up.

◎ CLINICAL SCENARIO (CONTINUED)

Follow-up of participants

In the CBT trial for depression in heart failure, participants were followed from baseline to 12 months post-randomisation. The flow of participants through the trial is clearly provided in Figure 1 of the article, which also lists the reasons for some people being unable to be followed up. Before the 6-month assessment, 16% of participants were lost to follow-up—that is, an 84% follow-up rate—which is around the 85% follow-up rate that is considered acceptable for trials. There were equal numbers lost from the two groups.

Loss to follow-up at the 9- and 12-month time points measures was higher. This trial used multiple imputation models to impute missing data so that analysis could use a full data set, consistent with analysis by intention to treat, which will now be examined.

Were participants analysed in the groups to which they were randomised using intention-to-treat analysis?

The final criterion for assessing a trial's risk of bias is whether data from all participants were analysed in the groups to which participants were initially randomised, regardless of whether they ended up receiving the treatment. This analysis principle is referred to as 'intention-to-treat analysis'. In other words, participants should be analysed in the group that corresponds to how they were *intended* to be treated, not how they were actually treated.

It is important that an intention-to-treat analysis is performed, because study participants may not always receive the intervention or control condition as it was allocated (that is, intended to be received). In general,

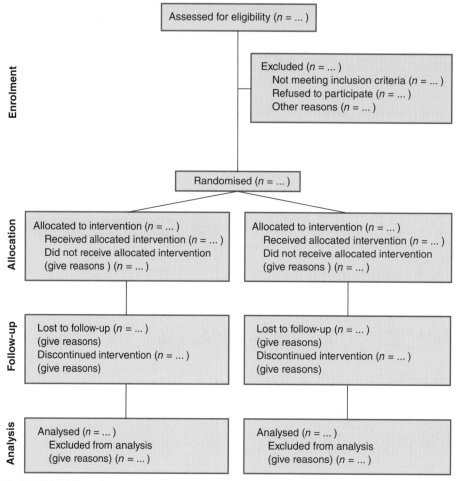

Fig 4.2 CONSORT flow diagram
From Schulz K et al. CONSORT 2010 statement: updated guidelines for reporting parallel group randomised trials. BMJ 2010;340:c332; reproduced with permission from BMJ Publishing Group Ltd.

participants may not receive the intervention (even though they were allocated to the intervention group) because they are either unwell or unmotivated, or for other reasons related to prognosis.[5] For example, in a study that is evaluating the effect of a medication, some participants in the intervention group may forget to take the medication and therefore do not actually receive the intervention as intended. In a study that is evaluating the effects of a home-based exercise program, some of the participants in the intervention group may not practise any of the exercises that are part of the intervention because they are not very motivated. Likewise, in a study that is evaluating a series of small-group education sessions for people who have had a heart attack, some participants in the intervention group

may decide not to attend some or all education sessions because they feel unwell. From these examples, you can see that even though these participants were in the intervention group of these studies, they did not actually receive the intervention (either at all or only partly).

It may be tempting for the researchers who are conducting these studies to analyse the data from these participants as if they were in the control group instead. However, doing this would increase the numbers in the control group who were either unmotivated or unwell. This would make the intervention appear more effective than it actually is, because there would be a greater number of participants in the control group who were likely to have unfavourable outcomes. It may also be tempting for researchers to discard the results from participants who did not receive the intervention (or control condition) as was intended. This is also an unsuitable way of dealing with this issue, as these participants would then be considered as lost to follow-up and we saw in the previous criterion why it is important that as few participants as possible are lost to follow-up.

For the sake of completeness, it is important to point out that it is not only participants who are allocated to the intervention group but do not receive the intervention that we should think about. The opposite can also happen. Participants who are allocated to the control group can inadvertently end up receiving the intervention. Again, intention-to-treat analysis should be used, and these participants should still be analysed as part of the control group.

The value of intention-to-treat analysis is that it preserves the value of randomisation. It helps to ensure that prognostic factors that we know about, and those that we do not know about, will still be, on average, equally distributed between the groups. Because of this, any effect that we see, such as improvement in participants' outcomes, is most likely to be because of the intervention rather than unrelated factors.

The difficulty in carrying out a true intention-to-treat analysis is that the data for *all* participants are needed. However, as we saw in the previous criterion about follow-up of participants, this is unrealistic to expect and most studies have missing data. There is currently no real agreement about how best to deal with such missing data, but researchers may sometimes estimate or impute data.[22–24] Data imputation is a statistical procedure that substitutes missing data in a data file with estimated data. Other studies may simply report that they have carried out an intention-to-treat analysis or that participants received the experimental or control conditions as allocated without providing details of what was actually done or how missing data were dealt with. In this case, as the reader of the article, you may choose to accept this at face value or to remain sceptical about how this issue was dealt with, depending on what other clues are available in the study report.

 CLINICAL SCENARIO (CONTINUED)

Intention-to-treat analysis
In the CBT trial for depression in heart failure, it is stated that data were analysed using intention to treat; and details about how missing data were imputed are provided in the statistical analysis section.

The role of chance

So far in this chapter, we have considered the potential for bias in randomised trials. Another aspect that is important to consider is the possibility that chance might be an alternative explanation for the findings. So, a further question that you may wish to consider when appraising a randomised trial is: did the study report a power calculation that might indicate what sample size would be necessary for the study to detect an effect if the effect actually exists? As we saw in Chapter 2, having an adequate sample size is important so that the study can avoid a Type 2 error occurring. You may remember that a Type 2 error is the failure to find and report a relationship when a relationship actually exists.[25]

CLINICAL SCENARIO (CONTINUED)

Did the study have enough participants to minimise the play of chance?
In the CBT trial for depression in heart failure, 158 participants were recruited. A power analysis had been performed. It had estimated that 240 participants would be needed to detect a between-group difference of 3 or more points on the BDI-II, previously determined as a clinically significant difference. The authors acknowledge the inability to recruit sufficient numbers but noted that this did not obscure the effect of the intervention on depression. However, small sample sizes (low power) can exaggerate the estimate of the magnitude of the effect[26] and this needs to be considered when interpreting the results.

COMPLETENESS OF REPORTING OF RANDOMISED CONTROLLED TRIALS

As we have seen in many places throughout this chapter, it can often be difficult for readers of research studies to know whether a study has met enough requirements to be considered a well-designed and well-conducted randomised trial that is relatively free of bias. To help overcome this problem and aid in the critical appraisal and interpretation of trials, an evidence-based initiative known as the CONSORT (Consolidated Standards of Reporting Trials) statement[15] has been developed to guide authors in how to completely report the details of a randomised controlled trial. The CONSORT statement is considered an evolving document and, at the time of writing, the most recent checklist contained 25 items (see Figure 4.2). Full details are available at www.consort-statement.org. The CONSORT statement is also used by peer reviewers of articles when the articles are being considered for publication, and many journals now insist that reports of randomised trials follow the CONSORT statement. The CONSORT statement also has a number of approved extensions—such as for particular trial designs (for example, cluster trials),[27] interventions (for example, Template for Intervention Description and Replication (TIDieR),[28] and types of data (such as harms data).[29] This is helping to improve the quality of reporting of trials but, unfortunately, many articles still do not contain all of the information that readers require. Some of the reasons are that not all journals require, or enforce, adherence to the CONSORT statement and older articles were published prior to CONSORT's development.

After appraising and determining that an article about the effects of an intervention appears to be reasonably free of bias, you then proceed to looking at the importance of the results.

UNDERSTANDING RESULTS

One of the fundamental concepts that you need to keep in mind when trying to make sense of the results of a randomised controlled trial is that clinical trials provide us with an *estimate* of the *average* effects of an intervention. Not every participant in the intervention group of a randomised trial is going to benefit from the intervention that is being studied—some may benefit a lot, some may benefit a little, some may experience no change, and some may even be worse (a little or a lot) as a result of receiving the intervention. The results from all participants are combined and the *average* effect of the intervention is what is reported.

Before getting into the details about how to interpret the results of a trial, the first thing that you need to look at is whether you are dealing with continuous or dichotomous data:

- **Variables with continuous data** can take any value along a continuum within a defined range. Examples of continuous variables are age, range of motion in a joint, walking speed, and score on a visual analogue scale.
- **Variables with dichotomous data** have only two possible values. For example, satisfied/not satisfied with treatment, or hip fracture/no hip fracture.

The way that you make sense of the results of a randomised trial depends on whether you are dealing with outcomes that were continuous or dichotomous. We will look at continuous data first. However, regardless of whether the results of the study were measured using continuous or dichotomous outcomes, we will be looking at how to answer two main questions:

1. What is the **size** of the intervention effect?
2. What is the **precision** of the intervention effect?

Continuous outcomes—size of the intervention effect

When you are trying to work out how much of a difference the intervention made, you are attempting to determine the size of the intervention effect. When you are dealing with continuous data, this is often quite a straightforward process.

The best estimate for the size of the intervention effect is the **difference in means** (or medians, if that is what is reported) **between the intervention and the control groups**. Many articles will already have done this for you and will report the difference. In other articles, you will have to do the simple subtraction calculation yourself. Figure 4.3 shows a hypothetical example in which the mean pain (on a 0–100 scale) experienced by the control group is higher (80 points) than the mean pain for the intervention group (50 points) when measured post-intervention. The effect size is simply the difference between these two means (80 – 50 = 30 points). Those in the intervention group had (on average) 30 points less than those in the control group.

Let us consider a real example from a randomised controlled trial. In a trial[30] of the efficacy of a self-management

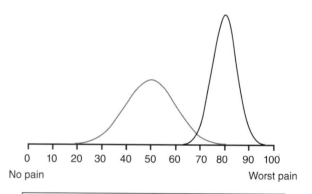

Difference in means
The black curve shows distribution of data for the **control** group, with a mean of 80 points.
The blue curve shows distribution of data for the **intervention** group, with a mean of 50 points.
Effect size = Difference between the two means (80 – 50 = 30)
Those in the intervention group had (on average) 30 points less than those in the control group.

Fig 4.3 Between-group effect size, illustrated as the difference between the means of two groups

program for people with knee osteoarthritis in addition to usual care, compared with usual care, one of the main outcome measures was pain, which was measured using a 0–10 cm visual analogue scale with 0 representing 'no pain at all' and 10 representing 'the worst pain imaginable'. At the 3-month follow-up, the mean reduction in knee pain was 0.67 cm (standard deviation [SD] = 2.10) in the intervention group and 0.01 cm (SD = 2.00) in the control group. This difference was statistically significant (p = 0.023). You can calculate the intervention effect size (difference in mean change between the groups) as: 0.67 cm minus 0.01 cm = 0.66 cm.

Note that, in this study, the authors reported the mean *improvement (reduction in pain) scores* at the 3-month follow-up (that is, the *change* in pain from baseline to the 3-month follow-up). Some studies report **change scores**; others report **end scores** (which are the scores at the end of the intervention period or follow-up period). Regardless of whether change scores or end scores are reported, the method of calculating the size of the intervention effect is the same. However, when dealing with change scores, you need the difference of the mean *change* between the intervention and control groups.

Clinical significance

Once you know the size of the intervention effect, you need to decide whether this result is clinically significant. As we saw in Chapter 2, just because a study finds a statistically significant result, it does not mean that the result is *clinically* significant. Deciding whether a result is clinically significant requires your judgment (and, ideally, your patient's, too) on whether the benefits of the intervention outweigh its costs. 'Costs' should be regarded in the broadest sense to be any inconveniences, discomforts or harms associated with the intervention, in addition to any monetary costs. To make decisions about clinical significance, it helps to determine what the smallest intervention effect is that you and your patient consider to be clinically worthwhile. Many trials do not comment on the clinical significance of the results, and when they do, it is often mentioned without any elaboration or justification.[31] This might be decided by the health professional based on their experience of using the measure, by using guidelines established by research on the particular measure being used (if available), by consulting with the patient, or by some combination of these approaches. Where possible, this decision is one that should be reached by discussion with the patient about their preferences in relation to the costs (including both financial costs and inconveniences) involved, compared to the potential size of improvement. The process

of doing this through shared decision making is described in Chapter 14.

One of the earliest methods for deciding important differences using effect sizes was developed by Cohen.[32] Effect sizes (represented by the symbol d) were calculated by taking the difference between group average scores and dividing it by the average of the standard deviation for both groups. This effect size is then compared with ranges classified intuitively by Cohen: 0.2 being a small effect size, 0.5 a moderate effect size and 0.8 a large effect size. This general rule of thumb has consequently been used to determine whether a change or difference was important.

A more direct approach is to simply compare the mean intervention effect with a nominated smallest clinically worthwhile difference. If the mean intervention effect lies below the smallest clinically worthwhile difference, we may consider it to be *not* clinically significant. For our knee osteoarthritis example, let us assume that in conjunction with our patient we nominate a 20% reduction of initial pain as the smallest difference that we would consider to be clinically worthwhile to add self-management to what the patient is already receiving. Our calculations show that a 20% reduction from the initial average pain of 4.05 cm experienced by participants in this study would be 0.8 cm. If the intervention has a greater effect than a 20% reduction in pain from baseline, we may consider that the benefits of it outweigh the costs and may therefore use it with our patient(s). In this study, the difference between groups in mean pain reduction (0.66 cm) is less than 0.8 cm, so we might be tempted to conclude that the result may not be clinically significant for this patient.

An alternative approach that is sometimes used for considering the effect size relative to baseline values involves comparing the effect size to the scale range of the outcome measure. In this example, we would simply compare the intervention effect size of 0.66 cm in relation to the overall possible score range of 0–10 cm and see that this between-group difference is not very large and therefore conclude that the result is unlikely to be considered clinically significant.

Note, however, that as this is an *average* effect there may be some patients who do much better than this and, for them, the intervention is clinically significant. Of course, conversely, there may be some patients who do much worse. This depends on the distribution of changes that occur in the two groups. One way of dealing with this is to look for the proportion of patients in both groups who improved, stayed the same or got worse relative to the nominated smallest clinically worthwhile difference. However, these data are often elusive, as they are often not reported in articles.

Another approach to determining clinical significance takes into account the uncertainty in measurement using the *confidence intervals* around the estimate. To understand this approach, we need first to look at confidence intervals in some detail.

Continuous outcomes—precision of the intervention effect

How are confidence intervals useful?

At the beginning of this results section, we highlighted that the results of a study are only an *estimate* of the true effect of the intervention. The size of the intervention effect in a study approximates but **does not equal** the true size of the intervention effect in the population represented by the study sample. As each study only involves a small sample of participants (regardless of the actual sample size, it is still just a *sample* of all the patients who meet the study's eligibility criteria and therefore is small in the grand scheme of things), the results of any study are just an estimate based on the sample of participants in that particular study. If we replicated the study with another sample of participants, we would (most likely) obtain a different estimate. As we saw in Chapter 2, the *true value* refers to the population value, not just the estimate of a value that has come from the sample of one study.

Confidence intervals are a way of describing how much uncertainty is associated with the estimate of the intervention effect (in other words, the precision or accuracy of the estimate). We saw in Chapter 2 how confidence intervals provide us with a range of values within which the true value lies. When dealing with 95% confidence intervals, what you are saying is that you are **95% certain that the true average intervention effect lies between the upper and the lower limits of the confidence interval**. In the knee osteoarthritis trial that we considered above, the 95% confidence interval for the difference of the mean change is 0.05 cm to 1.27 cm. (See Box 4.2 for how this was calculated.) So, we are 95% certain that the true average intervention effect (at 3 months follow-up) of the self-management program on knee pain in people with osteoarthritis lies between 0.05 cm and 1.27 cm.

How do I calculate a confidence interval?

Hopefully, the study that you are appraising will have included confidence intervals with the results in the results section. Fortunately, this is becoming increasingly common in research articles (probably because of the CONSORT statement and growing awareness of the usefulness of confidence intervals). If not, you may be able to calculate the confidence interval if the study provides you with the right information to do so. (See Box 4.2 for what you

---

BOX 4.2　How to calculate the confidence interval (CI) for the difference between the means of two groups

A formula[33] that can be used is:

$$95\% \, CI \approx Difference \pm 3 \times SD / \sqrt{n_{av}}$$

where:

Difference = difference between the two means
SD = average of the two standard deviations
n_{av} = average of the group sizes

For the knee osteoarthritis study, Difference = 0.66; SD = (2.10 + 2.00) ÷ 2 = 2.05; and n_{av} = (95 + 107) ÷ 2 = 101.

Therefore:

$$95\% \, CI \approx 0.66 \pm 0.61$$

$$\approx 0.05 \, to \, 1.27$$

When you calculate confidence intervals yourself, they will vary slightly depending on whether you use this formula or an online calculator. This formula is an approximation of the complex equation that researchers use to calculate confidence intervals for their study results, but it is

adequate for the purposes of health professionals who are considering using an intervention in clinical practice and wish to obtain information about the precision of the estimate of the intervention's effect.

Occasionally, you might calculate a confidence interval that is at odds with the *p* value reported in the paper (i.e. the confidence interval might indicate non-significance when in fact the *p* value in the paper is significant). This might occur because the test used by the researchers does not assume a normal distribution (as the 95% confidence interval does) or because the *p* value was close to 0.05 and the rough calculation of the confidence interval might end up including zero as it is a less precise calculation.

Note: if the study reports standard errors (SEs) instead of standard deviations, the formula to calculate the confidence interval is:

$$95\% \, CI = Difference \pm 3 \times SE$$

Herbert R. How to estimate treatment effects from reports of clinical trials I: continuous outcomes. Aust J Physiother 2000;46:229–35.

need.) An easy way of calculating confidence intervals is to use an online calculator. There are plenty available (for example: www.pedro.org.au/english/downloads/confidence-interval-calculator/). If the internet is not handy, you can use a simple formula to calculate the confidence interval for the difference between the means of two groups. (The formula is shown in Box 4.2.)

Confidence intervals and statistical significance

Confidence intervals can also be used to determine whether a result is statistically significant. Consider a randomised trial where two interventions were being evaluated and, at the end of the trial, it was found that, on average, participants in both groups improved by the same amount. If we were to calculate the size of the intervention effect for this trial it would be zero, as there would be no (0) difference between the means of the two groups. When referring to the difference between two groups with means, zero is considered a 'no effect' value. Therefore,

- if a confidence interval includes the 'no effect' value, the result is not statistically significant; and the opposite is also true:
- **if the confidence interval does *not* include the 'no effect' value, the result *is* statistically significant.**

In the knee osteoarthritis trial, we calculated the 95% confidence interval to be 0.05 cm to 1.27 cm. This interval does *not* include the 'no effect' value of zero, so we can therefore conclude that the result is **statistically significant** without needing to know the *p* value; although, in this case, the *p* value (0.023) was provided in the article and it also indicates a statistically significant result.

As an aside, if a result is *not* statistically significant, it is incorrect to refer to this as a 'negative' difference and to imply that the study has shown no difference and conclude that the intervention was not effective. It has not done this at all. All that the study has shown is an absence of evidence

of a difference.[34] A simple way to remember this is that **non-significance does not mean no effect**.

Confidence intervals and clinical significance

We now return to our previous discussion about clinical significance. Earlier we saw that there are a number of approaches that can be used to compare the effect estimate of a study to the smallest clinically worthwhile difference that is established by the health professional (and sometimes their patient as well). We will now explain a useful way of considering clinical significance that involves using confidence intervals to help make this decision.

Before we go on to explain the relationship between confidence intervals and clinical significance, you may find it easier to understand confidence intervals by viewing them on a **tree plot** (see Figure 4.4). A tree plot is a line along which varying intervention effects lie. The 'no effect' value is indicated in Figure 4.4 as the value 0 (that is, no difference between the groups). Effect estimates to the left of the 'no effect' value may indicate harm. Also marked on the figure is a dotted line that indicates the supposed smallest clinically worthwhile intervention effect. Anything to the left of this line but to the *right* of the 'no effect' value estimate represents effects of the intervention that are too small to be worthwhile. Conversely, anything to the right of this line indicates intervention effects that are clinically worthwhile.

In the situation where the **entire confidence interval is *below* the smallest clinically worthwhile effect**, this is a useful result. It is useful because at least we know with some certainty that the intervention is *not* likely to produce a clinically worthwhile effect. Similarly, when an **entire confidence interval is *above* the smallest clinically worthwhile effect**, this is a clear result, as we know with some certainty that the intervention is likely to produce a clinically worthwhile effect.

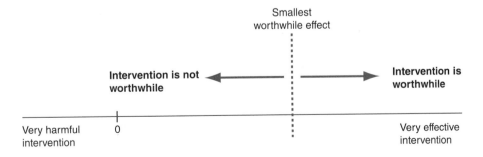

Effect of intervention

Fig 4.4 Tree plot of effect size
Adapted from Herbert R, Jamtvedt G, Hagen K, et al. Practice evidence-based physiotherapy. 2nd ed. Edinburgh: Elsevier; 2011. Reproduced with permission.

However, in the knee osteoarthritis trial, we calculated the 95% confidence interval to be 0.05 cm to 1.27 cm. The lower value is below 0.8 cm (20% of the initial pain level that we nominated as the smallest clinically worthwhile effect), but the upper value is above 0.8 cm. We can see this clearly if we mark the confidence interval on to a tree plot (see Figure 4.5, tree plot A). CI range indicates that there is uncertainty about whether a clinically worthwhile effect is occurring.

When the confidence interval *spans* the smallest clinically worthwhile effect, it is more difficult to interpret clinical significance. In this situation, the true effect of the intervention could lie either above the smallest clinically worthwhile effect or below it. In other words, there is a chance that the intervention may produce a clinically worthwhile effect, but there is also a chance that it may not. Another example of this is illustrated in tree plot B in Figure 4.5, using the data from a randomised controlled trial that investigated the efficacy of a guided self-management program for people with asthma compared with traditional asthma treatment.[35] One of the main outcome measures in this study was quality of life, which was measured using a section of the St George Respiratory Questionnaire. The total score for this outcome measure can range from −50 to +50, with positive scores indicating improvement and negative scores indicating deterioration in quality of life compared with one year ago. At the 12-month follow-up, the difference between the means of the two groups (that is, the intervention effect size) was 8 points (in favour of the self-management

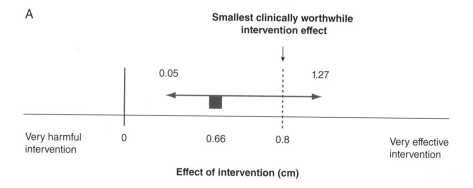

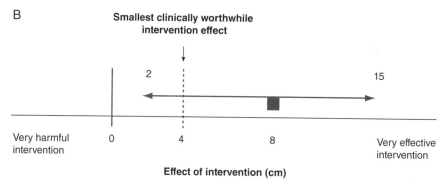

Fig 4.5 Tree plots showing the effect size, the smallest clinically worthwhile effect and the confidence interval associated with the effect size

In tree plot A, the estimate of the intervention effect size (0.66 cm) sits below the smallest clinically worthwhile effect of 0.8 cm and the confidence interval (0.05 cm to 1.27 cm) spans the smallest clinically worthwhile effect of 0.8 cm. The estimate of the intervention effect size is indicated as a small square, the 95% confidence interval about this estimate is shown as a horizontal line, and the dotted line indicates the supposed smallest clinically worthwhile intervention effect. In tree plot B, the estimate of the intervention effect size (8) is above the smallest clinically worthwhile effect (4) and the confidence interval (2 to 15) spans the smallest clinically worthwhile effect.

group), with a 95% confidence interval of 2 to 15. This difference was statistically significant ($p = 0.009$). Let us assume that we nominate a difference of 4 points to be the smallest clinically worthwhile effect for this example. In this example, the mean difference (8) is above what we have chosen as the smallest clinically worthwhile effect (4), but the confidence interval includes some values that are above the worthwhile effect and some values that are below it. If the true intervention effect was at the upper limit of the confidence interval (at 15), we would consider the intervention to be worthwhile, while if the true intervention effect was at the lower limit of the confidence interval (2), we may not. So, although we would probably conclude that the effect of this self-management intervention on quality of life was clinically significant, this conclusion would be made with a degree of uncertainty.

The situation of a confidence interval spanning the smallest clinically worthwhile effect is a common one, and there are two main reasons why it can occur. First, it can occur when a study has a small sample size and therefore low power. The concept of power was explained in Chapter 2. As we also saw in Chapter 2, the smaller the sample size of a study, the wider (that is, less precise) the confidence interval is, which makes it more likely that the confidence interval will span the worthwhile effect. Second, it can occur because many interventions only have fairly small intervention effects, meaning that their true effects are close to the smallest clinically worthwhile effect. As a consequence, they need to have very narrow confidence intervals if the confidence interval is going to avoid spanning the smallest worthwhile effect.[19] As we just discussed, this typically means that a very large sample size is needed. In some disciplines (such as allied health studies), this can be difficult to achieve.

There are two ways that you, as a health professional who is trying to decide whether to use an intervention with a patient, can deal with this uncertainty:[19]

- Accept the uncertainty and make your decision according to whether the difference between the group means is higher or lower than the smallest clinically worthwhile effect. However, keep the confidence interval in mind, as it indicates the degree of doubt that you should have about this estimate.
- Try to increase the certainty by searching for similar studies and establishing whether the findings are replicated in other studies. This is one of the advantages of a systematic review, in particular a meta-analysis, as combining the results from multiple trials increases the sample size. The consequence of this is usually a more narrow (more precise) confidence interval which is less likely to span the smallest clinically worthwhile effect. Systematic reviews and meta-analyses are discussed in detail in Chapter 12.

◎ CLINICAL SCENARIO (CONTINUED)

Main results—depression

In the CBT trial for depression in heart failure, depressive symptoms measured by the BDI-II are reported as means (and standard deviations) at each time point. At 6 months (the main time point of interest in this trial), the mean difference between the two groups was −4.43 points (95% CI −7.68 to −1.18), which was statistically significant. There are a few points to note about this. First, the negative sign indicates a *reduction* in depression (because, on this outcome measure, lower scores indicate less severe depression). Second, the confidence interval does not contain zero, and therefore this result was statistically significant.

Understanding the clinical significance of this result is more complex. A National Institute for Health and Care Excellence (NICE) guideline suggested that a difference of 3 or more BDI-II points is a clinically significant treatment effect for depression in the general population.[36] However, this has been subsequently questioned as not having empirical support[37] and is not included in an updated version of guidelines.[38] A more recent analysis examined the minimal clinically important difference (MCID) for the BDI-II by using data from three trials and anchoring the BDI-II change to patients' global report of improvement. It estimated an MCID of a 17.5% reduction in scores from baseline.[37] In our CBT trial, the baseline mean BDI-II score was approximately 30 in both groups, so this would be a reduction of approximately 5 points. The depressive symptoms in participants in both groups improved, on average; however, it is the between-group difference (a mean of −4.43) that we are really interested in. It is larger than the 3 points identified by the outdated NICE guidelines but not quite at the 17.5% reduction from baseline (about 5 points in this case) estimated by one MCID proposal. This suggests that this effect might be considered borderline clinically significant, although this might ultimately be determined by discussion between the clinician and each patient about what is acceptable. It also should be noted that the confidence interval for this mean change ranges from −7.68 to −1.18. This means that the effect may be as small as a 1.18 reduction for some patients, which some may consider to be not clinically significant, or it could be as large as a 7.68 reduction, which might be considered clinically significant.

On the Beck Anxiety Inventory, the mean difference between the two groups at 6 months was −4.47 (95% CI −7.70 to −1.25), which is statistically significant as the confidence interval does not contain zero. As the literature does not suggest what the smallest clinically worthwhile effect might be (particularly for people with heart disease), we could talk with our patients to see what amount of reduction in anxiety they would want to achieve.

Dichotomous outcomes—size of the treatment effect

Often the outcomes that are reported in a trial will be presented as dichotomous data. As we saw at the beginning of this results section, these are data for which there are only two possible values. It is worth being aware that data measured using a continuous scale can also be categorised, using a certain cut-off point on the scale, so that the data become dichotomised. For example, data on a 10-point visual analogue pain scale can be arbitrarily dichotomised around a cut-off point of 3 (or any point that the researchers choose), so that a pain score of 3 or less is categorised as mild pain and a score of above 3 is categorised as moderate/severe pain. By doing this, the researchers have converted continuous data into data that can be analysed as dichotomous data.

Health professionals and patients are often interested in *comparative* results—the outcome in one group relative to the outcome in the other group. This overall (comparative) consideration is one of risk. Before getting into the details, let us briefly review the concept of risk. *Risk* is simply the chance, or probability, of an event occurring. A probability can be described by numbers, ranging from 0 to 1, and is a proportion or ratio. Risks and probabilities are usually expressed as a decimal, such as 0.1667, which is the same as 16.67%. Risk can be expressed in various ways (but using the same data).[39,40] We will consider each of these in turn:

- relative risk (or the flip side of this, which is referred to as 'relative benefit')
- relative risk reduction (or relative benefit increase)
- absolute risk reduction (or absolute benefit increase)
- number needed to treat.

Risk and relative risk (or relative benefit)

Consider a hypothetical study that investigated an exercise intervention to prevent the occurrence of falls in older adults. The control group (*n* = 100) received no intervention and is compared with the intervention group (*n* = 100) who received the exercise intervention. Suppose that at the end of the 6-month trial, 25 of the participants in the control group had had a fall.

- The risk for occurrence of a fall in the control group can be calculated as 25/100, which can be expressed as 25%, or a risk of occurrence of 0.25. This is also known as the 'Control Event Rate' (CER).
- If, in the exercise group, only 5 participants had had a fall, the risk of occurrence would be 5% (5/100), or 0.05. This is sometimes referred to as the 'Experimental Event Rate' (EER).

These data can be represented graphically, as in Figure 4.6.

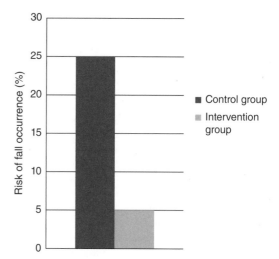

Fig 4.6 Risk of fall occurrence in the control group and intervention group in a hypothetical study

We are interested in the comparison between groups. One way of doing this is to consider the **relative risk**—a ratio of the probability of the event occurring in the intervention group versus in the control group.[41] In other words, **relative risk is the risk or probability of the event in the intervention group divided by that in the control group.** The term 'relative risk' is being increasingly replaced by 'risk ratio', which describes the same concept but reflects that it is a ratio that is being referred to. In the exercise for falls study, the relative risk (that is, the **risk ratio**) would be calculated by dividing the EER by the CER:

$$0.05/0.25 = 0.20 \text{ (or 20\%)}$$

This can be expressed as: 'The risk of having a fall for those in the exercise group is 20% of the risk in the control group.'

You may remember that when we were discussing continuous outcomes, the 'no effect' value was zero (when referring to the difference between group means). When referring to relative risk, the 'no effect' value (the value that indicates that there is no difference between groups) is 1. This is because if the risk is the same in both groups (for example, 0.25 in one group and 0.25 in the other group), there would be *no* difference and the relative risk (risk ratio) would be 0.25/0.25 = 1. Therefore, **a relative risk (risk ratio) of less than 1 indicates lower risk—that is, a benefit from the intervention.**[41]

If we are evaluating a study that aimed to improve an outcome (that is, make it more likely to occur) rather than reducing a risk, we might instead consider using the equivalent concept of **relative benefit**. For example, in a study that evaluated the effectiveness of phonological training to increase reading accuracy among children with learning disabilities, we could calculate relative benefit as the study was about improving an outcome, not reducing the risk of it happening.

Sometimes a study will report an **odds ratio** instead of relative risk. It is similar, except that an odds ratio refers to a ratio of odds, rather than a ratio of risks. The odds ratio is the ratio of the odds of an event for those in the intervention group compared with the odds of an event in the control group. Odds are derived by dividing the event rate by the non-event rate for each group. The odds ratio is calculated by the following formula, where, again, 'CER' refers to the Control Event Rate and 'EER' to the Experimental Event Rate:

$$\text{Odds ratio (OR)} = [\text{EER}/(1 - \text{EER})] \div [\text{CER}/(1 - \text{CER})]$$

Also, some studies may report the intervention effect as a **hazard ratio**. This typically occurs when a survival analysis has been performed. A hazard ratio is broadly similar in concept to a risk ratio (relative risk) and so can be interpreted in a similar manner—that is, it describes how many times more (or less) likely a participant is to experience the event at a particular point in time if they were in the intervention group rather than the control group.

Relative risk reduction (or relative benefit increase)

Relative risk reduction is another way of expressing the difference between the two groups and is simply the proportional reduction in an event of interest (for example, falls) in the intervention group compared with the control group, at a specified time point. Again, there is a flip side of this concept, which is known as 'relative benefit increase'. When appraising an article and using this concept, you need to keep in mind whether you are considering negative or positive outcomes:

- Relative risk reduction (RRR) is used to express the reduction in risk of a negative outcome (such as falling).
- Relative benefit increase (RBI) is used to express an increase in the probability of a beneficial outcome (such as returning to work).

The formula that can be used for calculating relative risk reduction or relative benefit increase is:

$$(\text{CER} - \text{EER}) \div \text{CER} \times 100$$

The CER is simply the proportion of participants in the control group who experienced the event of interest. In our study of exercise to prevent falls, this was 25% (or 0.25). Similarly, the EER is the proportion of participants in the

intervention (experimental) group who experienced the event of interest. This was 5% (or 0.05) in the exercise study.

Using our exercise study as an illustration, relative risk reduction can be calculated as: $(0.25 - 0.05) \div 0.25 = 0.80$. We could multiply this by 100 to get 80% and report that the participation in an exercise group reduced the risk of falls by 80%.

Alternatively, if you already know the relative risk, then the relative risk reduction can be calculated easily using the formula:

$$\text{RRR} = 1 - \text{RR}$$

In our example, where the relative risk (RR) is 0.20, the relative risk reduction is 0.80 or 80% (calculated as $1 - 0.20$).

The main difficulty in the use of relative risk reduction is that it does not reflect the baseline risk of the event.[42] This means that, as a reader, you are unable to discriminate between small intervention effects and large ones. **Baseline risk** has an important role to play. To understand this, you need to think about the risk in different populations. For example, in the general population the risk of falling might be between 8% and 40% (depending on factors such as gender, age, comorbidities and so on). Reducing the risk of falls in a population that has a low risk to start with is very hard to achieve, and any risk reduction that is found would be fairly small (and as you will see in the next section, absolute risk reduction would be smaller still). However, in a population of people who more commonly have falls (such as older adults and those who have previously fallen), the risk of recurrence is much higher and it would, therefore, be easier to achieve a larger relative risk reduction. Interventions that reduce the risk in populations who are at high risk of the event under consideration are likely to be clinically worthwhile.[43]

Another difficulty with the use of the relative risk reduction concept is that it can make results seem more impressive than they really are. Expressing the effects of an intervention in relative terms will result in larger percentages than when the same intervention is expressed in absolute terms. For example, suppose the use of a particular type of mattress reduced the risk of pressure sores from 0.05 to 0.025. In relative terms, the mattress reduces the risk by 50% (calculated by: $0.025 \div 0.05 = 0.5$, or 50%), while in absolute terms it reduces the risk by 2.5% (calculated by: $0.05 - 0.025 = 0.025$, or 2.5%). Similarly, in the hypothetical trial on exercise for reducing occurrence of falls the *relative* risk reduction seems an impressive 80% but, as we will see later, the *absolute* difference in the rate of events between groups is only 20%. So, we can see that the concept of relative risk reduction can inflate the appearance of intervention effectiveness.

You should also be aware that two studies might have the same relative risk reduction but there may be a large difference in the absolute risk reduction. As we saw in the example above about reducing the risk of pressure sores by using a particular type of mattress, a reduction in risk from 0.05 to 0.025 reduces the relative risk by 50%, while in absolute terms it reduces the risk by 2.5%. Let us say that another study found that the risk of pressure sores in a very high-risk group of people was reduced from 0.8 to 0.4 because of the intervention (the mattress). In relative terms, although the mattress reduced the relative risk by 50% (calculated by: 0.8 ÷ 0.4 = 0.5, or 50%), the absolute risk reduction is 40%, which is a more clinically valuable result than the absolute risk reduction of 2.5% that the first study found.

Absolute risk reduction (or absolute benefit increase)

Another way of presenting information about dichotomous outcomes is by referring to the absolute risk reduction. The *absolute risk reduction* is simply the absolute arithmetic difference in event rates between the experimental (intervention) and the control groups.[44] This is shown graphically in Figure 4.7. Absolute values are simply the value of a number, regardless of its sign (positive or negative sign). The notation used for absolute values is vertical bars either side of the value, for example: $|x|$. The absolute arithmetic difference for risk reduction is calculated as: $|EER - CER|$. As with the previous methods of calculating risk that we have explained,

there is a flip side to this concept. This is known as *absolute benefit increase* and is used when referring to a beneficial outcome (such as being discharged home instead of to residential care).

In our hypothetical exercise study for reducing the risk of falling, the absolute risk reduction would be 25% − 5% = 20%. This could be expressed as: 'the absolute risk of having a fall was 20% less in the people who were in the exercise group compared with those in the control group'.

A big absolute risk reduction indicates that the intervention is very effective, but how big is big enough to be considered clinically significant? A more meaningful measure, known as 'number needed to treat', can be used instead.

Number needed to treat

We saw that the absolute risk reduction of having a fall in the exercise study was calculated as 20%, but is this clinically worthwhile? Number needed to treat (NNT) is a method of making the magnitude of the absolute risk reduction more explicit and is a more clinically useful concept.[41] The number needed to treat is simply the inverse of absolute risk reduction[45] and is calculated as:

$$1 \div (EER - CER)$$

It tells you the number of people who would need to be treated to achieve the event of interest once. In the trial of exercise for preventing a fall, the number needed to treat is $1 \div (0.25 - 0.05) = 5$. So, in this example, you would have to treat 5 people for 6 months with the hypothetical exercise intervention to prevent *one* (extra) person from having a fall (when compared with the control group). Obviously, a smaller number needed to treat is better than a large one. An intervention that has a smaller number needed to treat is more effective than an intervention that has a larger number needed to treat.

This concept of number needed to treat makes it easier to consider clinical significance, as you can more easily weigh up the benefits of preventing the event in one person against the costs and harms of providing the intervention. The size of the smallest clinically worthwhile effect (that is, the smallest worthwhile number needed to treat) will then depend on the seriousness of the event and the costs and harms of the intervention.

Another handy feature when using number needed to treat is that you can compare two different interventions that are trying to achieve the same outcome that have the same number needed to treat but have other features that are different. For example, one of the interventions may have a shorter intervention time and/or result in fewer side effects and/or be more convenient to patients and/or be

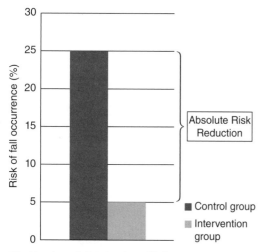

Fig 4.7 Absolute risk reduction of fall occurrence in a hypothetical study of an exercise intervention

less expensive. It is important to consider features such as these that a particular intervention has when deciding which intervention to use with a patient.

Applying results to your clinical situation

Most health professionals find it difficult to translate the results from studies to individual patients or to specific clinical situations, as studies usually only tell us about the *average* effects of the intervention. Further, the participants who took part in the study may be different from the patients that we see, and the intervention may differ from the intervention that we use. However, as a rough guide, if your patient is 'healthier' or the situation that you are considering is more optimistic than that in the study, the number needed to treat would be lower, the relative benefit increase would be higher, the mean difference would be larger and so on. If, however, your patient is 'worse off', or the situation that you are considering is worse than that in the study, the number needed to treat would be higher, the relative benefit increase would be lower, the mean difference would be smaller and so on. A solution to applying the results of a trial to patients with higher or lower levels of risk has been described by Straus and Sackett[46] and you may wish to read their article to learn more about this.

Dichotomous outcomes—precision of the treatment effect

Confidence intervals are also important to consider when examining dichotomous outcomes as, again, they indicate how much uncertainty is associated with the estimate of the intervention effect (in other words, the precision or accuracy of the estimate). The principles of confidence intervals associated with dichotomous data are similar to those for continuous data, but there is one very important difference to consider—what is the appropriate 'no effect' value to use?

- For effect size estimates where **subtraction is involved**, such as mean differences (for continuous outcomes) and absolute risk reductions, the **'no effect' value is 0**.
- For effect sizes that involve **division**, such as risk ratios and odds ratios, the **'no effect' value is 1**.

Therefore, you can see that it is important to consider the *type* of effect measure you are interpreting in order to reliably interpret the confidence interval. The same general principle applies, though—a 95% confidence interval that does *not* include the 'no effect' value indicates that the result is statistically significant. Table 4.1 presents a summary of the dichotomous effect measures, including what their 'no effect' value is, that have been discussed in this section of the chapter.

As we could do with continuous outcomes, if the confidence interval has not been provided by the authors of the article it is sometimes possible to calculate an approximate confidence interval. This is illustrated in Box 4.3. Again, a simplified version of the more complex equation is used, but the confidence interval that is calculated is sufficient for use by health professionals who wish to use the information to assist in clinical decision making. Once you know the confidence interval for the absolute risk reduction, if you wish you could plot it, the effect estimate and the smallest clinically worthwhile effect on a tree plot in the same way that we did for continuous outcomes in Figure 4.5.

Calculating the confidence intervals for number needed to treat is fairly straightforward, as you just use the inverse of the numbers in the confidence interval of the absolute risk reduction.[41] However, understanding how to interpret the confidence intervals for number needed to treat can be complicated, and the article by Altman[47] is recommended to understand this in detail.

◉ CLINICAL SCENARIO (CONTINUED)

Main results—dichotomous

In the CBT for depression for people with heart failure trial, the authors dichotomised the scores from the BDI-II so that participants with scores of ≤9 were considered to have achieved a remission from depression, while those scoring above this did not. Note that in using the data this way, achieving a remission is a *positive* change and therefore we need to think in terms of *benefit* rather than *risk*. The authors indicate that 46% of participants in the CBT group achieved remission from depression, compared with 19% in the control group. From this we can work out that the **absolute benefit increase** is |0.46 − 0.19| or 0.27 (27%). The **number needed to treat** is the inverse of the absolute benefit increase, so 1/0.27 = 3.70. The authors provide the 95% confidence interval of the number needed to treat as 3.62 to 3.90. Rounding the number needed to treat up to 4 (since you can't have 3.76 people) indicates that you would have to treat 4 people for 6 months with CBT for one extra person to achieve a remission from depression. With this information, you can, along with your patient, weigh up the likelihood of achieving remission from depression against the costs, risks and inconveniences of the intervention.

When making sense of the results of a randomised trial, one further issue that you should be aware of is that trials usually report results from many different outcomes. With so much information to process it may be helpful, in some cases, for you to focus your attention on the main

TABLE 4.1   Summary of dichotomous effect measures

Type of measure	Definition	Formula	'No effect' value
Relative risk (RR) (also called 'risk ratio')	The ratio of the probability of the event occurring in the intervention group versus the control group. Expressed as either a decimal proportion or a percentage.	The risk of an event in the intervention group divided by the risk in the control group: EER ÷ CER	1
Relative risk reduction (RRR)	The proportion of the risk that is removed by the intervention. That is, the proportional reduction in an event of interest in the intervention group compared with the control group. Usually expressed as a percentage.	(CER − EER) ÷ CER × 100 *or* 1 − RR	0
Absolute risk reduction (ARR)	The absolute arithmetic difference in event rates between the experimental (intervention) and control groups. Usually expressed as a percentage.	|EER − CER|	0
Number needed to treat (NNT)	The number of people that would need to be treated for the event of interest to occur in 1 person.	1 ÷ ARR *or* 1 ÷ (EER − CER)	Infinity. (Refer to article by Altman[47] for an explanation of why this is so.)
Odds ratio (OR)	The odds of an event in the intervention group divided by the odds of an event in the control group. Usually expressed as a decimal proportion.	[EER/(1 − EER)] ÷ [CER/(1 − CER)]	1

CER = Control Event Rate; EER = Experimental Event Rate.

BOX 4.3   How to calculate the confidence interval (CI) for absolute risk reduction

A formula[43] that can be used is:

$$95\% \, CI \approx \text{Difference in risk} \pm 1/\sqrt{n_{av}}$$

where n_{av} = average of the group sizes.

For our study of exercise, the 95% confidence interval for the absolute risk reduction would be:

$$\approx (30\% - 5\%) \pm 1/\sqrt{100} \approx 25\% \pm 0.1 \approx 25\% \pm 10\%$$

This tells us that the best estimate of the absolute risk reduction achieved from participating in an exercise group is 35% and that the 95% confidence interval extends from 15% to 35%.

Herbert R. How to estimate treatment effects from reports of clinical trials II: Dichotomous outcomes. Aust J Physiother 2000;46:309–13.

outcome(s) of the trial, the outcome(s) of interest to the question that you initially formed and/or the outcome that is of interest to your patient. If you have got to this point and determined that the article that you have been appraising not only appears to be reasonably free of bias but also contains some clinically important results, you then proceed to look at whether you can apply the results from the study to your patient or clinical situation. This is the third and final step of the critical appraisal process that we described in Chapter 1.

HOW CAN WE USE THIS EVIDENCE TO INFORM PRACTICE?

If you have decided that the validity of the study you are appraising is adequate and that the results are clinically important, the final step of the critical appraisal process is to consider the application of this information to the clinical situation that prompted your original clinical question. To do this, there are a few important questions that should be considered:

- Do the results apply to your patient or situation?
- Do the benefits found outweigh any harm, costs and/or inconveniences that are involved with the intervention?
- What other factors might need to be considered when applying this evidence?

Do the results apply to your patient or situation?

When considering whether the results apply to your patient or situation, you essentially need to assess whether your patient is so different from the participants in the study that you cannot apply the results of the study that you have been reading to your patient or situation. So, rather than just thinking about the study's eligibility criteria with respect to your patient, are the differences problematic enough that the results should not be applied? Further to this, results can sometimes be individualised to a particular patient by considering the individual benefit and harm for that patient. There is some complexity involved in doing so, which is beyond the scope of this book. If you wish to learn about this further, you are advised to read the article by Glasziou and Irwig[48] to understand how this may be done.

Do the benefits found outweigh any harm, costs and/or inconveniences that are involved with the intervention?

Understanding whether benefits outweigh harms, costs or inconveniences requires using information about benefits that is given in terms of the size of the intervention effect (for example, mean differences, relative risk reduction, number needed to treat) and comparing this against possible harms or even inconveniences. When information about harms and cost is provided in the article, this is relatively straightforward. However, this type of information is often not provided and some estimate of the costs associated with the intervention might need to be made. Information about harm is obviously more difficult to estimate,

and other sources might need to be consulted to get a sense of the potential harms involved. Clinical experience and discussion with patients about their preferences and values become very important at this stage and Chapter 14 discusses how this can occur through the process of shared decision making.

What other factors might need to be considered when applying this evidence?

A further important question to consider is: what other factors might need to be considered when applying this evidence? When you are thinking about what other factors affect the delivery of an intervention, there are a few key questions that you can ask, such as:

- How much does it cost?
- How many sessions might be involved or how long would the patient need to stay in hospital?
- How far would the patient (or the health professional) need to travel?
- Are the resources (for example, any equipment that is needed) available to deliver the intervention?
- Do you or other health professionals working with you have the skills to provide the intervention?
- Are the details of the intervention sufficiently described in the article or available elsewhere so that intervention can be accurately provided?

A central component of applying research evidence to your patient is discussing the information with them. The success of many interventions is dependent on the health professional successfully providing the patient with appropriate information.

Involving the patient in the decision-making process is important, and this is discussed further in Chapter 14. In Chapter 1, we emphasised the need for integrating information from patients, clinical experience, research and the practice context. To do so is the art of evidence-based practice. Integrating so many pieces of information from many different sources is certainly an art form and one that requires clinical reasoning and judgment. The roles of clinical reasoning and judgment are discussed further in Chapter 15.

◎ CLINICAL SCENARIO (CONTINUED)

Using the evidence to inform practice

So, what can we conclude from our reading of the CBT trial article? You know that depression is common among people with heart failure, that it is associated with an increased risk of mortality and poorer quality of life, and that tackling depression is an important issue. In summary, this trial[4] was well constructed, although it was unable to achieve

blinding of participants, health professionals or study personnel. This leads you, as the reader, to be a bit cautious of the results reported. For example, the depression data were collected by participant self-report, which would be subject not only to error but also to differential bias (that is, there could be systematic differences in the self-reports of people in the intervention compared with those in the

Continued

⊙ CLINICAL SCENARIO (CONTINUED)—cont'd

control group due to their knowledge about which group they were in). Participants in the intervention group also received more contact over the time of the trial, which makes you wonder what part that extra attention might have played in influencing outcomes.

At 6 months, the intervention group had lower levels of depressive symptoms than the control group (a mean between-group difference of −4.43) and this was sustained at the 9- and 12-month follow-ups. However, even though the 6-month result was statistically significant, you consider its clinical significance to be uncertain and you have similar concerns about the effect on anxiety at 6 months. Rates of remission from depression were higher in the intervention group than the control group, with an NNT of 4. As the reader of this article, you need to consider how the biases present in this study might have affected these results. You then also need to consider how to apply these results in your situation.

Do the results apply to our patient or situation?

The group of people that we were concerned about were people with heart failure who also had depression. The study that we looked at involved men and women with a mean age of 55.8 years who had a depression score of ≥14 on the BDI-II. It is likely that these results do apply to the group of people that we are concerned about.

Are the benefits worth the harms and costs?

While there are few 'harms' associated with this intervention, CBT can explore painful feelings, emotions and experiences that may, at times, make people feel emotionally uncomfortable. No details about costs of the intervention are provided in the article. All we know is that the intervention involved 1 hour of CBT per week and tapered off to monthly treatment towards the end of the 6 months, with a number needed to treat of 4. A very general idea of costs can be determined from this information. For individual patients, the 'cost' to them can be thought about in terms of the time commitment, inconvenience, potential disruption of other activities, and travel involved in attending weekly CBT sessions.

Other factors to consider

Other practical factors to consider are the availability of this type of CBT program in your clinical vicinity or, if you were to run it at the community health centre, the resources (such as staffing and space, or any training or intervention materials needed) and costs that would be involved. Data about the cost-effectiveness of this intervention would be valuable to further facilitate your team's decision making about whether to implement this intervention or not.

SUMMARY

- The effects of intervention are best determined through rigorous randomised controlled trials (or, better still, systematic reviews of randomised trials), as their methods best reduce the risk of bias.
- Most randomised controlled trials are not free from bias. Key questions that should be asked when appraising the risk of bias in a randomised trial are:
  - How were participants randomised to groups?
  - Was the allocation sequence concealed?
  - Were the groups similar at baseline?
  - Were participants, health professionals and study personnel blind to group allocation?
  - Was follow-up adequate?
  - Was intention-to-treat analysis used?
- Our understanding of the risk of bias that is present in a study is affected not just by the methods that the

researchers used, but also by how well these are reported in the article that describes the study.
- Two factors to consider when making sense of the results of a randomised trial are:
  - the size or magnitude of the intervention effect (this may be provided as continuous data or dichotomous data); and
  - the precision of the intervention effect (which can best be determined by inspecting the confidence interval for the intervention effect).
- Applying the results of the study requires thinking through whether the results apply to your patient or situation, identifying a range of logistical factors that can affect the delivery of the intervention and, in collaboration with your patient, discussing whether the possible benefits outweigh any harm, costs or inconveniences.

REFERENCES

1. Portney L, Watkins M. Foundations of clinical research: applications to practice. 4th ed. Philadelphia, PA: FA Davis Company; 2020.

2. Deeks J, Dinnes J, D'Amico R, et al. Evaluating non-randomised intervention studies. Health Technol Assess 2003;7:1–186.

3. Kariyawasam D, Morin C, Casteels K, et al. Hybrid closed-loop insulin delivery versus sensor-augmented pump therapy in children aged 6–12 years: a randomised, controlled, cross-over, non-inferiority trial. Lancet Digit Health 2022;4(3):e158–68.

4. Freedland K, Carney R, Rich M, et al. Cognitive behavior therapy for depression and self-care in heart failure patients: a randomized clinical trial. JAMA Intern Med 2015;175:1773–82.

5. Guyatt GH, Sackett DL, Cook DJ. Users' guides to the medical literature. II. How to use an article about therapy or prevention. A. Are the results of the study valid? JAMA 1993;270:2598–601.

6. Maher C, Sherrington C, Herbert R, et al. Reliability of the PEDro scale for rating quality of randomized controlled trials. Phys Ther 2003;83:713–21.

7. Shulz K, Chalmers I, Hayes R, et al. Empirical evidence of bias: dimensions of methodological quality associated with estimates of treatment effects in controlled trials. JAMA 1995;273:408–12.

8. Savović J, Jones H, Altman D, et al. Influence of reported study design characteristics on intervention effect estimates from randomised controlled trials: combined analysis of meta-epidemiological studies. Health Technol Assess 2012;16(35):1–82.

9. Page MJ, Higgins JP, Clayton G, et al. Empirical evidence of study design biases in randomized trials: systematic review of meta-epidemiological studies. PLoS One 2016 Jul 11;11(7):e0159267.

10. Odgaard-Jensen J, Vist GE, Timmer A, et al. Randomisation to protect against selection bias in healthcare trials. Cochrane Database Syst Rev 2011;(4):MR000012.

11. Hróbjartsson A, Thomsen AS, Emanuelsson F, et al. Observer bias in randomized clinical trials with measurement scale outcomes: a systematic review of trials with both blinded and nonblinded assessors. CMAJ 2013;185:E201–11.

12. Altman DG, Bland JM. Treatment allocation in controlled trials: why randomise? BMJ 1999;318:1209.

13. Hewitt C, Torgerson D. Is restricted randomisation necessary? BMJ 2006;332:1506–8.

14. Rababah JA, Al-Hammouri MM, AlNsour E. Effectiveness of an educational program on improving healthcare providers' knowledge of acute stroke: a randomized block design study. World J Emerg Med 2021;12(2):93–8.

15. Schulz K, Altman D, Moher D, et al. CONSORT 2010 statement: updated guidelines for reporting parallel group randomised trials. BMJ 2010;340:c332. doi:10.1136/bmj.c332.

16. Pildal J, Chan AW, Hróbjartsson A, et al. Comparison of descriptions of allocation concealment in trial protocols and the published reports: cohort study. BMJ 2005;330:1049–54.

17. Bennett S, McKenna K, McCluskey A, et al. Evidence for occupational therapy interventions: status of effectiveness research indexed in the OTseeker database. Br J Occup Ther 2007;70:426–30.

18. Roberts C, Torgerson D. Understanding controlled trials: baseline imbalance in randomised controlled trials. BMJ 1999;319:185.

19. Herbert R, Jamtvedt G, Hagen K, et al. Practical evidence-based physiotherapy. 2nd ed. Edinburgh: Elsevier; 2011.

20. Dumville J, Torgerson D, Hewitt CE. Reporting attrition in randomised controlled trials. BMJ 2006;332:969–71.

21. Higgins JPT, Savović J, Page MJ. Chapter 8: Assessing risk of bias in a randomised trial. In: Higgins JPT, Thomas J, Chandler J, et al., editors. Cochrane handbook for systematic reviews of interventions. The Cochrane Collaboration. Version 6.3 (updated February 2022); 2022. Online. Available: www.training.cochrane.org/handbook/ (accessed 17 March 2022).

22. Abraha I, Montedori A. Modified intention to treat reporting in randomised controlled trials: systematic review. BMJ 2010;340:c2697.

23. Bell ML, Fiero M, Horton NJ, et al. Handling missing data in RCTs; a review of the top medical journals. BMC Med Res Methodol 2014;14:118.

24. Altman DG. Missing outcomes in randomized trials: addressing the dilemma. Open Med 2009;3(2):e51–3.

25. Biau DJ, Kernéis S, Porcher R. Statistics in brief: the importance of sample size in the planning and interpretation of medical research. Clin Orthop Relat Res 2008;466(9):2282–8.

26. Button KS, Ioannidis JP, Mokrysz C, et al. Power failure: why small sample size undermines the reliability of neuroscience. Nat Rev Neurosci 2013;14(5):365–76.

27. Campbell M, Piaggio G, Elbourne DR, et al.; for the CONSORT Group. Consort 2010 statement: extension to cluster randomised trials. BMJ 2012;345:e5661.

28. Hoffmann T, Glasziou PP, Boutron I, et al. Better reporting of interventions: template for intervention description and replication (TIDieR) checklist and guide. BMJ 2014;348:g1687.

29. Ioannidis JP, Evans SJ, Gotzsche PC, et al. Better reporting of harms in randomized trials: an extension of the CONSORT statement. Ann Intern Med 2004;141(10):781–8.

30. Heuts P, de Bie R, Drietelaar M, et al. Self-management in osteoarthritis of hip or knee: a randomized clinical trial in a primary healthcare setting. J Rheumatol 2005;32:543–9.

31. Hoffmann T, Thomas S, Hung Shin P, et al. Cross-sectional analysis of the reporting of continuous outcome measures and clinical significance of results in randomized trials of non-pharmacological interventions. Trials 2014;15:362.

32. Cohen J. Statistical power analysis for the behavioral sciences. 2nd ed. Hillsdale, NJ: Lawrence Erlbaum; 1988.

33. Herbert R. How to estimate treatment effects from reports of clinical trials. I: continuous outcomes. Aust J Physiother 2000;46:229–35.

34. Altman D, Bland J. Absence of evidence is not evidence of absence. BMJ 1995;311:485.

35. Lahdensuo A, Haahtela T, Herrala J, et al. Randomised comparison of guided self-management and traditional treatment of asthma over one year. BMJ 1996;312:748–52.

36. NCCMH. Depression: management of depression in primary and secondary care. Leicester and London: British Psychological Society and Royal College of Psychiatrists; 2004.

37. Button KS, Kounali D, Thomas L, et al. Minimal clinically important difference on the Beck Depression Inventory—II according to the patient's perspective. Psychol Med 2015; 45(15):3269–79.

38. National Institute for Health and Care Excellence. Depression in adults: recognition and management. Clinical guideline. National Institute for Health and Care Excellence (updated May 2021); 2009. Online. Available: https://www.nice.org.uk/guidance/cg90 (accessed 17 March 2022).

39. Guyatt G, Sackett D, Cook D. Users' guide to the medical literature: II. How to use an article about therapy or prevention: B. What were the results and will they help me in caring for my patients? Evidence-Based Medicine Working Group. JAMA 1994;271:59–63.

40. George A, Stead TS, Ganti L. What's the risk: differentiating risk ratios, odds ratios, and hazard ratios? Cureus 2020; 12(8):e10047.

41. Cook R, Sackett D. The number needed to treat: a clinically useful measure of treatment effect. BMJ 1995;310:452–4.

42. Straus S, Glasziou P, Richardson WS, et al. Evidence-based medicine. How to practice and teach EBM. 5th ed. Edinburgh: Elsevier; 2018.

43. Herbert R. How to estimate treatment effects from reports of clinical trials. II: Dichotomous outcomes. Aust J Physiother 2000;46:309–13.

44. Centre for Evidence-Based Medicine. Glossary. Oxford: University of Oxford. Online. Available: https://www.cebm.ox.ac.uk/resources/ebm-tools/glossary (accessed 8 March 2022).

45. Laupacis A, Sackett D, Roberts R. An assessment of clinically useful measures of the consequences of treatment. N Engl J Med 1988;318:1728–33.

46. Straus S, Sackett D. Applying evidence to the individual patient. Ann Oncol 1999;10:29.

47. Altman D. Confidence intervals for the number needed to treat. BMJ 1998;317:1309–12.

48. Glasziou P, Irwig L. An evidence-based approach to individualising treatment. BMJ 1995;311:1356–9.

Questions about the Effects of Interventions
Examples of Appraisals from Different Health Professions

Elizabeth Gibson, Lauren Ball, John Bennett, Sally Bennett, Mary Bushell, Jeff Coombes, Fiona Dobson, Joanna Harnett, Isabel Jalbert, Nerida Klupp, David Long, Emma Power, Rachel Thompson, Cynthia Wensley and Caroline Wright

This chapter is an accompaniment to the previous chapter (Chapter 4) in which you learnt how to critically appraise evidence about the effects of interventions. To further illustrate the key points from Chapter 4, this chapter contains a number of worked examples of questions about the effects of interventions. As we mentioned earlier in the book, we believe that it can be easier to learn the process of critical appraisal when you see some worked examples of how it is done, and it is even better when the examples are from your own health profession. Therefore, this chapter (and likewise Chapters 7, 9 and 11) contains examples from a range of health professions. Some of the clinical examples are relevant to more than one health profession. Each example is formatted in a similar manner and contains the following elements:

- a brief clinical scenario that explains the origins of the clinical question
- the clinical question
- the search terms and databases used to find evidence to answer the clinical question
- a brief description of the search results and the reason for selecting the chosen article
- a structured abstract of the chosen article
- an appraisal of the risk of bias of the evidence
- a summary of the main results of the article that are relevant to the clinical question
- a brief discussion about how the evidence might be used to inform practice.

You will notice that in the examples, the type of article chosen to be appraised is a randomised controlled trial. You may wonder why this is the case when Chapters 2 and 12 explain that systematic reviews of randomised controlled trials should be the first choice of study design to answer questions about the effects of an intervention. There is a good reason behind this. The authors of the examples contained in this chapter were asked not to choose (or indeed, specifically search for) systematic reviews if these were available to answer their question. Why? Because it is easier to learn how to appraise a systematic review of randomised trials if you have first learnt how to appraise a randomised trial. This chapter and Chapter 4 are designed to help you learn how to appraise a randomised trial. Once you know how to do this, Chapter 12 will help you learn how to appraise a systematic review. In many of the examples the search was done in PubMed Clinical Queries, and while you may see that the search strategy sometimes yielded some systematic reviews (because of the use of the term 'randomised' in the title or abstract search), this will not yield all systematic reviews for the question.

As you read these examples, keep in mind that the suggestions the authors of these worked examples have provided in the 'How might we use this evidence to inform practice?' section have been drawn from only one study. In reality, additional studies (ideally in the form of a systematic review) would need to be located and appraised prior to drawing clear conclusions about what should be done in clinical practice.

When appraising an article, you need to obtain and carefully read the full text of the article. We have not included the full text of the articles that are appraised. However, for each of the examples in this chapter (and in Chapters 7, 9 and 11), the authors of the examples have prepared a structured abstract that summarises the article. This has been done so that you have some basic information about each article. As we mentioned in Chapter 1, the more you practise doing the steps of evidence-based practice, the easier it will become. This is particularly true of the critical appraisal step. You may find it useful if you approach these worked examples as a self-assessment activity and try to obtain a copy of some of the articles that are appraised in the examples (perhaps start with the ones that are most relevant to your health profession if you feel more comfortable with that). You can then critically appraise the articles for yourself and check your answers with those that are presented in the worked examples.

One other thing to note about the examples in this chapter (and in Chapters 7, 9 and 11) is that the appraisal of articles is not an exact science and sometimes there are no definite right or wrong answers. As with evidence-based practice in general, the health professional's clinical experience has an important role to play, particularly in deciding about issues such as baseline similarity (as we saw in Chapter 4) and clinical significance (as we saw in Chapters 2 and 4). Some of the examples may contain statements that you do not completely agree with and that you, as a health professional, would interpret a little differently. Also, the examples are provided to give you an overall sense of the general process of evidence-based practice. The content that is presented in the examples is not exhaustive (particularly in the 'How do we use this evidence to inform practice?' section). There may be other considerations raised by a patient that aren't captured here and there may be other factors or issues that you, as a health professional, would suggest or consider if you were in that situation. That is okay.

◎ OCCUPATIONAL THERAPY EXAMPLE

Clinical scenario

You are an occupational therapist working in the community and your caseload includes people who have dementia and live at home in the community. These people often have changes in their usual behaviour such as agitation, and commonly have difficulties with activities of daily living (ADLs). This can impact family or other carers' quality of life. For these people, you often provide advice about modifications to the home environment as well as education and support about dementia for the person's family or carers. You are aware there is a growing evidence base for training carers in the adaptation of meaningful activities to use with the person with dementia, which is not something that you often do because it takes more time. However, if there is good evidence available, you think you could discuss the need to offer this more intensive approach with your line manager. You decide to search the literature to inform this discussion and to understand how to explain this approach to the people you work with.

Clinical question

For people living with dementia and their families, does the use of meaningful activity reduce behaviours such as agitation and improve performance of ADLs for the person with dementia and improve caregiver quality of life?

Search terms and databases used to find the evidence
Database: PubMed—Clinical Queries (with 'therapy category' and 'narrow scope' selected).
Search terms: dementia AND "meaningful activity"
This search retrieves six hits, one of which looks relevant, so you retrieve its full text.

Article chosen
Gitlin LN, Marx K, Piersol CV, et al. Effects of the tailored activity program (TAP) on dementia-related symptoms, health events and caregiver wellbeing: a randomized controlled trial. BMC Geriatrics 2021;21(1):581. doi: 10.1186/s12877-021-02511-4.

Structured abstract (adapted from the above)
Study design: Randomised controlled trial.
Setting: Community, United States.
Participants: 250 dyads (persons with dementia and caregiver) were eligible if the person had been clinically diagnosed with dementia (mild, moderate or severe) and also had significant agitation or aggression, was able to participate in at least two ADLs, and was on a stable dose of psychotropic medications or anti-dementia medications. The caregiver could be family members, friends or neighbours who either lived with the person or nearby and was ≥21 years. Exclusion criteria were: previous

psychiatric history; dementia secondary to head trauma; planned placement in residential aged care within 6 months; or caregiver in poor health (e.g. being treated for cancer). People with dementia (mean age 81.4 years, 63.2% female) had a mean Mini Mental Status Examination (MMSE) score of 14.3. Caregivers' mean age was 65.4 years and 81.2% were female.

Intervention: The intervention and attention control were delivered by occupational therapists in the person's home for eight sessions across a 3-month period. The intervention was the Tailored Activity Program (TAP). TAP included assessment of the abilities and interests of the person with dementia as well as a range of caregiver assessments, followed by instructing caregivers in adapting both meaningful activities of interest for the person with dementia as well as the environment, planning use of activities as part of daily routines, and providing dementia education and stress reduction techniques for the caregiver. Caregivers in the attention control group were provided with education about dementia and advice about home safety.

Outcomes: *Primary outcome:* frequency multiplied by severity scores of agitated and aggressive behaviours at 3 months were measured by the relevant subscales of the Neuropsychiatric Inventory–Clinician version. *Secondary outcomes:* caregiver rating of ADL was measured with the Caregiver Assessment of Function and Upset which measured both instrumental (IADL) and basic ADLs, caregiver wellbeing (using the Perceived Change for Better Index), and the number and type of health-related events for people with dementia (death, hospitalisation, visits to emergency centres, and depression and/or suicidal ideation) and caregivers (hospital admission; depression scores ≥ 15 on the Patient Health Questionnaire [PHQ-9]).

Main results: There was no between-group improvement in agitation/aggression scores, but for those in the TAP group, less assistance was needed for IADLs and ADLs compared to those in the control group. Caregiver wellbeing also improved. At 6 months follow-up, fewer people with dementia who received TAP had ≥ 1 health-related event compared with the control group.

Conclusion: TAP did not improve the primary outcome of agitation/aggression, but it improved a number of other outcomes that could make a meaningful difference for people with dementia and their families.

Is this evidence likely to be biased?

- *Was the assignment of participants to groups randomised?*
  Yes. Participants were individually randomised (allocation by computer) 1:1 to intervention or attention control, with stratification by MMSE >10 or MMSE ≤ 10, in block sizes.
- *Was the allocation sequence concealed?*
  Yes. This was done by altering block sizes for stratification and using double opaque envelopes which were set up by a statistician and opened after the baseline interview by the project manager.
- *Were the groups similar at the baseline or start of the trial?*
  Yes. Detailed baseline characteristics are provided and the groups were largely similar.
- *Were participants blind to which study group they were in?*
  No. Because of the nature of the intervention in this study, it was not possible for participants to be blinded to group allocation.
- *Were the health professionals who provided the intervention blind to participants' study group?*
  No. This was not possible given the type of intervention being provided.
- *Were the assessors blind to participants' study group?*
  Yes. Outcome assessors were blinded to group allocation, although some outcomes were self-report for which participants were the assessors and were not blinded.
- *Were all participants who entered the trial properly accounted for at its conclusion, and how complete was follow-up?*
  Yes. A detailed flowchart with reasons for loss to follow-up is provided. At 3 months, 82.4% of participants were able to be followed up and 70.4% at 6 months. Caregivers reported lower cognitive status and poorer quality of life for the person with dementia, and a poorer relationship ($p < 0.05$) at baseline for those dyads who dropped out of the study compared to those who remained.
- *Was intention-to-treat analysis used?*
  Yes. Intention-to-treat analysis was conducted.
- *Did the study have enough participants to minimise the play of chance?*
  Yes. It was calculated, using data from a previous pilot study, that 250 participants (allowing for 20% dropout) were needed.

Continued

◎ OCCUPATIONAL THERAPY EXAMPLE—cont'd

TABLE 5.1   Three-month outcomes for people living with dementia and their caregivers

Outcome	Possible range of scores	Adjusted mean difference between groups (95% CI)	p value	Cohen's d*
People living with dementia				
Agitation / aggression	0–336 (higher is better)	3.14 (–4.71 to 10.99)	0.43	0.11
ADL independence	0–7 (higher is worse)	–0.59 (–1.15 to –0.03)	0.04	–0.30
IADL independence	0–8 (higher is worse)	–0.33 (–0.62 to –0.05)	0.02	–0.33
Caregivers of people with dementia				
Confidence using activities	0–10** (higher is better)	3.46 (0.42 to 6.50)	0.03	0.32
Perceived wellbeing	0–65 (higher is better)	3.50 (0.94 to 6.06)	0.01	0.39

*Note: A Cohen's d of 0.2 is considered a small effect size and 0.5 a moderate effect size.
**Total score of 50, but the score was averaged over five items scaled 0 to 10.

What are the main results?

As shown in Table 5.1, at 3 months there was no significant between-group improvement in agitation/aggression for people living with dementia. However, less assistance was needed for ADLs and IADLs for those receiving TAP compared to control. The between-group adjusted mean differences were statistically significant and, although small, the authors suggest that they may be clinically significant as it suggests caregiver assistance was not needed for close to one less daily ADL/IADL. Caregiver perceived wellbeing was also significantly higher in the intervention group, compared to the control, at 3 months.

How might we use this evidence to inform practice?

This trial is well designed and conducted and has a reasonably low risk of bias. It is also very well reported, which makes interpreting the results easier. Full details of the TAP intervention are contained in other publications which you intend to obtain. After looking carefully at this trial, you see the intervention had a small effect on ADLs and caregiver wellbeing. The reduction in health-related events is important as this could also impact on care costs. You decide to look at other trials of this same program before having a discussion with your line manager and with case managers about using this type of program on a more routine basis. Given that you would be providing more sessions for these clients than usual, you will also look for relevant cost-effectiveness studies. When talking with clients and their families about this intervention, you know that as well as explaining the options for care and support that you could provide, you need to discuss what is involved in TAP, the costs and potential benefits and harms, before deciding together whether that is something they would like to do.

◎ PHYSIOTHERAPY EXAMPLE

Clinical scenario

You are a physiotherapist working in a community setting. A 64-year-old woman with end-stage knee osteoarthritis (OA) who has been attending for physiotherapy has decided to have a unilateral total knee joint replacement. Her surgeon told her that she may require inpatient rehabilitation post-surgery or she could recover at home with an exercise program. She asks your advice on which option would be better to help her regain her mobility.

Clinical question

Is inpatient rehabilitation more effective than home-based rehabilitation at improving mobility following total knee arthroplasty?

Search terms and databases used to find the evidence

Database: PubMed—Clinical Queries (with 'therapy category' and 'narrow scope' selected). (You could have also chosen to search the PEDro database.)

Search terms: (((total knee arthroplasty) AND (inpatient rehabilitation)) AND (home-based rehabilitation)) AND (mobility)

After excluding protocols and a feasibility study, one primary article seems to be a good match for your patient scenario and setting.

Article chosen

Buhagiar MA, Naylor JM, Harris IA, et al. Effect of inpatient rehabilitation vs a monitored home-based program on mobility in patients with total knee arthroplasty: the HIHO randomized clinical trial. JAMA 2017;317(10): 1037–46.

Structured abstract (adapted from the above)

Study design: Multicentre, two parallel groups, concealed allocation, assessor-blinded randomised controlled trial with a third non-randomised observational group (results of which are not included here).

Setting: Two public, high-volume arthroplasty hospitals in Australia.

Participants: 165 participants presenting for primary, unilateral total knee arthroplasty with mean age 66.9 years (SD 8.4 years), 68% female. To be eligible, participants had to be >40 years, have a primary diagnosis of knee osteoarthritis, and be scheduled to undergo a primary total knee arthroplasty. Exclusion criteria included lack of social supports; other major coexisting physical impairments; inability to read English; and complications following surgery that interfered with participation in the planned programs.

Intervention: Participants were randomly allocated (1:1 ratio) to receive either (i) inpatient rehabilitation (n = 81), consisting of 10 days of public hospital inpatient rehabilitation followed by an 8-week clinician-monitored home-based program; or (ii) home-based rehabilitation (n = 84), consisting of one group-based hospital outpatient exercise session followed by an 8-week clinician-monitored home-based program. The inpatient rehabilitation group were provided with twice-daily physiotherapy sessions comprising 1 to 1.5 hours of 1:1 physiotherapy and 1 to 1.5 hours of class-based exercises. The home-based program included 40 minutes of structured exercises four times a week for an 8-week duration. Both inpatient and home programs included exercises designed to restore lower-limb mobility, strength and neuromuscular coordination.

Outcomes: *Primary outcome:* mobility at 26 weeks post-surgery using the 6-minute walk test recorded in distance walked (metres), minimum clinically important difference (MCID) 26–55 metres. *Secondary outcomes:* (i) patient-reported pain and physical function at 10, 26 and 52 weeks following surgery using the Knee injury and Osteoarthritis Outcome Score (KOOS), reported as 0 (worst) to 100 (best) points, MCID 8–10 points; and Oxford Knee Score reported as 0 (worst) to 48 (best) points, MCID 5 points; (ii) performance-based mobility tested at 10, 26 and 52 weeks following surgery using the 15-metre walk test (seconds); and (iii) quality of life at 10, 26 and 52 weeks. Patient satisfaction with rehabilitation at 10 weeks and the number of complications/adverse events were also recorded.

Main results: Intention-to-treat analysis found no significant difference between the inpatient and home-based groups for the primary 6-minute walk test (mean difference, –1.01 metres, 95% confidence interval [CI] –25.56 to 23.55) at 26 weeks post-surgery nor in any of the secondary outcomes.

Conclusion: For patients with uncomplicated knee arthroplasty and appropriate social supports for discharge directly home, a 10-day inpatient rehabilitation program followed by a monitored 8-week home-based program did not improve mobility more than a monitored 8-week home-based program alone.

Is this evidence likely to be biased?

- *Was the assignment of participants to groups randomised?*

  Yes. Participants were randomly assigned to groups in a 1:1 ratio using a centralised telephone-based randomisation service and a minimisation process which used age, height and sex to adaptively stratify the randomisation.

- *Was the allocation sequence concealed?*

  Yes. The allocation sequence was concealed using an off-site telephone-based randomisation service, reducing the potential for selection bias.

- *Were the groups similar at baseline or the start of the trial?*

  Yes. As adaptive stratified sampling was used, groups were similar on demographic factors and outcome measures at baseline. This demonstrated randomisation was preserved.

- *Were the participants blind to which study group they were in?*

  No. Due to the nature of the interventions, it was not possible to blind participants to group allocation. This

Continued

◎ PHYSIOTHERAPY EXAMPLE—cont'd

increases the potential for performance bias from participants as it may influence their volition during the intervention phase and outcome assessment, lowering the confidence in the study findings.

- *Were the health professionals who provided the intervention blind to the participants' study group?*

  No. Due to the nature of the interventions, it was not possible to blind the therapists to the participants' group allocation. This increases the potential for therapist performance bias as it can influence the way they deliver the intervention and/or interact with participants, lowering the confidence in the study findings.

- *Were the assessors blind to the participants' study group?*

  Yes for the primary outcome and no for self-reported outcomes. Assessors for the primary outcome (6-minute walk test) were unaware of the participants' group allocation and were not involved in providing the interventions. However, for the patient-reported secondary outcomes (such as pain), the participants, who were not blind to group allocation, were the assessors.

- *Were all participants who entered the trial properly accounted for at its conclusion, and how complete was follow-up?*

  Yes. The primary outcome was collected in 98% of the inpatient group and 95% for the home program. The characteristics of participants with missing data were similar to those with complete data, lowering the potential for attrition bias. A flow diagram is provided and it accounts for all participants and reasons for missing data.

- *Was intention-to-treat analysis used?*

  Yes. It is stated that an intention-to-treat analysis was conducted by a statistician who was blinded to group allocation in which all randomised participants were included.

- *Did the study have enough participants to minimise the play of chance?*

  Yes. An *a priori* sample size calculation estimated that 140 participants would be required to provide 80%

power at a significance level of 5% to detect a moderate effect size for the primary outcome. Data for 159/165 participants were available at follow-up, providing adequate power to detect a moderate effect size.

What are the main results?

Mobility: Both the inpatient and home-based groups had clinically worthwhile within-group increases in the mean walking distance on the 6-minute walk test at 26 weeks post-surgery. However, there was no significant difference between groups (mean difference, −1.01 metres, 95% CI, −25.56 to 23.55).

Secondary outcomes: Similarly, both groups had clinically worthwhile within-group increases in mean secondary mobility outcomes at 26 weeks following surgery; however, there were no statistically significant differences between the groups (KOOS mean difference, 1.99 points, 95% CI −3.68 to 7.67; OKS mean difference, 2.06 points, 95% CI −0.59 to 4.71; 15-metre walk test mean difference 0.50 seconds, 95% CI −1.01 to 2.01) (Figure 5.1). The number of post-discharge complications and adverse events were similar between the groups.

How might we use this evidence to inform practice?

On balance, you decide that the trial was at low risk of bias and was adequately powered. As the public inpatient rehabilitation program did not result in increased mobility following surgery compared to rehabilitation at home, and as complications and adverse events were similar in both groups, you discuss this with your patient. You explain that as long as her surgery is uncomplicated, the choice for rehabilitation in her home or an inpatient facility comes down to her preferences. An important factor that needs to be considered is whether she has adequate support in the home to be discharged directly home and to assist with a home-based program.

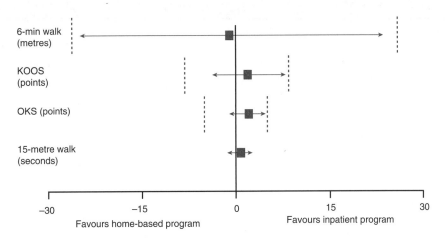

Fig 5.1 Mean differences in mobility outcomes between an inpatient program and a home-based program at 26 weeks flowing arthroplasty.

The small mean differences (boxes) for each outcome are non-significant, indicated by the 95% confidence intervals (arrows) crossing the zero line of no effect and unlikely to be meaningful for most patients as all sit below the known estimated minimum clinically important difference (MCID) (dashed lines). MCID not estimated for 15 m walk. KOOS = Knee injury and Osteoarthritis Outcome Score; OKS = Oxford Knee Score.

◎ PODIATRY EXAMPLE

Clinical scenario

You work as a podiatrist in private practice. A patient presents with unilateral Achilles pain that you diagnose as mid-portion Achilles tendinopathy. Your patient leads a busy life, has three children and works full-time as a teacher. You usually prescribe calf muscle eccentric exercise as this is the recommended first-line treatment. However, you are aware of the challenge of exercise compliance and although you have occasionally utilised heel lifts, you wonder if there has been any new research to evaluate their effectiveness as a treatment option for Achilles tendinopathy.

Clinical question

In people with Achilles tendinopathy, are heel raises as effective as calf eccentric muscle exercise (usual treatment) for reducing pain?

Search terms and databases used to find the evidence

Database: TRIP Medical Database PICO Search
Search terms: (achilles tendinopathy) AND (heel raise OR heel lift) AND exercise
This search returns 19 records. The first two results listed are the protocol and the full publication for a randomised

trial that evaluated the efficacy of heel lifts compared to eccentric exercise for Achilles tendinopathy. All other papers were not relevant to the PICO question.

Article chosen

Rabusin CL, Menz HB, McClelland JA, et al. Efficacy of heel lifts versus calf muscle eccentric exercise for mid-portion Achilles tendinopathy (HEALTHY): a randomised trial. Br J Sports Med 2021;55:486–92.
Website for full text: https://bjsm.bmj.com/content/55/9/486.long

Structured abstract (adapted from the above)

Study design: Randomised controlled trial.
Setting: Single university health clinic, Melbourne, Australia.
Participants: 100 adults (52% female, mean age 46 years) with a clinical and ultrasound-confirmed diagnosis of mid-portion Achilles tendinopathy present for at least 2 months. Exclusion criteria: previous Achilles tendon rupture or surgery, chronic ankle instability, tendinopathy secondary to underlying medical condition, or treatment with either trial intervention in previous 3 months.
Interventions: Participants in the intervention group received three pairs of 'Clearly Adjustable' 12 mm heel

Continued

PODIATRY EXAMPLE—cont'd

lifts (with 3.2 mm cover) for bilateral regular wear in shoes. Those in the comparison group followed a 12-week program of the Alfredson protocol of eccentric gastrocnemius/soleus exercises (15 reps twice daily) with resistance weight added incrementally.

Outcomes: The primary outcome was VISA–A (Victorian Institute of Sport Assessment—Achilles), a questionnaire (100-point scale, with lower scores representing greater severity) which measures self-reported pain, function, and activity measured at completion of the intervention period of 12 weeks.

Main results: The VISA–A score improved by 26 points (95% CI 19.6 to 32.4) in the heel lift group, and by 17.4 points (95% CI 9.5 to 25.3) in the eccentric exercise group. The between-group difference favoured the heel lift intervention (adjusted mean difference 9.6 points, 95% CI 1.8 to 17.4, $p = 0.016$), which was statistically significant.

Conclusion: Heel lifts were more effective than eccentric exercise for improving pain, function and activity in this study and may be considered first-line therapy for persons with mid-portion Achilles tendinopathy.

Is this evidence likely to be biased?

* *Was the assignment of participants to groups randomised?*
  Yes. Computer-generated (block) randomisation sequencing was used to assign participants to study groups.
* *Was the allocation sequence concealed?*
  Yes. The allocation sequence was concealed by being created and managed by an independent external service (online). Each participant's allocation was communicated to the study group after enrolment was confirmed.
* *Were the groups similar at the baseline or start of the trial?*
  Yes. The groups appear to be similar at baseline.
* *Were participants blind to which study group they were in?*
  No. Due to the nature of the intervention, participants were unable to be blinded.
* *Were the health professionals who provided the intervention blind to the participants' study group?*
  No. Due to the nature of the intervention, the clinicians providing the intervention were unable to be blinded.
* *Were the assessors blind to the participants' study group?*
  No. Due to the nature of the intervention, assessors were unable to be blinded. Also, the primary outcome measure (and most secondary measures) were self-reported questionnaires for which participants acted as their own assessors and could not be blinded.
* *Were all participants who entered the trial properly accounted for at its conclusion, and how complete was follow-up?*
  Yes. All participants were accounted for at study conclusion. The follow-up rate was 80%, with an equal number of participants in each group unable to be followed up at week 12.
* *Was intention-to-treat analysis used?*
  Yes. The authors state that an intention-to-treat analysis method was used.
* *Did the study have enough participants to minimise the play of chance?*
  Unclear. The sample size estimation was that 46 participants were needed in each group to detect a difference between groups (power 80% to detect a minimal important difference of 10 points, with alpha of 0.05). Even though 50 participants were randomised to each group, only 40 in each group completed the study.

What are the main results?

Table 5.2 shows the result for the primary outcome (VISA–A measuring Achilles pain, function and activity) at baseline and 12 weeks. Participants in both groups improved (represented by higher scores). The adjusted between-group mean difference was 9.61 points (95% CI 1.83 to 17.4) on a 100-point scale, in favour of heel raises. Whether this difference is clinically significant is unclear as it is about the same as the minimum clinically important difference (MCID) of 10 that was noted *a priori* by the authors and used in the power calculation. The authors note that while 10 is the most used MCID in the literature, its value ranges between 6.5 and 20 points.

There were no serious adverse events and no significant between-group differences for common adverse events or co-intervention use.

How might we use this evidence to inform practice?

This trial was conducted and reported to a high standard and appears to be at low risk of bias, notwithstanding the lack of blinding which was unavoidable. From the description of the participants, interventions and setting, it

TABLE 5.2   **Effect of heel lifts compared to eccentric calf exercises on pain, function and activity (VISA–A) at 12 weeks**

	Baseline	12 weeks	VISA–A SCORES	
			Adjusted mean difference (95% CI)	p value
Heel lifts	57 (15.4)	83 (16.9)	9.61 (1.83 to 17.4)	0.016
Eccentric exercise	53.3 (17.1)	70.7 (22.2)		

seems that the results can be reasonably generalised to your patient. You can explain to your patient that, in the study, those who received heel lifts increased their score, on average, by 9.6 points on the VISA–A scale (and you explain what this measures). You also explain there is uncertainty about predicting outcomes and that she could experience improvement of between about 2 to 17 points and discuss whether she would consider an improvement at the lower end of this range to be big enough to be worthwhile. You also mention that, from this study, the effects of using heel lifts beyond 12 weeks is not known. After discussing her goals, needs and preferences and considering how much less time and effort is required for the heel lift intervention compared to the exercises, she decides to try the heel lifts. Depending on her response to treatment, further evidence or information might need to be considered and discussed if the tendinopathy becomes a longer-term condition.

◎ **SPEECH PATHOLOGY EXAMPLE**

Clinical scenario
You are a speech pathologist in a metropolitan hospital, and you share the responsibility for service on the acute and subacute wards with your colleagues. Many of your patients are individuals who have had a stroke and have communication impairments such as aphasia. In the Stroke Guidelines, the treatment recommendation states: 'Treatment for aphasia should be offered as early as tolerated';[1] and the Aphasia Best Practice Statements suggest aphasia therapy *could* be provided in the very early stages.[2] Your team provide treatment to people with aphasia in the first week or two after the stroke depending on their medical conditions. You know that research in chronic aphasia has shown that more intensive treatment is more effective, and it appears that your team are providing therapy in the acute setting of varying intensity. You decide to search for evidence about the effectiveness of early aphasia treatment in terms of treatment intensity and dose to help inform your team's practice.

Clinical question
In adults with acute aphasia, is more intensive early aphasia therapy more effective than less intensive early aphasia therapy at improving language and communication skills?

Search terms and databases used to find the evidence
Database: PubMed—Clinical Queries (with 'therapy category' and 'narrow scope' selected).
Search terms: early AND (aphasia therapy) AND intens*
This search retrieved 14 publications. There is a trial that addresses very early aphasia therapy and examines intensity, so you retrieve its full text.

Article chosen
Godecke E, Armstrong E, Rai T, et al. A randomised control trial of intensive aphasia therapy after acute stroke: the Very Early Rehabilitation for SpEech (VERSE) study. Int J Stroke 2021;16(5):556–72.

Continued

◎ SPEECH PATHOLOGY EXAMPLE—cont'd

Structured abstract (adapted from the above)

Study design: A three-arm multicentre randomised controlled trial.

Setting: 17 acute care hospitals in Australia and New Zealand.

Participants: 245 patients (mean age 76 years, 51% female) with mild to severe aphasia (score of <93.7 on the Aphasia Quotient of the Western Aphasia Battery, WABAQ) following a stroke who were medically stable, were randomised at a median of 9 days after stroke onset. 91% of participants received therapy within 2 weeks of their stroke.

Intervention: Two treatment types were presented: the 'VERSE' treatment (Very Early Rehabilitation in SpEech, outlined in detail in the intervention protocol supplement) which is an impairment-focused treatment targeting verbal expression using errorless learning techniques; and usual care (a variety of current treatments utilised by speech pathologists targeting verbal and written expression and comprehension tasks). The key difference in the three intervention arms (usual care [UC], usual care-plus [UC-plus] and VERSE) was the intensity of the therapy provided. VERSE and UC-plus (usual care at the same high-intensity dose as VERSE) were prescribed at 20 sessions, 45–60 minutes per session in four–five sessions per week over 4 weeks. Usual care dose was not prescribed at any specific dose, but the type and dose of treatment for usual care was measured.

Outcomes: *Primary measures:* Improvement in communication at 12 weeks post-stroke as measured by the WABAQ. To compare change for participants with different baseline severities, the authors subtracted the WABAQ score at 12 weeks from the original WABAQ baseline score to get the outcome measure of Percentage of Maximal Potential Recovery achieved (%MPR). *Secondary outcomes:* included treatment effectiveness at 26 weeks and word naming, quality of life, and depression measures at 12 and 26 weeks post-stroke.

Follow-up period: Assessments were performed at baseline, 12 weeks and 26 weeks post-stroke.

Main results: Communication recovery based on the %MPR was 50.3% (95% CI 45.7 to 54.8) in the high-intensity group (VERSE group and UC-plus group) and 52.1% (95% CI 46.1 to 58.1) in the usual care lower intensity group. Comparing the two types of treatment in the high-intensity group (UC-plus and VERSE) showed no significant differences in outcomes based on type of aphasia treatment delivered.

Conclusion: Clinically meaningful changes in %MPR occurred in participants in all groups who were provided aphasia treatment very early after their stroke. However, the study did not demonstrate any benefit of providing higher intensity aphasia treatment with a greater overall dose than what was delivered as usual care.

Is the evidence likely to be biased?

- *Was the assignment of participants to groups randomised?*

  Yes. Participants were randomly allocated using a computer-generated block sequence to deliver a 1:1:1 ratio to the three arms, stratified by aphasia severity to maximise similarity of severity levels across the three arms and two final groups (low and high intensity).

- *Was the allocation sequence concealed?*

  Yes. Allocation occurred using a computer-generated randomised code by a baseline assessor who was not involved in the remainder of the trial.

- *Were the groups similar at the baseline or start of the trial?*

  Yes. The baseline characteristics were similar between the low- (UC) and high- (UC-plus and VERSE) intensity groups with one exception (increased concomitant dysarthria in the UC group).

- *Were participants blind to which study group they were in?*

  Unclear. None of the participants were told which group they were in and were asked not to discuss the study, although this may not have been sufficient to ensure participant blinding.

- *Were the health professionals who provided the intervention blind to the participants' study group?*

  No. It was not possible for this intervention.

- *Were the assessors blind to the participants' study group?*

  Yes. Outcome assessors were not provided information on which group the participant was allocated to, nor permitted to ask participants about treatment, and were not involved in their stroke care.

- *Were all participants who entered the trial properly accounted for at its conclusion, and how complete was follow-up?*

  Yes. The authors provided a CONSORT study flow diagram containing clear descriptions of the reasons for reduction in participant numbers. Follow-up was 88% at 12 weeks and 82% at 26 weeks.

- *Was intention-to-treat analysis used?*
  Yes. The paper states that intention-to-treat analysis was used to compare the high- versus lower intensity therapy.
- *Did the study have enough participants to minimise the play of chance?*
  Yes. The authors conducted an *a priori* sample size calculation and power analysis to detect a between-group difference of 20% on the %MPR (requiring 246 participants). The authors also allowed for an estimated 20% dropout rate.

What are the main results?

To answer the question of what level of intensity was most effective, results for the two high-intensity interventions (UC-plus and VERSE) were considered together and compared with the UC control. Over 28 days, the UC control group received a mean of 9.5 hours (SD 7.6) of aphasia treatment delivered 2–3 days per week in sessions lasting approximately 40 minutes (2.3 hours a week total). The high-intensity group received a mean of 22.7 hours (SD 8.4) of aphasia treatment over 32 days delivered 6 days a week with sessions lasting approximately 45 minutes (5 hours a week total).

At 12 weeks post-stroke, there was no significant difference between the low- and high-intensity groups on the primary outcome measure of %MPR (52.9% in low-intensity group; 50.5% in high-intensity group), with a non-significant between-group difference of −1.9 (95% CI −8.7 to −5.0; $p = 0.59$). There were also no significant between-group differences for any of the secondary outcomes. The mean %MPR improvement, regardless of group allocation, was large and clinically meaningful (>25 points on the WABQ; based on an established benchmark of ≥5 points). There was no significant difference in adverse outcomes between the groups.

How might we use this evidence to inform practice?

You consider the VERSE study to have low risk of bias and the results applicable to your setting and patients. The trial's groups contained roughly equal numbers of individuals with mild aphasia (approximately 30%), moderate aphasia (approximately 30%) and severe aphasia (approximately 40%) and almost half of participants had other communication impairments including dysarthria and apraxia of speech, and dysphagia. The results indicate no advantage from providing high-intensity treatment compared with the usual care treatment.

The trial's pilot study showed that 10 years ago, usual care consisted of only 15% of participants receiving any aphasia therapy. Those who received it did so for an average of 14 minutes in a single session over 3 weeks. You know your team provides more than this, with an audit of the treatment dose in your service finding that two staff provided 5–6 hours in 4 weeks, while one other provided 12 hours. Your team decides that within the first 2 weeks post-stroke, all patients (where tolerable) will receive a schedule of direct impairment-based intervention covering all relevant modalities of receptive and expressive language, totalling 9.5 hours over 4 weeks, with two–three sessions per week at 45 minutes. This calculation does not include the aspects of care excluded by the VERSE trial, and you agree that an additional 3–4 hours should be provided to address goal setting, education and counselling, and other aspects of care as required. You judge this schedule and dose to be feasible as it is close to what is already provided. With some students who begin placement next month, you will create some easy-to-use materials for your team that will enable more efficient planning and conducting of sessions so that the target dose of direct intervention can be obtained. You will also create a minimum standard checklist that is tied to your documentation requirements, referencing the stroke guidelines and the VERSE study. This checklist will ensure that your service delivery is somewhat standard across patients and documented in the hospital record. It will also allow auditing of progress in implementing this initiative across the team over time.

◎ MEDICINE EXAMPLE

Clinical scenario

You are a general practitioner in a city practice. One of your patients, Mary, aged 33, has had increasingly troubling chronic pelvic pain for over 5 years. The pain was initially treated as being due to endometriosis, but a laparoscopy 2 years ago did not find any evidence of this condition. She has also consulted a gastroenterologist and underwent a colonoscopy that was reported to be normal. She has trialled pelvic floor exercises from a physiotherapist with a special interest in pelvic floor dysfunction. Unfortunately, Mary has found the exercises are not helping much, nor is the paracetamol and ibuprofen she takes. She asks if gabapentin is worth trying, as she read on a Facebook group that this can work for women with chronic pelvic pain where other treatments have not helped. You decide to look at research examining the possible benefit of gabapentin in chronic pelvic pain.

Clinical question

In women with chronic pelvic pain, does gabapentin reduce pain?

Search terms and database used to find the evidence

Database: PubMed—Clinical Queries (with 'therapy category' and 'narrow scope' selected).

Search terms: "Chronic pelvic pain" AND gabapentin
The search retrieves seven results. Of the five randomised trials, two were pilot studies. You choose the largest randomised placebo-controlled trial, which was published in 2020.

Article chosen

Horne AW, Vincent K, Hewitt CA, et al. Gabapentin for chronic pelvic pain in women (GaPP2): a multicentre, randomised, double-blind, placebo-controlled trial. Lancet 2020;396(10255):909–17.

Structured abstract (adapted from the above)

Study design: A multicentre randomised, double-blind, placebo-controlled clinical trial.

Setting: 39 hospital centres in the United Kingdom.

Participants: 306 women, 18–50 years of age, with chronic pelvic pain (with or without dysmenorrhoea or dyspareunia) of at least 3 months duration. Participants were included if they were willing to use contraception to avoid pregnancy and had no pelvic pathology on laparoscopy.

Intervention: Daily treatment with gabapentin titrated to a maximum dose of 2,700 mg ($n = 153$) or a matching placebo ($n = 153$) for 16 weeks.

Outcomes: *Primary outcomes:* worst and average pain scores assessed on a numerical rating scale (NRS), with a 0–10 scale, at 13–16 weeks. *Secondary outcomes:* self-reported adverse events including dizziness, drowsiness and visual disturbances.

Main results: 246 people (80%) completed the study. There were no significant between-group differences in both worst and average numerical rating scale pain scores at 13–16 weeks. Dizziness, drowsiness and visual disturbances were more common in the gabapentin group.

Conclusion: Gabapentin did not significantly lower pain scores in women with chronic pelvic pain and was associated with higher rates of side effects than placebo. It is important for clinicians to consider alternative treatment options to gabapentin for the treatment of chronic pelvic pain.

Is this evidence likely to be biased?

- *Was the assignment of participants to groups randomised?*
  Yes. Participants were randomly allocated, at a ratio of 1:1, via a secure online randomisation system.
- *Was the allocation sequence concealed?*
  Yes, it seems likely that this could have been achieved. However, it is not completely clear who administered the online randomisation system.
- *Were the groups similar at the baseline or start of the trial?*
  Yes. Baseline characteristics were similar between the two study groups.
- *Were participants blind to which study group they were in?*
  Yes, this was a placebo-controlled trial with both groups receiving the assigned intervention that was identical in appearance, route and administration.
- *Were the health professionals who provided the intervention blind to the participants' study group?*
  Yes. The article states that patients, clinicians and research staff were unaware of the group assignments.
- *Were the assessors blind to the participants' study group?*
  Yes. The outcome was from participant self-report, but participants were blinded to group allocation.
- *Were all participants who entered the trial properly accounted for at its conclusion and how complete was follow-up?*
  Yes. The follow-up rate was 80%. Reasons are given as to why some participants were unable to be followed up, with approximately equal loss in both groups.

- *Was intention-to-treat analysis used?*
  Yes. The authors state that an intention-to-treat analysis was conducted.
- *Did the study have enough participants to minimise the play of chance?*
  Yes. The authors conducted a power analysis and determined that, with a sample size of 240, it would provide a power of 90% to detect a minimally important clinical difference in NRS pain scores of 1 point on a 0–10 scale.

What are the main results?

The intention-to-treat analysis showed no significant between-group differences in either worst or average NRS pain scores at weeks 13–16. The adjusted mean difference between groups for worst NRS pain score was −0.20 (97.5% CI −0.81 to 0.42; $p = 0.47$) and for average pain score it was −0.18 (97.5% CI −0.71 to 0.35; $p = 0.45$).

There were significantly more serious adverse events in the gabapentin group (7%) than in the placebo group (2%) $p = 0.04$; and there was a significantly higher risk for three of the nine milder adverse events investigated— that is, dizziness (risk ratio [RR], 1.91, 99% CI, 1.22 to 2.99), drowsiness (RR 1.71, 99% CI, 1.09 to 2.68), and visual disturbance (RR 2.25, 99% CI, 0.99 to 5.10).

How might we use this evidence to inform practice?

The results from this trial do not support the use of gabapentin in women with chronic pelvic pain. The low risk of bias of this trial means you can be reasonably confident of the results. You advise Mary that there is evidence that taking gabapentin will not decrease her pelvic pain and that the medication comes with the risk of potential harms. After discussing this new information, you decide together that she will see the physiotherapist again while considering other options for her, including specialist referral.

◎ NURSING EXAMPLE

Clinical scenario

You are a critical care nurse caring for adult patients with hypoxaemic respiratory failure due to COVID-19. Despite use of high-flow nasal oxygen (HFNO) or non-invasive ventilation (NIV), many patients eventually require ventilation for respiratory support. Once ventilated, these patients are nursed in the prone position to improve oxygenation. You have been wondering if using prone positioning in non-ventilated, awake patients could also improve oxygenation enough so that ventilation can be avoided. Currently, these patients are nursed lying on their back. You decide to search for evidence on the effectiveness of prone positioning in awake, spontaneously breathing patients.

Clinical question

Among adults with hypoxaemic respiratory failure due to COVID-19, does prone positioning in awake patients compared with usual care reduce the need for ventilation?

Search terms and databases used to find the evidence

Database: PubMed—Clinical Queries (with 'therapy category' and 'narrow scope' selected).

Search terms: (prone position*) AND covid-19 AND awake

This search located eight articles of which three were trial protocols. You select the largest randomised trial that has been conducted.

Article chosen

Rosén J, von Oelreich E, Fors D, et al. Awake prone positioning in patients with hypoxaemic respiratory failure due to COVID-19: the PROFLO multicentre randomised clinical trial. Crit Care 2021;25(1):209.

Structured abstract (adapted from the above)

Study design: A multicentre randomised controlled trial.
Setting: Two tertiary teaching hospitals and one county hospital in Sweden.
Participants: 75 hospitalised COVID-19 positive adults (mean age 65.5 years, 73% male) with hypoxaemic respiratory failure requiring HFNO or NIV for respiratory support and a PaO_2/FiO_2-ratio ≤20 kPa (or corresponding values of SpO_2 and FiO_2) for >1 hour. Exclusion criteria included oxygen supplementation with a device other than HFNO or NIV, inability to lie prone or semi-prone, immediate need for endotracheal intubation,

Continued

⊚ NURSING EXAMPLE—cont'd

severe haemodynamic instability, previous intubation for COVID-19 pneumonia, terminal illness or do not intubate order.

Intervention: The awake prone positioning (APP) protocol involved staff encouraging patients to assume a prone or semi-prone position for at least 16 hours per day. APP protocol discontinuation criteria were intubation, death, clinical improvement or safety concerns. In the usual care group, APP was not encouraged unless it was prescribed at the discretion of the attending clinician.

Outcomes: *Primary outcome:* intubation within 30 days after enrolment. *Secondary outcomes* included duration of APP, use of NIV and time to NIV for patients included with HFNO, use of vasopressors/inotropes, ventilator-free days, days free of NIV/HFNO for patients not intubated, hospital and intensive care unit (ICU) length of stay, 30-day mortality, World Health Organization (WHO) ordinal scale for clinical improvement at day 7 and 30, and adverse events, including pressure sores and death.

Main results: There was no difference in intubation within 30 days between the two groups and no significant between-group differences for the secondary outcomes, except for duration of APP (5.6 median hours higher in the prone group) and pressure sores (18% more patients in the control group developed these compared with the prone group, 95% CI –2 to –33%; $p = 0.032$). Mortality was higher in the prone group (17%) compared with the control group (8%), HR 2.29 (95% CI 0.57 to 9.14; $p = 0.30$) but the difference was not significant.

Conclusion: Prone positioning, compared to standard care, did not reduce the rate of intubation within 30 days or other clinical outcomes in hospitalised COVID-19 positive patients with hypoxaemic respiratory failure.

Is this evidence likely to be biased?

- *Was the assignment of participants randomised?*
  Yes. The randomisation sequence was generated using a centralised web-based system with an allocation ratio 1:1 and a block size of eight.
- *Was the allocation concealed?*
  Yes. A centralised web-based system was used so that allocation was concealed.
- *Were the groups similar at the baseline or start of the trial?*
  Partially. Age, haemodynamic status and some levels of respiratory support were similar. However, patients in the intervention group were more likely than those

in the control group to be receiving HFNO (86% vs 74%). There were also imbalances between the groups in the number of participants with various comorbidities.

- *Were participants blind to which study group they were in?*
  No. Because of the nature of the intervention, participants could not be blinded to group.
- *Were the health professionals who provided the intervention blind to the participants' study group?*
  No. Because of the nature of the intervention, healthcare staff were aware of the group allocation.
- *Were the assessors blind to the participants' study group?*
  No. All outcome data were recorded by non-blinded clinical staff.
- *Were all participants who entered the trial properly accounted for at its conclusion, and how complete was follow-up?*
  Yes. The flow of participants is clearly accounted for in the CONSORT flow diagram. There was no loss to follow-up.
- *Was intention-to-treat analysis used?*
  Yes. Intention-to-treat analysis occurred, with all participant data analysed in the groups to which they were initially allocated.
- *Did the study have enough participants to minimise the play of chance?*
  No. The authors conducted a power calculation and estimated that 224 participants would be required to detect a 20% decrease in intubation in the prone group, with 90% power at a type 1 error of 5%. A planned interim analysis was brought forward due to declining case numbers and re-estimation of the required sample size identified that at least 2,000 participants would be needed to detect a 20% decrease in intubation rates. As per protocol guidelines, the decision was made to terminate the trial early due to futility.

What are the main results?

Participants in the APP group had significantly more daily total prone time than those in the usual care group (median hours [interquartile range] 9.0 [4.4–10.6] vs 3.4 [1.8–8.4], $p = 0.014$). However, there was no difference in the number of participants who were intubated within 30 days between those in the APP group (12/36 [33%]) or usual care group (13/39 [33%]; HR 1.01, 95%

CI 0.46 to 2.21). There were also no significant between-group differences for any of the secondary outcomes, other than for pressure sores which were higher (9/39 [23%]) in the usual care group than the APP group (2/36 [6%]).

How might we use this evidence to inform practice?
You have concerns that this trial is very small and under-powered and has some risk of bias, particularly from baseline differences between the groups. You also have concerns about the duration of proning (only two patients met the target duration of 16 hours of daily APP, with no reasons given for why longer duration was not achieved) and contamination (as APP was also used in some control group participants). As this is a clinical question for which evidence is rapidly being generated, you decide to repeat the search monthly in anticipation of additional trials being published soon and you will appraise new evidence about APP as it emerges.

◎ DIETETICS EXAMPLE

Clinical scenario
You are a dietitian working in a primary care clinic. You receive a referral for a new female patient, aged 54 years, with type 2 diabetes and obesity (BMI >30 kg/m²). The patient wishes to lose weight and 'keep it off' and have better control of her blood glucose. She has heard about intermittent fasting and wants to know about it. Clinical guidelines for type 2 diabetes recommend weight management to improve health outcomes.

Clinical question
Is intermittent fasting (a very low energy diet of <500–600 kcal 2 days/week) more effective than a continuous low-energy diet (1,200–1,500 kcal 7 days a week) at facilitating sustained (≥24 months) weight loss and glycaemic control (glycated haemo-globin A1c (HbA1c)) for overweight and obese individuals with type 2 diabetes?

Search terms and databases used to find the evidence
Database: PubMed—Clinical Queries (with 'therapy category' and 'narrow scope' selected).
Search terms: ((type 2 diabetes) AND (very low energy diet)) AND (intermittent fasting) AND (continuous fasting) This search yielded 32 studies. You scan through the titles and abstracts and most do not match the intervention (such as carbohydrate restriction) or population (such as elderly) in your question. Of the relevant ones, you select the study with relevant outcome measures for your question and the longest follow-up period to examine sustained effect.

Article chosen
Carter S, Clifton PM, Keogh JB. The effect of intermittent compared with continuous energy restriction on glycaemic control in patients with type 2 diabetes: 24-month follow-up of a randomised noninferiority trial. Diabetes Res Clin Pract 2019;1(151):11–19.

Some details were obtained from the 2018 article[3] with 12-month trial results and trial protocol (in the supplement).

Structured abstract (adapted from the above)
Study design: Randomised non-inferiority trial.
Setting: A metropolitan university-based institute of health research. Participants were recruited using flyers posted in public places and via advertisements in print and broadcast media in South Australia.
Participants: 137 adults (mean age 61 years, 56% female) diagnosed with type 2 diabetes who were overweight or obese (BMI ≥27) and reported being otherwise healthy, not pregnant or breastfeeding, and had no previous weight loss surgery.
Interventions: One of two 12-month diets: (1) intermittent fasting diet: 2,100–2,500 kJ (500–600 kcal) 2 days/week and usual diet 5 days/week; or (2) continuous energy restriction: 5,000–6,300 kJ (1,200–1,500 kcal) diet for 7 days (30% protein, 45% carbohydrate and 25% fat). Dietary counselling was provided by a dietitian every 2 weeks for the first 3 months and then every 2–3 months for 9 months. Both groups received written dietary information booklets with portion advice and sample menus; no food or meal replacements were provided.
Outcomes: Follow-up was at 24 months. The primary outcome measure was a change in HbA1c; the secondary outcome was weight loss in the fasted state, minimum of 8 hours. Other outcomes included body composition, fasting glucose levels, lipid levels and total medication effect score.

Continued

◎ DIETETICS EXAMPLE—cont'd

Main results: Intention-to-treat analysis demonstrated no statistically significant between-group differences over 24 months in HbA1c or weight. At 24 months, both groups had slightly elevated HbA1c levels compared to baseline (start of intervention) and weight loss was maintained.

Conclusion: In both groups, adults with type 2 diabetes maintained their weight loss at 24 months and HbA1c was slightly higher than baseline levels. Ongoing dietary support may be more important than the type of dietary intervention.

Is this evidence likely to be biased?

* *Was the assignment of participants to groups randomised?*
  Yes. Participants were randomised, using an online-generated random number allocation sequence, 1:1 to treatment groups, stratified by sex and body mass index (as obese or non-obese).
* *Was the allocation sequence concealed?*
  Unclear. It is only stated that participants were allocated to groups by the study dietitian according to the randomisation schedule.
* *Were the groups similar at the baseline or start of the trial?*
  Yes. For the baseline characteristics that are provided, the groups were largely similar.
* *Were participants blind to which study group they were in?*
  No. Blinding was not possible because of the nature of the interventions.
* *Were the health professionals who provided the intervention blind to the participants' study group?*
  No. This was not possible because of the nature of the interventions.
* *Were the assessors blind to the participants' study group?*
  Unclear. For the outcomes of interest, it is not reported if the assessors who measured them were blind to group allocation. It may be possible to assume that, as weight loss and HbA1c do not involve assessor judgment, the assessor was blinded.
* *Were all participants who entered the trial properly accounted for at its conclusion, and how complete was follow-up?*
  Yes, all participants were accounted for, but there were some missing data. At 24 months, 84 (61%) participants were followed up (60% of the intermittent fasting group and 63% of the continuous energy group).

* *Was intention-to-treat analysis used?*
  Yes. It is stated that the data analysis was conducted on an intention-to-treat basis.
* *Did the study have enough participants to minimise the play of chance?*
  Unclear. The article reports the original trial, with the 12-month results, and states that it was calculated that 104 participants were needed to demonstrate equivalence between groups for HbA1c levels and weight. As fewer participants were retained by the 24-month follow-up, there is some concern about the results at that follow-up as the study may be underpowered.

What are the main results?

From baseline to 24 months, both groups experienced an increase in the mean (SEM) HbA1c level (continuous group 0.4% [0.3%] vs intermittent group 0.1% [0.2%], respectively) and both groups experienced a reduction in weight of −3.9 kg (1.1 kg). However, an intention-to-treat analysis found the between-group difference was not significant for HbA1c (0.3%, 90% CI −0.31 to 0.83%) or weight loss (0.07 kg, 90% CI −2.5 to 2.6 kg). Although some participants maintained their measures at 24-month follow-up and some had a decrease, over half of participants had an increase in HbA1c (68%) and weight (52%).

How might we use this evidence to inform practice?

When looking at the 24-month effect of intermittent fasting and continuous energy restriction on HbA1c and weight in adults with type 2 diabetes, this study does not provide support that one type of diet is superior to the other. It would be interesting to see what eating habits participants followed in the 12-month period between the intervention ending and the 24-month follow-up. The authors note that at the 24-month follow-up, none of the participants were still following the assigned diet, which may indicate that it is difficult to make these diets sustainable lifestyle behaviours. Most participants reported following parts or principles from the diets (such as occasionally using intermittent energy restriction or watching portion sizes in the continuous energy restriction group) to help maintain weight loss. Between 12 and 24 months, participants were under the care of their general practitioners or endocrinologists for medication management, which may suggest that additional ongoing counselling and contact with health professionals is needed to maintain HbA1c levels.

It is important to work with the patients' capacities to adopt the diet they prefer and work on the goals they have. Given your patient has requested an intermittent fasting diet, it may be safe and effective for her to pursue this style of diet initially as it is minimally invasive, and there is some chance that she will lose weight over the next 2 years. You also plan to discuss with her that sustained weight loss can be challenging and promote overall reduced energy intake to achieve weight loss, and the importance of ongoing health professional support. You may also like to use a peer-reviewed clinical resource and patient handout such as https://www.racgp.org.au/clinical-resources/clinical-guidelines/handi/conditions/diabetes/vled-for-type-2-diabetes.

◎ RADIATION THERAPY EXAMPLE

Clinical scenario

You are the radiation therapist representative involved in a weekly gastrointestinal multidisciplinary team meeting at your clinical centre. In today's meeting, the treatment options for patients with incurable oesophageal cancer are being discussed. A question is raised about how best to increase time to dysphagia deterioration, thereby enabling patients to maintain swallowing function for as long as possible. One of the cases being discussed is that of a 65-year-old man with late-stage oesophageal cancer. It has been decided that the patient will be referred for an insertion of a self-expanding metal stent (SEMS) to assist his swallowing and to improve his quality of life (QoL). The radiation oncologist has suggested that in addition to a SEMS, the patient could also be treated with a course of palliative external beam radiation therapy (EBRT) and that this may increase the time to dysphagia deterioration and reduce pain. The surgeon is not convinced that this is the best option and asks about the evidence for this prior to a decision being made. As you have recently been involved in the treatment of several patients receiving EBRT for oesophageal cancer, you offer to undertake a search of the evidence.

Clinical question

Is there a difference in time to dysphagia deterioration for patients with advanced oesophageal cancer who have a SEMS inserted and a course of external beam palliative radiation therapy (SEMS+EBRT), compared with patients who undergo SEMS insertion alone?

Search terms and databases used to find the evidence

Database: PubMed—Clinical Queries (with 'therapy category' and 'narrow scope' selected).

Search terms: ((self-expanding metal stent OR external beam radiation therapy) AND (oesophagus OR esophagus OR oesophageal OR esophageal) AND cancer AND dysphagia)

This search retrieves 27 articles and you choose one, a recent multicentre randomised trial, that most closely matches your PICO.

Article chosen

Adamson D, Byrne A, Porter C, et al. Palliative radiotherapy after oesophageal cancer stenting (ROCS): a multicentre, open-label, phase 3 randomised controlled trial. Lancet Gastroenterol Hepatol 2021;6(4):292–303. Erratum in: Lancet Gastroenterol Hepatol 2021 Apr;6(4):e3.

Structured abstract (adapted from the above)

Study design: Multicentre, parallel arm, open-label, phase 3 randomised controlled trial.

Setting: 23 cancer centres across England, Scotland and Wales.

Participants: 220 patients with incurable oesophageal cancer, aged ≥16 years, with an expected survival of ≥12 weeks. All patients had been referred for a SEMS as the primary management strategy to palliate their disease. Patients were considered as being clinically able to tolerate palliative radiation therapy and were unsuitable for radical radiation therapy either because of medical reasons or through personal choice.

Intervention: The intervention group received SEMS insertion, follow-up care and a course of palliative EBRT, to commence no later than 4 weeks post-SEMS insertion. The EBRT prescriptions and techniques were determined by the treating radiation oncologist, with the preferred dose and fractionation regimens being either 20 Gy in five

Continued

⊚ RADIATION THERAPY EXAMPLE—cont'd

fractions over one week or 30 Gy in ten fractions over 2 weeks. Control group: the SEMS and usual follow-up care.

Outcomes: *Primary outcome:* the difference in deterioration of dysphagia in patients within 12 weeks after stent insertion. Deterioration was defined as: two consecutive deteriorations of >11 points from baseline level on the European Organisation for Research and Treatment of Cancer Quality of Life Questionnaires (EORTC QLQ-C30 and QLQ-OG25), or a dysphagia-related event consistent with such a deterioration, or death by 12 weeks. The first deterioration was taken as the event time point. Consecutive deteriorations were specified because patients in the EBRT arm may have experienced dysphagia due to radiation toxicity. The pre-specified main patient reported outcomes were global health scores from the EORTC QLQC30, odynophagia, pain or discomfort, eating restrictions, and eating in front of others (dimensions from QLQ-OG25). Follow-up occurred at every 4 weeks for up to 1 year.

Secondary outcomes: overall survival (OS) which was calculated from the date of stent insertion to date of death, QoL (EORTC QLQ-C30 and QLQ-OG25), WHO Performance status, dysphagia-deterioration free survival, duration to first bleeding episode, hospital admission for a bleeding event, and first dysphagia-related stent complication or re-intervention.

Main results: 102 patients were assigned to SEMS alone and 97 to SEMS+EBRT (modified intention to treat [ITT] cohort sizes), with 74 and 75 patients, respectively, having complete data sets at the 12-week point. Dysphagia deterioration was reported in 36/74 (49%) of the patients in the SEMS only group and in 34/75 (45%) of patients in the SEMS+EBRT group, with no significant difference. There was no significant difference in OS. There was a significant between-group difference with the median time to first bleed or hospital admission for a bleeding event in the SEMS alone group at 49 weeks and 65.9 weeks in the SEMS+EBRT group (adjusted sub-hazard ratio 0.52, 95% CI 0.28 to 0.97, $p = 0.038$).

Conclusion: Patients who underwent SEMS+EBRT did not benefit from this additional management strategy in terms of dysphagia deterioration; thus, EBRT should not routinely be offered after SEMS insertion. There may be a benefit of EBRT for a small sub-group of patients who are at high risk of tumour bleeding.

Is the evidence likely to be biased?

- *Was the assignment of participants to groups randomised?*

  Yes. Participants were randomly allocated (1:1) to either the intervention or control group through a central telephone randomisation system developed by the trial centre.

- *Was the allocation sequence concealed?*

  Unclear. Although the article states that participants were randomly assigned via a central telephone randomisation system, it also states that the local principal investigator or research practitioner enrolled participants and assigned their trial group.

- *Were the groups similar at the baseline or start of the trial?*

  Yes. Minimisation was used, which is a method of stratified sampling used to ensure balanced treatment allocation by clinical centre, stage at diagnosis, histological variety of tumour and intent to manage with chemotherapy. Other characteristics appear balanced between the groups.

- *Were participants blind to which study group they were in?*

  No. Because of the intervention, it was not possible for participants to be blinded to group allocation.

- *Were the health professionals who provided the intervention blind to the participants' study group?*

  No. For this trial, it was not possible for the health professionals who provided the intervention to be blinded to group allocation.

- *Were the assessors blind to the participants' study group?*

  Yes for primary outcome. The chief investigators and independent gastroenterologist who reviewed patient event outcome data were masked to the groups, and issues such as dysphagia-related events were blindly assessed by them. It is not clear if assessment of other outcomes was blinded as the article states that 'the research practitioner was responsible for subsequent follow-up data collection'.

- *Were all participants who entered the trial properly accounted for at its conclusion, and how complete was follow-up?*

  Yes. The article includes a flowchart showing participant progression throughout the trial. Of the 220 participants randomised, 102 (91%) were analysed in the usual care group and 97 (89%) in the SEMS+EBRT group in the intention-to-treat analysis.

- *Was intention-to-treat analysis used?*
  Yes. The authors report conducting a modified intention-to-treat analysis. (This population was all patients who had a stent inserted and returned a baseline QoL questionnaire.)
- *Did the study have enough participants to minimise the play of chance?*
  Unclear. The initial number of participants calculated as needed was 496, based on a time-to-event analysis. As recruitment progressed, a lower than anticipated number of patients met the criteria and the required sample size was recalculated, with 164 patients (82 per study arm) calculated as needed to detect a reduction in the proportion of patients with deterioration from 40% to 20% (80% power at a two-sided α level of 5%), with a total of 220 participants to be recruited to account for 25% loss to follow-up.

What are the main results?

Deterioration of dysphagia: In the primary analysis of complete case data, 36/74 (49%) patients in the SEMS only group compared to 34/75 (45%) in the SEMS+EBRT group experienced dysphagia deterioration in the follow-up period with an adjusted odds ratio (OR) of 0.82 (95% CI 0.40 to 1.68; $p = 0.59$), indicating no significant difference between the groups.

Dysphagia-deterioration free survival: The median time to dysphagia event or death was 13.1 weeks (95% CI 10.0 to 17.9) in the SEMS alone group and 14.7 weeks (95% CI 12.1 to 17.4) for the SEMS+EBRT group, with an adjusted hazard ratio (HR) of 0.92 (95% CI 0.68 to 1.26; $p = 0.62$), indicating no significant between-group difference.

How do we use this evidence to inform practice?

This is a complex trial, but you appraise it to be at reasonably low risk of bias and it is the best available evidence to currently answer this question. For the outcomes that your team was particularly interested in (dysphagia deterioration and time to dysphagia event or survival), the results indicate no benefit of concurrent EBRT in addition to SEMS and supportive care for patients with advanced oesophageal cancer. You note that the trial found a significantly longer median time to first bleeding event in the SEMS+EBRT group and thus EBRT could be considered for patients who are at a higher risk of haemorrhage. There are other forms of radiation therapy that could be considered to treat dysphagia in late-stage oesophageal cancer such as intraluminal brachytherapy or endoluminal radiotherapy with a radioactive Iodine (I-125) particle-integrated covered stent; however, neither modality is used very frequently and you need to check for recent evidence about their effectiveness. You present the findings that you have so far at the next team meeting for consideration with the patient that was discussed previously, including discussion about whether he has a higher risk of haemorrhage.

◎ EXERCISE SCIENCE EXAMPLE

Clinical scenario

As a clinical exercise physiologist working in private practice, you have received a referral from a general practitioner for a 29-year-old female with polycystic ovarian syndrome (PCOS). The referral states that the woman has abdominal obesity, hypertension and a HbA1c of 5.7%. You undertake a fitness appraisal and determine she also has low cardiorespiratory fitness. During the consultation she indicates her desire to become pregnant. She hopes that improving her fitness and losing some weight will assist with this goal. The client tells you that she leads a busy life and would be keen to do higher intensity shorter duration exercise to fit in her schedule. She has heard that high-intensity interval training (HIT) is beneficial for protecting against heart disease but wants to know if HIT would impact on her reproductive health and her goal of becoming pregnant. Therefore, you search the research to investigate the effects of HIT on reproductive health in women with PCOS.

Clinical question

In females with polycystic ovarian syndrome, does high-intensity interval training improve reproductive health?

Search terms and databases used to find the evidence
Database: PubMed—Clinical Queries (with 'therapy category' and 'narrow scope' selected).

Continued

◎ EXERCISE SCIENCE EXAMPLE—cont'd

Search terms: (polycystic ovarian syndrome) AND (high intensity interval training)

This search retrieved four results. Of these, two were described as pilot trials and one was a trial protocol, leaving only one trial to appraise.

Article chosen

Kiel IA, Lionett S, Parr EB, et al. High-intensity interval training in polycystic ovary syndrome: a two-center, three-armed randomized controlled trial. Med Sci Sports Exerc 2022;54(5):717–27. doi:10.1249/MSS.0000000000002849.

Structured abstract (adapted from the above)

Study design: Randomised controlled trial.

Setting: Two metropolitan centres; one in Norway and one in Australia.

Participants: 64 women aged between 18 and 45 years old (mean age 30 years) with PCOS defined according to the Rotterdam criteria. Exclusion criteria included already doing endurance exercise two or more times per week; taking hormonal contraceptives, insulin sensitisers or drugs that affect gonadotropin or ovulation; pregnancy, known cardiovascular disease or other endocrine disorders.

Intervention: Participants were randomly assigned to either high-volume high-intensity interval training (HV-HIT), low-volume high-intensity interval training (LV-HIT) or a control group. Both HIT protocols consisted of three/week exercise sessions during the first 16 weeks; participants attended supervised exercise at the study centres at least once weekly and could choose to complete the other two weekly sessions either under supervision or unsupervised. For the remaining 36 weeks, participants were instructed to complete at least two weekly HIT sessions without any supervision or motivational support, according to the HIT protocol they were allocated to. All participants received a heart rate (HR) device to monitor intensity. The LV-HIT group completed 10x1-min workbouts at the maximal intensity the participants were able to sustain for 1 min, separated by 1 min at a low-to-moderate intensity. Participants in the HV-HIT protocol completed 4x4-min work-bouts at 90–95% of HRmax, separated by 3 min at a low-to-moderate intensity. A 10-minute warm-up at a low-to-moderate intensity preceded both HIT protocols. The control group received information about physical activity recommendations for health benefits.

Outcomes: *Primary outcome:* menstrual frequency as a proxy for reproductive function (ovulation), measured with a menstruation diary completed by the women over 12 months. *Secondary outcomes* included additional markers of reproductive health, pregnancy rates, quality of life, physical activity and physiological measures. Some secondary outcomes were only measured in Norwegian participants.

Main results: Menstrual frequency increased significantly ($p < 0.05$) in all groups from baseline to 12 months. There were no significant ($p < 0.05$) between-group differences in the changes in menstrual frequency. More participants became pregnant in the LV-HIT group ($n = 5$) than in the control group ($n = 0$).

Conclusion: In this trial, there was no impact on menstrual frequency in women with PCOS who undertook a semi-supervised HIT intervention compared with those who did not.

Is this evidence likely to be biased?

- *Was the assignment of participants to groups randomised?*

  Yes. Participants were randomised and the method of randomisation (computer random number generator) stated. Allocation was stratified based on BMI and study centre.

- *Was the allocation sequence concealed?*

  Yes. The article states that investigators were informed about group allocation result via email after enrolment of new participants.

- *Were the groups similar at the baseline or start of the trial?*

  Partially. The groups appear similar at baseline for most characteristics, although participants in the control group had lower insulin levels and participants in the LV-HIT group had the highest menstrual frequency at baseline (7.5 per year, compared with 5.2 in the HV-HIT and 6.3 in the control group). This group had the highest menstrual frequency over the 12 months and the authors suggest the higher frequency at baseline may help explain the increased pregnancy rate in this group. No adjustments appear to have been made for baseline differences.

- *Were participants blind to which study group they were in?*

  No. Participants were not blinded to group allocation due to the nature of the intervention.

- *Were the health professionals who provided the intervention blind to the participants' study group?*

  No. Health professionals were not blinded to group allocation due to the nature of the intervention.

- *Were the assessors blind to the participants' study group?*

  No. Although assessors were blinded to group allocation for some outcomes, the primary outcome was collected by a self-reported menstruation diary and the women were not blinded to group allocation.

- *Were all participants who entered the trial properly accounted for at its conclusion, and how complete was follow-up?*

  Yes. All participants who entered the trial were accounted for, with data on the primary outcome (menstrual frequency over 12 months) available for 90% of participants. Women who became pregnant did not continue with the exercise or complete outcome measures. Data completeness was much lower for secondary outcome measures.

- *Was intention-to-treat analysis used?*

  Unclear. The authors state that intention-to-treat analysis was done regardless of level of adherence to the intervention, but it is unclear how data from participants who withdrew was handled in the analysis.

- *Did the study have enough participants to minimise the play of chance?*

  Possibly not. The authors provide an *a priori* sample size calculation of needing 64 participants after accounting for attrition. While 64 participants were recruited, the primary outcome was only analysed for 58 participants.

What are the main results?

Table 5.3 shows the results of the outcome measures relevant to the clinical question. There were no significant between-group differences in the primary outcome measure of menstrual frequency.

How might we use this evidence to inform practice?

You have some concerns about the risk of bias in this trial, including that it may be underpowered, some aspects were unclear, adherence to the intervention protocol (and hence the 'dose' of the exercise) was reported as low and there were some differences in outcome measurement between the two countries. However, it appears to currently be the best available evidence for this question, although another trial with a published protocol will hopefully be available soon.

You will explain to your client that not much research has been done on HIT and its effect on reproductive health, but in the one study that you found, HIT had no effect on menstrual frequency (which was used as a proxy for reproductive health). However, you will discuss with her that HIT can improve other aspects of health that are relevant to her (such as cardiorespiratory fitness, weight) and see whether she would like to try this training approach designed to suit her fitness and time opportunities.

TABLE 5.3 **Outcomes of menstrual frequency, menstruations/year and pregnancy for all groups at baseline and 12-month follow-up.**

	BASELINE	12-MONTH FOLLOW-UP			FREQUENCY RATIO		
					LV-HIT vs Control	HV-HIT vs Control	LV-HIT vs Control
	All	Control	LV-HIT	HV-HIT			
Menstrual frequency: cycles during 12 months; observed/expected (95% CI)	0.49 (0.42 to 0.58)	0.67 (0.53 to 0.85)	0.68 (0.52 to 0.90)	0.62 (0.48 to 0.81)			
Menstruations/year—mean (95% CI)	6.4 (5.5 to 7.5)	8.7 (6.8 to 11.1)	8.9 (6.8 to 11.6)	8.1 (6.3 to 10.5)	1.02 (0.73 to 1.42)	0.93 (0.67 to 1.29)	1.09 (0.77 to 1.56)
Became pregnant, n (%)		0 (0%)	5/15 (33%)*	3/16 (19%)			

*Significantly ($p < 0.05$) greater than control.

◉ COMPLEMENTARY AND ALTERNATIVE MEDICINE EXAMPLE

Clinical scenario

As a naturopath working in the local pharmacy, you are regularly approached by consumers for your professional advice about the use of herbal products and nutritional supplements. A television advertisement was released last week making a claim that the advertiser's herbal product containing valerian (*Valeriana officinalis*) promotes 'restful sleep'. Since then, you have received multiple requests for the product. Most inquiries have been from postmenopausal women who are experiencing sleep disturbances. However, the manufacturers do not specify whether Valerian promotes restful sleep in postmenopausal women. Therefore, you conduct a search of the evidence so that you can provide your customers with evidence-based information.

Clinical question

Does valerian (*Valeriana officinalis*) improve sleep quality in postmenopausal women who are experiencing sleep disturbances?

Search terms and databases used to find the evidence

Database: PubMed—Clinical Queries (with 'therapy category' and 'narrow scope' selected).
Search terms: (sleep quality) AND menopaus* AND valerian
Only one article was directly relevant to the question.

Article chosen

Taavoni S, Ekbatani N, Kashaniyan M, et al. Effect of valerian on sleep quality in postmenopausal women: a randomised placebo-controlled clinical trial. Menopause 2011;18(9):951–5.

Structured abstract (adapted from the above)

Study design: A randomised, triple-blind, controlled trial.
Setting: Not specified. Authors from Tehran University of Medical Sciences, Iran.
Participants: 100 women (mean age 52.9 years) who were menopausal for at least 12 months, experiencing sleep disturbances, and with a Pittsburgh Sleep Quality Index (PSQI) score of ≥5.
Intervention: Each group received a product containing either 530 mg of concentrated valerian root extract or a placebo, twice a day for 4 weeks.
Outcomes: The primary outcome was improvement in sleep quality (defined as decrease in the PSQI score or a score of <5), from before until after the 4-week intervention, measured using the total score of the seven composite

scores obtained from the 19 items of the PSQI (range 0–21; lower scores indicate better sleep quality). The composite scores measure subjective sleep quality, latency, duration, disturbances, habitual sleep efficiency, use of sleeping medication, and daytime dysfunction.
Main results: 30% of participants receiving the valerian reported an improvement in sleep quality compared to 4% of those receiving the placebo ($p < 0.001$). The mean (SD) PSQI score reduction in the valerian group was 3.8 (1.7) and 1.7 (1.3) in the placebo group, and a significant difference between the groups ($p = 0.04$) was found.
Conclusion: Taking one capsule containing 530 mg of a valerian root extract twice daily over a 4-week period was superior to the placebo in improving sleep quality in postmenopausal women experiencing insomnia.

Is this evidence likely to be biased?

- *Was the assignment of participants to groups randomised?*
  Unclear. It is simply stated that participants were randomised, but no details for how this was done are reported.
- *Was the allocation sequence concealed?*
  Unclear. There is no mention in the article that concealed allocation occurred. The article reports that only the pharmacist knew the identity of each type of capsule, but their role is not clear. It is not clear who obtained consent from the participants and who held the randomisation sequence.
- *Were the groups similar at the baseline or start of the trial?*
  Unclear. The demographic characteristics appear to be largely similar between the groups. The baseline mean PSQI score was lower in the valerian group (9.8) than in the placebo group (11.1), indicating that the intervention group had better perceived sleep quality than the control group at baseline, but it is not clear whether a difference of this size is clinically important and could have biased the results.
- *Were participants blind to which study group they were in?*
  Yes, probably. The article reports that participants were blind to the study groups until the analysis was completed. The placebo had the same appearance as the herbal supplement. However, it was not reported if the placebo was identical in smell and taste, which is important to know as valerian has a distinctively strong smell and taste.

- *Were the health professionals who provided the intervention blind to the participants' study group?*

  Unclear. The article states that only the pharmacist knew the identity of each type of capsule, but it is unclear how much interaction the pharmacist had with the participants.
- *Were the assessors blind to the participants' study group?*

  Yes. As the outcome measure (PSQI) is a self-report measure and the participants were likely blind to their group allocation, this means that the assessors (who were the participants) were likely blinded.
- *Were all participants who entered the trial properly accounted for at its conclusion, and how complete was follow-up?*

  Yes. While the follow-up rate is not stated explicitly in the article and there is no CONSORT flow diagram, it appears that all 100 participants were followed up at week 4 as data from 100 participants is reported in a results table.
- *Was intention-to-treat analysis used?*

  Unclear. It is not stated if an intention-to-treat analysis was conducted.
- *Did the study have enough participants to minimise the play of chance?*

  Unclear. The article states that it was calculated that they would need to recruit 50 participants per group to detect a significant difference ($p = 0.05$) with a power of 80%. This number was recruited; however, what was used to inform this calculation was not explained.

What are the main results?

The mean (SD) PSQI of the valerian group after intervention was 6.02 (2.6) and 9.4 (3.9) for the placebo group, which was statistically significant ($p < 0.001$). Rather than interpret the *t*-test scores provided, you use an online calculator to calculate the between-group mean difference and confidence intervals at 4 weeks as 3.38 (95% CI 2.06 to 4.70). While this suggests improved sleep in the valerian group compared to the placebo group, you are unsure if this difference is a clinically significant amount. Also, you are aware that the calculation does not account for the difference in baseline PSQI scores between the groups, and that scores in neither group have decreased to <5 (which is the cut-off score for improvement that the authors mentioned in the Methods section of their article).

How might we use this evidence to inform practice?

The risk of bias in this study is high, with many aspects of it poorly reported. You have additional concerns about the study, including the short duration of intervention and follow-up, as both may be too short to provide useful information. Another concern is that during this study, no blood safety data were collected to monitor liver function and other important blood safety parameters. Additionally, no information was provided regarding the quality and regulation status of the valerian product used. Herbal products using the same species can vary between brands and from batch to batch. Where a herb is grown, and how it is stored, manufactured and formulated, influences the product quality. Such variations can result in different clinical outcomes (both in effectiveness and safety). Product-specific evidence is an important consideration in utilising herbal medicine evidence. In light of all these concerns, you will revisit your search strategy to see if there is other evidence about the use of valerian for sleep in post-menopausal women.

Clinical scenario

You are conducting a 'hot debrief' in the ambulance off-load bay of a major trauma centre with several of your paramedic colleagues. The patient is a 23-year-old male motorcycle rider who impacted a road barrier at high speed, sustaining a severe head injury. The patient was treated appropriately on scene following local clinical practice guidelines, with transport expedited to hospital. During the debrief, one paramedic remarked that tranexamic acid (TxA) is being introduced in other jurisdictions and wondered if its use could have made a difference to the patient's neurological outcome. Unsure of the answer, you decide to investigate and share your findings with the group.

Continued

◎ PARAMEDICINE EXAMPLE—cont'd

Clinical question

In adults experiencing severe traumatic brain injury, does prehospital administration of tranexamic acid improve neurological outcomes?

Search terms and databases used to find the evidence

Database: PubMed—Clinical Queries (with 'therapy category' and 'narrow scope' selected).

Search terms: (traumatic brain injury OR TBI) AND (out-of-hospital OR pre?hospital OR EMS OR ambulance OR paramedic) AND (tranexamic acid OR TXA)

This search returned four results, with one article appearing promising as it is a large multicentre, double-blinded randomised controlled trial. You repeat the search using 'broad scope' and get 12 results, but no articles that are a better match to your clinical question than the one already identified.

Article chosen

Rowell S, Meier E, McKnight B, et al. Effect of out-of-hospital tranexamic acid vs placebo on 6-month functional neurologic outcomes in patients with moderate or severe traumatic brain injury. JAMA 2020;324(10):961–74. doi:10.1001/jama.2020.8958.

Structured abstract (adapted from the above)

Study design: Three-group randomised controlled trial.

Setting: Multiple locations involving 20 trauma hospitals and 39 emergency medical services agencies across the United States and Canada between 2015 and 2017.

Participants: 966 participants aged 15 years or older (mean age 42 years, 74% male) presenting within 2 hours of sustaining an out-of-hospital TBI with a Glasgow Coma Score of ≤12 and a systolic blood pressure of ≥90 mmHg.

Intervention: Participants were randomly allocated to three groups. One intervention group ($n = 312$) was administered a 1g TxA bolus out-of-hospital followed by a 1 g TxA in-hospital via an 8-hour infusion (bolus maintenance group). Another intervention group ($n = 345$) received twice the out-of-hospital dose (2g bolus) as the bolus maintenance group and an in-hospital placebo infusion administered over 8 hours (bolus only group). A placebo group ($n = 309$) received both an out-of-hospital placebo and in-hospital 8-hour placebo infusion. For analysis, the results of the bolus maintenance and bolus only groups were combined and compared with the placebo group.

Outcomes: *Primary outcome:* neurological function at 6 months post-injury measured via the Glasgow Outcome Scale—Extended (GOSE), dichotomised into favourable (>4, indicating moderate disability or good recovery) or poor (≤4, indicating severe disability, vegetative state or death). *Secondary outcomes:* 28-day mortality, Disability Rating Scale (DRS) score and progression of intracranial haemorrhage.

Main results: Of the 1,063 participants randomised, 97 patients were not administered the study drug and not included in the analysis, leaving 966 participants. The adjusted difference for a favourable neurologic function at 6 months in the combined TxA group ($n = 657$) vs the placebo group ($n = 309$) was 3.5% (95% CI –0.9% to 10.2%; $p = 0.16$).

Conclusion: The administration of TxA, within 2 hours of injury, to patients 15 years or older with moderate or severe TBI did not significantly improve neurological outcomes at 6 months or 28-day mortality, disability and progression of intracranial haemorrhage.

Is the evidence likely to be biased?

- *Was the assignment of participants to groups randomised?*

  Yes. Randomisation was achieved via a computer-generated allocation sequence programmed by a data coordinating centre using a permuted block design.

- *Was the allocation sequence concealed?*

  Yes. Allocation was conducted off-site by a data coordinating centre; drug kits were identical and packaged in numerical order according to a permuted block design and shipped to emergency medical services (EMS) agencies for placement in EMS vehicles in random order.

- *Were the groups similar at the baseline or start of the trial?*

  Yes. Participants included in the analysis were generally well matched with respect to demographic and baseline anatomical and physiological characteristics, although there were fewer penetrating injuries in the bolus-only group.

- *Were participants blind to which study group they were in?*

  Yes. Drug kits were identical, so participants did not know which drug they were receiving.

- *Were the health professionals who provided the intervention blind to the participants' study group?*

  Yes. Paramedics, pharmacists and coordinators were blinded throughout the study. However, emergency unblinding was performed if it was determined by the treating doctor that TxA was clinically indicated in hospital. This occurred in 3% of patients, of whom 53% received open-label TxA.

- *Were the assessors blind to the participants' study group?*

  Unclear, but probably. The outcome assessment process is not described in detail in the article or supplement. It is only reported that structured telephone interviews with the patient or his or her caregiver were used for scoring the GOSE at follow-up. It is not clear if the interviewers were blind to the participants' group allocation, but as the participants were blinded and the GOSE is based on self-report, this may indicate that the outcome assessment was blinded.

- *Were all participants who entered the trial properly accounted for at its conclusion, and how complete was follow-up?*

  Yes. At 6 months, 77% of the randomised participants (85% of participants for whom the intervention was commenced) were able to be followed up (with similar percentages across the groups). For some participants, missing data for the primary outcome were imputed and data for 966 (90%) participants were included in the analysis. A detailed flowchart with reasons for drop-out is provided.

- *Was intention-to-treat analysis used?*

  Yes. Although it is not explicitly stated that intention-to-treat analysis was used, the flowchart indicates that the primary analysis was conducted according to randomised group.

- *Did the study have enough participants to minimise the play of chance?*

  Yes. The sample was greater than the planned size of 963 participants which was calculated as needed to provide 80% power.

What are the main results?

For the primary outcome of neurological function at 6 months post-TBI, a favourable outcome (GOSE >4) occurred in 65% of the combined TxA group and 62% of the placebo group, giving an absolute difference of 3.5% (90% 1-sided confidence limit for benefit −0.9%; $p = 0.16$). For the secondary outcomes, there were no statistically significant between-group differences for 28-day mortality (−2.9% difference, 95% CI −7.9% to 2.1%; $p = 0.26$), DRS scores (−0.9 difference, 95% CI −2.5 to 0.7; $p = 0.29$), or progression of intracranial haemorrhage (−5.4% difference, 95% CI −12.8% to 2.1%; $p = 0.16$).

How might we use this evidence to inform practice?

This is a well-designed and conducted trial that you judge to be at low risk of bias. You will present the findings to the group, including the result that out-of-hospital TxA does not appear to improve 6-month neurological recovery.

◎ PHARMACY EXAMPLE

Clinical scenario

Michael, a 65-year-old male, is a regular patient at the community pharmacy where you are a pharmacist. You notice him examining several different herbal preparations and looking confused, and ask him if he needs any help. Michael tells you he has just been diagnosed with mild benign prostatic hyperplasia (BPH). He says he has seen advertisements in his social media feed for *Serenoa repens* (saw palmetto) preparations that claim to reduce BPH symptoms. He would like to know if there is any 'real' evidence that *Serenoa repens* will reduce his BPH symptoms, especially a weak urine stream.

Clinical question

Does taking a herbal formula containing *Serenoa repens* assist in the reduction of symptoms of medically diagnosed mild benign prostatic hyperplasia (BPH)?

Search term and databases to find evidence

Database: PubMed—Clinical Queries (with 'therapy category' and 'narrow scope' selected).

Continued

◎ PHARMACY EXAMPLE—cont'd

Search terms: ((*Serenoa repens*) OR (saw palmetto)) AND (benign prostatic hyperplasia)

The search returns 63 hits. You screen the abstracts for relevance. You dismiss those with very small sample sizes, those that compare *Serenoa repens* in combination with other treatments, a trial in men with severe symptoms, and a trial that compares different doses. You select and appraise the following trial that seems to match your clinical question.

Article chosen

Ye Z, Huang J, Zhou L, et al. Efficacy and safety of *Serenoa repens* extract among patients with benign prostatic hyperplasia in China: a multicenter, randomised, double-blind, placebo-controlled trial. Urology 2019;129:172–9.

Structured abstract (adapted from above)

Study design: Double-blind randomised controlled trial.

Setting: Multicentre, across 19 institutions in China (no further setting details provided).

Participants: 354 males (50–70 years old) with clinically diagnosed BPH and an International Prostate Symptom Score (IPSS) of ≤19 (moderate to mild BPH).

Intervention: After a 2-week washout period, *Serenoa repens* extract 320 mg daily (160 mg capsule twice a day) for 24 weeks or a placebo twice daily for 24 weeks.

Outcomes: *Primary outcome:* change in IPSS and peak urinary flow between assessments (baseline, and week 2, 4, 12 and 24). *Secondary outcomes:* improvement of storage symptom and voiding symptoms scores, prostate volume, urinary frequency and total prostate specific antigen level.

Main results: There was a statistically significant improvement in the primary outcomes of IPSS scores (total symptom score decreased) and peak urinary flow and in the secondary outcomes of storage and voiding symptoms and quality of life scores.

Conclusion: Compared to the placebo, the use of *Serenoa repens* extract was associated with statistically and clinically significant BPH symptom alleviation.

Is this evidence likely to be biased?

* *Was the assignment of participants to groups randomised?*
  Yes, probably. The authors state that the participants were 'randomly assigned (1:1)', but the method of randomisation is not reported.

* *Was the allocation sequence concealed?*
  Unclear. It is not reported if concealed allocation occurred.

* *Were the groups similar at baseline or start of the trial?*
  Partially. However, there is a difference in peak urinary flow (mean higher in the placebo group [13.6] compared to the intervention group [11.3]) which may be important, but any possible clinical relevance or implication of this size difference is not discussed.

* *Were participants blind to which study group they were in?*
  Yes. It is stated that the trial was double-blind, and all participants took capsules (although it is not stated if the two types of capsules looked, smelled and tasted similar).

* *Were the health professionals who provided the intervention blind to the participants' study group?*
  Unclear. It is stated that the trial was double-blind, but it is not explicitly stated which trial personnel were blinded.

* *Were the assessors blind to the participants' study group?*
  Yes. The outcome measures were either self-report measures (and participants were therefore the 'assessors' and were blinded) or conducted during 'double-blind visits', implying the assessors were blind to group allocation.

* *Were all participants who entered the trial properly accounted for at its conclusion, and how complete was follow-up?*
  Yes. It appears that 92% of participants were followed up, with a simplified flowchart provided. Loss to follow-up is similar between the groups, but reasons (other than loss to follow-up) are not provided and follow-up rates at only one timepoint are provided (presumably, 24 weeks).

* *Was intention-to-treat-analysis used?*
  Unclear. The article states that a modified intention-to-treat analysis was conducted, but no further details are provided. The flowchart in the online supplement indicates that 29 participants were excluded from the ITT analysis, due to either loss to follow-up from the first visit ($n = 26$) or protocol violation ($n = 3$). Although 354 participants were randomised, it is reported that only 325 'met the criteria for inclusion in the intent-to-treat population' and baseline data were provided for 325.

- *Did the study have enough participants to minimise the play of chance?*

  Unclear. There is no mention of an *a priori* sample size calculation being performed.

What are the main results?

Table 5.4 shows the results for the primary outcomes, with participants in the *Serenoa repens* group experiencing greater improvement in the IPSS score (mean difference in change scores of 2.77) and peak urinary flow (mean difference in change score of 3.16 mL/s) from baseline to 24 weeks than participants in the placebo group. You cannot determine the precision around this effect size estimate, as no confidence intervals are reported, nor does the data provided enable their calculation. While the between-group differences for both these outcomes are statistically significant, the authors also conclude that the improvements are clinically significant but provide no justification or reference for this claim.

How might we use this evidence to inform practice?

You have some concerns about the risk of bias in this trial, especially around its lack of concealed allocation, lack

of clarity around the intention-to-treat analysis, and baseline difference in peak flow rate. You also have concerns about whether the size of the change in the primary outcomes is clinically important. For example, you search the literature on IPSS use and find that other studies have considered change of 3.1 and 5.2 on the IPSS as clinically important.[4]

From the search you did, there appear to be few multicentre double-blind randomised trials in men with mild symptoms. When Michael returns to the pharmacy after doing his grocery shop, you will explain to him that you have examined a randomised trial that compared a herbal preparation containing *Serena repens* with a placebo and found that it may reduce the symptoms of BPH, including improving urinary flow. However, you would like to search for and examine additional trials (such as the one that compared different doses with a placebo) as there is some uncertainty about the effect. He needs to come back to the shopping centre in a few days' time and will stop back in then to continue his discussion with you. You will also counsel him that if he decides to commence taking a herbal preparation, he needs to inform his doctor about this at his next visit.

TABLE 5.4 Results of primary outcomes for *Serenoa repens* versus placebo

	Serenoa repens group (*n* = 150)	Placebo group (*n* = 154)	*p* value
	Change scores (SD) from baseline to 24 weeks		
IPSS score	4.39 (4.38)	1.62 (3.92)	<0.001
Peak urinary flow	4.09 (7.55) mL/s	0.93 (7.46) mL/s	0.008

◎ OPTOMETRY EXAMPLE

Clinical scenario

You are an optometrist working in a major city. In your practice, you routinely see children with myopia who display rapid myopia progression. You use the broad range of available treatments, including daily low-dose atropine eyedrops, orthokeratology, or dual-focus soft contact lenses.

During a consultation, one parent mentioned a news report about a 'breakthrough' spectacle lens tested in Hong Kong and asked if you can prescribe them. A quick search of the popular press reveals that these are called

'DIMS lenses'. You learn that DIMS stands for Defocus-Incorporated Multiple Segments and that the DIMS lens is a custom-made plastic spectacle lens. It comprises a central optical zone (9 mm in diameter) for correcting distance vision and an annular zone (33 mm in diameter) with multiple (approximately 400) segments (each segment 1.03 mm in diameter) having a relative positive power of +3.50 dioptres (D), with the aim of creating myopic defocus to inhibit eye growth. You decide to see if there is any evidence of its effectiveness.

Continued

OPTOMETRY EXAMPLE—cont'd

Clinical question

In children with myopia, does prescribing Defocus-Incorporated Multiple Segments lenses reduce myopia progression?

Search terms and databases used to find the evidence

Database: PubMed—Clinical Queries (with 'therapy category' and 'narrow scope' selected).

Search terms: (myopia) AND (Defocus-Incorporated Multiple Segments)

You exclude articles that are a protocol or focused on different outcomes. The remaining study appears to match your question.

Article chosen

Lam CSY, Tan WC, Tse DYY, et al. Defocus Incorporated Multiple Segments (DIMS) spectacle lenses slow myopia progression: a 2-year randomised clinical trial. Br J Ophthalmol 2020;104:363–8.

Structured abstract (adapted from the above)

Study design: Prospective randomised double-masked controlled trial.

Setting: Centre for Myopia Research at the Hong Kong Polytechnic University, China.

Participants: 183 children aged 8–13 years, with low to moderate myopia (spherical equivalent refraction [SER] of −1.00 to −5.00 D) in both eyes, low refractive astigmatism and anisometropia (≤1.50 D), and best corrected visual acuity of 0.00 logMAR (6/6) or better in both eyes. Exclusion criteria: strabismus or binocular vision abnormalities, previous myopia control treatment, ocular and systemic abnormalities.

Intervention: Defocus Incorporated Multiple Segments (DIMS) spectacle lenses. Participants in the control group were prescribed single-vision distance correction spectacles.

Outcomes: *Primary outcome:* myopia progression defined as the difference between the mean cycloplegic spherical equivalent objective refraction measured with an open-field autorefractor at baseline and subsequent 6-monthly visits for 24 months. *Secondary outcome:* change in axial length defined as the difference between the mean axial length at baseline and subsequent 6-monthly visits for 24 months.

Follow-up period: 2 years (24 months) with 6-monthly visits for cycloplegic refraction and axial length. The current study reports the 2-year results; however, the study is ongoing and planned to continue for another year.

Main results: Over the 2 years, myopia progression reduced by 52% in the DIMS group compared to the control group (mean difference −0.44±0.09 D, 95% CI −0.73 to −0.37, $p < 0.0001$) and axial elongation was 62% less in the DIMS group compared to the control group (mean difference 0.34±0.04 mm, 95% CI 0.22 to 0.37, $p < 0.0001$) in the DIMS group compared to controls.

Conclusion: At 2 years, children with myopia who were prescribed DIMS spectacle lenses had a slower myopia progression and axial elongation compared to those wearing single-vision spectacles. Younger children may be at risk for more progression and may benefit from early DIMS treatment.

Is this evidence likely to be biased?

* *Was the assignment of participants to groups randomised?*

  Yes. Participants were randomly allocated using a sequence generated with randomisation software. Randomisation was not stratified.

* *Was the allocation sequence concealed?*

  Unclear. It is unclear if concealed allocation occurred.

* *Were the groups similar at the baseline or start of the trial?*

  Yes. The baseline characteristics and scores of the outcome measures were similar between the two groups.

* *Were participants blind to which study group they were in?*

  Unclear. Children and their parents were described as masked to group allocation until data analysis was completed. However, DIMS spectacle lenses can potentially be differentiated by their appearance when the lens is tilted, making the multiple segments observable from the reflection of a light source. It cannot be ruled out that a few children and their parents in the DIMS group may have recognised the multiple segments in the spectacle lens.

* *Were the health professionals who provided the intervention blind to the participants' study group?*

  No.

* *Were the assessors blind to the participants' study group?*

  Yes. A masked investigator was responsible for measurement of refraction and axial length. Spectacles were removed from the children by the unmasked investigator prior to any data measurement by the masked investigator.

- *Were all participants who entered the trial properly accounted for at its conclusion, and how complete was follow-up?*

  Yes. The follow-up rate was 90% at 6 and 12 months, and 87% at 18 and 24 months, with reasons provided for the attrition and which group they were in.

- *Was intention-to-treat analysis used?*

  Yes. The authors state that data analysis followed the intention-to-treat approach for participants lost to follow-up.

- *Did the study have enough participants to minimise the play of chance?*

  Yes. The authors undertook a power analysis based on data from a pilot study involving defocus incorporated soft contact lenses and calculated that 118 participants (59 per group) were needed to detect a 0.50 ± 0.70 D difference in myopia progression, with a power of 90% and a significance level of 0.01 (2-tailed). Assuming a dropout rate of 15%, they calculated that 140 participants (70 per group) were required.

What are the main results?

The changes in outcomes measures (myopia progression and axial length) over 24 months are shown in Table 5.5. The data are for the participants who completed the study, not for all enrolled participants. Ideally, we would like to use the enrolled data, but not all data were presented in the article. The effect sizes are similar between the completed and enrolled results.

One in five children (22%) in the DIMS group had no myopia progression over the 2-year study period compared to less than one in 10 (7%) in the control group. 13% of children in the DIMS group showed significant progression (>1 D) over 24 months compared with 42% in the control group.

A change of −0.50 D in refraction is routinely considered clinically significant. An average annual growth of 0.18 mm axial elongation corresponds to an increase in myopia of ~0.50 D, and 0.36 mm axial elongation to an increase in myopia of ~1.00 D. On that basis, the refraction changes are probably large enough to be considered significant at 24 months and the axial length changes at 12, 18 and 24 months. No treatment-related adverse events were reported.

How might we use this evidence to inform practice?

The trial appears to be at quite low risk of bias and the results are important. Most of the children with progressive myopia that you see in your practice are Caucasian. Children in the study were Chinese and you note that the effectiveness of DIMS lenses in Caucasian children has yet to be confirmed. You verify that DIMS lenses have recently become available in Australia. There are unanswered questions, though. What might happen in the final year of the trial or when treatment is stopped? To what age will children be required to continue to wear DIMS lenses? Will axial length and myopia suddenly accelerate if DIMS wear is ceased, and will this negate any gains achieved? This has been shown to occur for other types of myopia control interventions and you are aware that it is important to manage this possible rebound.

You are also aware of other effective interventions for myopia progression, such as dual-focus contact lenses, orthokeratology and daily low-dose atropine eyedrops. You wonder how DIMS might compare to these and whether it could be combined with some of them. These unanswered questions make you hesitant to offer this

TABLE 5.5 Changes in outcome measures from baseline over 24 months (mean ± standard error) (completed participants)

Time/Visit	Change in cycloplegic SER, D			Change in axial length, mm		
	DIMS (n = 79)	Control (n = 81)	Mean difference	DIMS (n = 79)	Control (n = 81)	Mean difference
6 months	−0.13±0.03	−0.37±0.04	−0.24±0.05*	0.03±0.01	0.20±0.01	0.16±0.02*
12 months	−0.17±0.05	−0.55±0.04	−0.38±0.07*	0.11±0.02	0.32±0.02	0.21±0.02*
18 months	−0.31±0.06	−0.72±0.05	−0.42±0.08*	0.15±0.02	0.43±0.02	0.27±0.03*
24 months	−0.38±0.06	−0.93±0.06	−0.55±0.09*	0.21±0.02	0.53±0.03	0.32±0.04*

*Statistically significant difference between two groups (unpaired *t*-tests, $p < 0.0001$).

Continued

intervention to your patients. Before deciding whether to become accredited and to equip your practice for DIMS fitting, you will need to calculate the likely retail cost of DIMS spectacles in your practice and estimate the demand by assessing the number of myopic children in your neighbourhood who may benefit and whose parents might be interested in purchasing this treatment relative to other treatments. When the parent returns with their child for their next visit, you will discuss the findings with them, explaining that this may be an option for their child but there are currently some uncertainties.

◎ PSYCHOLOGY EXAMPLE

Clinical scenario

You are the psychologist on a multidisciplinary team in the gynaecology department of a large public hospital. In response to feedback from patients, one of your team's goals is to adopt a more systematic approach to preparing patients who are awaiting surgical procedures. As part of this effort, you are responsible for identifying evidence-based non-pharmacological strategies for reducing preoperative anxiety. You recall hearing a presentation at a conference recently which suggested that a commercial musical therapy application reduced patients' preoperative anxiety. You wonder if encouraging patients to bring their own device and playlist would also be beneficial and you search for evidence about this.

Clinical question

In people in hospital awaiting a gynaecological surgical procedure, is listening to a self-curated music playlist as effective as listening to a commercial musical therapy application at reducing preoperative anxiety?

Search terms and databases used to find the evidence

Database: PubMed—Clinical Queries (with 'therapy category' and 'narrow scope' selected).
Search terms: music AND (surg* OR operat*) AND (gynaecological OR gynecological) AND anxiety
The search yields 12 articles. You screen them. Some are trials focused on specific surgeries. You choose a trial in which various gynaecological procedures were performed, as this is the most relevant to your clinical question.

Article chosen

Reynaud D, Bouscaren N, Lenclume V, et al. Comparing the effects of self-selected MUsic versus predetermined music on patient ANXiety prior to gynaecological surgery: the MUANX randomised controlled trial. Trials 2021;22(1): 535. Open access at: https://doi.org/10.1186/s13063-021-05511-2.

Structured abstract (adapted from the above)
Study design: Parallel group superiority randomised controlled trial.
Setting: Gynaecological surgery department of the South Reunion Island University Hospital, France.
Participants: Eligible were patients aged 18–70 years who were scheduled to undergo gynaecological surgery under general anaesthesia or spinal anaesthesia and not taking anxiety medication. Exclusion criteria included people with generalised anxiety disorder, depression, dementia or neuromotor disabilities. 171 women (mean age 41.5 years) of 174 randomised were included in analyses.
Intervention: In the intervention group, within the hour preceding surgery, patients listened to a 20-minute self-curated music playlist on a device of their choice, with or without headphones. Patients created the playlist prior to hospitalisation and based on their personal taste. In both groups, patients listened to the playlist while alone in an individual room and either sitting in an armchair or lying supine. In the control group, within the hour preceding surgery, patients listened to a 20-minute predetermined playlist on the MUSIC CARE® music therapy application using a MUSIC CARE® tablet and provided headphones. Patients selected the playlist from among 25 options prior to randomisation.
Outcomes: *Primary outcome:* change in state anxiety (measured using the Spielberger State-Trait Anxiety Inventory [STAI] Form Y-A) from before to after the music session. *Secondary outcomes:* change in anxiety (measured using a visual analogue scale, VAS), pulse rate and systolic and diastolic blood pressure from

before to after the music session, postoperative pain intensity and duration of hospitalisation.

Main results: There was no significant difference in the mean change in state anxiety between the intervention group (mean change −5.5 [SD 6.6]) and control group (mean change −7.2 [SD 9.0]) ($p = 0.215$). There were also no significant between-group differences for any of the secondary outcomes.

Conclusion: Among patients scheduled to undergo gynaecological surgery, listening to a self-curated music playlist was as effective for reducing preoperative anxiety as listening to a predetermined playlist in a music therapy application.

Is this evidence likely to be biased?
- *Was the assignment of participants to groups randomised?*
  Yes. Patients were randomly allocated to one of two groups using clinical data management software.
- *Was the allocation sequence concealed?*
  Unclear. It is not reported if concealed allocation occurred.
- *Were the groups similar at the baseline or start of the trial?*
  Yes. The groups appear similar at baseline with respect to socio-demographic characteristics, musical habits, medical history, surgery types, anxiety scores and physiological parameters.
- *Were participants blind to which study group they were in?*
  No. Patients were told which group they had been allocated to. They were asked not to report their group allocation to their health professionals.

- *Were the health professionals who provided the intervention blind to the participants' study group?*
  Yes. It is stated that healthcare team members were blind to group allocation, although the intervention did not really involve delivery from a health professional.
- *Were the assessors blind to the participants' study group?*
  No for the primary outcome. For the outcomes of state anxiety, anxiety and postoperative pain intensity, the assessors were the patients (as these are self-report measures) and hence were not blind to group allocation. For the other outcomes, assessors were blind to group allocation.
- *Were all participants who entered the trial properly accounted for at its conclusion, and how complete was follow-up?*
  Yes. All patients who were randomised were accounted for and reported in a flowchart. Loss to follow-up was low at 2%.
- *Was intention-to-treat analysis used?*
  No. It is not mentioned if intention-to-treat analysis occurred. The flowchart shows that 1 patient who had an interruption while listening to music and 2 who refused to listen to music were excluded from analyses.
- *Did the study have enough participants to minimise the play of chance?*
  Probably. The authors reported that a sample size of 85 per group was calculated as being needed, which was similar to the number analysed ($n = 84$ intervention group; $n = 87$ in control group).

What are the main results?
Table 5.6 shows the mean change in anxiety from pre- to post-intervention for both groups. There was no significant

TABLE 5.6 Mean change in anxiety from pre- to post-intervention for both groups

| | MEAN CHANGE (SD) FROM PRE- TO POST-INTERVENTION | | |
	Intervention group (self-developed playlist)	Control group (predetermined playlist)	Absolute difference (*p* value)
State anxiety (STAI) (range 20–80; higher indicates greater anxiety)*	−5.5 (6.6)	−7.2 (9.0)	1.7 ($p = 0.215$)
Anxiety (VAS) (range 0–10; higher indicates greater anxiety)	−1.1(1.8)	−1.1(2.0)	0 ($p = 0.798$)

*A reduction >3 was considered clinically important.

Continued

◉ PSYCHOLOGY EXAMPLE—cont'd

between-group difference for any of the outcomes. The decrease in anxiety within each group from before to after the music session was significant.

How might we use this evidence to inform practice?
You consider that this study was conducted in a different country and that some aspects of the design may have introduced bias but that the evidence is relevant to inform your team's efforts to improve preoperative care. You arrange to meet with clinical and administrative staff who interact with patients awaiting gynaecological surgical procedures both before and while they are in hospital. You explain the interventions evaluated in the study and the results and ask for input on whether and how it could be

implemented locally. You also arrange to meet with the hospital's consumer advisory group to discuss the idea of encouraging patients to bring a music playlist on their own device (your hospital does not have access to a commercial music therapy service) and identify any important implementation considerations. In your next team meeting, you present a summary of the evidence and the subsequent input from the clinical and administrative staff and the consumer advisory group. The team agrees that the intervention has no cost or adverse effects and decide to begin encouraging and enabling patients to listen to a self-curated playlist while awaiting a surgical procedure. The team also plans to monitor this implementation and discuss it again in a few months' time.

REFERENCES

1. Stroke Foundation. Clinical guidelines for stroke management. Melbourne; 2022. Online. Available: https://informme. org.au/guidelines/clinical-guidelines-for-stroke-management.
2. Power E, Thomas E, Worrall L, et al. Development and validation of Australian aphasia rehabilitation best practice statements using the RAND/UCLA appropriateness method. BMJ Open 2015;5:e007641.
3. Carter S, Clifton PM, Keogh JB. Effect of intermittent compared with continuous energy restricted diet on glycemic control in patients with type 2 diabetes: a randomized noninferiority trial. JAMA Netw Open 2018;1(3):e180756.
4. Blanker MH, Alma HJ, Devji TS, et al. Determining the minimal important differences in the International Prostate Symptom Score and Overactive Bladder Questionnaire: results from an observational cohort study in Dutch primary care. BMJ Open 2019;9:e032795.

Evidence about Diagnosis

Sharon Sanders and Jenny Doust

LEARNING OBJECTIVES

After reading this chapter, you should be able to:
- Generate a structured clinical question about diagnosis for a clinical scenario
- Appraise the risk of bias (validity) in studies of diagnostic test accuracy
- Understand how to interpret the results from diagnostic test accuracy studies and calculate additional results (such as positive and negative predictive values and likelihood ratios) where possible

- Describe how evidence from diagnostic test accuracy studies can be used to inform practice
- Understand what diagnostic clinical prediction rules are, how and why they are developed, and how to determine the readiness of published diagnostic clinical prediction rules for clinical practice

This chapter will begin with describing and explaining how to appraise and interpret research studies that are concerned with determining the accuracy of diagnostic tests. Later sections of the chapter will touch on other types of diagnostic test research, including research that assesses the impact or utility of diagnostic tests and their reliability.

Let us consider a clinical scenario that will be useful for illustrating the concepts of diagnostic test accuracy that are the focus of this chapter. The scenario relates to testing for the virus (severe acute respiratory syndrome coronavirus 2, SARS-CoV-2) that causes COVID-19. Given the evolving nature of this coronavirus and the rapid, ongoing development of testing technologies, the clinical scenario and test referred to in this chapter should be considered indicative of the situation at the time the chapter was written.

Diagnosis classifies an individual as having, or not having, a particular condition and can provide crucial information for clinical decisions that influence health outcomes for an individual. The diagnostic tests we use might lead to a patient being given a broad diagnostic label or sometimes to patients being classified into various categories and

◎ CLINICAL SCENARIO

You are a clinician working in a ward of a major city hospital. You have just been advised that you will be required to undergo testing for severe acute respiratory syndrome coronavirus (SARS-CoV-2) infection before each shift. SARS-CoV-2 is the coronavirus that has caused the pandemic of acute respiratory disease, named coronavirus disease 2019—or COVID-19. A rapid antigen test, a test that detects virus particles present in a sample from a swab inserted into your nose or pharynx and provides a result within 15 minutes, will be used. You have heard mixed reports about the ability of these tests to detect SARS-CoV-2 infection. You decide to find out about the accuracy of rapid antigen tests for confirming or ruling out SARS-CoV-2 infection.

stratifications within a diagnostic label that can be used to assist with decisions about management. However, as explained in earlier chapters of the book, and as can be seen in some of the worked scenarios in Chapter 7, studies of 'diagnostic test accuracy' are not just about identifying the presence or absence of a condition. When we refer to 'diagnosis' in this chapter, we are also referring to assessing aspects of body structure, function or task performance.

Using the COVID-19 scenario, this chapter will examine and explain how to assess the diagnostic accuracy of rapid antigen tests to detect SARS-CoV-2 infection. We will start by defining the components of a structured clinical question about diagnosis. We will then see how to appraise the evidence to determine its likely risk of bias. Subsequent sections of the chapter will review how to understand the results of a study that tells us about the accuracy of a diagnostic test and how to use the evidence to inform practice.

While the example used in this chapter focuses on a single diagnostic test (in this case, a pathology test), we can also assess the accuracy of combinations of diagnostic tests. Clinical examination is an example of this. Clinical examination is usually an iterative process of data collection that generally begins with the history of the presenting condition, recording an individual's symptoms and signs and then performing physical examination. Each piece of information collected may be viewed as a diagnostic 'test' with a measurable diagnostic power. Though comprised of many individual 'tests', clinical examination itself may be considered a diagnostic 'test', akin to a laboratory test, that helps health professionals to decide whether a patient has a disease, impairment or disability.

STUDY DESIGNS THAT CAN BE USED FOR ANSWERING QUESTIONS ABOUT DIAGNOSTIC TEST ACCURACY

Studies of diagnostic tests generally measure how accurately a test can detect the presence or absence of a disease by comparing the test with a reference standard. The reference standard is considered the best available method for finding out whether an individual has the condition and may sometimes be referred to as the 'gold standard'. The reference standard may be a single test or a combination of 'tests'. For example, in studies of the accuracy of ultrasound for the diagnosis of acute appendicitis, in order to ascertain all cases of appendicitis in the tested population, the reference standard not only needs to be the findings at surgery in those who test positive and subsequently have surgery, but also needs to consider any cases of appendicitis in those individuals who test negative and who do not have surgery, at least initially. The reference standard in this case will therefore be a composite of the findings at surgery and clinical follow-up. As we saw in Chapter 2 (Table 2.5), the best type of study to estimate diagnostic accuracy is a study of test accuracy conducted in a consecutive or random

sample of individuals suspected of having the condition of interest. Every eligible individual who presents with a similar type of clinical problem in a particular setting (or a random sample of eligible individuals) over a particular time period should be tested with both the test of interest (the index test) and the reference standard. The index test result of each study participant is then compared with the reference standard result. Again, as we saw in Chapter 2, systematic reviews are even better than an individual study or trying to read all the studies that are available. Systematic reviews are discussed further in Chapter 12.

Other study designs are also possible. For example, the study may compare the test results in patients who are selected into the study by convenience or arbitrary methods rather than by selecting consecutive patients. This is a weaker study design because the selection of participants might introduce selection bias. For example, the most conveniently enrolled patients might be those who are generally sicker. Another alternative is the diagnostic 'two-gate' (or two-group) study design, which compares the test results of the index test and reference standard in two separate groups of patients: the first is a group who are known to have the condition of interest (for example, they have tested positive on the reference standard) and a group of patients who are known or assumed not to have the condition of interest, generally because they have no symptoms of the disease in question (often referred to as 'healthy controls').[1] Some studies may enrol several groups of people—for example, a group with no symptoms, a group with symptoms but known to have another disease, and people known to have the disease—and such studies are termed 'multiple-gate' (or multiple-group). Two-gate and multiple-gate studies are also a weak study design because, apart from the participant selection bias, they are unlikely to enrol patients with the whole spectrum of the condition seen in clinical practice. Spectrum bias can result in the test's diagnostic accuracy being overestimated as the patients who are known to have disease and known to not have disease are often patients who are 'easier' to diagnose.[2]

HOW TO STRUCTURE A DIAGNOSTIC TEST ACCURACY QUESTION

 CLINICAL SCENARIO (CONTINUED)

Structuring the clinical question
As with clinical questions about the effectiveness of interventions, we can define the clinical question for diagnostic questions using the PICO format that was outlined in Chapter 2. For questions about diagnosis,

the 'I' (Intervention/Issue) component of PICO is the diagnostic test you are interested in, and the Comparison is the reference standard. The Outcome is the diagnosis in question.

Using the PICO format for questions about test accuracy is sometimes not straightforward, as there may be more than one test of interest and because of the alternative ways a test might be used in practice (for example, as a replacement for an existing test, as an add-on to an existing test or as a triage test before an existing test[3]). Consequently, an alternative format for defining questions about diagnostic test accuracy has been recently proposed by the Cochrane Collaboration.[4] This approach is known as 'PIT', where P describes the people or populations in whom the test may be used, I is the index test, or the test we wish to evaluate, and T is the target condition, or the condition we are trying to diagnose. There may be more than one index test of interest. For example, we might be interested in knowing the accuracy of different urinary biomarkers (separately or in combination) for detecting endometriosis. With the PIT approach, the reference test is not considered to be the comparator in the PICO sense, but rather, something that is used to establish how well the index test performs in detecting the target condition. As the PICO format is still the most widely recognised format for creating a focused clinical question, we have used it in this chapter.

Patient/population

In the clinical scenario described at the beginning of this chapter, the population that we are interested in is clinicians working in a hospital ward who have no symptoms of SARS-CoV-2 infection. When considering the patient/population component of PICO, it may be important to specify the setting you are interested in, as diagnostic tests may have different accuracy in different settings. For example, the accuracy of a test may vary in primary and secondary care settings due to the different types of patients that present in these settings. Test accuracy may also vary depending on characteristics of the population (for example, age, gender or ethnicity, or the prior testing individuals may have had). In the clinical scenario above, it may be important to consider if tests perform differently in people who are symptomatic and those who are asymptomatic. If you think the diagnostic test may perform differently in different sub-groups of patients, you may wish to define the population of interest more narrowly. Remember, though, that if you make the population too specific, you may not find any studies.

Intervention

For a diagnostic question, this component of PICO relates to the diagnostic test you are interested in. In the clinical scenario discussed in this chapter, the test of interest (or index test) is a single rapid antigen test for detecting infection with the SARS-CoV-2 virus. Antigens are structures on the surface of a virus that are recognised by the body's immune system and can trigger an immune response in an individual. When a sample taken from the nose or throat is mixed with a solution, viral antigens in the solution are unleashed. A small quantity of the solution is placed on a test cartridge and the presence of the antigens can then be 'captured' by the test containing antibodies specific to the viral antigen. In the setting where this test will be used (testing large numbers of healthcare workers), the collection of the sample by the individual being tested will be supervised by another health professional and the sample analysed in an onsite immunofluorescence analyser. The analyser provides a qualitative result (the test is either positive or negative) and the result is documented and reported by the testing supervisor. The result is usually available after about 15–20 minutes.

In our example, we are considering only a single test, but you may also be interested in the accuracy of a combination of tests, such as a rapid antigen test performed each day for three days. In other diagnostic scenarios, a combination of different tests may be used to identify a condition. For example, if you are interested in the diagnostic accuracy of physical examination for the presence of an anterior cruciate ligament injury of the knee, you may consider a combination of the anterior drawer test, Lachman's test and the pivot shift test. Another form of diagnostic test is a more formal combination of 'tests', such as a clinical prediction rule (which we discuss later in this chapter).

Comparison

The comparator test should be the most accurate method of diagnosing the condition of interest. The most accurate test available for detecting SARS-CoV-2 infection is the Reverse Transcription Polymerase Chain Reaction (RT-PCR) test. A PCR test detects the presence of a part of the genome of the virus, and in SARS-CoV-2 tests the test is often trying to detect the part of the viral RNA that codes for the spike protein that allows the virus to enter host cells. Again, the sample is usually taken from the nose and/or throat. The test uses a polymerase chain reaction to produce a reverse transcription of the viral RNA, resulting in a DNA sample. The test is run over several cycles, with each cycle amplifying the quantity of DNA present. When a large quantity of virus is present, the test will only require a few cycles to detect the presence of the virus, but if only a small amount of virus is present, the test requires more cycles to detect the virus. The sample is analysed in a laboratory using complex techniques and by trained technicians and takes longer to obtain a result than the rapid antigen test—generally, several hours.

Outcome

This component of PICO relates to the target condition—that is, the disease or condition we want the index test to detect. The study should specify how the condition is defined by the reference standard.

For SARS-CoV-2 tests, there are a number of possible target conditions that might be relevant for different settings. These include if a person is infected with the virus, if they have COVID-19 disease caused by the virus, if they are infectious, if they have had a past or recent infection with

the virus and if they have immunity to infection. To make decisions about the opening of businesses and public gatherings, for example, testing for infectiousness (whether an individual can spread the virus to other people) rather than for the presence of infection may be more useful.[5] Infectiousness may also be of value in the setting of interest; however, as there is currently no reliable reference standard for infectiousness, the outcome we will use is the presence of SARS-CoV-2 infection denoted by the presence of viral RNA.

You decide on the following question:

- **In clinicians working in a hospital ward with no symptoms of COVID-19, how accurate is rapid antigen testing compared to RT-PCR testing as a reference standard for detecting SARS-CoV-2 infection?**

◎ CLINICAL SCENARIO (CONTINUED)

Finding the evidence to answer your question

As we saw in Chapter 3, one of the best options for finding diagnostic accuracy studies is PubMed—Clinical Queries. If you are looking for studies on a particular test, you may type in the name of the test and select 'diagnosis' and 'narrow scope'. This may be enough to find what you want. If you do not find anything with a narrow search, you can then look for more studies by selecting 'broad scope'. If the test is used for diagnosing more than one condition, you will also need to type in the name of the condition to narrow the search to only the condition that you are considering (for example, ultrasound AND breast cancer).

In the current scenario, the test of interest is the rapid antigen test. As these types of tests may be used for detecting other conditions, you will need also to enter terms related to the condition you are trying to detect—infection with the SARS-CoV-2 virus that causes COVID-19 disease. You would need to think about synonyms used to describe the test of interest, including 'RAT', 'RADT', 'antigen test', 'lateral flow' and 'rapid test' and consider how these would be included in your search.

You go to PubMed's Clinical Queries section and notice there is a filter for COVID-19 studies. You decide to

use this filter and the one for 'Diagnosis' studies and enter the terms 'antigen test' OR 'rapid test' OR RAT OR RADT into the search box. Your search retrieves just over 2,400 studies. You know this is too many results to look through, so while trying to think of a way to revise your search, you look through the first dozen results that come up. You notice several systematic reviews of the accuracy of rapid antigen tests in different settings and population groups, including a living systematic review (these are discussed in Chapter 12). After having a quick look at this review, you realise there are many different types of rapid tests available and that their accuracy varies. You recall the name of the particular rapid antigen test proposed for use in your hospital and go back to your PubMed search. Adding the term 'Elecsys' with an AND—for example ('antigen test' OR 'rapid test' OR RAT OR RADT) AND Elecsys with the COVID-19 and Diagnosis filter—retrieves 32 results. You look through these and find a study that appears to be just what you are looking for—a study of the diagnostic accuracy of the Elecsys antigen test for detecting SARS-CoV-2 infection.[6] You obtain the full text of this study for further appraisal.

◎ CLINICAL SCENARIO (CONTINUED)

Structured abstract of the chosen article
Citation: Adapted from Montalvo Villalba MC, Sosa Glaria E, et al. Performance evaluation of Elecsys SARS-CoV-2 antigen immunoassay for diagnostic of COVID-19. J Med

Virol 2021;Oct 2. doi: 10.1002/jmv.27412.[6] The structured abstract is adapted from this reference.

Question: In nasopharyngeal swabs sent to the national laboratory in Cuba, what is the diagnostic performance of the Elecsys SARS-CoV-2 antigen test compared with the SARS-CoV-2 RT-PCR test for detecting SARS-CoV-2 infection?

Design: Nasopharyngeal swabs obtained from individuals meeting 5 different epidemiological definitions of samples used at the laboratory (see 'Participants' section below) are tested with the test of interest – the rapid antigen test, and the reference standard test (RT-PCR) for detecting SARS-CoV-2 infection. As there are more than two groups of study participants (in this case, samples), the study may be described as a 'multiple-group' or 'multiple-gate' diagnostic accuracy study. The study also evaluated the cross-reactivity of the antigen test—that is, whether the test identifying the SARS-CoV-2 virus proteins also detects other viral proteins it is not intended to detect.

Setting: National Reference Laboratory for Respiratory Virus in Havana, Cuba.

Participants: The study included 523 randomly selected nasopharyngeal swab samples received at the laboratory from individuals who were classified as (1) being a case of COVID-19 based on having a positive RT-PCR test for SARS-CoV-2, (2) having contact with a confirmed or suspected COVID-19 case, (3) being a case of COVID-19 5 days after diagnosis, (4) having met the clinical criteria of COVID-19 and contact with a probable case, and (5) being an international traveller arriving in Cuba.

Test: Elecsys SARS-CoV-2 antigen test.

Diagnostic (reference) standard: SARS-CoV-2 RT-PCR test.

Main results: The sensitivity of the Elecsys SARS-CoV-2 antigen test for identifying non-SARS-CoV-2 infection across all samples was 89.7% and specificity was 90.6%. Cross-reactivity to other respiratory viruses was not detected. Sensitivity of the test ranged from 78.4% in samples taken from travellers returning to Cuba (known as the 'surveillance' samples in the study) to 94.2% in samples taken from people tested 5 days after a positive RT-PCR test for SARS-CoV-2. Specificity ranged from 86.8% in surveillance samples to 97.1% in samples collected from people who had had contact with a confirmed or suspected COVID-19 case (referred to as 'contact cases' in the study).

Conclusions: Elecsys SARS-CoV-2 antigen immunoassay may be used as an alternative to RT-PCR testing or in complement with it.

IS THIS EVIDENCE LIKELY TO BE BIASED?

As we saw in Chapter 4 for studies about the effectiveness of interventions, it is important to critically appraise the diagnostic test studies that you find to determine whether each study is adequate to inform your clinical practice. As with the other types of study designs, the main elements to consider are: (1) internal validity (that is, the risk of bias); (2) the results (the estimates of diagnostic accuracy); and (3) whether or how the evidence might be applicable to your patient or clinical practice.

We will use the Critical Appraisal Skills Program (CASP) checklist for appraising a diagnostic test study to explain how to assess the likelihood of bias in this type of study. The key questions to ask when appraising the risk of bias (validity) of a diagnostic study are shown in Box 6.1. The checklist begins with two simple screening criteria (not shown in Box 6.1) that, if not met, indicate that the article is unlikely to be helpful and that further assessment of potential bias is probably unwarranted. The reporting statement for diagnostic accuracy studies is the STARD (STAndards for the Reporting of Diagnostic accuracy studies) statement. Further details are available at: https://www.equator-network.org/reporting-guidelines/stard/.

> **BOX 6.1 Key questions to ask when appraising the risk of bias (validity) of a diagnostic accuracy study**
>
> 1. Did all participants get the diagnostic test and the reference standard?
> 2. Could the results of the test of interest have been influenced by the results of the reference standard, or vice versa?
> 3. Was there a clear description of the disease/condition status of the tested population?
> 4. Was there sufficient description of the methods for performing the test?

Was there a clear question for the study to address?

The first screening criterion on the checklist is whether there was a clear question for the study to address. For diagnostic evidence, the study should clearly define the population, the index and comparator tests, the setting and the outcomes considered.

⊚ **CLINICAL SCENARIO (CONTINUED)**

Did the study address a clearly focused issue?

The study addressed a clearly focused question. The study's aim of evaluating the accuracy of the Elecsys SARS-CoV-2 rapid antigen test in nasopharyngeal swab samples received by a large national laboratory using RT-PCR as the reference standard is clearly outlined. There are, however, some differences between the study and the clinical scenario that you will need to keep in mind when interpreting the study results. In the study, the 'population' is not people as such, but samples from individuals who have received the index test for various reasons. The test is likely to perform differently in these distinct groups. The setting in which the study was conducted is a large laboratory with highly experienced staff handling and analysing the samples. You would need to consider if the skills and experience of the staff handling and analysing the sample in this study are similar to the situation in your own clinical setting. The target condition, infection with SARS-CoV-2, is the same in the study and the scenario.

Is the comparison with an appropriate reference standard?

The second screening criterion is whether there was a comparison with an appropriate reference standard. The reference standard should, in general, be the most accurate method available to diagnose, or test for, the target disorder(s). If the reference test used in the study is not 100% accurate, the diagnostic accuracy of the index test may be either over- or underestimated.

Sometimes, the reference standard will be a combination of a number of tests. This is often called a 'composite reference standard'. With this type of reference standard, multiple methods/procedures/tests are used and a rule based on these procedures defines who has or does not have the condition of interest. For example, a test for diagnosing heart failure may be assessed against the combined results of clinical examination and echocardiography. If the index test is included in the reference standard (this is called *incorporation bias*), the diagnostic accuracy of the test is likely to be overestimated.

A reference standard may also include follow-up. Using follow-up to confirm a diagnosis at the time of testing is known as *delayed verification*. An example is a 30-day follow-up of individuals with suspected appendicitis. If a clinical event related to appendicitis (for example, re-presentation in the emergency department and subsequent surgery) occurs during the follow-up period, appendicitis is presumed to have been present at the time of index testing.

⊚ **CLINICAL SCENARIO (CONTINUED)**

Comparison with an appropriate reference standard

The reference standard in this study was the SARS-CoV-2 RT-PCR test. This is widely considered the best available test for detecting SARS-CoV-2 infection. However, even RT-PCR tests may not detect infection in the first few days after infection, as the test requires a certain level of viral load to be present in the throat or nose to be positive.[5] It is important to consider how soon after the exposure to potential SARS-CoV-2 infection the swab was taken for the RT-PCR test.

Did all participants get the diagnostic test and the reference standard?

As we explained earlier in this chapter, the best type of study to estimate diagnostic accuracy is a study of test accuracy in a consecutive sample of eligible individuals. In a well-designed study, *every* individual who presents with a similar type of clinical problem in a particular setting over a particular time period receives both the test of interest and the reference standard, and the results are compared. In a study looking at the diagnostic accuracy for appendicitis, if we were to only assess the accuracy of the test in those individuals who have surgery, and not those who did not need surgery, we will have a biased estimate of the accuracy of the test. This type of bias is known as *verification bias*.

A common form of verification bias occurs when the authors of a study use patient records to select patients to include in the study who have had both the index test and the reference test. For example, in a study of the accuracy of physical signs versus the reference standard of arthroscopy or MRI for diagnosing anterior cruciate ligament injury of the knee, individuals were included in the study if they attended an orthopaedic clinic and had *both* a physical examination and an MRI scan. Further, when patient records are used to select patients for a study, study participants are likely to be different from the type of patients who present to a clinic with a particular clinical problem and the sample is therefore likely to provide a biased estimate of the accuracy of the diagnostic test. This is a form of *spectrum bias*. For example, patients who had both a suspected anterior cruciate ligament injury and an MRI scan are likely to be a different spectrum of patients from all patients who present to an orthopaedic clinic with a suspected anterior cruciate ligament injury. Patients who had both a physical examination and an MRI may, for example, have more severe injuries.

The timing of the reference standard is also important. Ideally, the results of the test of interest and the reference standard are obtained from the same patients at the same time. If this does not occur and the time between the performance of the index and reference standard test is too long (what is too long will depend on the clinical condition), individuals may be misclassified due to spontaneous recovery, response to treatment or progression to a more advanced stage of the condition that can occur during this delay.

 CLINICAL SCENARIO (CONTINUED)

Did all participants get the diagnostic test and the reference standard?

For this study, which used nasopharyngeal samples sent to a national laboratory for the diagnosis of SARS-CoV-2 infection, it is likely both the index and the reference standards would have been performed on all the included samples. It is also likely they would have been performed at the same or very similar time, though neither point is clearly reported in this study. The same type of PCR assay was conducted for all samples.

Could the results of the test of interest have been influenced by the results of the reference standard, or vice versa?

The results of the index test and the reference test should each be decided without knowledge of the results of the other test. That is, the person who interprets the test should be blinded to the results of the other test. Knowledge of one test result may bias the reading of the other, particularly where the reading is subjective, such as physical examination or the interpretation of imaging results (this is known as *review bias*).

CLINICAL SCENARIO (CONTINUED)

Could the results of the test of interest have been influenced by the results of the reference standard, or vice versa?

No. It is unlikely that the results of one test would have influenced the results of the other.

This study took place in a laboratory where specialised automated machinery was used to analyse the samples and provide a result based on pre-specified thresholds/cut-offs for positive and negative results on both the rapid test and the reference standard test. It is not likely that laboratory staff knowing the result of the index test would have been able to influence the result of the reference standard, or vice versa. Ideally, though, the study would provide some statement about blinding or reassurance that test results could not influence each other.

Was there a clear description of the disease/condition status of the tested population?

Studies of test accuracy inform us about the behaviour of a test under particular circumstances. As diagnostic accuracy is very much dependent upon the spectrum of included participants, a clear description of the disease stage and severity of the tested population helps us to understand study findings and how they may apply to our situation. The test should be investigated in a clinical setting that is as close as possible to the clinical setting in which it will be used. The spectrum of patients included in the study can affect the sensitivity or specificity, or both, and therefore may affect the observed accuracy of the test. For example, if the study is conducted in a tertiary referral centre (as compared with a general practitioner's office, say), patients may have more severe symptoms, and this may affect the sensitivity and/or the specificity of the physical examination.

CLINICAL SCENARIO (CONTINUED)

Clear description of the disease/condition status of the tested population

Yes. The study describes the samples as being from individuals who were (1) a confirmed case of COVID-19, (2) a contact of a confirmed or suspected COVID-19 case (that is, contact cases), (3) a case of COVID-19 5 days after diagnosis, (4) meeting the clinical criteria of COVID-19 and had contact with a probable case (that is, suspected cases), and (5) an international traveller arriving in Cuba (that is, surveillance cases). The samples used in the study were a random selection of samples received at the laboratory.

Was there sufficient description of the methods for performing the test?

Both the index test and the reference standard test should be described in sufficient detail so that it is possible to: (1) reproduce the test; and (2) determine whether the test was performed adequately and is similar to the test being conducted in your own clinical setting.

CLINICAL SCENARIO (CONTINUED)

Sufficient description of the methods for performing the test

Yes. The study reports specific details of the assays used, the machinery (analysers) models employed and the procedures followed (for example, as per manufacturer's

Continued

If you have determined that the article about diagnostic accuracy you have been appraising is valid, you can then consider the importance and applicability of the results.

WHAT ARE THE RESULTS?

Diagnostic accuracy studies may report the results in a variety of ways. Most studies will report the sensitivity and specificity of the index test. These metrics tell us about the properties of the diagnostic test—that is, its ability to identify who tests positive (in people with the disease or condition) and who tests negative (in those who are disease free)—and help us determine the test's appropriateness. No test is 100% accurate; there will always be false-positive and false-negative results.

However, the most useful measures for you as a health professional are the post-test probabilities of a positive and negative test. In practice, we do not know whether an individual has the disease or condition of interest (that is why we are doing the test!). When we do the test and receive the results, the post-test probabilities help us interpret that result—how likely it is that the individual actually has the disease when the test is positive and does not have the disease when the test is negative. Post-test probabilities are dependent on the prevalence or pre-test probability of the disease in the population of interest and on the sensitivity and specificity of the test.

The measures of test accuracy—sensitivity, specificity and post-test probabilities—are obtained from the cross-classification of the reference standard result and the index test result and are commonly presented in the form of a 2×2 table. All study participants are classified into one of the four cells of the 2×2 table depending on their index and reference test result. An example of a 2×2 table showing data from our clinical scenario study is in Table 6.1. The true positives (the upper left cell of the 2×2 table) have a positive index test result *and* are classified by the reference standard as having the disease. The true negatives (lower right cell of the 2×2 table) have a negative index test result *and* are negative on the reference standard. The false positive (upper right cell) and false negatives (lower left cell) are the number of individuals misclassified by the index test.

We will now look at how to interpret and calculate measures of test accuracy.

Sensitivity and specificity

- The **sensitivity** of a test measures how well it performs in detecting a condition in people who have the condition. It is the probability that a test is positive in people who have a condition (true positives ÷ [true positives + false negatives]). This is represented graphically in Figure 6.1.
- The **specificity** of a test measures how well it performs in determining that a condition is *not* present in people who do not have the condition. It is the probability

TABLE 6.1 2×2 cross-classification of the index test (the rapid antigen test) for detecting SARS-CoV-2 infection and the reference standard (RT-PCR test) in samples collected from returning international travellers (i.e. the surveillance samples)

		REFERENCE STANDARD RESULT		
		SARS-CoV-2 infection	No SARS-CoV-2 infection	Total
Index test result	Rapid antigen test positive	True positives	False positives	49
		40	9	
	Rapid antigen test negative	False negatives	True negatives	70
		11	59	
	Total	**51**	**68**	**119**

Montalvo Villalba MC, Sosa Glaria E, Rodriguez Lay L, et al. Performance evaluation of Elecsys SARS-CoV-2 Antigen immunoassay for diagnostic of COVID-19. J Med Virol 2022;94:1001–8. doi:10.1002/jmv.27412.

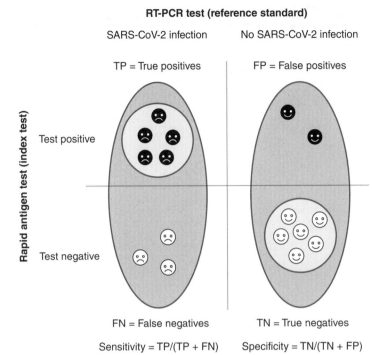

RT-PCR test (reference standard)

SARS-CoV-2 infection   No SARS-CoV-2 infection

TP = True positives   FP = False positives

Rapid antigen test (index test)

Test positive

Test negative

FN = False negatives   TN = True negatives

Sensitivity = TP/(TP + FN)   Specificity = TN/(TN + FP)

Key
- The sad smiley faces represent those who have the condition according to the reference standard (RT-PCR test in this example).
- The happy faces represent those who do not have the condition according to the reference standard.
- The dark faces represent those who are positive on the index test (a rapid antigen test in this example) and the light faces represent those who are negative on the index test.

Fig 6.1 Graphical representation of sensitivity and specificity

that a test is negative in people who do not have the condition (true negatives ÷ [true negatives + false positives]). This is represented graphically in Figure 6.1. Box 6.2 shows how to calculate the sensitivity and specificity of the rapid antigen test being evaluated in the clinical scenario article.

Post-test probabilities of a positive and a negative test

These values tell us about the clinical relevance of a test and are the most useful way of interpreting the results of a test accuracy study for you as a health professional:

- The **post-test probability of a positive test** (also known as **positive predictive value**) tells you the probability that a patient has the condition if they have a positive test result. The closer this number is to 100%, the better the test is at ruling in the condition. Its calculation (true positives ÷ [true positives + false positives]) is represented graphically in Figure 6.2.
- Conversely, the **post-test probability of a negative test** (which is the *complement* of the **negative predictive value**) tells you the probability that a patient has the condition if they have a negative test result. The closer this number is to 0%, the better the test is at ruling out the condition (as there will be few false negatives). Its

calculation (false negatives ÷ [false negatives + true negatives]) is represented graphically in Figure 6.2. The closer a *negative predictive value* approaches 100%, the better the test is at ruling out the condition. Its calculation is true negatives ÷ (false negatives + true negatives).

The difficulty with post-test probabilities (positive and negative predictive values) is that you need to have an estimate of the pre-test probability of the condition (that is, the likelihood of having the condition before having the test) in order to be able to calculate them. In testing for SARS-CoV-2 infection, for example, the pre-test probability of infection will depend on the rate of new diagnosis of COVID-19 in the community at the time of testing and the level of clinical suspicion that a person has been infected (for example, whether symptoms are present in an individual or there has been a close contact). The pre-test probability of being infected will be higher for a person with a fever, sore throat and exposure to another infected individual, than for a person who has no symptoms and when there is low rate of new cases of infection in the community at the time.

When more individuals in the study have the condition, the post-test probability of both positive and negative tests will increase.[7] So, if you use post-test probabilities to guide

BOX 6.2 Measuring diagnostic accuracy: sensitivity and specificity

This box uses data (see Table 6.1) about the diagnostic accuracy of the rapid antigen test for detecting SARS-CoV-2 infection in the samples collected from returned international travellers from our clinical scenario article as an example.

$$\text{The sensitivity of the rapid antigen test} = \frac{\text{true positives}}{\text{true positives} + \text{false negatives}} = \frac{40}{(40+11)} = \frac{40}{51} = 78.4\%$$

$$\text{The specificity of the rapid antigen test} = \frac{\text{true negatives}}{\text{true negatives} + \text{false positives}} = \frac{59}{(59+9)} = \frac{59}{68} = 86.8\%$$

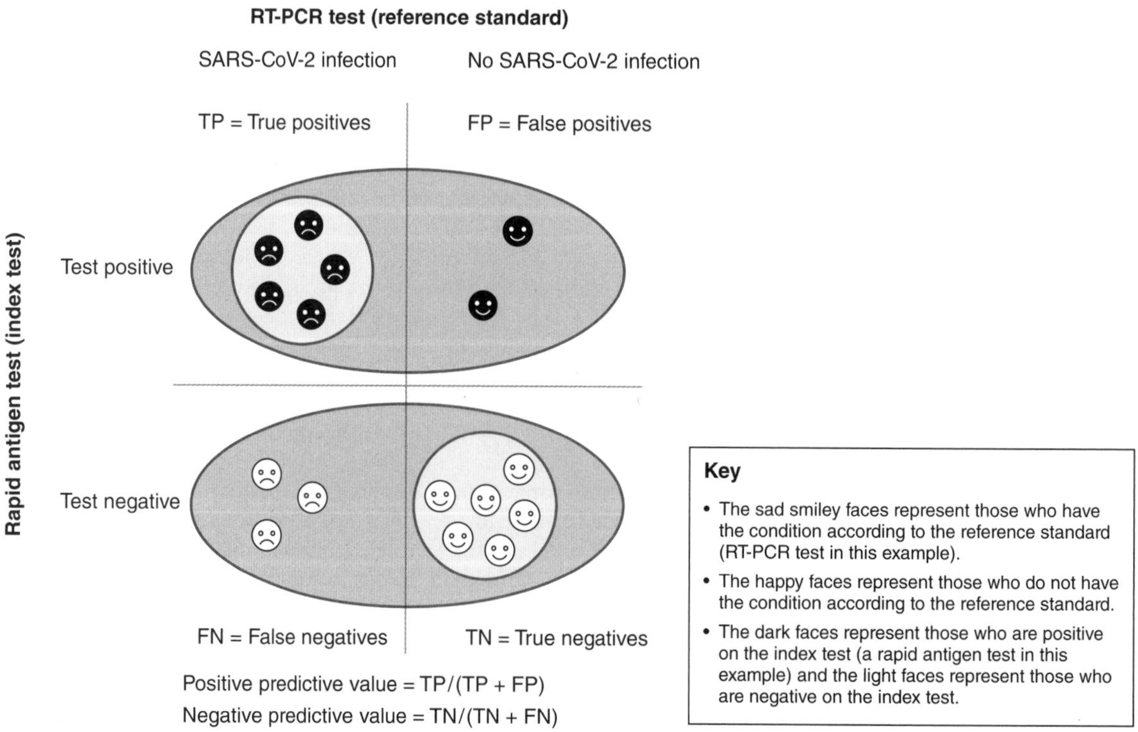
RT-PCR test (reference standard)
SARS-CoV-2 infection
No SARS-CoV-2 infection
TP = True positives
FP = False positives
Rapid antigen test (index test)
Test positive
Test negative
FN = False negatives
TN = True negatives
Positive predictive value = TP/(TP + FP)
Negative predictive value = TN/(TN + FN)
Key
• The sad smiley faces represent those who have the condition according to the reference standard (RT-PCR test in this example).
• The happy faces represent those who do not have the condition according to the reference standard.
• The dark faces represent those who are positive on the index test (a rapid antigen test in this example) and the light faces represent those who are negative on the index test.

Fig 6.2 Graphical representation of post-test probabilities of positive and negative tests

BOX 6.3 Measuring diagnostic accuracy: post-test probabilities of a positive and a negative test result

As a health professional, what you want to know is the probability that a patient has a condition if you receive a positive or a negative test result for them. These values are the post-test probabilities of a positive and a negative test. However, most diagnostic accuracy studies report the sensitivity and the specificity of a diagnostic test. The probability of a condition after a positive or a negative test result requires further calculation, and we also need to consider the *prevalence* (also called the 'pre-test probability') of the condition.

Using some of the data from our clinical scenario article as an example:

The rapid antigen test in the samples collected from returned international travellers (the surveillance samples) had a sensitivity of 78.4% and a specificity of 86.8%. The study reports that 51 of 119 of these samples had a positive RT-PCT test for SARS-CoV-2 infection. The **prevalence or pre-test probability** of SARS-CoV-2 infection in this population is therefore 51 ÷ 119 = 42.9%.

The post-test probability of a positive test (also known as the 'positive predictive value')

= the probability of SARS-CoV-2 infection with a positive rapid antigen test

$$= \frac{\text{true positives}}{(\text{true positives} + \text{false positives})}$$

$$= \frac{40}{(40 + 9)}$$

$$= \frac{40}{49}$$

$$= 81.6\%$$

The post-test probability of a negative test (the *complement* of the negative predictive value)

= the probability of having SARS-CoV-2 infection given a negative rapid antigen test

$$= \frac{\text{false negatives}}{(\text{false negatives} + \text{true negatives})}$$

$$= \frac{11}{(11 + 59)}$$

$$= 11/70$$

$$= 15.7\%$$

To help people remember whether tests rule in or rule out a condition, the following mnemonics may be helpful:
- **SpPIn** (Specificity-Positive-In) = if a test has a high specificity and the result is positive, it rules the condition in.
- **SnNOut** (Sensitivity-Negative-Out) = if a test has a high sensitivity and the result is negative, it rules the condition out.
  Note that this is a generalisation, and that the post-test probability depends on both sensitivity and specificity, and on the prevalence of the condition.[8]

Note: When the pre-test probability is low—for example, in screening programs—even tests with high sensitivity and specificity will have a low positive predictive value; that is, most positive test results will be false positives.

your decision about whether to use a diagnostic test or not, this means it is particularly important that you check the spectrum of patients that were included in the diagnostic accuracy study to ensure they match the sort of patients you see in your practice. Box 6.3 explains how to calculate post-test probabilities of positive and negative test results, as well as the pre-test probability of the condition.

Positive and negative likelihood ratios

Another pair of values that can be used to report the results of diagnostic test accuracy studies is the **positive and negative likelihood ratios**. Box 6.4 shows how likelihood ratios can be calculated. These results have the advantage of being relatively stable across different clinical settings, but also give an indication of how well the test rules in or rules out a condition.

BOX 6.4   Measuring diagnostic accuracy: positive and negative likelihood ratios

The *positive likelihood ratio* is the probability that a test is positive in people with the condition divided by the probability that the test is positive in people without the condition.

The *negative likelihood ratio* is the probability that a test is negative in people with the condition divided by the probability that the test is negative in people without the condition.

Using some of the data from our chosen article as an example:

The positive likelihood ratio for the rapid antigen test

$$= \frac{(\text{true positives} / \text{people who have the condition})}{(\text{false positives} / \text{people who do not have the condition})}$$

$$= \frac{(40 / 51)}{(9 / 68)}$$

$$= 0.784 / 0.132$$

$$= 5.9$$

The negative likelihood ratio for the rapid antigen test

$$= \frac{(\text{false negatives} / \text{people who have the condition})}{(\text{true negatives} / \text{people who do not have the condition})}$$

$$= \frac{(11 / 51)}{(59 / 68)}$$

$$= 0.216 / 0.867$$

$$= 0.25$$

If the article only reports the sensitivity and specificity of the tests, another way to calculate likelihood ratios is:
- Positive likelihood ratio (LR+) = sensitivity/(100 − specificity)
- Negative likelihood ratio (LR−) = (100 − sensitivity)/specificity

When interpreting likelihood ratios, as a rough guide:
- A positive likelihood ratio >2 indicates a test that helps rule in the condition.
- A positive likelihood ratio >10 is an extremely good test for ruling in the condition.
- A negative likelihood ratio of <0.5 indicates a test that helps rule out the condition.
- A negative likelihood ratio of <0.1 is an extremely good test for ruling out the condition.

◎ CLINICAL SCENARIO (CONTINUED)

What are the results?

We will focus our attention on the results for the samples taken for screening international travellers returning to Cuba (this group of samples is referred to as 'surveillance' samples in the study), as this is the scenario that is closest to our clinical scenario. These samples were from people who were not known to have had contact with other people who had had CO-VID-19. The study analysed 119 samples collected from returned travellers.

In this group of samples, RT-PCR identified SARS-CoV-2 infections in 51 of the 119 samples (42.9%). In these samples, the rapid antigen test performed reasonably well for ruling in (positive likelihood ratio of 5.9) and ruling out (negative likelihood ratio of 0.25) SARS-CoV-2 infection. The sensitivity of the rapid antigen test, or the ability of the test to yield a positive result when an individual had SARS-CoV-2, in the samples of returned travellers was 78.4%. Specificity, or the ability of the test to obtain a negative result for an individual who did not have SARS-CoV-2 infection, was 86.8% (Table 6.2). Cross-reactivity with other respiratory viruses was not detected.

TABLE 6.2 Estimates of the diagnostic accuracy of the rapid antigen test for the detection of SARS-CoV-2 infection in samples collected from returning international travellers (i.e. the surveillance samples)

	Sensitivity	Specificity	Positive likelihood ratio	Negative likelihood ratio	Positive predictive value	Negative predictive value
Rapid antigen test	78.4%	86.8%	5.9	0.25	81.6%	84.3%

Montalvo Villalba MC, Sosa Glaria E, Rodriguez Lay L, et al. Performance evaluation of Elecsys SARS-CoV-2 Antigen immunoassay for diagnostic of COVID-19. J Med Virol 2022;94:1001–8. doi:10.1002/jmv.27412.

How changes in cut-off will affect the test

For many conditions, there is no clear threshold between the presence and absence of a condition. For example, blood pressure and blood glucose levels exist on a spectrum, and the cut-offs that have been chosen to define hypertension or diabetes are, to some extent, arbitrary. In cases where the cut-off for normal/abnormal levels can be raised or lowered, this will affect the test characteristics, and the choice of cut-off will involve a trade-off between the sensitivity and the specificity of the test. If higher values indicate more-abnormal test results, and the cut-off point is raised, there will be fewer false positives (increased specificity) but more false negatives (reduced sensitivity). If the cut-off point is lowered, there are fewer false negatives but more false positives (increased sensitivity but reduced specificity) (see Figure 6.3). A receiver operating characteristic (ROC) curve (see Figure 6.4) plots this trade-off between sensitivity and specificity with changes in the cut-off. The curve demonstrates the trade-off between sensitivity and specificity of a test as the cut-off point changes. A test that performs no better than a coin toss would have a ROC curve that traces a straight (diagonal) line from the bottom left to the top right-hand corner of the ROC box. The top left-hand corner of the ROC box is the point where sensitivity = 100% and specificity = 100% (1 – specificity = 0%). This represents a perfect test. The closer the ROC curve is to the top left-hand corner of the ROC box, the better the test overall.

How can we use this evidence to inform practice?

As part of our judgment about whether to use the results of this study in our own practice, we need to think about

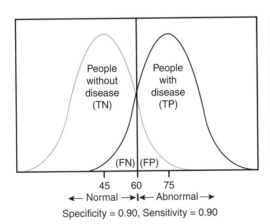

Panel A: two hypothetical distributions with test cut-off at 60

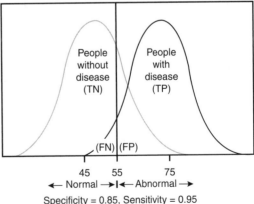

Panel B: two hypothetical distributions with test cut-off lowered to 55 increases sensitivity but decreases specificity

TN = true negative, TP = true positive, FN = false negative, FP = false positive

Fig 6.3 The effect of lowering test cut-off on sensitivity and specificity
From Dawson B, Trapp RG. Basic and clinical biostatistics. 4th ed. New York: McGraw-Hill Education; 2004, Ch 12, p 314.

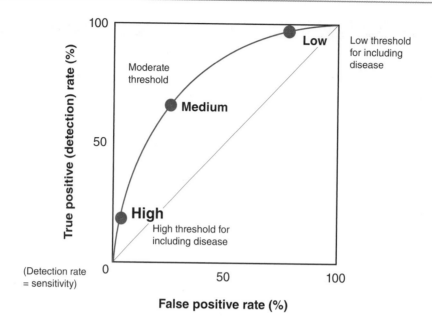

(False positive rate = 1 – specificity)

Fig 6.4 Receiver operating characteristic (ROC) curve

how likely it is that the test performs in a similar way in our own clinical setting to the diagnostic accuracy in this study.[9] We need to consider:

1. Is the spectrum of patients in the diagnostic study similar to the spectrum of patients in the clinical setting in which you are working?
2. Is the prevalence of the condition in the diagnostic study similar to the prevalence of the condition in the clinical setting in which you are working?
3. Is the method for using the index test similar in the diagnostic study and the clinical setting in which you are working? This includes both the method for performing the index test and the person performing the test.
4. Is the method for using the reference test similar in the diagnostic study and the clinical setting in which you are working?
5. Is the study defining the target disorder in the same way as in your own clinical setting?

◎ CLINICAL SCENARIO (CONTINUED)

Using the evidence to inform practice

Tests that provide accurate results within a short time frame may facilitate timely decisions around the need for isolation and contact tracing activities, ultimately reducing transmission of SARS-CoV-2 infection. Because of the time delay in receiving results and the resource constraints involved with PCR testing, rapid antigen testing may be a good substitute for PCR testing.

The findings from the group of returning travellers show that this particular rapid antigen test is reasonably good at detecting the presence and confirming the absence of SARS-CoV-2 infection but will miss some who actually have a SARS-CoV-2 infection and label

some who truly do not have SARS-CoV-2 infection as positive.

An important consideration is the timing of the rapid antigen and reference standard tests in relation to when a person may have been exposed to the virus. People who are infected with SARS-CoV-2 will have a positive PCR test earlier than a rapid antigen test (about 2–3 days after exposure for a PCR test and 4–5 days for a rapid antigen test).[5] This is because the rapid antigen test requires a higher viral load before it is able to detect the infection. This may be appropriate in a workplace setting, where it is more important to determine if someone is infectious (which is a risk to other people in the workplace) rather than if someone is infected. It is important to remember that a person who tests negative one day may be in the early stages of infection, so repeat testing may be required. If someone has symptoms, it is therefore more important to determine if they have the infection and not just if they are possibly infectious, a RT-PCR test may be more appropriate where available.

As described above, the post-test probability of disease is greatly affected by the pre-test probability of disease. Table 6.3 shows the probabilities of infection given a positive and negative rapid antigen test result when the probability of infection prior to doing the test is low (1%) and higher at 10% and at 43% (the proportion of samples from the returned travellers tested in the study that were positive on RT-PCR testing). As can be seen from the table, when the pre-test probability of infection is low, the positive predictive value will be low and most positive tests will be false positives. When the pre-test probability is 1%, the probability that a person with a positive rapid antigen test is actually infected is only 5.6%. Even when the pre-test probability is higher at 43%, and the positive predictive value is therefore higher at 81.7%, this means approximately 2 in 10 rapid antigen positive results will be falsely positive. In this situation, repeat rapid antigen testing or RT-PCR testing will be necessary to confirm infection and avoid unnecessary exclusion from the workplace.

False negatives are also of concern. At 43% pre-test probability in the surveillance sample, and negative predictive value of 84.2%, 15.8% of those with negative rapid antigen test results are missed cases of SARS-CoV-2. The potential effect on transmission of infection from missed cases needs to be considered. The role and position of the rapid antigen test in the clinical scenario of interest should be specified and leads to the following further questions. What tolerance is there for false positive and false negative results in the hospital setting of interest? What further testing (if any) happens or what action is taken, given a positive and negative result?

Could the quality of the study have biased the results?
Our earlier appraisal of this study suggests that the risk of bias is likely to be low. It is likely all samples were tested with both the rapid antigen test and the reference standard test, and that the results of one would not influence the results of the other. The samples are clearly described according to type of sample, which facilitates understanding of the risk of infection and the methods for performing the tests are clearly described. It is unlikely the quality of the study will have biased the results.

Could other factors have affected the results—for example, the setting of the study?
Other factors which may affect the results of the rapid antigen tests include whether the person taking the sample and performing the test is trained, and whether the sample is taken from the nose or the throat. The accuracy of the rapid antigen test may also vary with the procedure used to store and transport the test. When thinking about the possible consequences of testing, it is important to consider how likely it is that the person has been exposed to possible infection, and whether there is potential for repeat testing using either rapid antigen tests or RT-PCR.

Should I use these tests?
As a healthcare worker who will be required to undergo rapid antigen testing before each shift, understanding the accuracy of the test being used is important. The rapid time to a result is a key driver for use of the test in this setting, but the trade-off is the possibility of false positive and negative results.

TABLE 6.3 Post-test probabilities of rapid antigen testing based on the pre-test probability of infection and sensitivity and specificity of the test

Pretest probability (the likelihood of infection before having the rapid antigen test)	Sensitivity of the rapid antigen test	Specificity of the rapid antigen test	Positive predictive value/post-test probability of a positive test	Negative predictive value	Post-test probability of a negative test*
1%	78.4%	86.8%	5.6%	99.8%	0.2%
10%	78.4%	86.8%	39.7%	97.3%	2.7%
43%	78.4%	86.8%	81.7%	84.2%	15.8%

*The post-test probability of a negative test is the complement of the negative predictive value. It is the probability of SARS-CoV-2 infection when a negative rapid antigen test result is received.

OTHER TYPES OF TEST STUDIES

So far, we have considered diagnostic test accuracy. Studies of diagnostic test accuracy measure how well a test can correctly identify or rule out a disease. But not all studies about tests aim to measure accuracy. Some studies measure the *reliability* of a test; that is, whether you get the same test result when the test is done by different health professionals or by the same health professional at different times. The first are usually called *studies of inter-observer reliability* and the latter *studies of intra-observer reliability*.[10] The agreement between different operators of the test (or different groups of operators) can be assessed using measures of agreement such as Cohen's kappa scores. These scores measure the agreement that is seen beyond that expected by chance.

Other clinical tests are used for assessing or monitoring patients. For example, haemoglobin A_{1c} (HbA_{1c}) can be used to monitor glycaemic control in patients with diabetes. Other monitoring tests, such as assessments of ability to perform self-care skills or assessments of pain, can be used to monitor a patient's progress, predict the likelihood of their needing further treatment, and/or monitor their response to intervention and whether adjustments to intervention are needed.

Tests that are used for monitoring need to be reliable, and they are evaluated using measures of reliability such as those described above. Sometimes in clinical practice we use the *average* of several measures to improve the reliability of a test. For example, by taking an average of several blood pressure measurements, we reduce the random error that would be seen in a single measurement. When tests are used to monitor a patient, the most appropriate study design is a randomised controlled trial. In these clinical settings, the test is being used as part of a strategy to intervene in the patient's clinical course. Therefore, these tests should be evaluated in the same way as other interventions (see Chapter 4), and preferably by using outcomes that are clinically relevant to the patient.[11]

Studies may also be undertaken to determine the clinical utility of tests—that is, the ability of a test to improve clinical outcomes.[12] The availability of an accurate and reliable test does not necessarily translate into better outcomes for people. This is because there are many 'mechanisms' that affect health outcomes once a diagnosis is made, including the degree to which the diagnosis affects treatment plans and the certainty with which a course of treatment is pursued, and the treatment implemented (its timing, efficacy and adherence to it). The test-treatment randomised controlled trial is regarded as the ideal study design for evaluating the clinical utility of a test. In these studies, participants are randomised to the new or existing test, followed by management based on the test results with measurement of patient outcomes.[13]

DIAGNOSTIC CLINICAL PREDICTION RULES

Making a diagnosis usually involves the interpretation of multiple 'pieces' of information obtained through questioning the patient about signs and symptoms, performing an examination and/or conducting laboratory or imaging tests. In assessing children with fever for the presence of serious bacterial infection, for example, over 40 clinical signs and symptoms may be considered.[14] However, assimilating and interpreting the often large amount of diagnostic information we collect is challenging and error prone. We may discount some of the diagnostic information we have when the amount of it is overwhelming, or we may misunderstand or misinterpret the 'diagnosticity' or diagnostic value of the information. This may occur because diagnostic test results are often mutually dependent. In other words, the diagnostic information conveyed by the results of different tests is, to varying extents, overlapping and dependent on the information obtained from previous tests. For example, consider two tests—test A and test B—that might be used in the assessment of individuals with chest pain presenting to the emergency department. Both tests measure enzymes found in the blood that are released when there is damage to heart muscle cells. When evaluated on their own (that is, test A is compared to a reference standard and test B is compared to a reference standard), both tests show diagnostic value. However, because the enzymes occur through a related pathological mechanism, the two tests are not independent, and the value of a positive test B is influenced by a positive test A. This means that, in a diagnostic workup, test B has little or no diagnostic value when test A has already been performed. Knowing just which pieces of information have true diagnostic value, and the relative contribution or 'diagnostic power' each test or piece of information makes towards the diagnosis, is a challenge.

Diagnostic clinical prediction rules are tools that have been developed to assist clinicians to efficiently and objectively combine multiple pieces of diagnostic information. Essentially, clinical prediction rules are combinations of features, or 'predictors' (such as patient characteristics including age and sex, items from the patient's history, physical examination or imaging or laboratory test results), that provide the probability of a 'diagnosis' for an individual. The predicted probabilities assist diagnostic decision making, helping to rule in a condition by identifying individuals very likely to have it (and who thus may require further testing or treatment), or to rule out a condition by identifying those very unlikely to have it (thereby reducing unnecessary testing or treatment).

Contemporary diagnostic prediction rules are typically developed by applying multivariable statistical techniques (usually, logistic regression) to patient datasets where both the possible predictors and outcome (the presence or absence of the condition of interest) are measured in each participant at the same time (a type of cross-sectional study). The statistical techniques used identify only the predictors that are truly predictive of, or most useful for identifying, the condition of interest in view of other test results (in a way, 'accounting' for the mutual dependency between tests). By entering data from an individual on these predictors, we can obtain an estimate of the probability of a condition (0–100%) for that individual. We may use this objective estimate of the probability in combination with our clinical judgment to assist in reaching a diagnosis when we are uncertain, or as a sort of 'second opinion' when a diagnosis or decision has already been reached. Using a diagnostic prediction rule may also help you to focus on the predictors/features/diagnostic information that are truly useful for identifying the condition of interest, and to give less importance to features that have less predictive power, making the diagnostic process simpler and more efficient. Earlier clinical prediction rules were predominantly developed based on expert opinion. The well-known APGAR score for assessing the health of newborns (developed in the 1950s) is an example of this type of clinical prediction rule.

Diagnostic clinical prediction rules are often presented as scoring systems, where each predictor in the prediction rule is assigned a point value if present or absent. The points are then summed to give a 'score' which corresponds to a risk probability estimate. Sometimes developers of clinical prediction rules apply cut-offs to the probability estimate provided by the clinical prediction rule, so the prediction rule classifies individuals into risk groups—for example, high, intermediate or low risk of a condition being present. The diagnostic clinical prediction rule may further recommend a course of action based on these groups. This may be a recommendation on further testing or treatment, or both. In some cases, the cut-off may be set at a point that the prediction rule effectively rules out a condition when certain criteria are met (or alternatively rules in a diagnosis, though these are less common). A well-known diagnostic clinical prediction rule using this approach is the Ottawa Ankle Rules (Figure 6.5), which recommends that a foot or ankle X-ray series be performed

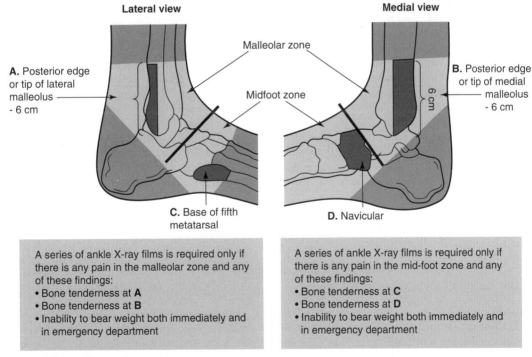

Lateral view   **Medial view**

Malleolar zone

A. Posterior edge or tip of lateral malleolus - 6 cm

Midfoot zone

B. Posterior edge or tip of medial malleolus - 6 cm

6 cm

C. Base of fifth metatarsal

D. Navicular

A series of ankle X-ray films is required only if there is any pain in the malleolar zone and any of these findings:
• Bone tenderness at **A**
• Bone tenderness at **B**
• Inability to bear weight both immediately and in emergency department

A series of ankle X-ray films is required only if there is any pain in the mid-foot zone and any of these findings:
• Bone tenderness at **C**
• Bone tenderness at **D**
• Inability to bear weight both immediately and in emergency department

Fig 6.5 The Ottawa Ankle Rules
Bachmann LM, Kolb E, Koller MT, et al. Accuracy of Ottawa Ankle Rules to exclude fractures of the ankle and mid-foot: systematic review BMJ 2003;326:417. doi:10.1136/bmj.326.7386.417.

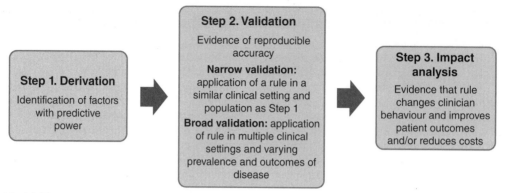

Fig 6.6 The stages of evaluation of a diagnostic prediction rule
Adapted from McGinn T. Putting meaning into meaningful use a roadmap to successful integration of evidence at the point of care. JMIR Med Inform. 2016;4(2):e16.

only when certain findings are present. For example, a series of ankle x-rays is only necessary if there is pain near the malleoli, the patient is unable to bear weight and has bone tenderness at specific sites.[15] If one of these findings is not present, an ankle X-ray series is not required.

Before a diagnostic clinical prediction rule can be considered for use in practice it should have been through three main stages of development and evaluation. It is important to know the stage of evaluation of the rule, as it gives an indication of the 'readiness' of the rule for application in clinical practice. These main stages are: derivation, validation and impact analysis (Figure 6.6).[16] Others have identified a further three stages: the need for a prediction rule, determining the cost-effectiveness of a prediction rule, and long-term dissemination and implementation of the clinical prediction rule.[17] In the derivation phase, the diagnostic clinical prediction rule is developed by applying statistical modelling techniques (often logistic regression modelling) to data obtained from individuals suspected of having the condition and in which the presence of the condition of interest is reported. These statistical techniques identify the predictor variables (characteristics, signs, symptoms or diagnostic tests) statistically related to the presence or absence of the condition of interest. The diagnostic performance of this combination of predictors compared to a reference test is then evaluated. Because the performance of prediction rules is usually overestimated when the rule is used in the same data in which it was developed, its performance should be evaluated in other patient data than was used for the rule derivation. Such validation studies may use participant data collected by the same investigators but at a later time period (temporal or narrow validation) or by other investigators in a different geographical location (geographic or broad validation) or setting (model developed in secondary care and used in a primary care population). A diagnostic prediction rule

may also be validated in other types of participants entirely (for example, a model developed for adults but validated in a population of children).

The performance of prediction rules in validation studies is typically measured in terms of calibration—the agreement between the predictions of the rule and the observed outcomes, and discrimination—the ability of the rule to differentiate between those who do and who do not have the outcome of interest. A widely reported measure of discrimination of a prediction rule is the area under the receiver curve. The AUROC is a measure of the Area Underneath the ROC curve (seen earlier in the chapter) that represents how likely it is that the prediction rule will rank two individuals, one with and one without the condition, in the correct order across all possible thresholds. An AUROC of 1 represents a perfect test, while 0.5 represents a test no better than a coin toss and therefore not worth doing. Sensitivity and specificity and predictive values might also be used to quantify the performance of a diagnostic clinical prediction rule; however, as with other diagnostic tests with continuous outcomes, a cut-off point must be applied to the probability provided by the diagnostic prediction rule to classify individuals as high or low risk.

The final stage is to evaluate the use of the clinical prediction rule and the effect of its use on patient outcomes. This step generally requires a comparative study. A randomised controlled trial is ideal. At minimum, the diagnostic clinical prediction rule should demonstrate good performance in broad validation studies before being considered for use in practice. But caution should be exercised if incorporating the diagnostic clinical prediction rule into the clinical decision-making process without careful evaluation of its effects on patient outcomes.

Diagnostic clinical prediction rules are also called prediction models or guides, decision rules or guides, scoring systems, algorithms, decision support systems or risk scores. This can make it difficult to locate studies of clinical prediction rules in the literature. Studies of diagnostic clinical prediction rules may be found in the clinical literature by searching in resources such as syntheses such as Evidence Updates where they are appraised and rated for relevancy and newsworthiness (see Chapter 3). Appraised studies of diagnostic prediction rules may also appear in specific discipline databases such as the Diagnostic Test Accuracy database for physiotherapists (www.dita.org.au), which was described in Chapter 3. If searching for studies of diagnostic clinical prediction rules in bibliographic databases such as Medline via Ovid or PubMed, you can limit your search to studies of clinical prediction guides using the 'Clinical Queries' feature and for PubMed by using the 'Clinical Queries' screen, 'clinical prediction rule' filter.

When you find a study of a clinical prediction rule, you may need to appraise it (if it has not already been appraised by synopses or pre-appraised sources) to determine the stage of evaluation of the rule and the rigour of the methods used to derive and validate it. The Critical Appraisal Skills Program (CASP) has produced a checklist for appraising a study about a clinical prediction rule. The key questions to ask when appraising the validity of a study of a clinical prediction rule are summarised in Box 6.5. The checklist begins with three simple screening criteria. The first two questions ask about the clinical prediction rule under study: whether it is adequately presented in the paper with regard to how and with whom to use it, and the population in which the rule was derived. If the study you have describes the derivation of a clinical prediction rule, this should be easy to answer. If, instead, the study you have is a validation or impact study, to answer this question you may need to check the references and obtain the derivation study if detail about the derivation is not given in the

---

BOX 6.5 Key questions to ask when appraising the risk of bias (validity) of a clinical prediction rule study

1. Is the clinical prediction rule clearly defined?
2. Did the population from which the rule was derived include an appropriate spectrum of patients?
3. Was the rule validated in a different group of patients?
4. Were the predictor variables and the outcome evaluated in a blinded fashion?
5. Were the predictor variables and the outcome evaluated in the whole sample selected initially?
6. Are the statistical methods used to construct and validate the rule clearly described?
7. Can the performance of the rule be calculated?
8. How precise are the results?

---

paper. The third question—Was the rule validated in a different group of patients?—assists in determining the level of evaluation of the clinical prediction rule—that is, whether it is a study of the development of the clinical prediction rule, or a validation study assessing the performance of the rule in a population other than that in which it was developed. If these screening criteria are not met, further assessment of potential bias may not be warranted. If you find a study of the impact of a clinical prediction rule, you may need to use a different appraisal checklist depending on the design of the impact study. The CASP checklist we saw in Chapter 4 would be suitable to appraise a randomised controlled trial of the impact of a clinical prediction rule. If you have located a systematic review of clinical prediction rules, appraise the study using the checklist for systematic reviews presented in Chapter 12.

SUMMARY

- The diagnostic accuracy of a test is best assessed by a study of the test against a 'gold-standard' reference test in a consecutive series of patients presenting with a clinical problem.
- The accuracy of single tests (for example, an X-ray) or combinations of tests (for example, clinical examination which usually incorporates information from the patient's history and physical examination) can be assessed.
- Some of the main risks of bias in a diagnostic accuracy study are: (1) only a selected portion of the patients who receive the index test also receive the reference test (a form of *verification bias*); (2) the study does not include patients with the whole spectrum of the condition

that would be seen in clinical practice (*spectrum bias*); (3) not all patients suspected of having the condition are included in the study consecutively or via a process of random selection (*selection bias*); (4) when the results of the test and reference standard are not interpreted independently from the other test or blinded to the results of the other test (*review bias*); and (5) when the test of interest is part of the reference standard (*incorporation bias*).

- The most common methods for reporting the results of a diagnostic accuracy study are the sensitivity and specificity of a test. However, the most useful results for a health professional are the post-test probabilities

Continued

SUMMARY—cont'd

of a positive and a negative test, or the positive and negative likelihood ratios.

- Along with the assessment of the risk of bias in a diagnostic accuracy test, it is also necessary to think how the results may be affected by the setting of the study and the types of patients included in it.
- Using the results of a diagnostic accuracy study can help you to decide whether the test is useful at ruling in or ruling out the diagnosis, or both.

- Tests are also used for assessing and/or monitoring patients, and studies reporting about tests used for this purpose should also be critically appraised.
- Diagnostic clinical prediction rules can be used to assist you during the process of making a diagnosis. Studies of diagnostic clinical prediction rules should be appraised to determine their readiness for clinical use.

REFERENCES

1. Bossuyt PMM. Chapter 3: Understanding the designs of test accuracy studies. In: Deeks JJ, Bossuyt PMM, Leeflant MMG, et al., editors. Cochrane handbook for systematic reviews of diagnostic test accuracy. Draft version for Version 2 (Oct 2022); 2022. Online. Available: https://methods.cochrane.org/sdt/handbook-dta-reviews.
2. Rutjes A, Reitsma J, Di Nisio M, et al. Evidence of bias and variation in diagnostic accuracy studies. CMAJ 2006;1744:469–76.
3. Bossuyt PM, Irwig L, Craig J, et al. Comparative accuracy: assessing new tests against existing diagnostic pathways. BMJ 2006;332(7549):1089–92. doi: 10.1136/bmj.332.7549.1089. Erratum in: BMJ 2006;332(7554):1368.
4. Leeflang MM, Davenport C, Bossuyt PM. Chapter 5: Defining the review question. In: Deeks JJ, Bossuyt PM, Leeflang MM, et al., editors. Cochrane handbook for systematic reviews of diagnostic test accuracy. Draft version for Version 2 (Oct 2022); 2022. Online. Available: https://methods.cochrane.org/sdt/handbookdta-reviews.
5. Doust JA, Bell KJL, Leeflang MMG, et al. Guidance for the design and reporting of studies evaluating the clinical performance of tests for present or past SARS-CoV-2 infection. BMJ 2021;372:n568. doi: 10.1136/bmj.n568.
6. Montalvo Villalba MC, Sosa Glaria E, Rodriguez Lay L, et al. Performance evaluation of Elecsys SARS-CoV-2 Antigen immunoassay for diagnostic of COVID-19. J Med Virol 2022;94:1001–8. doi:10.1002/jmv.27412.
7. Peat J, Barton B, Elliott E. Statistics workbook for evidence-based healthcare. Chichester, UK: Wiley-Blackwell; 2008.

8. Pewsner D, Battaglia M, Minder C, et al. Ruling a diagnosis in or out with 'SpPIn' and 'SnNOut': a note of caution. BMJ 2004;329:209–13.
9. Deeks J. Using evaluations of diagnostic tests: understanding their limitations and making the most of available evidence. Ann Oncol 1999;10:761–8.
10. Byrt T, Bishop J, Carlin J. Bias, prevalence and kappa. J Clin Epidemiol 1993;46:423–9.
11. Glasziou P, Irwig L, Mant D. Monitoring in chronic disease: a rational approach. BMJ 2005;330(7492):644–8.
12. Bossuyt PM, Reitsma JB, Linnet K, et al. Beyond diagnostic accuracy: the clinical utility of diagnostic tests. Clin Chem 2012;58(12):1636–43.
13. Ferrante di Ruffano L, Hyde CJ, McCaffery KJ, et al. Assessing the value of diagnostic tests: a framework for designing and evaluating trials. BMJ 2012;344:e686.
14. Craig J, Williams G, Jones M, et al. The accuracy of clinical symptoms and signs for the diagnosis of serious bacterial infection in young febrile children: prospective cohort study of 15,781 febrile illnesses. BMJ 2010;340:c1594.
15. Stiell I, Greenberg G, McKnight R, et al. Decision rules for the use of radiography in acute ankle injuries. Refinement and prospective validation. JAMA 1993;269:1127–30.
16. McGinn T. Putting meaning into meaningful use: a roadmap to successful integration of evidence at the point of care. JMIF Med Inform 2016;4(2):e16.
17. Stiell I, Wells G. Methodologic standards for the development of clinical decision rules in emergency medicine. Ann Emerg Med. 1999;33(4):437–47.

Questions about Diagnosis
Examples of Appraisals from Different Health Professions

Loai Albarqouni, Bridget Abell, Sally Bennett, Malcolm Boyle, Kylie Hill, John Pierce, Claire Rickard, Sharon Sanders, Katrina Schmid, Michal Schneider, Adam Vogel, Kylie Williams and Tammy Hoffmann

This chapter accompanies the previous chapter (Chapter 6), where the steps involved in answering a clinical question about diagnosis or assessment were explained. To further help you learn how to appraise the evidence for this type of question, this chapter contains a number of worked examples of questions about diagnosis from a range of health professions. These worked examples follow the same format as those in Chapter 5. (Note that the screening criteria from the relevant CASP checklist are not presented for each example and were considered as part of the step of selecting which article to appraise.) As with the worked examples in Chapter 5, the authors of the worked examples

in this chapter were asked not to choose a systematic review, but instead to find and use the next best available level of evidence to answer the clinical question that is in the worked example. This is because it is easier to learn how to appraise a systematic review of test accuracy studies if you have first learnt how to appraise a primary study about test accuracy. Chapter 12 will help you to learn how to appraise a systematic review. All the other caveats about these worked examples (such as using more than one study prior to deciding about how the evidence might inform practice) that were presented at the beginning of Chapter 5 also apply to the worked examples in this chapter.

◎ OCCUPATIONAL THERAPY EXAMPLE

Clinical scenario

As a new occupational therapist in a busy stroke rehabilitation unit, you are often required to screen patients for cognitive impairments. You have been using the Montreal Cognitive Assessment (MoCA) because it is known to have good sensitivity and modest specificity for identifying cognitive impairment post-stroke. However, you find that it takes about 20 minutes to complete. You wonder about using a briefer version of the MoCA, known as the miniMOCA, and decide to search for research about its accuracy compared with the full MoCA.

Clinical question

For people with cognitive impairment post-stroke, how accurate is the miniMoCA for detecting cognitive impairment?

Search terms and databases used to find the evidence

Database: PubMed—Clinical Queries (with 'diagnosis category' and 'narrow scope' selected).

Search terms: MiniMOCA AND Stroke

Continued

⊚ OCCUPATIONAL THERAPY EXAMPLE—cont'd

This search retrieved only two articles. You repeat the search using the 'broad scope', and the same two articles are returned, with one appearing highly relevant.

Article chosen

Campbell N, Rice D, Friedman L, et al. Screening and facilitating further assessment for cognitive impairment after stroke: application of a shortened Montreal Cognitive Assessment (miniMoCA). Disabil Rehabil 2016;38:601–4.

Structured abstract (adapted from the above)

Although this article examines the miniMoCA against the MoCA—which is what you are interested in—it also includes another gold standard (Cognistat test). You disregard the information about the Cognistat because it is not the test of interest to your clinical question.

Study design: Cross-sectional design, comparing the Montreal Cognitive Assessment with the miniMOCA.

Setting: Stroke rehabilitation inpatient unit in Ontario, Canada.

Participants: 72 people with stroke (51% female, mean age 68 years), with a mean education level of 11 years.

Description of test: The Mini Montreal Cognitive Assessment test (miniMoCA) consists of five of eight MoCA sub-test items (verbal fluency, cube copy, trail making, five-word recall and abstraction) with a maximum possible total score of 10. A cut-off score for detecting cognitive impairment had been set at <7/10.

Reference standard: The full MoCA.

Main results: There was a significant level of agreement between the MoCA and miniMoCA in classifying patients according to cognitive function. The MoCA found that 51% of participants had cognitive impairment. The miniMoCA had a sensitivity of 93% and specificity of 92% to abnormal MoCA scores (<26).

Conclusion: The miniMoCA provides good prediction for abnormal full MoCA scores. Further research is needed to determine the accuracy of the miniMoCA against a neuropsychological test.

Is the evidence likely to be biased?

- *Did all participants get the diagnostic test and the reference standard?*

  Yes. Each patient was screened for cognitive deficits using the MoCA. The miniMOCA score was derived from the full MOCA score.

- *Could the results of the test of interest have been influenced by the results of the reference standard, or vice versa?*

  Yes. Although the MoCA was administered to patients during two separate sessions by an occupational therapist and trained student investigator, since the miniMOCA score was derived from the full MOCA score, the result of the miniMOCA might have been influenced by the full MOCA. That is, doing the miniMOCA separately might have derived a different result.

- *Was there a clear description of the disease status of the tested population?*

  Unclear. Some participant characteristics were well described. However, time since stroke and severity of stroke were not reported.

- *Was there sufficient description of the methods for performing the test?*

  Yes. The cut-off points are described. The specific sub-tests of the MOCA used in the miniMOCA were identified.

What are the main results?

You focus on the comparison between the miniMOCA and the results of the full MOCA (which has already been shown in previous research to have high levels of sensitivity for identifying cognitive impairment post-stroke). Against the full MOCA, the miniMOCA had a high sensitivity (93%), meaning that the test was good at detecting cognitive impairment, and a high specificity (92%), which means that it was good at detecting true negatives (people without cognitive impairment) (see Table 7.1).

The post-test probability of a positive test was 98%. This is the same as saying that out of 100 people who

TABLE 7.1   Summary of the test accuracy of the miniMoCA compared to the full MoCA

Test	Sensitivity	Specificity	POST-TEST PROBABILITY FOR A		Positive Likelihood Ratio	Negative Likelihood Ratio
			Positive Test	**Negative Test**		
MiniMoCA	93%	92%	98%	75%	11.6	0.076

test as positive (in this case, as having a cognitive impairment) by the miniMOCA, two would be false positive. Similarly, using the post-test probability of a negative test, the chance of a person with stroke actually *not* having cognitive impairment with a negative test is 75%. This is the same as saying that out of 100 people who test negative by the miniMOCA, 25 would be false (that is, they actually would have cognitive impairment if tested by the MOCA).

As you saw in Chapter 6, two things contribute to the post-test probabilities: the *quality of the test* (how well it performs as described by the sensitivity and specificity); and the *prevalence of the disorders*, so you would need to obtain data about the prevalence of post-stroke cognitive impairment in a rehabilitation setting.

Another way to deal with this is to look at likelihood ratios, which enable us to not have to rely on prevalence to describe the usefulness of a test, yet also to employ both sensitivity and specificity. The positive likelihood ratio is the likelihood of a positive test result in a person with the condition compared with the same likelihood in one without the condition. In this study, the positive likelihood ratio is 11.6 (calculated as sensitivity ÷ [100 − specificity]). Using the approximate guide values that were presented in Chapter 6, a positive likelihood ratio over 10 indicates that the MiniMOCA is extremely good for ruling in the presence of cognitive impairment if it is present. The negative likelihood ratio was 0.07 (calculated as [100 − sensitivity] ÷ specificity), which, again using the values in Chapter 6, indicates that it is a test that can also help rule out the presence of cognitive impairment.

How might we use this evidence to inform practice?
Your main concern about risk of bias in this study is that the accuracy of the miniMOCA was evaluated against the full MOCA, rather than against a gold-standard neuropsychological test. Although the brevity of the miniMOCA is appealing, comparison with a more comprehensive neuropsychological examination is needed to confirm the accuracy of the miniMOCA.

You think back to your original dilemma. Can you use the miniMOCA for identifying cognitive impairment in people who have had a stroke? The study focused on people with stroke who were inpatients of a stroke rehabilitation unit, so the results from this study could be applied to some of the patients you work with. However, the study did exclude those with aphasia and dysphasia, as well as those with severe hearing or visual impairments, so the miniMOCA could not reasonably be used with this sub-group. However, you are not really confident of the accuracy of the miniMOCA because of the weak post-test probability of a negative test (75%), which means that 25% of patients with a negative test will have missed cognitive impairment. You decide to continue using the full MOCA.

◎ PHYSIOTHERAPY EXAMPLE

Clinical scenario
A 57-year-old male who works as a plumber attends your outpatient clinic to manage shoulder pain and weakness in his dominant arm. The onset of pain was gradual and he first noticed it after lifting heavy machinery at work about 2 months ago. He has noticed increased pain and weakness during overhead arm activity over the past 2 weeks. He is now experiencing pain at night when lying on the affected shoulder. This history and the location of the pain make you suspect an injury to the rotator cuff, particularly the supraspinatus tendon. You are aware of two manual tests that identify injury to the supraspinatus tendon—the 'empty-can' and the 'full-can'—but you wonder if they have a similar level of diagnostic accuracy.

Clinical question
In middle-aged men, what is the diagnostic accuracy of the 'empty-can' test versus the 'full-can' test at identifying supraspinatus tendon injury?

Search terms and databases used to find the evidence
Database: DiTA (diagnostic test accuracy): https://dita.org.au/. This is a free database that includes tests of diagnostic accuracy that are likely to be relevant to physiotherapy practice.
Search terms: Subdiscipline: musculoskeletal; Type of index test: physical examination; Name of index test: empty can; Type of reference test: surgery; Method: primary study.

Continued

⊚ PHYSIOTHERAPY EXAMPLE—cont'd

The search returns 10 records. One of these articles looks promising as it describes the use of both the 'empty-can' and the 'full-can' tests to identify supraspinatus tendon tears. The accuracy of these tests was established using a robust gold standard—direct arthroscopic visualisation. It looks highly relevant, but you are concerned that your search is too narrow and may have missed something. You subsequently undertake a search of PubMed—Clinical Queries (with 'diagnosis category' and 'broad scope' selected) using search terms 'supraspinatus' AND 'empty can'. This returns 28 records. You scan these records and notice the same article identified in the DiTA search.

Article chosen

Ackmann J, Schneider KN, Schorn D, et al. Comparison of efficacy of supraspinatus tendon tears diagnostic tests: a prospective study on the 'full-can', the 'empty-can' and the 'Whipple' tests. Musculoskelet Surg 2021;105:149–53.

Structured abstract (adapted from above)

Study design: Prospective single-centre cohort.
Setting: University Hospital in Munster, Germany.
Participants: 61 adults (mean age 60.2 years) presenting for arthroscopic shoulder surgery for suspected rotator cuff tears based on physical examination and MRI scan findings. Exclusion criteria comprised any history of shoulder surgery or adhesive capsulitis.
Description of tests: *Empty-can:* in a standing position, the patient is required to hold their shoulder near 90 degrees flexion, 20 degrees of horizontal abduction and full internal rotation (the thumb is pointing towards the ground). *Full-can:* in a standing position, the patient is required to hold their shoulder near 90 degrees flexion, 20 degrees of horizontal abduction without full internal rotation (the thumb is pointing towards the ceiling). For both tests, the patient is required to resist a downward force applied by the examiner. For both tests, a positive result is recorded if it produces pain in the shoulder and/ or was weaker against the downward force when compared with the contralateral arm.
Reference standard: Shoulder arthroscopy.
Main results: Data were available on 61 participants. Arthroscopic examination showed full- or partial-thickness supraspinatus tendon tears in 44 participants (46%). The empty-can test had a sensitivity of 89% and a specificity of 59% to detect a full- or partial-thickness supraspinatus tendon tear. The positive predictive value was 0.85 and the negative predictive value was 0.67. The full-can test

had a sensitivity of 75% and a specificity of 47% to detect a full- or partial-thickness supraspinatus tendon tear. The positive predictive value was 0.79 and the negative predictive value was 0.42. The 95% confidence intervals for these values were not reported.
Conclusion: Both tests had better sensitivity than specificity. The empty-can test appears to be more accurate than the full-can test when identifying full- or partial-thickness supraspinatus tendon tears in people seeking treatment for shoulder dysfunction.

Is the evidence likely to be biased?

- *Did all participants get the diagnostic test and the reference standard?*
  Yes. All 61 participants were examined using both manual tests before undergoing shoulder arthroscopy.
- *Could the results of the test of interest have been influenced by the results of the reference standard, or vice versa?*
  Unclear. Although the manual tests were performed on the day before the arthroscopy, it is not clear if the examiner who recorded the results of the shoulder arthroscopy was blinded to the results of the manual tests. The examiner who assessed the indication for surgery was the examiner who performed the manual tests. It is not reported whether the order of the manual tests was randomised.
- *Was there a clear description of the disease status of the tested population?*
  Yes. There is detailed information regarding inclusion and exclusion criteria for this study.
- *Was there sufficient description of the methods for performing the test?*
  Probably. The description of the tests was a little confusing, but these tests are generally well known by physiotherapists.

What are the main results?

In this sample, 44 (46%) participants had a full- or partial-thickness supraspinatus tendon tear. The article reports the sensitivity, specificity, positive predictive value and negative predictive value of both tests. The positive predictive value (that is, post-test probability of a positive test) for the 'empty-can' and 'full-can' tests were 85% and 79%, respectively. This indicates that, on average, 85% of people with a positive test empty-can test and 79% of people with a positive full-can test result will actually have a full- or partial-thickness supraspinatus tendon tear. The negative predictive value (that is, post-test probability of a negative test) for the empty-can and full-can tests were 67% and 42%, respectively. This indicates that, on average, 67% of people with a negative empty-can test and 42% of people with a negative full-can test will actually have no tear of their supraspinatus tendon.

Using the data presented in the article and following the method presented in Chapter 6, for the empty-can test, the positive and negative likelihood ratio were calculated to be 2.17 and 0.19, respectively. Using the data presented in the article, for the full-can test, the positive and negative likelihood ratio were calculated to be 1.42 and 0.53, respectively. Using the rough guide that is presented in Chapter 6, a positive likelihood ratio of >2 indicates that a positive test result is helpful at ruling in the condition. This is because the test result has a high true positive rate and a low false positive rate. The negative likelihood ratio of <0.5 indicates that a negative test result is helpful at ruling out the condition. This is because this test has a low false negative rate and a high true negative rate.

How might we use this evidence to inform practice?
You judge the study to be at low risk of bias and the results to be clinically useful. The study population is reasonably similar to the patient in whom you are considering applying the test (although your patient has not had any investigation of his shoulder pain to date, so he might be at lower risk of supraspinatus tear). Both tests can be performed quickly and easily, without any specialised equipment. You decide to perform the empty-can test described in this article and use the results to help inform the diagnosis and subsequent management plan.

◎ PODIATRY EXAMPLE

Clinical scenario
You are a podiatrist who has just started working in a major urban hospital high-risk foot service. As part of an interdisciplinary team, you perform neurovascular assessments in people at risk of foot complications, with the aim of preventing or reducing the impact of foot ulcerations. The ankle-brachial pressure index (ABPI) is one of the tests conducted to determine the presence of peripheral arterial disease (PAD). Obtained by comparing systolic blood pressure measured at the ankle with blood pressure measured in the arm, the test informs of the patency of the large arteries supplying blood to the foot. You know that many of the people attending the service have diabetes. You also recall from university that diabetes can stiffen the blood vessel walls, preventing vessel compression. This may affect the pressure measurements taken and used to calculate the ABPI. You begin to wonder about the accuracy of the ABPI for detecting peripheral arterial disease in people with diabetes.

Clinical question
For people with diabetes, how accurate is the ankle-brachial pressure index (ABPI) for detecting peripheral arterial disease (PAD)?

Search terms and databases used to find the evidence
Database: PubMed—Clinical Queries (with 'diagnosis category' and 'narrow scope' selected).

Search terms: (ankle brachial pressure index) AND diabetes
The search retrieves 117 articles. You scan through the first five shown and find two articles that look relevant. The first is a systematic review of point-of-care tests (including ABPI), used for the detection of peripheral arterial disease in people with diabetes. The second is a recent study reporting the diagnostic accuracy of a novel test for the detection of PAD also in people with diabetes. As well as evaluating the accuracy of a new novel test, this study also considers the accuracy of common currently used tests to detect PAD, including the ABPI. As explained in this chapter's introduction, as the chapter's focus is learning how to appraise primary studies, you choose the primary study to appraise (and will consider its findings in conjunction with the systematic review).

Article chosen
Normahani P, Poushpas S, Alaa M, et al. Diagnostic accuracy of point-of-care tests used to detect arterial disease in diabetes: Testing for Arterial disease in Diabetes (TrEAD) study. Ann Surg 2022 Nov 1;276(5):e605–12.

Structured abstract (adapted from the above)
Although this article is primarily interested in the performance of a novel test (the podiatry ankle duplex scan [PAD scan]), commonly used bedside tests for the detection of PAD such as the ABPI, the toe-brachial pressure

Continued

⦿ PODIATRY EXAMPLE—cont'd

index, transcutaneous pressure of oxygen, pulse palpation, and audible and visual ultrasound waveform assessment were also assessed. You focus your attention on the performance of the ABPI.

Study design: Cross-sectional design comparing the ABPI (and other tests) with full lower limb arterial duplex ultrasound.

Setting: Two diabetic foot clinics in the United Kingdom.

Participants: 305 adults with a known history of diabetes (median age 72 years). Two-thirds had evidence of peripheral neuropathy and 40% had an active foot ulceration. The mean duration of diabetes was 17 years.

Description of test: The ABPI is calculated using systolic blood pressure measurements taken at the ankle and arm. Using a sphygmomanometer cuff at the ankle and a handheld audible Doppler device, dorsalis pedis and posterior tibial artery systolic pressure were determined. Brachial artery pressures from both arms were taken and the highest reading was used to calculate the ABPI. The ABPI was calculated using the equation: ankle systolic pressure/brachial systolic pressure. Cut-off values for detecting PAD were set at ≤0.9 (primary cut-off) for either dorsalis pedis or posterior tibial vessels and at ≤0.9 or >1.3 (as a secondary cut-off) in either vessel.

Reference standard: Full lower limb Doppler ultrasound.

Main results: Two-thirds (66%) of participants had PAD by the full lower limb duplex ultrasound (reference test). ABPI (at cut-off ≤0.9) had a sensitivity of 60% and a specificity of 75%. The ABPI could not be determined for 25% of participants because the foot vessels could not be compressed.

Conclusion: ABPI performed poorly for the detection of PAD in people with diabetes. A high number of indeterminate results further limits the utility of this test in clinical practice.

Is the evidence likely to be biased?

- *Did all participants get the diagnostic test and the reference standard?*
  Yes. Each participant had the ABPI performed and underwent the reference test in the same day.
- *Could the results of the test of interest have been influenced by the results of the reference standard, or vice versa?*
  No. Two vascular scientists performed the index and reference tests. For each participant, a different scientist performed the index and reference test. The scientists were blinded to the findings of the other.

- *Was there a clear description of the disease status of the tested population?*
  Yes. Participants are clearly described as having a known history of diabetes. The type and duration of diabetes are reported, as is the occurrence of diabetic complications (for example, retinopathy, chronic kidney disease, amputations). The study was performed in settings similar to where the test will be used and participants were a consecutive sample of people attending the study clinics.
- *Were the methods for performing the test described in sufficient detail?*
  No. The method of performing the ABPI is clearly described (in supplemental material) and the cut-offs used to detect PAD are stated. However, participant positioning and preparation are not described. The test was performed by experienced vascular scientists who may be more skilled and possibly obtain more reproducible measures than less experienced and trained clinicians.

What are the main results?

Based on the reference test, two-thirds (66%) of participants had PAD. Table 7.2 shows the results of the index test cross classified with the reference test for both the primary and secondary cut-off values.

Against the reference test, full lower limb arterial Doppler ultrasound, ABPI (using the primary cut-off ≤0.9) had a sensitivity of only 60% (95% CI 53 to 67), meaning many cases of PAD were missed. Specificity was 75% (95% CI 66 to 83), meaning that quite a number of people who do not actually have PAD will be found to have PAD with the ABPI (they are false positives). Sensitivity was slightly improved with the cut-off ≤0.9 or >1.3, but this was at the expense of specificity which was only 49%.

The post-test probabilities presented in Table 7.2 tell us how likely it is a person has PAD based on the test result and prevalence of the disease within the study population. The post-test probability of a positive test is the same as the positive predictive value (PPV) and the post-test probability of a negative result is the complement of the negative predictive value (NPV) (100-NPV), as was explained in Chapter 6. In this population of people attending diabetic foot clinics (where the prevalence of PAD is 66%), the probability of actually having PAD when the ABPI (using the ≤0.9 cut-off) is positive is 83%. When the ABPI test is negative, the probability that a person will not

TABLE 7.2 **Comparing ABPI with primary study cut-off (≤0.9) and secondary study cut off (≤0.9 or >1.3)**

		PAD		Total			PAD		Total
		+	−				+	−	
ABPI (cut-off	+	118	25	143	ABPI (cut-off	+	143	52	195
≤0.9)	−	78	77	155	≤0.9 or >1.3)	−	53	50	103
		196	102	298			196	102	298

ABPI (cut-off ≤0.9)
Sensitivity = 60%
Specificity = 75%
Post-test probability of:
    a positive test = 83%
    a negative test = 50% (i.e. 100 − NPV)

ABPI (cut-off ≤0.9 or >1.3)
Sensitivity = 73%
Specificity = 49%
Post-test probability of:
    a positive test = 73%
    a negative test = 51% (i.e. 100 − NPV)

have PAD is 50%. In other words, out of 100 people who have a negative ABPI, 50 would be a false negative—they would be shown to actually have PAD if tested by the reference standard.

For one-quarter (25.3%) of ABPI tests performed, a result could not be determined. This was due to incompressible vessels or absent Doppler signal.

How might we use this evidence to inform practice?

You are satisfied that the study is valid and that the results are useful. Further, the study population is similar to the people you expect to see in your high-risk foot clinic. Based on the results of this study, you do not think the ABPI test is particularly helpful for detecting PAD in people with diabetes. The low sensitivity means that many cases of PAD will be missed if ABPI is the only test used.

After appraising the systematic review of the accuracy of ABPI for detecting PAD in people with diabetes, you learn the results are similar. This systematic review, which does not include the recent study discussed above (as the review searched for studies prior to its publication), found that ABPI generally had low sensitivity against a range of reference standards, with the review authors concluding the test has limited effectiveness for the detection of PAD in people with diabetes.

You return to your original article to consider the performance of other tests for detecting PAD that were evaluated. You note the much higher sensitivity, reasonable specificity and absence of indeterminate results with the novel PAD scan test and decide to look into this further to discuss with your colleagues later. For the time being, you will use the ABPI as part of the suite of tests you are required to perform during your assessment, keeping in mind what you have learnt.

◎ SPEECH PATHOLOGY EXAMPLE

Clinical scenario

You are a speech pathologist working in an outpatient movement disorders clinic. You are treating Mr Bruce, who was referred to the program by a neurologist. Mr Bruce has a provisional diagnosis of Parkinson's disease. In the weekly team meeting, the physiotherapist described some concerns, reporting that Mr Bruce was progressing rapidly for someone who has only been symptomatic for a year. The patient had also described worsening of symptoms over the last 3 months. Your assessment found that Mr Bruce presented with a mild–moderate rough voice, moderately reduced loudness, slightly slowed articulation rate and masked face. He was also dysfluent and presented with syllable repetition at

Continued

◎ SPEECH PATHOLOGY EXAMPLE—cont'd

the beginning of an utterance. Severity varied, with up to ten repetitions. You and the physiotherapist wondered whether Mr Bruce might have an atypical parkinsonian syndrome (for example, progressive supranuclear palsy [PSP] or multiple system atrophy [MSA]) rather than Parkinson's disease. You both plan to provide your opinion to the neurologist for consideration, but prior to this, you are unsure whether dysarthria differs between Parkinson's disease and atypical parkinsonism.

Clinical question

Is speech presentation sensitive in differentiating atypical parkinsonism from Parkinson's disease?

Search terms and databases used to find the evidence

Database: PubMed—Clinical Queries (with 'diagnosis category' and 'broad scope' selected).
Search terms: ((speech) AND (atypical parkinsonism)) AND (parkinson's) AND (differential diagnosis)

The search identified 15 studies. Two of the articles relate specifically to speech, but one requires acoustic analysis software that you do not have in your clinic.

Article chosen

Rusz J, Bonnet C, Klempíř J, et al. Speech disorders reflect differing pathophysiology in Parkinson's disease, progressive supranuclear palsy and multiple system atrophy. J Neurol 2015;262:992–1001.

Structured abstract (adapted from the above)

Study design: Prospective cross-sectional study.
Setting: Laboratory testing.
Participants: 77 participants consisting of 40 consecutive patients: 12 with a diagnosis of probable PSP (ten men, two women); 13 with a diagnosis of probable MSA (six men, seven women); 15 with Parkinson's disease (nine men, six women) matched to the PSP and MSA groups by disease duration (based on self-report of onset) and 37 healthy controls (21 men, 16 women) matched by age.
Description of tests: Participants completed three speech tasks: a 90-second monologue, sustained phonation of /a/ and sequential motion rates (SMR; that is, /pataka/). Sixteen acoustic dimensions were measured using purpose-built scripts. Features were selected based on their sensitivity to ataxic, hypokinetic and spastic dysarthria subtypes. To calculate the type and severity of dysarthria, dimensions were first compared to the normal

range of healthy controls—any measurements in the top or bottom 5% of controls were considered abnormal. Different combinations of dimensions were then weighted to develop scores out of 100 for spastic, hypokinetic and ataxic dysarthria. Finally, the sensitivity and specificity of each dimension within diagnosis groups were calculated.
Reference standard: Formal diagnostic criteria were applied and further confirmed by two expert neurologists.
Main results: Dysarthria was present in all participants with parkinsonism. Speech deficits were more severe in patients with PSP and MSA than those with Parkinson's disease. Participants with Parkinson's disease presented with pure hypokinetic dysarthria. Participants with MSA were more likely to have hypokinetic and ataxic dysarthria. Participants with PSP were more likely to present with hypokinetic and spastic dysarthria. In those with PSP, dysfluency, slow rate, inappropriate silences, vowel distortions and harsh voice quality were common features. In those with MSA, pitch fluctuations, excess loudness variation, prolonged phonemes, vocal tremor and strained–strangled voice quality were more common.
Conclusion: The speech dimensions explored in this study were highly sensitive (75–95%) to underlying aetiology.

Is the evidence likely to be biased?

- *Did all participants get the diagnostic test and the reference standard?*
  Unclear. Although it appears that all participants received the diagnostic test and the reference standard, there is no explicit reporting about this, nor if there were any missing data.
- *Could the results of the test of interest have been influenced by the results of the reference standard, or vice versa?*
  Unclear. The dimensions measured in this study were acoustic, with a clear and mostly objective method for calculating each feature using validated software. However, the analysis was not fully automated, introducing the potential for bias. For example, dysfluencies require manual identification and categorisation. Regarding the reference standard, atypical parkinsonian syndromes are difficult to diagnose and often require post-mortem confirmation. This prospective study involved living participants, making definitive diagnosis challenging, so the reference standard was appropriate. However, blinding is not mentioned, so the assessors may have been privy to the diagnosis of participants. Two neurologists

confirmed the initial diagnosis using disease-specific consensus-based criteria. It is not stated whether the neurologists were blinded to the other's conclusions and whether this confirmation was made independently. There is no comment about the order in which the diagnosis and speech assessments occurred.

- *Was there a clear description of the disease status of the tested population?*

  Yes. The article provides a clear description of participant characteristics, including scores for speech, and disease features derived from standardised rating scales.

- *Was there sufficient description of the methods for performing the test?*

  Yes. The method of recording the speech samples was clearly described, although it is not clear if the monologue topic was the same between each participant (semantic or emotional differences can alter aspects of speech production such as timing). The article's supplementary material describes the analysis of samples in sufficient detail to replicate procedures.

What are the main results?

The group with Parkinson's disease presented with milder dysarthria and with hypokinetic features only. In contrast, participants with PSP or MSA presented with more severe dysarthria (relative to symptom duration—that is, faster progression) and features of spastic and/or ataxic dysarthria. The combination of six acoustic features that measured five speech dimensions differentiated Parkinson's disease from atypical parkinsonian syndromes with 93.4% sensitivity and 99.5% specificity. These dimensions are listed in Table 7.3.

Dysfluency was the only feature that significantly (Cohen's $d = 1.06$, $p < 0.05$) differentiated MSA from PSP in isolation. Four speech dimensions taken together (see Table 7.3) could differentiate MSA from PSP with 74.3% sensitivity and 81.2% specificity. Considering overall dysarthria profiles, participants with MSA commonly presented with either ataxic dysarthria (43%) or ataxic and spastic/hypokinetic (15%). Participants with PSP typically presented with hypokinetic, spastic or mixed hypokinetic–spastic dysarthria (83%). However, these summary labels appear less accurate than considering individual features.

How might we use the evidence to inform practice?

This study appears to be at low risk of bias, except for some concerns about blinding, and while its sample size is small, PSP and MSA are uncommon diseases, making this study one of the larger cohorts in these disease groups. In patients with suspected atypical parkinsonism, there are two diagnostic questions important for a speech pathologist: (1) Is the patient's speech consistent with idiopathic (that is, 'typical') Parkinson's disease or with atypical parkinsonism? (2) If atypical, does this patient present with features to suggest a specific atypical parkinsonian syndrome?

For the first question, you are now aware that more severe dysarthria relative to symptom onset and features of ataxic or spastic dysarthria suggest a diagnosis of an atypical parkinsonian syndrome. A patient with pure hypokinetic dysarthria and a gradual progression may be more likely to have Parkinson's disease.

To differentiate the atypical parkinsonian syndrome (PSP and MSA), PSP appears more likely to present with

TABLE 7.3   **Features that may assist in differential diagnosis of Parkinson's disease and atypical parkinsonian syndromes**

Features that may differentiate Parkinson's disease from atypical parkinsonian syndromes	Features that may differentiate between two atypical parkinsonian syndromes (PSP and MSA)
Harsh voice (jitter)	Harsh voice (harmonics to noise ratio)
Inappropriate silences (% pause time, no. of pauses)	Fluency (% dysfluent words)
Slow AMR (syllables/sec)	Slow rate (articulation rate)
Excess loudness variation (intensity variation)	Vocal tremor (frequency tremor intensity index)
Excess pitch fluctuation (pitch variation)	

Continued

◎ SPEECH PATHOLOGY EXAMPLE—cont'd

hypokinetic and/or spastic dysarthria and MSA appears more likely to present with ataxic ± spastic or hypokinetic dysarthria. Mr Bruce's slow rate of speech and relatively rapid progression in only 12 months supports the opinion that he could have an atypical parkinsonian syndrome. His significant dysfluency makes you think that PSP is the most likely diagnosis.

You think it could be worthwhile learning some of the acoustic measurements from this article as the software used is free and was more accurate than the dysarthria subtype labels. While you cannot diagnose the neurological disease of Mr Bruce, nor of other patients, you report your findings from the speech assessment to the neurologist.

◎ MEDICINE EXAMPLE

Clinical scenario

You are an emergency physician working in the emergency department of an urban university hospital. A 63-year-old woman with a history of high blood pressure and a previous myocardial infarction presents to the emergency department with a 3-day history of worsening shortness of breath at rest, orthopnoea and paroxysmal nocturnal dyspnoea. She also reports mild fatigue, increased urinary frequency and leg swelling. Physical examination reveals bilateral basal lung fine crepitations (or rales) and bilateral pedal oedema up to her knees. The clinical presentation make you suspect that she has symptoms suggestive of acute heart failure. At a recent conference, you heard a presentation suggesting that a blood test (B-type natriuretic peptides [BNP]) is a useful test for diagnosing patients with suspected acute heart failure. You are unsure about the diagnostic performance of this test and decide to search for research studies examining the diagnostic accuracy of BNP, or N-terminal pro-B-type natriuretic peptide (NT-proBNP), in identifying patients with acute heart failure.

Clinical question

For adult patients who present to the emergency department with symptoms suggestive of acute heart failure, how accurate is BNP or NT-proBNP for diagnosing acute heart failure, compared to standard clinical assessment?

Search terms and databases used to find the evidence

Database: PubMed—Clinical Queries (with 'diagnosis category' and 'narrow scope' selected).
Search terms: (("natriuretic peptide" OR "NT-proBNP" OR "BNP") AND "emergency department" AND "acute heart failure")

This search yielded 23 citations. The first is the most relevant and recent article; checking the title and abstract of the other citations showed that they were evaluating other diagnostic modalities (for example, ultrasound), different question types (for example, prediction model studies) or specific patient sub-groups (such as patients with previous obstructive airway disease).

Article chosen

Januzzi JL Jr, Chen-Tournoux AA, Christenson RH, et al. N-terminal pro-B-type natriuretic peptide in the emergency department: the ICON-RELOADED study. J Am Coll Cardiol 2018;71(11):1191–200.

Structured abstract (adapted from the above)

Study design: Prospective multi-centre cohort study.
Setting: Emergency departments of 19 sites in the United States and Canada.
Participants: 1,461 patients presenting to emergency with dyspnoea (49% women, mean age 56.4 years, 37% African American, 63% had hypertension, 25% with previous history of heart failure, and 13% had a previous history of myocardial infarction). Patients with severe renal insufficiency, dyspnoea secondary to chest trauma, pregnancy or unable to cooperate were excluded.
Description of test: N-terminal pro-B-type natriuretic peptide (NT-proBNP)—a blood sample was taken from each patient at enrolment and analysed using a cobase 601 analyser (Roche Diagnostics). Age-stratified cut-offs of 450, 900 and 1,800 pg/mL were used for diagnosis of acute heart failure among patients <50, 50–75 and >75 years old, respectively. The rule-out cut-off value used for the exclusion of acute heart failure is 300 pg/mL—irrespective of the age of patients.

Reference standard: A clinical events adjudication committee (including a minimum of two emergency physicians and a cardiologist), blinded to NT-proBNP results (obtained either by the hospital or by the study), independently reviewed and adjudicated the diagnosis of acute heart failure.

Main results: Of 1,461 included patients, 277 (19%) were adjudicated as having acute heart failure. The median NTproBNP concentration of patients with acute heart failure (2,844 pg/mL; interquartile range [IQR], 1,247 to 5,976) was higher than those without it (98 pg/mL; IQR 35 to 369, $p < 0.001$). ROC curve analysis indicated an AUC of 0.91 (95% CI 0.90 to 0.93). Sensitivity for age-stratified cut-offs of 450, 900 and 1,800 pg/mL was 85.7%, 79.3% and 75.9%, respectively; and the specificity was 93.9%, 84.0% and 75.0%, respectively. The sensitivity for the rule-out cut-off of 300 pg/mL was 93.9%.

Conclusion: An NT-proBNP <300 pg/mL strongly excludes the presence of acute heart failure in patients who present to emergency with acute dyspnoea, while age-stratified NT-proBNP cut-offs may be helpful in the diagnosis of acute heart failure.

Is the evidence likely to be biased?

- *Did all participants get the diagnostic test and the reference standard?*
  Yes. The authors reported that NT-proBNP was measured and the clinical events adjudication committee reviewed and adjudicated the diagnosis of acute heart failure for each enrolled patient.
- *Could the results of the test of interest have been influenced by the results of the reference standard, or vice versa?*
  No. The authors reported that the NT-proBNP was measured at enrolment and the clinical events adjudication committee, blinded to NT-proBNP results, independently reviewed and adjudicated the diagnosis of acute heart failure for each patient.
- *Was there a clear description of the disease status of the tested population?*
  Yes. The authors provided a clear description of the disease status in the main article and the protocol.[1]
- *Was there sufficient description of the method for performing the test?*
  Yes. The method for performing the test was clearly described so that it could be replicated.

TABLE 7.4 A 2 × 2 table of true and false positive and negative results for acute heart failure using serum NT-proBNP

	ACUTE HEART FAILURE		
	+ve	−ve	Total
Age-stratified rule-in cut-offs			
<50 yrs (450 pg/mL)			
Test +ve	30	26	56
Test −ve	5	401	406
Total	35	427	462
50–75 yrs (900 pg/mL)			
Test +ve	146	104	250
Test −ve	38	545	583
Total	184	649	833
>75 yrs (1,800 pg/mL)			
Test +ve	44	27	71
Test −ve	14	81	95
Total	58	108	166
Rule-in, overall			
Test +ve	220	157	377
Test −ve	57	1,027	1,084
Total	277	1,184	1,461
Rule-out (300 pg/mL), overall			
Test +ve	260	335	377
Test −ve	17	849	1,084
Total	277	1,184	1,461

What are the main results?

In this study, 277 (19%) of 1,461 included patients were adjudicated as having acute heart failure. Using data presented in the article, you construct a 2 × 2 table for each age-stratified rule-in cut-offs as well as rule-out cut-offs (see Table 7.4). Using the methods outlined in Chapter 6, you calculate the sensitivity, specificity, positive and negative predictive values, and positive and negative likelihood ratios (see Table 7.5).

Continued

◎ MEDICINE EXAMPLE—cont'd

TABLE 7.5   Comparison of serum NT-proBNP and clinical events adjudication committee for diagnosing acute heart failure

Test	Sensitivity	Specificity	Positive predictive value	Negative predictive value	Positive likelihood ratio	Negative likelihood ratio
Age stratified rule-in cut-offs						
<50 yrs	85.7	93.9	53.6	98.8	14.08	0.15
(450 pg/mL)	(74.1–97.3)	(91.6–96.2)	(43.7–63.2)	(97.3–99.4)	(8.48–19.7)	(0.03–0.28)
50–75 yrs	79.3	84.0	58.4	93.5	4.95	0.25
(900 pg/mL)	(73.5–85.2)	(81.2–86.8)	(53.7–63.0)	(91.5–95.0)	(4.00–5.90)	(0.18–0.32)
>75 yrs	75.9	75.0	62.0	85.3	3.03	0.32
(1,800 pg/mL)	(64.8–86.9)	(66.8–83.2)	(53.3–70.0)	(78.4–90.2)	(1.94–4.13)	(0.17–0.47)
Rule-in, overall	79.4	86.7	58.4	94.7	5.99	0.24
	(74.7–84.2)	(84.8–88.7)	(54.5–62.1)	(93.5–95.8)	(5.05–6.93)	(0.18–0.29)
Rule-out	93.9	71.7	43.7	98.0	3.32	0.09
(300 pg/mL), overall	(91.0–96.7)	(69.1–74.3)	(41.4–46.1)	(96.9–98.8)	(3.00–3.63)	(0.05–0.13)

How might we use this evidence to inform practice?
This is a well-conducted diagnostic accuracy study that you assess to be at minimal risk of bias. While the clinical events adjudication committee was a reasonable reference standard, it is worth noting that it is not a true, objective criterion. The study demonstrated that serum NT-proBNP might be useful in identifying patients with acute heart failure in emergency departments, with a positive predictive value of 58.4% and a positive likelihood ratio of 6. However, the high negative predictive value (98%) of a normal-level NT-proBNP and negative likelihood ratio of 0.09 indicate that the test is more powerful for ruling out acute heart failure in patients suspected of it in emergency departments.

◎ NURSING EXAMPLE

Clinical scenario
You are a nurse who works in an intensive care unit (ICU) of a large tertiary hospital. Many of the patients you care for require the placement of a central venous catheter (CVC) into a large vein for invasive monitoring and administration of medications such as inotropes, as well as blood and fluids. CVC insertions are performed using equipment that monitors electrocardiographic (ECG) status, with amplitude changes in the P-wave on the ECG used to guide correct positioning of the CVC tip. Because it is unsafe to use a CVC if the tip is not in the correct place, your unit's practice is to request the radiography department to visit the ICU and take a chest X-ray. Use of the CVC for therapy is postponed until the X-ray results show the tip is correctly positioned. This means typically 1–2 hours' delay in starting treatment.

You wonder whether the amplitude changes in the P-wave of intra-cavity electrocardiography are adequate in assessing correct tip location of CVCs without the chest X-ray confirmation.

Clinical question
Among critically ill patients who need a central venous catheter, are amplitude changes in the P-wave of intra-cavity electrocardiography a reliable method to assess correct tip placement of the central venous catheter, in comparison to a chest X-ray?

Search terms and databases used to find the evidence
Database: PubMed—Clinical Queries (with 'diagnosis category' and 'narrow scope' selected).

Search terms: (central venous catheter) AND (*P*-wave) AND X-ray

This search yields two hits. You choose the one that more closely matches your question.

Article chosen

Wang G, Guo L, Jiang B, et al. Factors influencing intra-cavitary electrocardiographic *P*-wave changes during central venous catheter placement. PLOS One 2015; 10(4):e0124846.

Structured abstract (adapted from the above)

Study design: Prospective cohort study.
Setting: Oncology hospital in China.
Participants: 1,160 cancer patients ≥16 years (mean age 54 years, 51% male) with normal sinus rhythm on baseline ECG and needing a central venous catheter (CVC) (peripherally inserted, typically through the arm, or centrally inserted through the internal jugular vein).
Description of test: *P*-wave changes on intra-cavity ECG-guided tip location.
Reference standard: Postero-anterior chest X-ray.
Main results: Compared with X-ray diagnosis of correct CVC tip location, ECG-guided diagnosis had a sensitivity of 97.3%, with a false negative rate of 2.7%. Its specificity was 1, with no false positive cases. Patient characteristics including age, gender, height, body weight and heart rate were not significantly associated with *P*-wave amplitude changes.
Conclusion: Intra-cavity electrocardiography with ultrasound inspection is an accurate method of checking the placement of a central venous catheter tip.

Is this evidence likely to be biased?

- *Did all participants get the diagnostic test and the reference standard?*
  Yes. All participants were assessed by the intra-cavity ECG during CVC placement, and by the gold standard (chest X-ray). Any cases initially malpositioned were corrected during the procedure.
- *Could the results of the test of interest have been influenced by the results of the reference standard, or vice versa?*
  Unclear. It does not state whether the tests results were concealed, so it is possible that the radiologist assessing the X-ray knew about concerns from the inserting team.

- *Was there a clear description of the disease status of the tested population?*
  Yes. Participants were clearly described as adult cancer patients who underwent CVC insertion. Other specific inclusion criteria (such as confirmation of sinus rhythm before the procedure and planned access via PICC, or CICC) and exclusion criteria (for example, patients with a cardiac pacemaker, or unstable base ECG) were also clearly stated.
- *Was there sufficient description of the methods for performing the test?*
  Yes. There was a clear description of a positive tip location on both ECG placement and chest X-ray, materials used, as well as the access team, operational procedures and lead connection for ECG monitoring.

What are the main results?

Tip location results from intra-cavity electrocardiography were compared with the results of X-ray examination. Table 7.6 shows the number of patients with correct tip location diagnosed by each method.

The sensitivity of the intra-cavity ECG method was 97.3% (true positives/[true positives + false negatives] = 1,119/[1,119 + 31] = 0.973).

The specificity was 1. Calculated as: true negatives/[true negatives + false positives] = 10/[10 + 0].

The post-test probability of a positive (correct tip location) identified correctly via the intra-cavity ECG was 1.0. This means that no false positive cases were observed: 100% of patients diagnosed with a correct CVC tip location using intra-cavity ECG were correctly placed.

The post-test negative value was 0.756. Calculated as: false negatives/[false negatives + true negatives] or 31/[31 + 10]. This means that 76% of those diagnosed as having incorrect CVC tip position were actually correctly placed.

TABLE 7.6   Number of patients with correct tip location diagnosed by each method (chest X-ray and ECG)

		Correct by chest X-ray		
		+	−	Total
Correct by chest ECG	+	1,119	0	1,119
	−	31	10	41
Total		1,150	10	1,160

Continued

◎ NURSING EXAMPLE—cont'd

How might we use this evidence to inform practice?
The current practice in your unit is to use the intra-cavity ECG method to guide tip placement during CVC insertion, and then an X-ray procedure to confirm correct placement. It is more important clinically that the ECG 'rules out' incorrectly placed catheter tips (that is, has minimal false positives) than 'rules in' (has minimal false negatives) correctly placed ones. The results of this study, which you appraise as having a low risk of bias, suggest this, and therefore confirmation by chest X-ray appears unnecessary. Not doing this will reduce waiting time for medications, infusions and haemodynamic monitoring (as well as reducing costs, workload for radiology and ICU staff, and exposure to ionising radiation for patients and staff).

One concern is about the generalisability of the results of this study, as it involved cancer patients who typically had normal sinus rhythm, while you work with ICU patients, some of whom may have abnormal ECGs (for example, sinus tachycardia or bradycardia). Nevertheless, you decide to speak to the senior ICU and radiology staff about considering not conducting the confirmatory chest X-ray in eligible patients who have normal ECGs.

◎ MEDICAL IMAGING EXAMPLE

Clinical scenario
The SARS COVID-19 pandemic has, at times, necessitated urgent diagnosis and evaluation of disease severity for patients presenting to emergency departments. Traditionally, patients presenting with respiratory symptoms were referred for a chest computed tomography (CT) to explore the presence of disease. CT has excellent sensitivity and specificity in detecting and stratifying moderate to severe lung disease. However, machine availability, exposure to radiation and costs limit its application, especially during high workloads such as those seen during the pandemic. Lung ultrasound is an alternative imaging tool to assist in the diagnosis of pneumonia associated with COVID-19. It is readily available, not associated with radiation and is relatively cheap to perform. Furthermore, it can be performed at the bedside or wherever required in the hospital. You work in medical imaging in a major metropolitan hospital with a very busy emergency department and are asked about the accuracy of lung ultrasound compared to chest CT for quickly diagnosing COVID-19 pneumonia, as a way of aiding the diagnosis of COVID-19, in an emergency setting.

Clinical question
What is the diagnostic performance of lung ultrasound compared to chest CT, when each is compared to the reference standard for COVID-19, for detecting COVID-19 pneumonia among adults who present to the emergency department with symptoms suggestive of COVID-19?

Search terms and database used to find the evidence
Database: PubMed—Clinical Queries (with 'diagnosis category' and 'narrow search' selected).
Search terms: COVID-19 AND ultrasound AND emergency AND (chest CT OR chest computed tomography)

The search yielded 32 articles. Only one appeared to address your specific question.

Article chosen
Lieveld AWE, Kok B, Schuit FH, et al. Diagnosing COVID-19 pneumonia in a pandemic setting: Lung ultrasound versus CT (LUVCT)—a multicentre, prospective, observational study. ERJ Open Res 2020;6:00539-2020. https://openres.ersjournals.com/content/early/2020/10/08/23120541.00539-2020.

Structured abstract (adapted from the above)
Study design: Prospective, multi-centre study.
Setting: Three academic hospitals in The Netherlands.
Participants: 187 adult patients (mean age 63 years, 58% male) referred to the emergency department with suspected COVID-19 who had interpretable CT and lung ultrasound, and PCR performed, as well as a multidisciplinary team (MDT) diagnosis.
Description of tests: Both the ultrasound and the CT were performed at presentation or within 24 hours of admission. Ultrasound scans were performed using a handheld system. Cases were deemed positive if there were three or more B-lines and/or consolidation in two or more zones unilaterally or in one or more zones bilaterally. The chest CTs were reported by radiologists using the

COVID-19 pneumonia Reporting and Data systems (CO-RADS) to score pre-specified criteria for diagnosis. Equivocal CTs were considered negative for COVID-19.

Reference standard: PCR tests were used as the reference standard according to World Health Organization (WHO) recommendations. PCR tests were performed as per WHO guidelines using an oropharynx or nasopharynx swab. Negative or indeterminate results were repeated. A daily MDT review was performed for all patients and in patients with negative PCR but high clinical suspicion of COVID-19; diagnosis could be made by the MDT (a team comprising consultants in infectious diseases, respiratory disease and microbiology based on clinical, laboratory, microbiological and CT data). No clinical decisions were made based on lung ultrasound as all MDT members were blinded to the ultrasound findings.

Main results: 86 patients (46%) were PCR positive. There were no significant differences in sensitivity and specificity between ultrasound and CT. Agreement between ultrasound and CT was interpreted as substantial (Cohen's kappa = 0.65). When assessed against the reference standard PCR, lung ultrasound had a sensitivity of 92% and a specificity of 71%. Positive and negative likelihood ratios were 3.2 and 0.1, respectively. When assessed against PCR, CT had a sensitivity of 88% and a specificity of 82%. Positive and negative likelihood ratios were 4.9 and 0.1, respectively. When ultrasound was compared to the MDT diagnosis reference standard, sensitivity was 90%, specificity was 80%, and positive and negative likelihood ratios were 4.5 and 0.1, respectively.

Conclusion: The accuracy of lung ultrasound is comparable to chest CT when used to diagnose COVID-19 pneumonia among patients presenting with pulmonary involvement to the emergency department. It may be useful as an extension of the clinical examination, especially in settings where CT or PCR are not readily available.

Is this evidence likely to be biased?

- *Did all the patients get the diagnostic test and the reference standard?*

  Yes. All adults with suspected COVID-19 who were referred to the emergency department for internal medicine were eligible and consenting patients with interpretable CT and lung ultrasound were included. All recruited patients received all three diagnostic tests (PCR, lung ultrasound and chest CT) and MDT assessment; however, it is not clear if consecutive patients were recruited and then had all tests performed, or if the sample was created from an existing group of patients who had had all the tests conducted. All tests were performed within 24 hours of presentation or admission to the hospital.

- *Could the results of the test have been influenced by the results of the reference standard, or vice versa?*

  Unclear, but probably not. The treating doctors and sonographers who performed the lung ultrasound tests were blinded to the CT and PCR results but knew patients' clinical histories. The radiologists who reported on the CT scans were blinded to the ultrasound and PCR results but were aware of clinical histories. The MDT diagnosis was made without knowledge of the ultrasound findings. It was not stated how much time lapsed between the imaging tests and the PCR and in what order these tests were performed. This could have impacted on the PCR results, especially given the large variation in duration of symptoms at the time of presentation (mean days 6.5 ± 5.1).

- *Was there a clear description of the disease status of the tested population?*

  Yes. Comorbidities and demographic characteristics are well documented.

- *Was there sufficient description of the methods for performing the tests?*

  No. The equipment (and manufacturer) was not described for any of the three tests performed (PCR, ultrasound and CT). Further, the protocols for ultrasound and CT were not outlined, although the scanning zones and technique for ultrasound and images and videos showing examples of COVID-19 sonographic features are provided in the supplement. It is not known if the three hospitals used a standardised approach for these tests.

What are the main results?

Table 7.7 presents a summary of the results relevant to this clinical question. When compared to PCR reference standard, the sensitivity of ultrasound was comparable to CT (92% vs 88%). However, the specificity was lower (71% vs 82%). This means that there will be more false positives (people who do not have the disease and who should have tested negative) with ultrasound. Both the ultrasound and the CT had a positive likelihood ratio > 2, indicating they are tests that help rule in the condition, and a negative likelihood ratio around 0.1, which is the cut-off guide used to indicate that a test is good for helping to rule out a condition. When each was compared with PCR, the positive predictive value for ultrasound was not as good as CT (73.2 versus 80.9), with the closer the

Continued

⊚ MEDICAL IMAGING EXAMPLE—cont'd

TABLE 7.7 Summary of diagnostic accuracy results of lung ultrasound and chest CT with each compared to PCR for COVID-19, and lung ultrasound compared with MDT diagnosis

	REFERENCE STANDARD: PCR		REFERENCE STANDARD: MDT COVID-19 DIAGNOSIS*
	Lung ultrasound	CT	Lung ultrasound
Sensitivity % (95% CI)	91.9 (84.0–96.7)	88.4 (79.7–94.3)	90.1 (82.5–95.2)
Specificity % (95% CI)	71.0 (61.1–79.6)	82.0 (73.1–89.0)	80.0 (69.9–87.9)
Positive likelihood ratio (95% CI)	3.2 (2.3–4.3)	4.9 (3.2–7.5)	4.5 (2.9–6.9)
Negative likelihood ratio (95% CI)	0.1 (0.06–0.24)	0.1 (0.08–0.26)	0.1 (0.07–0.2)
PPV % (95% CI)	73.2 (66.6–78.8)	80.9 (73.4–86.6)	84.2 (77.7–89.2)
NPV % (95% CI)	91.0 (83.1–95.4)	89.1 (82.0–93.7)	90.8 (81.7–95.6)

*It is not possible to compare the diagnostic accuracy of CT with the MDT diagnosis reference standard because that reference standard included CT (which means incorporation bias is present and that would lead to an overestimate of accuracy).

value is to 100%, the better a test is at ruling in a condition. This means that in this population where COVID-19 is prevalent (46%), 73% with a positive ultrasound and 81% with a positive CT will have COVID-19.

How might we use this evidence to inform practice?
This is an area of rapidly emerging evidence. Despite some concerns about the risk of bias of this study, it is useful to inform current applications of lung ultrasound in your hospital and provide confidence in its application, especially where CT and/or PCR is not available or not quickly available. You will continue to monitor for new research and additional research with larger patient populations to help establish guidelines for its use in your setting.

⊚ HUMAN MOVEMENTS EXAMPLE

Clinical scenario
You have recently started conducting exercise training sessions in your clinic specifically targeting adults who are 70 years and older. To tailor exercise programs for these clients, you need to evaluate their physical activity levels on a regular basis. At present you use the International Physical Activity Questionnaire (IPAQ)—short form. You could use a modified version of Physical Activity Questionnaire (IPAQ), the IPAQ-E, which was developed for an older population. However, older adults may find it difficult to answer these types of physical activity questionnaires due to recall challenges, lower intensities of exercise and performing larger amounts of unstructured physical activity. A colleague tells you about another tool—the Single Item Measure (SIM)—which can be used to assess physical activity with just one self-reported question about the number of days in the last week a person has been active. You read a bit about it and learn that the SIM has appropriate reliability and validity for measuring physical activity at one point in time, and that it is suitable for use with older adults. However, before adopting this measure in your clinic you want to make sure it can also effectively classify changes in physical activity levels over time.

Clinical question
For older adults participating in an exercise program, is a self-reported single item measure of physical activity accurate in measuring changes in physical activity levels?

Search terms and databases used to find the evidence
Database: PubMed (general database, as not a clear diagnostic question for PubMed—Clinical Queries)

Search terms: (single item measure) AND (physical activity change) AND exercise

The search identified 47 articles. You examine the abstract of several which report use of a single item measure and may be relevant. However, only a couple of studies compare this measure to accelerometry (the reference standard) and/or examine the ability of the measure to classify changes in physical activity (rather than measure physical activity at one point in time). You decide to look at the most recent study that meets these criteria.

Article chosen

O'Halloran P, Kingsley M, Nicholson M, et al. Responsiveness of the single item measure to detect change in physical activity. PLOS One 2020;15(6):e0234420. Accessed via https://doi.org/10.1371/journal.pone.0234420.

Structured abstract (adapted from the above)

Study design: Repeated measure cross-sectional design, comparing the SIM with a hip-worn accelerometer for detecting increases in levels of moderate-to-vigorous physical activity.

Setting: Regional campus of an Australian university.

Participants: 90 adults (mean age 47 years, 79% females) comprising university staff members and their family members and housemates. All had passed pre-exercise screening with the Physical Activity Readiness Questionnaire (PAQ).

Description of tests: The SIM asks participants to report the number of days in the last week that they undertook at least 30 minutes of activity which was enough to raise their breathing rate (moderate-to-vigorous physical activity) for either leisure or transport purposes. Participants answered this question retrospectively at the end of week 1 (baseline), and again at the end of week 2 (follow-up). During this same 2-week period, all participants wore a triaxial accelerometer during waking hours. Participants were asked to maintain their routines in week 1 but were encouraged to increase physical activity during the second 7-day period of monitoring.

Reference standard: Triaxial accelerometry via the Actigraph device. This device is worn on the hip, and measures the quality and intensity of movement, providing information about energy expenditure, steps and physical activity intensity.

Main results: The SIM displayed moderate sensitivity (63%) in detecting participants who increased the number of days they spent doing 30 minutes or more of moderate-to-vigorous physical activity from week 1 to week 2. These findings did not vary when moderate-to-vigorous physical activity was analysed as total minutes per day or in 10-minute bouts. Over three-quarters of those who self-reported increases in physical activity via the SIM also had increased accelerometry activity levels (positive predictive value of 78%). Specificity of the SIM for detecting changes in moderate-to-vigorous physical activity was low (52%).

Conclusion: The SIM may have potential as an assessment tool for evaluating change in moderate-to-vigorous physical activity, particularly for evaluating the impact of community-based programs when device-based measures or longer self-report measures are not feasible.

Is this evidence likely to be biased?

• *Did all participants get the diagnostic test and reference standard?*

   Yes. The authors state that all participants wore an accelerometer (reference standard) and completed a SIM (diagnostic test) for the same weekly period, thereby reducing the chance of verification bias. However, only 70% of recruited participants had valid data from both tests which could be used to analyse change in physical activity from one week to the next. As no information is given about these excluded participants, the impact of this on the study is unclear.

• *Could the results of the test of interest have been influenced by the results of the reference standard, or vice versa?*

   Unclear, but unlikely. It is not reported who analysed the accelerometer data or if they were blinded to the results of the SIM. If the researchers who analysed the accelerometry data were aware of the results and physical activity classifications from the SIM, it could have biased how they interpreted data downloaded from the accelerometer devices. However, the authors provide a clear objective methodology for their accelerometer data analysis and classification, which greatly reduces the chance of measurement bias. It is also unlikely that those conducting the SIM with participants would have had knowledge of accelerometry results due to the concurrent timing of both assessments.

• *Was there a description of the disease status of the tested population?*

   Unclear. The study participants were all recruited from a regional Australian university campus. They are

Continued

◎ HUMAN MOVEMENTS EXAMPLE—cont'd

described as being staff members or household members who were over 18 years old and capable of performing physical activity according to the PAQ. These selection criteria may have introduced bias in that the participants included may have been better educated and generally healthier and fitter than the underlying population from which they were selected. The population is described in terms of age, sex and body mass index. Participants tended to be female, middle-aged and slightly overweight, which is comparable to study populations in Australia.

- *Was there sufficient description of the methods for performing the test?*

For the accelerometers, yes. The protocol for setting up and wearing the accelerometers is well described, including calibration, placement on the right hip, wearing during waking hours, when to change/not change routine and removal when in water. The analysis and interpretation of this data is clearly described. However, description of the methods for performing the SIM is lacking. It is not clear whether the questionnaire was self-administered by participants or conducted by a researcher, and the format of the questionnaire (for example, paper, online, verbal) is not specified.

What are the main results?

Accelerometry identified that 53 (59%) participants had increased the total number of days that they spent doing more than 30 minutes in moderate-to-vigorous physical activity (MVPA) during the second week of the study. When MVPA was counted via 10-minute bouts of activity, 58 (64%) participants were classified as having increased physical activity levels during the week.

The sensitivity, specificity and post-test probabilities of the single item measure for identifying participants who

increased either total MVPA or bouts of MVPA over 1 week are reported in Table 7.8. The SIM had moderate sensitivity for this identification as it correctly classified 63% of those who had increased their total physical activity. It performed slightly better when considering MVPA bouts, with 69% sensitivity. The post-test probability values indicate that, on average, 77% of participants who registered an increase in physical activity via the SIM actually did so. In other words, the SIM may return some false positives, recording almost one-quarter of participants as increasing physical activity when they may not have done so. On the other hand, a failure to increase MVPA on the SIM does not mean that we can rule out an increase in MVPA due to its low specificity and negative predictive value.

How might we use this evidence to inform practice?

You appraise this study's risk of bias as quite low. While the reference (gold) standard for measuring physical activity is calorimetry, the Actigraph is cheaper and practical and has been validated as the reference standard for physical activity measurement in free-living situations. However, you are not sure how the findings could be used to inform your practice in a meaningful way. While the SIM is simple, fast and practical, you have identified several important considerations when applying it to your client population.

First, the study only assessed changes in MVPA, rather than total physical activity levels. Given you are working with an older population, you are interested in tracking changes across the physical activity spectrum. By using the SIM, you will neglect to capture changes in lower intensity exercise which may be important to your clients' health and goal setting. Study participants were younger and potentially more educated than those you see in practice. This may mean they are better able to understand the

TABLE 7.8 **Sensitivity, specificity, post-test probabilities and likelihood ratios of the SIM for identifying participants who increased their physical activity levels**

	Sensitivity % (95% CI)	Specificity % (95% CI)	Positive predictive value % (95% CI)	Negative predictive value % (95% CI)	Positive likelihood ratio	Negative likelihood ratio
Total MVPA	63 (50–75)	52 (31–72)	77 (69–84)	35 (25–47)	1.31	0.71
Bouts of MVPA	69 (57–80)	48 (21–69)	78 (70–84)	38 (26–51)	1.33	0.65

SIM question and recall weekly activities for the self-assessment. Study participants were also fitter than your clients, with more than half increasing physical activity during the monitoring period. While the sensitivity and specificity of the SIM should not change with differences in group physical activity levels (as they are independent of the incidence of the condition), the positive predictive value of the SIM may be reduced in a population with lower physical activity levels (such as your clients). Also, while you like the SIM's simplicity, you are not sure how it was administered to participants, and if the results may differ when a client self-completes it versus being guided by a clinician.

Your main concern, however, is that the primary use of physical activity assessment in your program is to identify clients who are not meeting their activity goals, so you can provide them with targeted motivation, exercise tailoring and prescription. The SIM is unable to correctly identify many of these clients due to its low specificity and negative predictive value. In other words, if you targeted all those who did not increase physical activity on the SIM from one visit to the next, this may be an inefficient use of time and resources given that only 35% of negative results on the SIM are true negatives. Moreover, you would miss targeting clients who were classified as false positives by the SIM. The SIM also does not give you any indication of the total time spent in physical activity, or the types of activities undertaken, which may be helpful in your program planning. Therefore, you decide that it is not currently appropriate to use the SIM with your older clients and continue seeking other methods of tracking changes in physical activity.

◎ PARAMEDICINE EXAMPLE

Clinical scenario

You work as a paramedic for an Australian ambulance service. You are on a scene with a patient who appears to have had a stroke. Your assessment with the modified National Institutes of Health Stroke Scale (NIHSS) leads you to believe the patient may have had a large vessel occlusion (LVO). Understanding that delay in receipt of treatment may result in unfavourable outcomes for the patient, you discuss with the family and your paramedic partner whether to travel further to a hospital that provides endovascular thrombectomy (EVT), which is part of the optimal standard of care of a LVO, or just to go directly to the closest hospital. Later, when reflecting on this case with your partner, your partner questions how well a stroke screening tool can identify LVO.

Clinical question

In patients who appear to have had a stroke and are receiving emergency prehospital care, how accurate is a stroke screening tool for detecting large vessel occlusion (LVO) so that early bypass to a hospital with capability for endovascular thrombectomy (EVT) can be considered?

Search terms and databases used to find the evidence
Database: PubMed—Clinical Queries (with 'diagnosis category' and 'narrow scope' selected).

Search terms: (prehospital) AND ((stroke assessment) OR (stroke screen*)) and (large vessel occlusion)

The search identified 53 articles, with a few articles describing prehospital care. You choose an Australian study looking at the accuracy of a screening tool so you can have a good understanding of how well the tool may perform in a setting that may be similar to yours.

Article chosen

Zhao H, Smith K, Bernard S, et al. Utility of severity-based prehospital triage for endovascular thrombectomy. Stroke 2021;52(1):70–9. https://www.ahajournals.org/doi/full/10.1161/STROKEAHA.120.031467.

Structured abstract (adapted from the above)
Study design: Prospective observational design.
Setting: Initially metropolitan Melbourne and then statewide Victoria, Australia.
Participants: 517 patients (50.2% male, mean age 72.3 years) who were assessed by a paramedic for suspected stroke and transported to the nearest stroke management–capable hospital.
Description of test: The ACT-FAST (Ambulance Clinical Triage for Acute Stroke Treatment) algorithm consists of the following steps: check for arm weakness (either side) (ARM); if right arm weakness, check for severe speech deficit (CHAT); if left arm weakness, shoulder tap and

Continued

◉ PARAMEDICINE EXAMPLE—cont'd

check patient gaze (TAP); if yes to previous, check eligibility criteria for EVT (<24 hours onset, independent at home with minimal assistance, mimics excluded, no rapid spontaneous improvement at the scene) (ACT-FAST positive). If no to any step, result is ACT-FAST negative. The article and its supplement contain the full algorithm.

Reference standard: In-hospital cerebral imaging which determined LVO status. Three reference standards were applied: (1) intracranial internal carotid artery (ICA), first segment middle cerebral artery (M1), and basilar artery occlusions—those typically eligible for EVT; (2) extended definition which includes additional occlusions and large vessel conditions—representing developing EVT eligibility worldwide; (3) all LVO. Details are described in full in the article. If no imaging was performed, the discharge diagnosis was used.

Main results: In the prehospital setting, 168 (32.5%) patients were assessed as ACT-FAST positive. 132 (25.5%) had LVO according to the extended definition. Using the extended definition for LVO, the positive predictive value of ACT-FAST was 58.8% and the negative predictive value was 90.8%. Sensitivity of ACT-FAST for detecting LVO was 75.8% and specificity was 81.8%. Modelling indicated that 52 minutes to EVT commencement was saved by avoidance of secondary transfers with use of ACT-FAST.

Conclusion: The findings suggest a reasonable overall benefit of using the ACT-FAST algorithm to triage patients to an EVT-capable hospital.

Is this evidence likely to be biased?

* *Did all participants get the diagnostic test and the reference standard?*

   Yes. All participants received both the diagnostic test and a reference standard, but the reference standard was different for some. For 22 (4.3%) patients, cerebral imaging was not performed and the reference standard was the (non-stroke) diagnosis made by the hospital. For these patients, the discharge diagnosis was used as the reference standard. As the discharge diagnosis may be less accurate than imaging, bias in estimates of accuracy may have been introduced.

* *Could the results of the test of interest have been influenced by the results of the reference standard, or vice versa?*

   No. The ACT-FAST assessment form had already been completed electronically prior to the cerebral imaging being completed. It is not mentioned if those interpreting the imaging or providing the discharge diagno-

sis could have been aware of the ACT-FAST result, but this is probably unlikely.

* *Was there a clear description of the disease status of the tested population?*

   Yes. Patients who met stroke criteria (from the Melbourne Acute Stroke Screen) then had the ACT-FAST assessment conducted. Hospital imaging results are summarised in the article.

* *Were the methods for performing the test described in sufficient detail?*

   Yes. The assessment is summarised in the article, with the full algorithm provided in the article's supplementary materials.

What are the main results?

ACT-FAST accuracy: 32.5% (168/517) of participants were assessed as positive with the ACT-FAST. ACT-FAST had a sensitivity of 75.8% and specificity of 81.8% when compared to the hospital imaging extended definition of LVO. The study also reported the sensitivity and specificity of ACT-FAST for identifying participants who required EVT. Sensitivity of the ACT-FAST for this reference standard was greater at 82.4%, but specificity was lower at 75.4%. In this population where prevalence of LVO was 25.5% by the extended definition on hospital imaging, the probability that participants with positive ACT-FAST had LVO on hospital imaging or required EVT (the positive predictive value) was low (35.9% for EVT, 58.8% for LVO). The probability of ACT-FAST positive participants requiring an EVT-capable hospital was higher at 80%. Table 7.9 summarises the diagnostic performance of ACT-FAST compared to in-hospital imaging, need for being taken to a EVT-capable hospital and EVT being performed.

Consequences of incorrect triage with ACT-FAST: Of the 168 ACT-FAST positive patients, 21 did not have an LVO using the base or extended definition. ACT-FAST was false-positive for eight patients who received thrombolysis and false-negative in four patients, who needed EVT (5.4% of 74 EVT cases) and required secondary transfer. Of 68 metropolitan patients who needed EVT, ACT-FAST correctly identified 55/68 (80.9%), including 29/55 patients (52.7%) who were transported to a non-EVT-capable hospital and for whom bypass could have avoided secondary transfer.

Transfer time: When difference in time to intervention from direct transport to an EVT-capable hospital was compared to a secondary transport to one, the resulting difference estimated, from modelling, was an overall scene time to EVT arterial access median time saving of

TABLE 7.9 **Diagnostic performance of ACT-FAST in prehospital care, compared to in-hospital imaging, to determine LVO status**

	EVT-capable hospital need (LVO/ICH or tumour present)	LVO on in-hospital imaging (ICA/M1/ basilar)	LVO on in-hospital imaging (extended definition)	EVT
Sensitivity	70.1	82.6	75.8	82.4
Specificity	89.5	77.9	81.8	75.4
Positive predictive value	80.0	44.7	58.8	35.9
Negative predictive value	83.3	95.4	90.8	96.3
Area under the curve (ROC)	0.798 (95% CI 0.76 to 0.84)	0.802 (95% CI 0.75 to 0.85)	0.788 (95% CI 0.74 to 0.84)	0.789 (95% CI 0.73 to 0.85)

52.0 minutes (95% CI 40.0 to 61.5) in favour of the direct bypass strategy.

How might we use this evidence to inform practice?
This study appears to have a low risk of bias. The results suggest that if a patient is ACT-FAST positive, then it may be reasonable to bypass a non-EVT-capable hospital and transport to an EVT-capable hospital if the bypass time does not exceed the approximate time to commence EVT for beneficial patient outcomes. You plan to discuss this study with the director of your service. Prior to this, you will search for studies evaluating alternative stroke screening tools and their accuracy in identifying LVO.

◉ PHARMACY EXAMPLE

Clinical scenario
As the senior pharmacist in a regional hospital, you are responsible for conducting medication reviews which aim to prevent drug-related problems. When reviewing patients admitted to the hospital you are considering asking some standard questions that might help you determine the patient's risk of experiencing medication-related harm. This includes questions about the types and number of medications patients are taking, the route of administration and previous adverse drug reactions. However, many of the patients are elderly and often have memory problems. You wonder about the likely accuracy of patients' responses to such questions.

Clinical question
When talking with elderly hospitalised patients about their medications to try to identify drug-related problems, how accurately do they answer questions about their medications, in comparison to objective information (such as that found in medical records)?

Search terms and databases used to find the evidence
Database: PubMed—Clinical Queries (with 'diagnosis category' and 'narrow scope' selected).
Search terms: (drug-related problems OR medication-related harms) AND (patient report OR questions)

This search retrieved 14 hits. You choose the one that most closely matches your clinical question.

Article chosen
Kaufmann CP, Stampfil D, Mory N, et al. Drug-Associated Risk Tool: development and validation of a self-assessment questionnaire to screen for hospitalised patients at risk for drug-related problems. BMJ Open 2018;8(3): e016610.

Continued

◎ PHARMACY EXAMPLE—cont'd

Structured abstract (adapted from the above)
Study design: Prospective validation study.
Setting: Two hospitals in Switzerland.
Participants: 195 adult patients on orthopaedic, geriatric and internal medicine wards who could communicate meaningfully in German.
Description of tests: The Drug-Associated Risk Tool (DART) is a self-assessment questionnaire which is based on 27 risk factors for the development of drug-related problems that were identified in a previous study. Two versions of the tool were tested in this study: DART version 1.0 and a revised version (DART version 2.0), which consists of questions related to the patient's state of health, medications used, concerns around medications and application of medication.
Reference standard: For questions/statements in DART V.2.0, the reference standard was data obtained from the medical record (including diagnosis, laboratory values and medicines at entry). The investigators determined the accuracy of each question by comparing the question responses to information in the medical record. (For example, the accuracy of the patient's response to the statement 'I am suffering from diabetes' was compared to the information in the medical record.)
Main results: 164 patients (median age 74 years, 49% women) completed the DART V.1.0. Statements with low sensitivity and possible poor patient understanding were revised. DART V.2.0 was validated in 31 patients. The investigators examined the mean sensitivity, specificity and predictive values (the average of the values obtained for each question) of the DART V.2.0. The average specificity of the questions was 88% (range of specificities 27–100) and average sensitivity of 67% (range of sensitivity 21–100).
Conclusion: The specificity of DART V.2.0 statements was mostly high, while sensitivity was lower and more variable.

Is this evidence likely to be biased?

- *Did all participants get the diagnostic test and the reference standard?*

  Yes. Every hospitalised patient who met the inclusion criteria on the included wards was seen by investigators and, if consented, completed the DART. It appears that the medical records (the reference standard) were reviewed for all of the consenting patients. However, missing data (9–10%) was a concern for some of the DART statements and the authors state that missing data were excluded from analysis.

- *Could the results of the test of interest have been influenced by the results of the reference standard, or vice versa?*

  Unclear. The article does not describe when the medical records were reviewed in relation to the completion of the DART by the patient, if this was done by the same investigators who approached the patients, or whether the investigators were blinded to the DART responses.

- *Was there a clear description of the disease status of the tested population?*

  Unclear. The study describes the participants as adult patients on the orthopaedic, geriatric and internal medicine wards in two hospitals who could communicate meaningfully to be able to complete the self-administered questionnaire (that is, in German and without conditions such as delirium, acute psychosis, advanced dementia, aphasia, clouded consciousness state) and who were not palliative or terminally ill patients. Basic demographic information such as median age, gender and number of drugs on admission was outlined, along with ward type. The eligibility criteria suggest that the sample may not be representative of all elderly hospitalised patients. All patients on the specified wards meeting the inclusion criteria during a predefined period were asked to participate. However, the article does not indicate what this time period was, what proportion of patients on each ward were eligible and reasons for not consenting (21% declined).

- *Was there sufficient description of the methods for performing the test?*

  Unclear. The article includes a copy of the questionnaire (DART), describes some of the procedure for administering it and notes that patients received it after giving informed consent and completed it independently. Investigators only assisted if the patient needed assistance with writing. It appears that patients completed a paper version of the questionnaire, although this is not stated explicitly. The reference standard was objective data from medical records, and it is not clear how the data were collected, by whom, and if a standardised data collection form was used.

What are the main results?

The article presents the sensitivity, specificity, positive predictive value and negative predictive value for each statement in the DART, and as averages (see Table 7.10). The large range for individual statements is of concern.

How might we use this evidence to inform practice?

The investigators do not provide information about the overall performance of the tool—that is, the sensitivity and specificity of the tool itself (the combination of all the questions) at various tool cut-offs for detecting a drug-related problem—which is a major limitation of the study. Your appraisal of it also raised some concerns about the risk of bias in the study and whether its findings are generalisable to your patients. It does not appear that this tool has been externally validated in other populations. Given these concerns and

TABLE 7.10 **Average (range) sensitivity, specificity, positive predictive values and negative predictive values of the DART statements**

Sensitivity	Specificity	PPV	NPV
Average % (range)			
67 (21–100)	88 (27–100)	74 (26–100)	86 (20–100)

limitations of the tool to identify drug-related problems, you decide to search further for other ways that might more accurately identify patients at risk of drug-related problems.

◎ OPTOMETRY EXAMPLE

Clinical scenario

You are an optometrist in a suburban practice and are seeing an increasing number of patients with dry eye. It is an age-related problem that affects about 1 in 3 people aged over 50 years, has a range of causes and is of many different types. You wonder what is the best test for differentiating dry eye caused by meibomian gland dysfunction (small lipid-producing glands in the lids) from other types. You know that the meibomian glands can be imaged using meibography, but you do not have access to the equipment needed for that. You know that the meibomian glands produce the tear lipids and decide to search for research to determine if meibomian gland dysfunction (MGD) can be diagnosed by a clinical assessment of tear quality that is dependent on tear lipids.

Clinical question

In people with symptoms of dry eye, can clinical tests that assess tear lipids quality be used to diagnose meibomian gland dysfunction?

Search terms and databases used to find the evidence

Database: PubMed—Clinical Queries (with 'diagnosis category' and 'narrow scope' selected).
Search terms: ((meibomian gland (disease OR dysfunction)) AND (tear lipids)

This search gives 16 results. You choose the one article that most closely matches your clinical question.

Article chosen

Giannaccare G, Vigo L, Pellegrini M, et al. Ocular surface workup with automated noninvasive measurements for the diagnosis of meibomian gland dysfunction. Cornea 2018;37(6):740–5.

Structured abstract (adapted from the above)

Study design: Case-control cross-sectional, with comparison of ocular surface measures in patients with and without a diagnosis of meibomian gland dysfunction (MGD).
Setting: Ophthalmology centre in Milan, Italy.
Participants: 149 participants with MGD and 27 control participants. MGD diagnosis was based on a validated ocular discomfort symptom survey (ocular surface disease index, OSDI; score $\geq$ 13) and at least one clinical lid or gland sign of MGD. The healthy control group were age balanced to the MGD group (mean age MGD 53.4±15.5 years vs control 52.9±15.2 years).
Description of tests: All participants undertook the following tests. The OSDI survey, tear quality assessment (tear breakup time, tear lipid layer thickness, tear osmolarity) and imaging of the meibomian glands of the lower eyelid. The order of tests was from least to most invasive—that is, with potential to affect the ocular surface.
Reference standard: Meibography is a non-contact method for imaging the meibomian glands in situ within the eyelid. An infrared light source and infrared light-sensitive camera system are required. The area of the lid occupied by the glands versus the total lid area can be

Continued

◎ OPTOMETRY EXAMPLE—cont'd

determined from the images. The degree of gland drop-out can also be calculated.

Main results: OSDI scores, tear breakup time and meibomian gland area were significantly different in the two groups. Based on the area under the receiver operating characteristics (ROC) curve analysis, tear breakup time, followed by meibomian gland loss, had the highest diagnostic accuracy. From this analysis, cut-off values to diagnose MGD were breakup time ≤9.6 seconds, lipid layer thickness grade ≤2, meibomian gland loss >20%, and tear osmolarity >303 mOsm/L.

Conclusion: Assessment of tear quality, particularly tear breakup time, is a useful screening test to diagnose MGD.

Is this evidence likely to be biased?

- *Did all participants get the diagnostic test and the reference standard?*

  Yes. All the participants had all the tests performed.

- *Could the results of the test of interest have been influenced by the results of the reference standard, or vice versa?*

  Yes. A potential issue is that the tests used to initially diagnose MGD (OSDI score, a lid or gland sign of MGD) are then used again within the results. This means that, because of the nature of the participant selection criteria, significant differences in these will occur and thus outcome bias is likely. This means the findings could be affected by the selection criteria.

- *Was there a clear description of the disease status of the tested population?*

  No. The severity of the MGD in the test population is not clear. The severity of the lid and gland signs used to diagnose the MGD are not provided. There are many more participants in the MGD group than in the healthy control group (and no details about their recruitment are provided) and this has the potential to affect the outcomes. A small control group may not adequately reflect the range of normal values.

- *Was there sufficient description of the methods for performing the tests?*

  Mostly. However, related data are included—that is, both eyes of participants were measured (298 eyes in the MGD group and 54 in the control group). It is not clear if or how the fact that right and left eye data are not independent was dealt with.

What are the main results?

The mean OSDI score was significantly higher in the MGD group than in the control group (MGD 37.9±19.6 vs control 7.1±2.8; $p < 0.001$). The tear breakup time was significantly shorter in the MGD group (8.8±3.6 vs 11.0±3.0 seconds; $p < 0.001$). Meibomian gland loss was significantly higher in the MGD group (28.0±17.6 vs 21.2±13.0; $p = 0.029$). There were no significant group differences for the other measures.

There were significant positive correlations between lipid layer thickness and tear breakup time (the tear breakup time was shorter when the lipid layer was thinner, $r = 0.169$, $p = 0.004$) and between meibomian gland loss and OSDI score (the greater the meibomian gland loss, the higher the symptom score, $r = 0.187$, $p = 0.004$). These were calculated using Spearman correlation analysis which assumes a monotonic relationship between paired data; that is, one variable always increases or always decreases as the other variable increases. However, the statistical significance of these relationships is considered 'very weak' ($r = <0.2$).

Comparisons of each diagnostic test at differentiating MGD from controls are provided by the authors, with ROC curves provided for each diagnostic test. By looking at the curves for each test on one figure (as shown in the article), we can compare the performance of each test. The ROC curves show, in a graphical way, the sensitivity and specificity (represented by the false positive rate 1 – specificity) of the test at each possible cut-off point (the point at which a test result is considered normal/negative or abnormal/positive). For example, the sensitivity and specificity of the breakup time test at different cut-off values (for example, at 4 seconds, 9 seconds, 12 seconds, etc.). The curve displays the trade-off between sensitivity and specificity (how one value increases while the other decreases) at the varying test cut-offs.

The ROC curve informs us of the overall performance of each diagnostic test by estimating the area under the curve (AUC). The higher the AUC, the better the test is at distinguishing between people who do and do not have the disease. For a test with very high sensitivity and specificity, the curve would reach closer to the left upper corner of the plot and the AUC would be close to 1. An AUC of 0.5 means the test has no ability to discriminate between people with and without the disease; a value of 0.6 to 0.7 (as observed for tear breakup time) indicates acceptable discrimination.

The ROC curve and AUC values show that tear breakup time had the highest diagnostic power as a single parameter, followed by meibomian gland loss, tear osmolarity and lipid layer thickness. The plot may also be used to

TABLE 7.11 Areas under the ROC curves (AUCs), sensitivity and specificity for the calculated cut-off values* of each parameter

Characteristic	AUC (95% CI)	Cut-off	Sensitivity (%)	Specificity (%)
Non-invasive breakup time	0.69 (0.64–0.73)	≤9.6 sec	65.8	63.0
Meibomian gland loss	0.60 (0.54–0.65)	>20%	59.7	61.1
Lipid layer thickness	0.55 (0.49–0.60)	≤2	57.7	33.3
Tear osmolarity	0.55 (0.50–0.61)	>303 mOsm/L	49.3	53.7

*Determined as the value whose corresponding point on the ROC curve was nearest to the coordinate (0,1).

identify the best cut-off value for each test—that is, the cut-off value with the highest sensitivity and specificity (the point of the curve closest to the top left-hand corner of the plot). Cut-off values to diagnose MGD were breakup time ≤9.6 seconds, lipid layer thickness grade ≤2, meibomian gland loss > 20% and tear osmolarity >303 mOsm/L. The AUC values and values for sensitivity and specificity for each test at these cut-off values are also shown in Table 7.11. These were highest for tear breakup time.

A value of 0.69 means the tear breakup time test would be able to correctly identify the person who has MGD (out of two people, one who does and one who does not have MGD) 69% of the time (at a cut-off score of 9.6 seconds).

How might we use this evidence to inform practice?

After appraising the study, you have some concerns about its risk of bias, particularly around sampling and recruiting both participants with and without the condition of interest. (This 'two-gate' study design was explained in Chapter 6.) This is a key limitation, as spectrum bias is likely and tends to result in overestimation of diagnostic accuracy. You keep this in mind when interpreting the results. It appears the tear breakup time is the best first test to perform to assist in the diagnosis of dry eye due to MGD. This is a simple, fast, non-invasive clinical test that can be easily performed. The data indicate that if the breakup time is less than 9.6 seconds, this is suggestive of MGD. Of course, patients with longer breakup times could still have this condition, but values shorter than this are unlikely to be normal. A battery of tests is likely to have better diagnostic ability than a single test, but the best combination of tests is not known or has not been tested.

A key issue in the diagnosis of MGD is that it is a slowly progressive condition with a continuum from clearly normal glands to slightly impaired glands to very abnormal glands (maybe even non-existent due to severe atrophy). Thus, test values will be reliably altered only when the gland function is sufficiently impaired for tear quality to be greatly affected. However, a screening test needs to be able to detect a condition early in the pathological process so that treatments can be instigated at a point when they are useful and able to slow progression. Imaging of the glands with meibography is a direct way of determining if normal gland anatomy is present or not. Current tests may suggest a problem, especially in severe disease, but meibography clearly remains the reference standard test for early detection of gland dropout and thus for diagnosis of early MGD.

REFERENCE

1. Gaggin HK, Chen-Tournoux AA, Christenson RH, et al. Rationale and design of the ICON-RELOADED study: International Collaborative of N-terminal pro-B-type Natriuretic Peptide Re-evaluation of Acute Diagnostic Cut-Offs in the Emergency Department. Am Heart J 2017 Oct;192:26–37.

Evidence about Prognosis

Adrian Traeger

LEARNING OBJECTIVES

After reading this chapter, you should be able to:
- Generate a structured clinical question about prognosis for a clinical scenario
- Appraise the validity (risk of bias) of prognostic evidence

- Understand how to interpret the results from prognostic studies and calculate confidence intervals when needed
- Describe how prognostic evidence can be used to inform practice
- Explain prognostic information to a patient

Let us consider a clinical scenario that will be useful for illustrating the concepts of evidence about prognosis that are the focus of this chapter.

◎ CLINICAL SCENARIO

Mrs Lee is a 55-year-old woman who recently presented to her general practitioner with a 1-week history of moderate intensity (5/10 on a pain intensity scale) sciatica in her right leg. She was initially prescribed a non-steroidal anti-inflammatory medicine and advised to remain as active as possible. However, due to pain, she is currently unable to work. She cannot sit comfortably for more than 10 minutes, has difficulty getting out of chairs, and finds it difficult to bend and kneel down. She is unable to walk at her normal pace, and her sleep is disrupted due to pain. Her Roland-Morris Low Back Pain and Disability Questionnaire (RMDQ) was 14/23 (higher scores indicate higher levels of pain-related physical disability). She has symptoms predominantly in the right leg but also has low back pain. On neurological examination, her reflexes and sensation are slightly reduced indicating a right-sided L5 nerve root compression, but there is no detectable myotomal weakness. Mrs Lee works 3 days per week as a human resources manager, which often involves prolonged periods of sitting. Prior to the episode she exercised regularly, including daily walks, and engaged in her community without limitations.

The clinical scenario presented here raises several questions about the future for Mrs Lee. Some of these are: How well is Mrs Lee likely to recover from her sciatica? Will she be able to continue to work? How long will it take for her to recover? What is her risk of prolonged disability? These types of questions will be the focus of this chapter on prognosis.

Prognosis is about predicting the future—the future of a patient's condition. While it is impossible for anyone to predict the future with absolute certainty, we can use evidence from prognostic studies to make informed predictions about the future. These evidence-based predictions about the future can be useful in many ways. They can help to reassure patients by removing some doubt about the future, especially if their expectations are unjustifiably pessimistic. Predictions about natural recovery can help you and your patient to jointly decide whether any interventions need to be considered. Sometimes the type of intervention that is being considered is typically applied only once, such as a joint replacement or organ transplant. In such cases, the optimal time to intervene can be determined by predictions about the rate of deterioration before the intervention and the rate of recovery afterwards. Predictions about the average course of a particular condition can also be adjusted for individual patients. This adjustment is possible when other features about a patient or the patient's health or management, besides the primary diagnosis, have been shown to affect outcomes. Prognostic information can be about the likely course and duration of a condition, the likelihood of various outcomes (which can include cure, recovery or complications) either with intervention or without. If it is the latter, then this is often referred to as the natural history of a condition.

This chapter will address the process of using prognostic evidence to make these predictions and of incorporating them into clinical practice. We will start by defining the components of a structured clinical question about prognosis. Then we will see how to appraise the evidence to determine its risk of bias (validity). Subsequent sections of the chapter will review how to understand the results of a prognostic study, how to use the evidence to inform practice and how to explain prognostic information clearly to patients.

HOW TO STRUCTURE A PROGNOSTIC QUESTION

You will recall from Chapter 2 that clinical questions can be structured using the PICO format: Patient/Problem, Intervention/Issue, Comparison (if relevant) and Outcomes. When our question was about the effect of an intervention, the comparison was an important component. The effect of an intervention was always estimated by comparison against this component. Questions about prognosis are questions about expected outcomes over time and what factors might be associated with (but not necessarily the cause of) certain outcomes. Therefore, the comparison component is not used in questions about prognosis. Let us look at each of the remaining components in more detail.

Patient/problem

The patient/problem component can be specified as previously described—for example: 'In patients with coronary heart disease . . .', 'Among children with epilepsy . . .' or, using our scenario, 'In adults who present to primary care with sciatica . . .'. Sometimes, the prognosis for typical patients with the condition is quite different from the prognosis for patients with some additional characteristic. For example, the prognosis for patients with cystic fibrosis who become infected with the bacteria *Burkholderia cepacia* is worse than for those without this infection.[1] Characteristics that influence outcomes are known as **prognostic factors**. If you suspect that some characteristic of your patient might be a prognostic factor, this can be incorporated into the patient/problem component. Let us assume for a moment that Mrs Lee, the patient in our scenario at the beginning of this

chapter, is obese. This may be a prognostic factor, so we could incorporate this into our clinical question: 'In adults who present to primary care with sciatica and who are obese . . .'

In addition to comorbidities such as obesity, prognostic factors can also relate to the severity of the condition—for example: 'In patients with coronary heart disease (New York Heart Association Functional Class IV) . . .'. The New York Heart Association functional classification is a simple way of describing the extent of heart disease. It places patients in one of four categories based on the severity of their symptoms and how much they are limited during exercise. The history of the condition can also be a prognostic factor. For example: 'Among children who have had their first epileptic seizure . . .'.

Intervention/issue

The next component of the question is the intervention/issue of interest, or 'exposure'. If you are interested in the natural course of a condition, then you can simply add the term 'untreated' to your clinical question—for example: 'In children with untreated nocturnal enuresis . . .'—to remind you to search for prognostic evidence about untreated patients. However, you might instead be interested in a patient's prognosis with an intervention. In this case, your clinical question about prognosis should specify what intervention a patient has received or is receiving for their condition. Some questions are only relevant to a population that has received an intervention, as in these two examples: 'In patients undergoing surgical skin grafts for major burns, what is the risk of postoperative infection?' and 'Among patients who no longer stutter at the end of a course of intensive therapy, what is the probability that their stuttering will relapse in the next year?'

Outcomes

It is important to consider outcomes that are measurable and, where possible, quantifiable. Outcomes such as 'better' or 'improved' are usually too vague. We also need to select outcomes that are important to the patient's goals and priorities.

Time

For some prognostic scenarios, you may be interested in adding time as a component of the clinical question (a PICOT question). This may be particularly relevant if the outcome changes with time. For example, in women with postpartum depression, rates of psychosocial recovery will be different at 3 months after giving birth, than they will at 9 months.[2]

CLINICAL SCENARIO (CONTINUED)

Structuring the clinical question

Several prognostic questions can be drawn from our scenario. Let us assume that we focus on Mrs Lee's restricted function and inability to sit, bend or work comfortably, as these issues are concerning her. If she is likely to regain her function in a few weeks, she would need to make only minimal alterations regarding her work duties. However, if she is likely to have a prolonged recovery, or not regain her prior level of function, she might need to make more substantial work alterations. Critical to these concerns is when or if Mrs Lee will recover her physical function. A suitable prognostic question might be:

In adults who present to primary care with sciatica, what factors are predictive of physical function in the short and long term?

CLINICAL SCENARIO (CONTINUED)

Finding the evidence to answer your question

You start by looking for a prospective cohort study in PubMed—Clinical Queries, using the search terms *sciatica AND (primary care) AND function**, and filtering your search by selecting the 'prognosis' and 'narrow' options. This search results in about 14 articles. A quick scan of the titles confirms that several of the articles are probably relevant. A recent study appears to match your clinical question and provides data about function at 4 months and 1 year after an episode of sciatica.[3] Throughout the rest of this chapter, we will refer to this study as the 'sciatica study'.

A number of additional search techniques could have been employed if the previous search had not identified a helpful article, such as: selecting the 'broad' search option may help if few articles had been retrieved; or modifying and/or adding search terms may help if the original search retrieved too many irrelevant or too few articles.

CLINICAL SCENARIO (CONTINUED)

Structured abstract of our chosen article

Citation: Konstantinou K, Dunn KM, Ogollah R, et al. Prognosis of sciatica and back-related leg pain in primary care: the ATLAS cohort. Spine J 2018;18(6):1030–40. doi: 10.1016/j.spinee.2017.10.071. The structured abstract has been adapted from this reference.

Question: For patients with back-related leg pain and sciatica seeing their primary care physicians, what factors are predictive of function at 4 and 12 months following the episode?

Design: Cohort followed prospectively for 1 year.

Setting: Primary care practices in the United Kingdom.

Participants: 609 adult patients (mean age 50.2 years, 63% female) who presented to primary care with back-related leg pain ($n = 157$) or sciatica ($n = 452$).

Prognostic factors: The factors considered as possible prognostic factors were: duration of pain, pain intensity, neuropathic pain features, psychological perceptions (for example, symptoms contributing to an 'illness identity', recovery expectations), clinical examination features and imaging (MRI) examination features.

Outcome: Good outcome was defined as 30% or more reduction in disability (Roland-Morris Disability Questionnaire—23 items, with total score from 0 to 23, with higher scores indicating poorer function).

Main results: At 12 months, 55% of patients improved in both the total sample and the sciatica group. For the whole cohort, longer leg pain duration (odds ratio [OR] 0.41; confidence interval [CI] 0.19 to 0.90), higher 'illness identity' score (OR 0.70; CI 0.53 to 0.93), and a patient's belief that the problem will last a long time (OR 0.27; CI 0.13 to 0.57) were the strongest independent prognostic factors negatively associated with improvement. These last two factors were similarly negatively associated with improvement in the sciatica sub-group.

Conclusions: Just over half of patients had improved function at 12 months. Patient's belief of recovery time scale and number of other symptoms attributed to the pain are independent prognostic factors. These factors can be used to inform and direct decisions about timing and intensity of available therapeutic options.

IS THIS EVIDENCE LIKELY TO BE BIASED?

As you saw in Chapters 4 and 6, there are standards for reporting of randomised controlled trials (CONSORT statement) and diagnostic accuracy studies (STARD statement). The reporting standard for observational studies in epidemiological studies is known as the STROBE statement, and there is a particular checklist for cohort studies (and checklists for other study designs such as case-control studies and cross-sectional studies). Further details are available at www.strobe-statement.org. A well-reported study typically makes critically appraising the study easier.

We will use questions drawn from the Critical Appraisal Skills Program (CASP) and associated checklists for appraising a *cohort* study to explain how to assess the likelihood of bias in a prognostic study. Note that there is a separate CASP checklist for case-control studies. The key questions to ask when appraising the risk of bias of a prognostic study are summarised in Box 8.1. The checklist begins with screening criteria that, if not met, indicate that the article is unlikely to be helpful and that further assessment of potential bias is probably unwarranted.

Did the study address a clearly focused issue?

The screening question on the CASP checklist is: Did the study address a clearly focused issue? For prognostic evidence, the article should clearly define the population, potential prognostic factors and the outcomes considered.

◎ CLINICAL SCENARIO (CONTINUED)

Did the study address a clearly focused question?

Use the PICO(T) mnemonic to help you decide this. In this study, yes, the question is focused. The authors define the **P**opulation (individuals with back-related leg pain and sciatica, presenting to primary care), **I**ntervention/**I**ssue (episode of back-related leg pain or sciatica), and a relevant **O**utcome (function). They also specify the **T**ime component (4 and 12 months). Remember that if you *only* want the overall prognosis (without the embellishment of the prognostic factors), this could simply be a **PO** question (just the **P**opulation and **O**utcome).

Was an appropriate study type used?

Another screening question that is good to consider before appraising the rest of the article (and to help you determine if the cohort checklist is the most appropriate one) is whether the method used was appropriate to answer the question posed by the authors. In Chapter 2, we saw that longitudinal studies, particularly prospective cohort

---

BOX 8.1 Key questions to ask when appraising the validity (risk of bias) of a prognostic study

1. Was there a representative and well-defined sample of participants?
2. Were participants recruited at a common point in the disease or condition?
3. Was exposure measured accurately?
4. Were the outcomes measured accurately?
5. Were important confounding factors considered?
6. Was the follow-up of participants sufficiently long and complete?

---

studies, provide the best evidence about prognosis. Even better than that is a systematic review of several prospective cohort studies. This chapter appraises an individual prognostic cohort study.

Although prospective cohort studies are typically the study type that you should aim to use to answer prognostic questions, prognostic information can also be generated by other study designs. For example, if you are interested in the natural history (that is, without intervention) of a condition, then the outcomes of an untreated control group in a randomised controlled trial can provide this. However, an important caveat here is that randomised trials often impose additional eligibility criteria (such as criteria to ensure that the participants are suitable/willing to receive either intervention, undergo all outcome measurements and provide responses to all the patient-reported outcomes). Therefore, the data from an untreated control group may not be as representative as the data from a prospective cohort study.

◎ CLINICAL SCENARIO (CONTINUED)

Was an appropriate study type used?

The researchers in the sciatica study wanted to answer a prognostic question and they used the ideal study design for this: a prospective, longitudinal study of an inception cohort of patients who had just presented to primary care with back-related leg pain or sciatica. Because this article satisfies the two screening questions, we can move on to the more detailed appraisal criteria.

Was the cohort recruited in an acceptable way?

The broad criterion in CASP is whether the cohort was recruited in an acceptable way—ensuring that it is representative of the larger population of interest. Its importance lies in the study's ability to generalise to the wider population. Two questions that should be considered under this criterion are: (1) 'Was there a representative and well-defined sample of participants?'; and (2) 'Were participants recruited at a common point in the disease or condition?'

Was there a representative and well-defined sample of participants?

A study's estimate of prognosis will be biased if its sample is systematically different from (and therefore not representative of) the larger population of interest. It is important that a study clearly defines its inclusion and exclusion criteria, as this can clarify the representative nature of the sample. Clearly defined criteria help make it clear to everyone (researchers, participants, you) just what the target population of the study was. A representative sample is also more likely to be obtained if the study recruits all of the eligible patients who presented at the recruitment site into the study. When appraising a study, look for a statement in the article that describes either recruiting 'all patients' or recruiting 'consecutive cases'. Recruiting all eligible patients prevents bias in the data that could arise if some eligible patients avoided, or were missed, in recruitment and these patients differ in some systematic way from those who were recruited. The greater the proportion of eligible patients that are recruited into the study, the more representative of the target population the sample is likely to be.

◎ CLINICAL SCENARIO (CONTINUED)

Representative and well-defined sample
In the sciatica study, participants were consecutively recruited from primary care practices in the United Kingdom. Additionally, the inclusion and exclusion criteria of the study are clearly defined. We conclude that the cohort is likely to be representative of the target population with the caveat that the participants are receiving care in the United Kingdom. Some countries and regions may have sufficiently different healthcare systems or resources as to make this a limitation.

The weaknesses of retrospective studies

As we saw in Chapter 2, cohort studies can be either prospective or retrospective, with retrospective studies being lower down the hierarchy of evidence for prognostic questions. Retrospective studies are more likely to have incomplete and inaccurate data sets because a plan for collecting the needed data was not (by definition) implemented prior to its collection. Additionally, retrospective cohort studies are more prone to recruitment bias because patients with a particular characteristic may be systematically missed. For example, a retrospective cohort study examining 81 patients with infections after total knee arthroplasty[4] could not be used to determine the risk of joint infection (because everyone was selected to have an infection), nor used to determine the likelihood of independent mobility at 1 year after surgery, as the mobility of individuals with infections may differ from those of the total (including not having an infection).

Were participants recruited at a common point in the disease or condition?

Although it is not explicitly mentioned on the CASP checklist, one of the things that will help you to determine whether the cohort was recruited in an acceptable way is whether participants were recruited at a common well-described point in the disease or condition of interest. This is important, as a group of people with the same condition may vary in their prognoses depending on the length of time they have had the condition. Consider the scenario of a disease that is sometimes fatal, with the deaths that do occur usually being within 2 years of its onset. If we consider the prognosis for short-term mortality, it is likely to be worse in newly diagnosed patients than in those who have had the disease for 5 years. This is because the 5-year survivors have survived the 'danger period' and now have a short-term mortality that is similar to people without the disease. This means that, in a cohort study that recruited people with this disease, the average prognosis could be greatly affected by the proportions of participants who are newly diagnosed and participants who are chronic (that is, diagnosed some time ago). This problem is minimised by recruiting participants at a consistent and defined point in their disease. When this point is very early in the disease process the cohort is called an **'inception' cohort**. Some studies recruit participants at diagnosis. However, the point of diagnosis is not always at an early or a uniform point in the disease process. This is particularly the case for chronic conditions such as rheumatoid arthritis or low back pain. You must therefore consider carefully whether a true inception cohort has been identified when recruitment occurs at diagnosis.

◎ CLINICAL SCENARIO (CONTINUED)

Were participants recruited at a common point in the disease or condition?
In the sciatica study, participants were recruited when they had symptoms of any duration. Although the majority (63.7%) of participants had symptoms for fewer than 12 weeks (acute or subacute pain), a substantial proportion (36.4%) had chronic symptoms, so we cannot consider that all participants were recruited at a common point.

Was the exposure measured accurately?

Exposure in a prognostic cohort study refers to the event or experience of interest that the whole cohort has had. (In other types of studies that might be used to provide prognostic information, such as case-control studies, only some of the participants will have had the exposure of interest.) This is the 'I' (intervention/issue) of the study's PICO. Some appraisal checklists consider the exposure and potential prognostic factors (for example, age or comorbid conditions) that might influence the outcome of interest together in this one question. However, in this chapter, we will explain the role of prognostic factors separately under the appraisal question, 'Were all confounding factors considered?' As long as prognostic factors are considered somewhere as part of the appraisal process, it does not matter under which item of the checklist this occurs.

In some prognostic cohort studies, individuals are selected for having had a particular exposure—say, caesarean section delivery among new mothers. In these studies, a particular outcome, such as exclusive breastfeeding, is measured over time. We can think of exposure measurement as whether participants' eligibility criteria were determined accurately. In the case of new mothers having had caesarean section, we need to assess whether the surgery was accurately documented—which is relatively straightforward. However, if the exposure was 'use of a trained doula throughout the birthing process', it would be important that the study provide a clear definition of 'trained doula' and 'throughout the birthing process' to ensure accurate measurement of the exposure.

⊚ CLINICAL SCENARIO (CONTINUED)

Was the exposure measured accurately?

In the sciatica study, the exposure was whether the participants had back-related leg pain or sciatica. Participants were recruited during a primary care visit and then had their pain and leg symptoms assessed by a physiotherapist. It is unlikely that there were errors in measuring this exposure; however, because the diagnosis of 'back-related leg pain' or 'sciatica' involves clinical opinion, there is more potential for bias than if the exposure was measured objectively (for example, if a diagnosis of sciatica could be based purely on diagnostic imaging [MRI] features, which is not possible using current technology). Notably, the sciatica study included a nested study assessing the reliability of physiotherapists making a sciatica diagnosis and found acceptable agreement. This improves confidence that the exposure was measured accurately.

Were the outcomes measured accurately?

Accuracy is important not only in the measurement of exposure, but also in the measurement of outcomes (that is, what the study is trying to predict). Researchers should specify and clearly define their outcomes at the start of the study. We must consider whether the outcome measures have been **validated**—that is, do they measure what they claim to measure? The article that you are appraising should provide details about the validity of the outcome measures that were used. The CASP checklist also suggests that we consider whether the outcomes are *objective* (for example, a fall) or *subjective* (for example, pain). Although it is not always possible, outcomes should be measured using **objective criteria** where possible. As the subjectivity of the outcome measures increases, the risk of bias increases. When the outcome requires a degree of judgment on the part of the person doing the assessing (the researcher or the participant), it is important that the **assessor be blinded to the participant's exposure/prognostic factors**. In some cases, the outcome assessor is the participant, as with Patient Reported Outcome Measures (PROMs) such as pain or quality of life, and so blinding of the assessor is not possible. If studies use PROMs, blinding patients to the study hypotheses and prognostic factors of interest could theoretically reduce bias, but this has not been explored empirically. It can be difficult to blind assessors to certain prognostic factors such as age and gender.

When prognostic studies report dichotomous outcomes, the criterion of accuracy is that the events have been clearly defined and a reliable system for identifying them has been implemented. For example, consider a cohort study of patients receiving non-invasive ventilation for acute respiratory failure that reports the number of patients that died during that hospital admission. As this study involved hospitalised patients, the death of a patient would have been recorded in the medical record, so we can be confident about the accuracy of this dichotomous outcome (alive or dead). Now consider a cohort study that followed up older people who had received a multidisciplinary intervention to prevent falls in the home and evaluated whether the patients sustained a fall in the year following the intervention. This dichotomous outcome (did or did not fall) is more difficult to measure accurately than the outcome of death in the above cohort study. Even if a fall was well defined and explained to patients, and strategies used such as a diary to record falls and a monthly telephone call to ask about falls, such events may not be reported if a patient misjudged whether the incident was a fall or forgot that it occurred or to make a record of it.

Were the outcomes measured accurately?

In the sciatica study, function was measured using the Roland-Morris Disability Questionnaire, which participants completed via a self-reported questionnaire. A strength of this outcome measure is that it is a valid and reliable outcome measure for people with low back pain, with or without leg pain. Because the assessors were the participants themselves (providing self-reported measures of function) it is likely that they were blind to the prognostic factors of interest measured in the study. Overall, the assessment of outcome measures in the sciatica study is sufficient to provide useful information.

Were important confounding factors considered?

We saw in Chapter 2 how confounding factors are anything that can become confused with the outcome of interest and bias the results. Although the CASP checklist explicitly mentions confounding factors, in studies of prognostic factors, it may be useful also to consider the full range of factors that may influence how well individual factors *predict* the outcome of interest, and to check whether the study has considered those factors.

A **prognostic factor** is any characteristic that is associated strongly enough with the outcome that it can accurately predict the eventual development of the outcome. Note that this does not necessarily mean that the prognostic factor causes the outcome. As mentioned previously, cohort prognostic studies only establish that a prognostic factor is associated with a given outcome. Prognostic factors, in some cases referred to as 'risk factors', can include demographic characteristics (such as age), disease-specific characteristics (for example, severity of a head injury) or whether the patient has any comorbid conditions. Accurate measurement of these factors is essential to the validity of the study. Objective and prospective collection of prognostic factor information is optimal but not always possible. When prognostic factors such as 'balance ability' or 'fear of falling' are assessed as potential factors for the risk of falling, for example, we must consider whether validated standardised measures were used; that is, do the study's measures measure what they claim to measure? Although it is not always possible, measurements should include **objective criteria** where possible. As the subjectivity of the measure increases, the risk of bias increases.

Many prognostic studies will report results for various sub-groups of participants who differ because of the presence of a certain prognostic factor (or factors), and the prognosis that is reported for each sub-group may be different. Once again, poorer outcomes in a group with a specific prognostic factor do not necessarily mean that the factor *caused* the outcome. A prognostic factor is *not* a target for treatment, unless there is evidence of a causal relationship. Herbert (2014) has written more on the important differences between studies of prognostic factors and aetiological factors.[5] When a study reports sub-group results, you need to check whether the researchers did an adjusted analysis. By this, we mean: did they check that these sub-group differences and predictions are not the result of another important prognostic factor? Information about any adjusted analysis that was done is usually presented in the data analysis section of an article. It is beyond the scope of this book to explain the statistical methods that are involved with adjusted analysis.

Prognostic factors

In the sciatica study, six sets of potential confounding or prognostic factors were considered for entry into each of the stepwise multiple linear regression analyses. They are a combination of standardised measures of pain and function (for example, leg pain intensity and the Hospital Anxiety and Depression scale [HADs] for depressive symptoms) and objective measures (such as clinical examination findings and imaging [MRI] examination findings). A broad array of factors was considered, making it unlikely that important factors were missed. Most of the factors were assessed by self-report questionnaire or in a standardised clinical examination by a physiotherapist with experience in the assessment and management of low back pain and sciatica. However, no data are provided on how many therapists were involved in data collection or how well standardised the collection of prognostic factors really was. All participants underwent an MRI within 2 weeks of their clinical assessment, and data on whether there was any relevant nerve root compression—an imaging finding sometimes associated with back-related leg pain and sciatica—were collected from participants' diagnostic imaging reports.

Was the follow-up of participants sufficiently long and complete?

There are two elements to this criterion, and you should assess whether the study meets both. You must use your knowledge about the condition of interest to judge whether the follow-up period was long enough for clinically important changes or events to occur. Consider a cohort study to determine the proportion of patients with a tracheostomy who can manage a speaking valve after weaning off a ventilator. This outcome (using a speaking valve) can be determined in minutes, meaning only a very short follow-up period is necessary. Conversely, another cohort study of very low birthweight infants to assess the onset of neurodevelopmental delay will need to follow participants for a decade or more to accurately assess the extent of neurodevelopmental delay.

The next issue is whether the follow-up was complete enough. We saw with randomised controlled trials in Chapter 4 that as loss to follow-up increases, so the risk for bias of the results increases (especially if there is something systematic about those who drop out). Some experts suggest the '5 and 20' rule: a loss to follow-up of less than 5% is unlikely to influence the results much, while a loss greater than 20% seriously threatens the risk of bias in a study.[6] The same rule-of-thumb guide can be used to determine whether follow-up in a prognostic study was sufficiently complete. As with randomised controlled trials, a study should also state the reasons why participants were lost to follow-up. It can also be helpful if a study provides a comparison of baseline potential prognostic factors for participants who were lost to follow-up and those who were not. This information can help you to determine whether there were certain types of participants who were selectively lost to follow-up.

◎ CLINICAL SCENARIO (CONTINUED)

Follow-up of participants
The sciatica study reports relatively poor follow-up of participants over 1 year: 73.9% of 609 participants had follow-up data. The clinical nature of sciatica means that a 1-year follow-up is sufficiently long to capture sustained and important changes in the primary outcome measures (pain and function).

If at this point you determine that the article about prognosis that you have been appraising is reasonably valid, you can proceed to look at the importance and applicability of the results.

WHAT ARE THE RESULTS?

Prognostic data can be presented in several ways, and studies commonly report continuous or dichotomous outcomes. Similar to the approach used to assess results of randomised trials in Chapter 4, we will look at two main questions for prognostic studies:
1. How **likely** are the outcomes over time?
2. How **precise** are the estimates of likelihood?

Likelihood of the outcomes over time

Prognostic data are usually only relevant to a particular time period (for example, 1 year post hip fracture or 1 week post total knee arthroplasty). Continuous outcomes measures are usually reported as a mean value at a certain time period. For example, men with aphasia after their first stroke showed an average improvement of 12.3 on the Aphasia Quotient 1 year after stroke.[7] The Aphasia Quotient is a measure of the severity of aphasia, rated from 0 (worst) to 100 (best).

Dichotomous and ordinal outcomes are usually reported as the proportion of patients who experienced the outcome (that is, the risk of the event) at a particular point in time. For example, among adults over 65 years who present to primary care with back pain, 60% reported persistent disability (Roland-Morris Disability Questionnaire score of ≥4) at 6 months.[8] The same information can be reported from the viewpoint of an individual patient: for an older adult who presents to primary care with a new episode of back pain, the risk of having persistent disability 6 months later is 60%. Such information over several time intervals can be evaluated in a *survival analysis*.

Survival analyses were originally used to evaluate time from treatment until death, but survival analysis is now applied to other areas and outcomes, including in studies of prognosis. In some prognostic studies, a survival analysis might be used to compare outcomes in people (such as whether they experience the event/outcome of interest) and when that occurs. Some studies might examine outcomes in people, over time, with and without a prognostic factor. One common statistic in survival analysis is *median survival time,* which refers to the shortest time at which the probability of the outcome drops to 0.5 or 50% or below. In other words, it is the length of time from study entry to when half of the participants in the study experience the outcome of interest (for example, death, persistent disability, recovery). In intervention studies, differences in median survival time can be used to examine intervention effectiveness, but in prognostic studies, median survival time can be used to evaluate the influence of prognostic factors.

A study about risk factors for women experiencing a hip fracture provides an example of how a prognostic factor from continuous data can be reported as ordinal data.[9] In this study, increasing age (continuous data) was reported as a risk factor for hip fracture in women over 65 years of age. For every 5-year increment in age (ordinal data), the

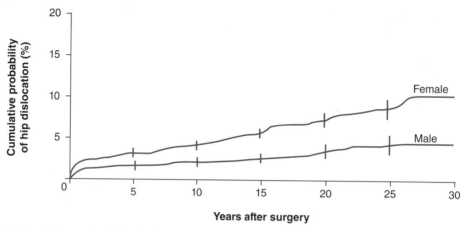

Fig 8.1 Cumulative probability of a first-time hip dislocation for female and male patients.
Reproduced with permission from Berry DJ, von Knoch M, Schleck CD, et al. The cumulative long-term risk of dislocation after primary Charnley total hip arthroplasty. J Bone Joint Surg Am 2004;86:9–14.

risk of a hip fracture increased 1.5 times. This study also treated some risk factors dichotomously. For example, having a maternal history of hip fracture was found to double a woman's risk for hip fracture.

Survival curves are often used to visually present prognostic data and they show how the likelihood of an event changes over time. A Kaplan-Meier curve is a common method used in survival analysis. Figure 8.1 shows a survival curve from a study that examined the long-term risk of dislocation following total hip arthroplasty (replacement).[10] In this particular survival curve, the cumulative risk of hip dislocation following hip replacement is presented separately for females and males. You can see that at 25 years, the risk of dislocation for females was 8.9% (the authors also provide the 95% confidence interval [CI] for this: 7.7 to 10.2), whereas the risk for males was 4.5% (95% CI 3.3 to 5.8). You can also see, by looking at the slope of the curve, that female participants had both a higher early and a higher late risk of dislocation compared to male participants.

It is possible to calculate the magnitude of the difference between the two curves in a Kaplan-Meier survival plot; this is known as the *hazard ratio*. A hazard ratio of 1 means there is no difference in outcomes in those with or without the prognostic factor. Values above or below 1 mean that outcomes were better in people with the prognostic factor, or vice versa. Interpretation of the hazard ratio is therefore like a risk ratio. That is, it describes how many times more (or less) likely a participant was to experience an event at a given time point if they were exposed to the prognostic factor or not. For example, in a study of frailty and risk of mortality from COVID-19, a hazard ratio of 2.39 was reported, meaning that those with frailty

were 2.39 times more likely to die during the study period than those who were not classified as frail.[11]

Precision of the estimates of likelihood

To properly interpret a prognostic study, it is necessary to know how much uncertainty is associated with its results. Just as we saw for estimating the effect of an intervention in Chapter 4, a 95% confidence interval indicates the precision of an estimate of prognosis. As with the confidence intervals for randomised controlled trials, the larger the size of the prognostic study, the narrower (and more precise) the confidence interval will be. Confidence intervals can often be calculated if the authors of an article have not provided them.

Calculating a confidence interval for continuous outcomes

For continuous outcomes, the 95% confidence interval provides the range of average values within which we are 95% certain that the true average value lies. It can be calculated approximately using an online calculator (https://sample-size.net/confidence-interval-mean/).[12,13]

You will need to enter values for N (sample size), m (sample mean) and S (sample standard deviation). Let us assume in our example of aphasia in men after their first stroke that the mean improvement of 12.3 on the Aphasia Quotient had a standard deviation of 18 and was determined using data from 83 patients. Entering these values into the calculator, it provides a lower bound CI of 8.37 and an upper bound of 16.23. Therefore, we could expect that, in men with aphasia after their first stroke, the average level of improvement would be between 8 and 16 on the Aphasia Quotient 1 year post-stroke.

Calculating a confidence interval for dichotomous outcomes

For dichotomous outcomes, which are reported as the risk of (or proportion of people experiencing) an event, the 95% confidence interval provides the range of risks within which we are 95% certain that the true risk lies. It can be calculated approximately using an online calculator (https://sample-size.net/confidence-interval-proportion/).[12] Let us assume, in our example of back pain, that the 60% risk of having persistent disability 6 months later was determined using data from 1,080 patients. You just need to enter values for N (1080) and x (number in the sample with the result or finding in question—that is, 648 [60% of 1,080]) and this gives a lower bound of 0.570 and an upper bound of 0.629. Therefore, we can assume that the risk of persistent disability at 6 months is between 57% and 63%.

Identification and analysis of prognostic factors

In prognostic studies, data about the likelihood of the outcome are typically presented first, and then an analysis of prognostic factors is presented, if the study conducts such an analysis. Such data may be presented by simply reporting the prognosis for various sub-groups of participants, where each sub-group has a certain prognostic factor (or if dealing with a continuous variable, varying degrees of the factor). Data about prognostic factors may also be presented in a more complex way using multivariate predictive models that assess how each prognostic factor is associated with each other prognostic factor and the overall prognosis. An explanation of multivariate analysis techniques is beyond the scope of this book.

◎ CLINICAL SCENARIO (CONTINUED)

What are the results?
In the sciatica study, of the individuals ($n = 452$) who were diagnosed with sciatica, 55% reported improvement by 12 months. At 12 months after presenting to primary care, leg pain had reduced from a mean (SD) numeric rating scale score of 5.2 (2.4) at baseline to 2.4 (2.7), and function had improved from a mean (SD) Roland-Morris Disability Questionnaire score of 12.6 (5.7) at baseline to 7.8 (7.0), which would be classified as 'persistent disability/functional limitation'.

A patient's pain duration, pain intensity and psychological factors, including whether the symptoms were contributing to an illness identity, and the belief that the problem will last a long time, were the best predictors of poor physical function outcome at 12 months. Perhaps unexpectedly, nerve-related muscle weakness, which is often associated with more serious neurological compromise in patients with sciatica,[14] was associated with a *higher* likelihood of functional improvement at 12 months.

This suggests that Mrs Lee has about a 55% chance of being improved at 4 and 12 months. She has had the pain for a relatively short period, her pain intensity is moderate and, although her HADs score suggests she has some depressive symptoms, overall the association of HADs with poor outcome is weak. So, her prognosis for improved physical function by 4 months is fair, although it should be explained that this is not certain and that about 45% of patients like her will still have symptoms after a year.

HOW CAN WE USE THIS EVIDENCE TO INFORM PRACTICE?

As we saw in Chapter 4 in the section on using evidence about interventions, before applying the evidence from a study, you need to consider whether your patient is similar to the participants in the study. The same consideration needs to occur before applying the results from a prognostic study to your patient.

Prognostic information has several uses in clinical practice. Having information about the likely clinical course of a condition can help you to determine whether an intervention is needed. If the prognosis for natural recovery is very good, there may be little point in providing any intervention. Similarly, if the prognosis for a cohort treated with a particular intervention is very good, then alternative or additional interventions may not need to be considered. In such cases, using the information to counsel patients and provide them with explanation and reassurance may be all that is necessary.

Prognostic information can be valuable in educating patients. For example, if the prognosis for the condition may be able to be improved by intervention and there are available interventions that are likely to make a clinically important difference, the information that you have about prognosis can form the starting point for a discussion with your patient. Additionally, shared decision making (see Chapter 14) can be supported by discussing the prognosis associated with various intervention options (which may include the option of 'doing nothing'). Shared decision making is an important component of evidence-based practice (and indeed, clinical practice in general) and further information about this and strategies to facilitate shared decision making are discussed in Chapter 14.

Central to facilitating patient engagement in decision making is communicating with patients effectively. Again, Chapter 14 provides you with several practical strategies that you can use to ensure that you are communicating effectively with your patients. When explaining prognostic information to a patient, do so in a way that the patient can understand and communicate what is relevant to the patient's goals and priorities, and use visual tools where appropriate.[15] Focus on the outcomes and time frames that matter most to the patient. In addition, if the patient has particular factors that affect their prognosis, it is reasonable to consider explaining their influence especially if any of them have evidence of a causal association with outcomes and are modifiable (for example, smoking). It is also important to remember that each patient has their own course of recovery (or decline). Whether the prognostic evidence that you have reviewed for the patient is positive or negative, the individual nature of each person's experience requires consideration for, and acknowledgment of, the possibility that that individual might have a different experience than any group of individuals described in a prognostic research study.

◎ CLINICAL SCENARIO (CONTINUED)

Using the evidence to inform practice
After reading about the characteristics of the study participants, you decide that Mrs Lee is similar enough to the study participants that the results could apply to her. We could begin by explaining that her predicted function at 4 and 12 months after presenting is likely to be mainly influenced by how long she has had the pain, but that psychological factors such as her outlook for the future may also play a role. Given that her main concern is her capacity to return to work, it needs to be explained that her recovery may occur slowly (over the course of 12 months), but she has a reasonable chance at recovery over the coming months. It is not possible from the results in this study to estimate Mrs Lee's likelihood of returning to desk work in the short term, because this outcome was not measured in the sciatica study.

Ultimately, although Mrs Lee has several indicators of a good recovery, she is likely to need some level of on-going care and timely review. Because it is not possible to estimate Mrs Lee's likelihood of returning to work in the short term based on the sciatica study alone, this makes timely follow-up to monitor her progress important. All participants in the sciatica fracture study received rehabilitation. Most had brief physiotherapy (47%) or extended physiotherapy (42%), and a smaller percentage (12%) were also referred for secondary care. Thus, to achieve similar outcomes to the participants in the study, you should discuss the option of rehabilitation with Mrs Lee.

SUMMARY

- Evidence about prognosis is traditionally found in cohort studies, with prospective cohort studies a stronger study design than retrospective cohort studies.
- Systematic reviews of data from several studies are usually even better.
- When searching for prognostic studies, include terms for the patient's problem, the intervention they receive (unless you are interested in the prognosis of the untreated condition) and the outcomes that are most important to the patient.
- The participants included in the study should be representative of the population from which they were sampled, and their condition should have been accurately diagnosed.
- The most valid prognostic evidence comes from cohort studies in which the participants were identified at an early and uniform point in their disease.
- Exposures and their outcomes should have been accurately measured with an appropriate and valid tool.

- Follow-up of the participants in the study should have been sufficiently long and complete to identify the outcome of interest.
- The two main questions that you need to ask when considering the results of a prognostic study are: (1) How likely are the outcomes over time? (2) How precise are the estimates of likelihood?
- The average prognostic estimate for patients in the study can often be tailored to your particular patient by considering factors that influence the prognosis.
- Many patients require help in interpreting prognostic estimates. This can sometimes be done by relating predicted outcomes to threshold values, such as the patient's current value or the average value for healthy people, and the values required for functional activities that are important to the patient.

ACKNOWLEDGMENTS

The updated version of this chapter for this edition is based on Chapter 8 in the first three editions of this book, which were authored by Professor Mark Elkins (University of Sydney) and Professor Julie Tilson (University of Southern California). We gratefully acknowledge their valuable contribution to the structure and content of this chapter.

REFERENCES

1. Liou T, Adler S, FitzSimmons B, et al. Predictive 5-year survivorship model of cystic fibrosis. Am J Epidemiol 2001;153: 345–52.
2. Burgerhout K, Kamperman A, Roza S, et al. Functional recovery after postpartum psychosis: a prospective longitudinal study. J Clin Psychiatry 2017;78(1):122–8.
3. Konstantinou K, Dunn KM, Ogollah R, et al. Prognosis of sciatica and back-related leg pain in primary care: the ATLAS cohort. Spine J 2018;18(6):1030–40.
4. Segawa H, Tsukayama D, Kyle R, et al. Infection after total knee arthroplasty: a retrospective study of the treatment of eighty-one infections. J Bone Joint Surg Am 1999;81:1434–45.
5. Herbert RD. Cohort studies of aetiology and prognosis: they're different. J Physiother 2014;60(4):241–4.
6. Straus S, Richardson W, Glasziou P, et al. Evidence-based medicine: how to practice and teach EBM. 5th ed. Edinburgh: Elsevier; 2018.
7. Pedersen P, Vinter K, Olsen T. Aphasia after stroke: type, severity and prognosis. Cerebrovasc Dis 2004;17:35–43.
8. Rundell S, Sherman K, Heagerty P, et al. Predictors of persistent disability and back pain in older adults with a new episode of care for back pain. Pain Med 2017;18(6): 1049–62.
9. Cummings S, Nevitt M, Browner W, et al. Risk factors for hip fracture in white women. N Engl J Med 1995;332: 767–74.
10. Berry J, Von Knoch M, Schleck C, et al. The cumulative long-term risk of dislocation after primary Charnley total hip arthroplasty. J Bone Joint Surg Am 2004;86:9–14.
11. Hewitt J, Carter B, Vilches-Moraga A, et al. The effect of frailty on survival in patients with COVID-19 (COPE): a multicentre, European, observational cohort study. Lancet Public Health 2020;5(8):e444–51.
12. Kohn MA, Senyak J. Sample Size Calculators (website). UCSF CTSI; 20 December 2021. Online. Available: https://www.sample-size.net/ (accessed 2 March 2022).
13. Hulley SB, Cummings SR, Browner WS, et al. Designing clinical research: an epidemiologic approach. 4th ed. Philadelphia, PA: Lippincott Williams & Wilkins; 2013. Appendix 6A, p. 73.
14. Grotle M, Brox JI, Veierød MB, et al. Clinical course and prognostic factors in acute low back pain: patients consulting primary care for the first time. Spine 2005;30(8):976–82.
15. Abukmail E, Bakhit M, Del Mar C, et al. Effect of different visual presentations on the comprehension of prognostic information: a systematic review. BMC Med Inform Decis Mak 2021;21(1):249.

9

Questions about Prognosis
Examples of Appraisals from Different Health Professions

Mina Bakhit, Malcolm Boyle, Elizabeth Gibson, Isabel Jalbert, Jacqueline Jauncey-Cooke, Sohil Khan, Karl Landorf, Amary Mey, Natalie Munro, Shannon Munteanu, Toby Pavey, Nicola Shelton, Josh Zadro and Tammy Hoffmann

This chapter is an accompaniment to the previous chapter (Chapter 8), where the steps involved in answering a clinical question about prognosis were explained. To further help you learn how to deal with prognostic clinical questions when they arise and appraise the evidence, this chapter contains a number of worked examples of questions about prognosis from a range of health professions. The worked examples in this chapter follow the same format as the examples in Chapters 5 and 7 (and note that the screening criteria from the relevant CASP checklist are not presented for each example and were considered as part of the step of selecting which article to appraise). As with the worked examples that were written for Chapters 5 and 7, the authors of the worked examples in this chapter were asked not to choose a systematic review (for the reason explained in Chapter 5), but instead to find the next best available level of evidence to answer the prognostic question that was generated from the clinical scenario. All the other caveats about these worked examples (such as using more than one study prior to deciding about how the evidence might inform practice) that were presented at the beginning of Chapter 5 also apply to the worked examples in this chapter.

◎ OCCUPATIONAL THERAPY EXAMPLE

Clinical scenario

You are an occupational therapist working in a neurological rehabilitation unit of a large metropolitan hospital. A 50-year-old woman, Maria, who had an ischaemic stroke 3 weeks ago, has been referred to the unit from acute care for rehabilitation. At your initial goal-setting interview, Maria identifies that one of her main goals is to return to work in a part-time administration job in a government agency. Although she is keen to return to work and her employer is keeping her job available for her while she is on sick leave, she is also increasingly worried about how realistic a goal it is given her residual impairments. These include hemiparesis and difficulty concentrating and remembering things, which are affecting some basic and instrumental activities of daily living. She is walking independently. She was discharged from acute care with a score of 3 on the modified Rankin Scale, indicating moderate disability, and a score of 10 on the Hospital Anxiety and Depression Scale, indicating possible mild depression. You assure her that you can work with her to assess her functional abilities and consider her return-to-work goal. You decide to search the evidence about return to work for people post-stroke to assist your discussion with Maria.

Clinical question

For an employed middle-aged woman with a recent stroke and who has mild to moderate disability in activities of daily living, how likely is it that she will return to work within the next 6 months and what factors are predictive of returning to work?

Search terms and databases used to find the evidence

Database: PubMed—Clinical Queries (with 'prognosis category' and 'narrow scope' selected).
Search terms: stroke AND (return to work)

This search retrieves 107 records. You find several possibly relevant studies, but you first look at a study from Brazil which notes the differences about stroke in developing countries, including lower age of occurrence, which is applicable to your patient.

Article chosen

Nascimento LR, Scianni AA, Ada L, et al. Predictors of return to work after stroke: a prospective, observational cohort study with 6 months follow-up. Disabil Rehabil 2021;43(4):525–9.

Structured abstract (adapted from above)

Study design: Prospective observational cohort study.
Setting: Four public hospitals in Brazil.
Participants: 117 of an initial 142 adults (≥18 years) with a clinical diagnosis of a stroke within 28 days and who had undertaken any paid employment in the month before the stroke. Exclusion criteria included severe cognitive or language deficits.
Outcome: Return to full-time or part-time work (yes or no).
Prognostic factors studied: Age, gender, education (dichotomised into low [none or primary school] or high [≥secondary school]), marital status, contribution to household income (main contributor or partial contributor ≤50%), type of work (blue- or white-collar), independence in activities of daily living (ADL; dependent, ≥3/6 on the Modified Rankin Scale [mRS] or independent, <3/6 on mRS), depression (depressed, ≥8/21 on Hospital and Anxiety Depression Scale or not depressed, <8/21).
Follow-up period: 3 and 6 months after stroke onset.
Main results: Of the 117 participants (mean age 57 years) who were contactable at follow-up, 20 (17%) had returned to work immediately (<28 days), 45 (38%) by 3 months and 52 (44%) by 6 months. Being the major contributor to household income, a white-collar worker, independent in ADL and not depressed at 3 months after stroke, predicted return to work at 6 months, with independence in ADL the greatest predictor.

Conclusion: Interventions aimed at improving independence in ADL may increase return to work after stroke.

Is the evidence likely to be biased?

- *Was there a representative and well-defined sample?*
  Unclear. Although it was a prospective study, the period of recruitment was clear ('over the course of a year') and the sample was well-defined—for example, in terms of stroke, definition of employment, work status and clear exclusion criteria (severe cognitive or language deficits)—it was not clear if all or consecutive patients were screened for eligibility, as a reported limitation of the study was that 'the recruitment was conducted on a volunteer basis'.
- *Were participants recruited at a common point in their disease or condition?*
  Yes. Participants were recruited at a common point after stroke onset (within 28 days).
- *Was exposure determined accurately?*
  Yes. A clinical diagnosis of stroke was required.
- *Were the outcomes measured accurately?*
  Probably. Although a definition of return to paid work was provided, it was based on self-report so may not be as reliable as registry data or other more objective measures.
- *Were important confounding factors considered?*
  Yes. Important potentially confounding factors were measured, including demographic factors and disability-related factors. The demographic factors were measured by self-report, but ADL and depression were measured by validated and reliable instruments.
- *Was the follow-up of participants sufficiently long and complete?*
  Unclear. Although early return to work after illness can be promising for sustaining longer term employment, the follow-up was only 3 and 6 months, so we cannot make any conclusions about the likely sustainability of the return-to-work outcomes. However, for your patient and clinical question, which involved a 6-month time frame, it is sufficient. Follow-up at 3 months was 82% (n = 117) with reasons provided for participant drop-out (three had died, 17 were uncontactable). Results for follow-up at 6 months are reported for all the remaining participants, so it appears no further participants were lost to follow-up between 3 and 6 months.

What are the main results?

By 28 days, 17% of participants had returned to work, 38% by 3 months and 44% by 6 months. Being independent with ADLs at 3 months (scoring <3 on mRS) meant participants were nearly 11 times more likely to return to work at 6 months than to be dependent (odds ratio [OR]

Continued

⊚ OCCUPATIONAL THERAPY EXAMPLE—cont'd

10.6, 95% confidence interval [CI] 2.9 to 38.3). Not being depressed at 3 months (<8 on the HADs) meant participants were nearly five times more likely to return to work at 6 months than someone who had depression (OR 4.92, 95% CI 1.69 to 14.37). Being a white-collar worker meant participants were four times more likely as a blue-collar worker to return to work (OR 4.0, 95% CI 1.80 to 8.57). Making more than 50% of the household income meant participants were more than twice as likely to return to work at 6 months than someone making less than 50% (OR 2.41, 95% CI 0.99 to 5.89).

How might we use this evidence to inform practice?

In your assessment with Maria, you briefly tell her about this research and note that while some of the results may not apply to her due to circumstances such as where she lives and works, the study can be useful as reassurance that return to work is possible for some people after stroke, especially in a white-collar job such as hers. You work with her to set goals about improving her ADL independence and mental health, conduct a detailed assessment of her basic and instrumental ADL, and obtain a report of her work tasks and environment. You encourage Maria that return to work is a realistic goal, given that she has a white-collar job and especially if you and she can work together on improving her independence and increasing her engagement in meaningful activities, obtain psychological support and strategies for her mild depression, and liaise with her workplace about potential modifications to her work tasks and environment, at least in the short term.

⊚ PHYSIOTHERAPY EXAMPLE

Clinical scenario

Jonathan Kelly is a 67-year-old man who retired 10 years ago after working as a carpenter for most of his life. He has been a pack-a-day smoker for the last 30 years. Mr Kelly's work required a significant amount of heavy lifting and sustained awkward positions, which he believes contributed to persistent bilateral shoulder pain. He is scheduled to undergo rotator cuff repair surgery for a right full-thickness supraspinatus tear next week. He has been referred to you for preoperative care and to explain to him what postoperative rehabilitation will involve. Mr Kelly had a similar surgery on his left side 10 years ago when he retired. Over the last 2 years, worsening pain in his right shoulder has prevented him from playing golf and doing work in the garden. This prompted him to go back to the orthopaedic surgeon who operated previously on his left shoulder. An MRI showed a full-thickness supraspinatus tear and significant atrophy of the supraspinatus and infraspinatus muscles. Mr Kelly took 2 years to get back to his usual activities following surgery on his left shoulder. The pain in his right shoulder is not as bad as his left shoulder pain was before surgery but Mr Kelly is worried that being older now will prolong his recovery from this surgery.

Clinical question

In adults scheduled to undergo rotator cuff repair surgery, are any preoperative factors associated with poor postoperative shoulder function at 2 years?

Search terms and databases used to find the evidence

Database: PubMed—Clinical Queries (with 'prognosis category' and 'narrow scope' selected).

Search terms: (rotator cuff repair) AND (function OR (functional outcome)) AND (prognostic factors) AND (adults) AND (2-year OR 2 year)

The search returns 23 records. You scan the titles of the articles and read the abstracts of several studies that seem like they could be relevant. Of these, one is highly relevant as it is a large prospective cohort study of people after rotator cuff repair surgery with a 2-year follow-up.

Article chosen

Jenssen KK, Lundgreen K, Madsen JE, et al. Prognostic factors for functional outcome after rotator cuff repair: a prospective cohort study with 2-year follow-up. Am J Sports Med 2018;46(14):3463–70.

Structured abstract (adapted from the above)

Study design: Prognostic cohort study.

Setting: Consecutive participants treated with rotator cuff repair surgery between 2010 and 2014 at a single orthopaedic unit in Norway.

Participants: 733 participants (647 followed up, mean age 58 years, 39% female) who underwent rotator cuff repair surgery due to a dysfunctional and painful shoulder attributed to an acute or chronic rotator cuff tear that was non-responsive to a minimum of 3 months' exercise therapy. The rotator cuff tear needed to be repairable or partially repairable as diagnosed by clinical examination and confirmed on MRI.

Outcomes: Shoulder function assessed by the Western Ontario Rotator Cuff Index (WORC) and expressed as a percentage. Higher scores indicate better shoulder function.

Prognostic factors: Divided into pre- and perioperative factors. Examples of preoperative factors include age, gender, body mass index (BMI), smoking, duration of symptoms, previous shoulder surgery, shoulder function, and muscle atrophy and fatty infiltration on MRI. Examples of perioperative factors include number of tendons ruptured, revision rotator cuff repair, partial repairs for massive cuff tears not amenable to complete repair, and other concomitant surgical procedures.

Follow-up period: 2 years.

Main results: Of the 647 (88%) participants who completed the follow-up, mean WORC scores were 81% (increased from 44% preoperatively). In a multivariate analysis, the strongest positive independent predictors of shoulder function at 2 years were preoperative WORC and Constant-Murley score in the contralateral shoulder. Factors with independent positive associations with better shoulder function at 2 years included ADL, age, subacromial decompression and biceps surgery. Those with negative associations with shoulder function after 2 years were previous surgery in the ipsilateral or contralateral shoulder, smoking, partial rotator cuff repair, preoperative pain, and atrophy in the infraspinatus.

Conclusion: Several pre- and perioperative factors were predictive of worse shoulder function at 2 years, with the finding that better preoperative shoulder function in the contralateral shoulder was the best prognostic factor of shoulder function in the operated shoulder at 2 years follow-up.

Is this evidence likely to be biased?

- *Was there a representative and well-defined sample?*
  Yes. The participants, as defined by the inclusion criteria, are representative of the type of patients who undergo rotator cuff repair surgery. Participants were recruited prospectively and consecutively, suggesting a low risk of selection bias.

- *Were participants recruited at a common point in their disease or condition?*
  Unclear. All participants were recruited at a single orthopaedic unit before undergoing rotator cuff repair surgery. Although the preoperative recruitment time frame is unclear, it is highly likely all participants were recruited within a few weeks of the surgery due to the nature of the clinic. There is a wide range in duration (0 to 120 months) from time of shoulder trauma to surgery and while this is probably representative of patients having this surgery, it is unclear if this duration range may have influenced the results.

- *Was the exposure measured accurately?*
  Unclear. Numerous pre- and perioperative exposure (prognostic) variables are listed, but the accuracy of the tools used to assess many of them is not reported in the article.

- *Were the outcomes measured accurately?*
  Unclear. The main outcome was shoulder function assessed by the WORC. Accuracy for the method of data collection is unknown, since how it was administered is not reported.

- *Were important confounding factors considered?*
  Yes. The researchers identified a range of possible prognostic factors (see abstract). Potential confounding factors (including pre- and perioperative factors) were included as prognostic factors.

- *Was the follow-up of participants sufficiently long and complete?*
  Yes. The duration was sufficient, as 2 years postoperatively is sufficient to see improvements in shoulder function following surgery. The follow-up rate is reasonably high (88%), indicating low risk of attrition bias.

What are the main results?

Of the 647 participants who completed the 2-year follow-up, mean shoulder function scores were 81% (improved from 44% preoperatively). Table 9.1 shows preoperative prognostic factors significantly associated with shoulder function at the 2-year follow-up. Perioperative factors are not reported here as these were not part of our PICO question. Preoperative factors independently predictive of worse postoperative shoulder function included previous surgery on the same or contralateral shoulder, smoking, atrophy of the infraspinatus on MRI and worse preoperative shoulder function (including on the contralateral side) and younger age. For continuous prognostic factors, the

Continued

PHYSIOTHERAPY EXAMPLE—cont'd

TABLE 9.1   Multivariate analysis of preoperative prognostic factors significantly associated with shoulder function (measured by WORC) at 2-year follow-up

Preoperative prognostic factors, ranked in order of relative effect of each factor on the outcome	Unstandardised coefficient B values (95% CIs)	p-value
Previous surgery: same shoulder	−7.14 (−12.01 to −2.27)	0.004
Smoking	−6.04 (−10.8 to 1.27)	0.013
Previous surgery: Contralateral shoulder	−5.84 (−9.79 to −1.88)	0.004
Atrophy of the infraspinatus on MRI	−4.47 (−7.05 to −1.89)	0.01
CM score: ADL sub-score	0.79 (0.24 to 1.34)	0.005
CM score: pain sub-score	−0.75 (−1.3 to −0.19)	0.009
WORC index	0.42 (0.32 to 0.52)	<0.001
Age	0.37 (0.21 to 0.53)	<0.001
CM score contralateral shoulder	0.20 (0.14 to 0.27)	<0.001

CM: Constant-Murley is an objective measure of shoulder function with four sub-scales: strength, pain, activities of daily living (ADL), magnetic resonance imaging (MRI).
B represents the difference in the number of points on the outcome variable for each unit change in the independent variable.

change in shoulder function score at 2 years is based on a one-unit change in the prognostic factor. For example, a one-point increase in preoperative WORC score translates to a 0.4-point increase in postoperative WORC score. For dichotomous prognostic factors, the change in shoulder function score at 2 years is based on moving from the reference category to the case category. For example, people who smoked preoperatively experienced, on average, 6 points worse shoulder function postoperatively compared to those who were non-smokers preoperatively.

How might we use this evidence to inform practice?
This prognostic evidence seems to have a reasonably low risk of bias and the sample size is quite large. Mr Kelly's clinical presentation does not seem so vastly different

from the study participants' that the evidence would not apply to him. To apply the evidence, you will need to assess the preoperative prognostic factors used in the study for Mr Kelly, as the presence of some of these factors may suggest he will experience worse function postoperatively (for example, if his preoperative WORC score is low). You plan to explain this evidence to Mr Kelly carefully, as he is already anxious about his prognosis due to his age, and to help him have realistic postoperative expectations. The design of this study does not provide information about whether changing any of these factors will improve shoulder function postoperatively, so you next plan is to search for evidence about postoperative rehabilitation protocols that might be able to increase Mr Kelly's postoperative shoulder function.

PODIATRY EXAMPLE

Clinical scenario
You are a podiatrist working in a diabetic foot service in a regional hospital in northern Australia. You have just seen a 39-year-old man, who was referred by his general practitioner for assessment and management of an ulcer on the plantar aspect of the first metatarsophalangeal joint of his left foot. It has been present for about 2 months. He has had type 2 diabetes for

about 12 years and advises that his blood glucose control has 'not been very good'. He is a long-term smoker.

Your initial examination indicates that in addition to the ulcer, there is some foot deformity (that is, a plantarflexed first ray and clawing of the lesser digits), neuropathy is present and vascular assessment is satisfactory. The ulceration has white, macerated margins, the base is clean and pink to red and there is no exudate. The ulcer is round with a surface area of 2 cm^2 and its depth extends to the subcutaneous tissue but not tendon or bone. There do not appear to be any sinuses and you cannot probe to bone, suggesting it is not infected.

While discussing an intervention plan with the patient, you observe that he does not consider his poor diabetes control and foot ulcer to be an issue. He jokingly says, 'I'm young . . . My ulcer will heal fine in no time!' You know that foot ulceration is a serious complication of diabetes, but you are not sure of the prognosis for healing, especially in someone so young. You decide to conduct a search to see if you can find some evidence to guide your answer to the question before you see the patient again in a few days' time.

Clinical question
In a person with a diabetes-related foot ulcer, what factors predict healing?

Search terms and databases used to find the evidence
Database: PubMed—Clinical Queries (with 'prognosis category' and 'narrow scope' selected).
Search terms: (diabetes-related foot ulcer*) AND heal*

Your search finds about 30 studies, including some studies in Australian populations and some in non-Australian populations. Because there are some unique issues related to healing diabetic foot ulcers in northern Australia, you scan the titles and choose the following article, which most closely matches your clinical question and context.

Article chosen
Zhang Y, Cramb S, McPhail SM, et al. Factors associated with healing of diabetes-related foot ulcers: observations from a large prospective real-world cohort. Diabetes Care 2021;44(7):e143–5.

Structured abstract (adapted from the above)
Study design: Prospective cohort study.
Setting: Diabetic foot services across 15 of 17 regions in Queensland, Australia.
Participants: 4,832 patients that presented to a diabetic foot service for their first visit with a diabetic foot ulcer. Data were available for analysis at 3 months and 12 months for 4,709 people (median age 63 years; 69.5% male; 10.5% Indigenous Australians; 91.0% with type 2 diabetes). Where patients had multiple ulcers, researchers used the most severe score for each factor and combined the ulcer size from all ulcers.

Outcomes: Diabetic foot ulcers healed.
Prognostic factors studied: Several prognostic factors were measured at the first visit using the Queensland High Risk Foot Form.[1] Factors related to: demographics (age, sex, Indigenous status and residential postcode), presence of comorbidity (diabetes type, diabetes duration, glycated haemoglobin [HbA1c], blood glucose levels, hypertension, dyslipidaemia, cardiovascular disease, chronic kidney disease, and smoking status), the lower limb (previous foot ulcer, previous amputation, foot deformity, peripheral neuropathy, peripheral arterial disease, suspected Charcot foot), ulcer characteristics (surface area, grade and depth, presence of infection), recent provider of treatment at the first visit or preceding week (podiatrist, general practitioner, surgeon, physician, nurse, orthotists or other) and treatment type at the first visit (sharp debridement, appropriate wound dressings, prescribed antibiotics; optimum offloading using a cast walker, appropriate footwear, patient education).
Follow-up period: 12 months (with assessments at 3 and 12 months).
Main results: Of 4,709 patients available at 12 months follow-up, the ulcers of 1,956 (42%) patients had healed within 3 months and 3,012 (64%) within 12 months. Factors negatively associated with foot ulcer healing, at both 3 and 12 months, included younger age (<50 years), geographical remoteness, smoking, peripheral arterial disease, large ulcer sizes, deep ulcers and infection. Neuropathy was negatively associated with ulcer healing at 3 months only. Previous amputation as well as recent surgical and medical specialist treatment were negatively associated with healing at 12 months. Only one factor (receiving knee-high offloading treatment at the first visit) was positively associated with foot ulcer healing by 3 and 12 months.
Conclusion: This study confirms the negative influence of smoking and ulcer-related and limb factors that affect healing of diabetic foot ulcers. It provides evidence of additional negative factors for healing, including being of a younger age and living in regional or remote geographical areas.

Is the evidence likely to be biased?
* *Was there a representative and well-defined sample?*
  Yes. The target population is well-defined, and the sample is likely to be representative of the broader population with this condition in this geographical region. Consecutive patients with a diabetic foot

Continued

◎ PODIATRY EXAMPLE—cont'd

ulcer who attended each of the 65 diabetic foot services across 15 Queensland regions between July 2011 and December 2017 were recruited. The definition used for a foot ulcer is appropriate. The characteristics of the patients attending the diabetic foot services are representative of those with a diabetic foot ulcer.

- *Were participants recruited at a common point in their disease or condition?*
  Unclear. The range of time over which the foot ulcers had been present is not reported. As participants may not have been recruited at a similar point during this condition, it is possible that bias due to variable disease duration within the cohort may exist.
- *Was exposure measured accurately?*
  Yes. A diabetic foot ulcer was clearly defined (a full-thickness wound below the ankle on a person with diabetes), with assessments performed by foot-related health professionals.
- *Were the outcomes measured accurately?*
  Probably. The outcome of diabetic foot ulcer healing was clearly defined (complete epithelialisation of all ulcers without amputation, death, or recurrence within 1 month) and measured using a validated outcome measure. It is not clear whether the outcome assessors were blind to clinical characteristics or prognostic factors when measuring the outcome, although as the outcome is quite objective this is of less concern.

- *Were important prognostic factors considered?*
  Yes. The researchers identified an extensive range of factors that could have potential prognostic value and controlled for these in their statistical analyses. Prognostic factors were assessed using the Queensland High Risk Foot Form,[1] which is a valid and reliable tool to assess relevant aspects of foot disease in at-risk populations, including individuals with diabetes.
- *Was the follow-up of participants sufficiently long and complete?*
  Yes. The follow-up of 12 months is an adequate duration to observe ulcer healing. Of the 4,832 patients originally enrolled, 123 were lost to follow-up, providing a follow-up of 97%.

What are the main results?

By 3 months, 42% of the ulcers had healed and by 12 months, 64% had healed. Seven factors were negatively associated with healing (that is, made healing less likely) at 3 and 12 months and one was positively associated. Table 9.2 lists the prognostic factors relevant to your patient, including younger age (<50 years), being a smoker and being from a regional area. Receiving a knee-high offloading treatment at the first visit meant that the odds of healing is 1.34 times higher at 3 months and 1.21 at 12 months.

How might we use this evidence to inform practice?

The study seems to have a low risk of bias. Your patient is similar to the study participants in some respects (type

TABLE 9.2   Relevant prognostic factors significantly associated with healing of diabetic foot ulcers

Prognostic factor	ODDS RATIO (OR) (95% CI)	
	Healing within 3 months	Healing within 12 months
Age (< 50 years)	0.77 (0.63 to 0.95)	0.72 (0.57 to 0.90)
Regional area	0.65 (0.56 to 0.75)	0.67 (0.56 to 0.79)
Smoker	0.76 (0.61 to 0.95)	0.71 (0.56 to 0.89)
Neuropathy	0.76 (0.62 to 0.93)	(not significant)
Ulcer size 1 to 3 cm²	0.59 (0.49 to 0.72)	0.72 (0.58 to 0.90)
Treatment with knee-high offloading (cast walker)	1.34 (1.17 to 1.53)	1.21 (1.04 to 1.41)

Note: An OR <1 means that having this factor is less likely to result in the ulcer not healing in the given time frame. An OR >1 means that having this factor is more likely to result in the ulcer healing in the time frame provided.

of diabetes, living in regional area of northern Australia, ulcer characteristics), although he is younger (39 years, whereas the study participants' mean age was 63 years). You will use the study results to inform your discussion with the patient. As part of this, you will encourage your patient to seek support to quit smoking and liaise with his GP about this. You may also discuss the option of treatment with a knee-high offloading device (a cast walker) as, although use of a cast walker can cause some inconvenience for the patient, this treatment may also improve the likelihood of the ulcer healing. (However, you will search for specific evidence on this first.)

◎ SPEECH PATHOLOGY EXAMPLE

Clinical scenario

Mr and Mrs Li have brought their 4-year-old son, Lucas, to see you in your community speech pathology clinic. Lucas attends preschool and staff there have raised with his parents that Lucas's speech is occasionally hard to understand. Mr and Mrs Li have no difficulties understanding Lucas's speech production but acknowledge he has speech errors, which include pronouncing 'k' as 't' (for example, saying 'tar' for 'car') and pronouncing 'r' as 'w' (for example, saying 'wabbit' for 'rabbit'). The family speak only English at home. Lucas has a large vocabulary, enjoys talking with family and friends and his development is otherwise typical. There is no family history of speech production difficulties or spoken language skills, although Mr Li was diagnosed with dyslexia during high school. Mr and Mrs Li are wondering whether Lucas's acquisition of literacy skills during primary school might be impacted. You assess Lucas's speech and language skills and determine that he has a speech sound disorder (SSD), but not a language impairment. You decide to search the literature to obtain information that will inform your answer to Mr and Mrs Li's question.

Clinical question

In children with a history of speech sound disorder, what is the effect of a family history of dyslexia on the development of literacy skills?

Search terms and databases used to find the evidence

Database: PubMed—Clinical Queries (with 'prognosis category' and 'narrow scope' selected).
Search terms: (speech sound disorder) AND literacy AND dyslexia

This search retrieves one article, but it did not include discussion of the impact of a family history of dyslexia.

You repeat the search with the 'broad scope' selected and retrieve more articles. Reviewing the abstracts, you find only one that includes family history of dyslexia as a variable. You select this article as being relevant to your clinical question.

Article chosen

Hayiou-Thomas ME, Carroll JM, Leavett R, et al. When does speech sound disorder matter for literacy? The role of disordered speech errors, co-occurring language impairment and family risk of dyslexia. J Child Psychol Psychiatry 2017;58(2):197–205.

Structured abstract (adapted from the above)

Study design: Longitudinal cohort study.
Setting: Community-dwelling families in the United Kingdom.
Participants: 245 children recruited at 3.5 years of age (and a parent or full sibling).
Outcomes: Literacy outcomes (phoneme awareness, word reading, spelling, reading comprehension).
Prognostic factors studied: Family risk of dyslexia (biological parent or full sibling) status, language impairment status, SSD.
Follow-up period: Children were tested six times (approximately annually) between the ages of 3.5 and 9 years. Results at three time points are reported: T1 (age 3.5), T3 (age 5.5) and T5 (age 8).
Main results: SSD presents a small but significant risk of poor literacy skills acquisition at age 5.5 (phonemic skills and spelling) and 8 (word reading). Persistent SSD to school entry was also associated with poorer literacy skills. However, the severity of SSD did not predict reading development. A family risk of dyslexia predicted additional variance in literacy skills at both 5.5 and 8 years.

Continued

SPEECH PATHOLOGY EXAMPLE—cont'd

Conclusion: By itself, SSD has modest effects on literacy development; however, a family history of dyslexia increases the risk of negative literacy consequences. As such, a collection of multiple risks predicts reading disorders.

Is the evidence likely to be biased?

- *Was there a representative and well-defined sample?*

  Probably not. A convenience sample of participants was recruited and while exclusion criteria were specified, children were not originally recruited based on having an SSD, with those who met criteria for SSD (see below) identified via assessment at Time 1. Further, several children fulfilled criteria for more than one risk category (family risk of dyslexia, language impairment, SSD).

- *Were participants recruited at a common point in their disease or condition?*

  No. The children were all recruited at approximately 3.5 years of age. However, the nature of the children's SSD (that is, the pattern of their speech sound errors) varied.

- *Was exposure determined accurately?*

  Yes. Details of how SSD status and family risk of dyslexia status were ascertained were reported, including use of assessments and practices which are standard in the field, such as the Diagnostic Evaluation of Articulation and Phonology screener and articulation measure for SSD status and established measures of family risk of dyslexia status.

- *Were the outcomes measured accurately?*

  Yes. Outcomes were mainly measured with both well-established standardised and criterion-referenced assessments: the York Assessment of Reading Comprehension (YARC), the Test of Word Reading Efficiency (TOWRE), the Wechsler Individual Ability Test (WIAT II) and the Single Word Reading Test. A small number of bespoke tasks were also used.

- *Were important confounding factors considered?*

  No. Environmental influences that may affect literacy development, such as socio-economic status and home literacy environment, were not considered.

- *Was the follow-up of participants sufficiently long and complete?*

  Unclear. 245 children were recruited aged 3.5 years. The results presented cover a period of approximately 5 years, to when the children were aged 8. By age 8 in the UK, the children would likely have been in Year 3 or 4 at school, and this is a long enough period to determine the development of the identified literacy outcomes. However, although data are included for a minimum of 212 children (87% of participants) at this age point for the total sample, only 68 of the initial 245 had SSD at baseline and reporting of the dropouts in this sub-sample is unclear. It appears that only 33 of the children in the original sample with SSD were available at the last follow-up point (age 8), so follow-up data may not be sufficiently complete.

What are the main results?

The authors used regression models to examine SSD status and family risk of dyslexia status as predictors of continuous literacy outcomes. Of the initial sample of 245 children, 68 had SSD diagnosed at baseline. Linear regression models for examining predictors of literacy outcomes were based on samples of 222 to 224 at age 5.5 follow-up and 212 to 218 at age 8 follow-up. Literacy outcome analysis was conducted with the sub-sample of children with SSD (n = 68), compared to a control group (n = 68), and correlational analysis was conducted with just the sub-sample of children with SSD.

Effect of SSD status on literacy outcomes

Children identified with SSD at 3.5 years of age performed more poorly than typically developing peers in phoneme awareness and spelling outcomes at age 5.5. SSD status accounted for a small amount of variance in literacy outcomes (for example, 5.8% for phoneme awareness, 3.4% for spelling skills and 0.9% for word reading) at this age, and smaller amounts at age 8 (1.9% for word reading, 0.4% for spelling and 0.8% for reading comprehension). These results suggest that the risk of poor literacy in children with isolated SSD is low, with only modest and short-term effects on literacy development.

Effect of family risk of dyslexia status on literacy outcomes

Family risk of dyslexia status had effects that were stronger than the effects of SSD, accounting for statistically significant unique variance (3.3%) in word reading at age 5.5 and word reading, spelling and reading comprehension at age 8 (3.2% to 3.8% variance). Family risk of dyslexia status did not predict phoneme awareness or spelling at age 5.5, which may be because most variance in these skills is associated with SSD status at 3.5 years.

Effect of severity and persistence of SSD on literacy outcomes

For the sub-sample of children with SSD ($n = 68$), severity of SSD at age 3.5 did not correlate highly with any of the literacy outcomes. Persistence of SSD to age 5.5 significantly predicted phoneme awareness (16% of the variance) and word reading (21% of the variance) at this age. However, none of the predictors were significantly associated with literacy outcomes at age 8. The effects of SSD may be short-lived because children are able to draw on compensatory mechanisms to support their literacy development.

How might we use this evidence to inform practice?

Despite being at some risk of bias, it appears that this study provides the current best available evidence to inform your clinical question. Encouragingly, the influence of SSD status at age 3.5 was a weak predictor of literacy outcomes. However, family risk of dyslexia status accounted for statistically significant unique variance in word reading, spelling, and reading comprehension at age 8. Further, while severity of SSD at age 3.5 did not correlate with any of the literacy outcome measures, the persistence of SSD to age 5.5 correlated significantly with phoneme awareness and word reading outcomes at 5.5.

Additionally, you consider that during your assessment of Lucas you learnt that while the Li home literacy environment has some supportive elements, Mr Li reported that he often finds reading to Lucas uncomfortable because of his dyslexia. You consider various factors, including that Lucas is 4 years old and will be starting primary school soon, he has an SSD (which might persist if untreated) and there is a family history of dyslexia. Together, these factors may impact Lucas's acquisition of literacy skills during primary school. You discuss your findings with Mr and Mrs Li and possible next steps, including collaborating with Lucas's kindergarten teacher to monitor his literacy development when Lucas does begin school, and beginning therapy with Lucas for his SSD.

◎ MEDICINE EXAMPLE

Clinical scenario

You are a general practitioner (GP) with a 55-year-old male patient who was discharged after presenting to the emergency department 2 weeks ago while experiencing an acute coronary syndrome (ACS) episode. His fasting LDL cholesterol was >6.5 mmol/L when measured 2 months ago. Since then, he has been taking a statin for primary prevention of cardiovascular disease. His blood pressure is within normal range. Your patient has familial hypercholesterolaemia, and his father had a coronary heart disease diagnosis in his fifties and high LDL cholesterol levels. The patient asks you whether he is at an increased risk of heart attack in the next year or so now that he has had an ACS episode. You search the research for relevant evidence.

Clinical question

In patients hospitalised with chest pain due to acute coronary syndrome and with familial hypercholesterolaemia, how likely is a cardiovascular event within the following 12 months compared to patients without a familial hypercholesterolaemia history?

Search terms and databases used to find the evidence

Database: PubMed—Clinical Queries (with 'prognosis category' and 'narrow scope' selected).

Search terms: (acute coronary syndrome) AND (familial hypercholesterolaemia)

This search returned 25 records. You scan the titles of the articles, read the abstract of several and choose one that appears to be a highly relevant prospective cohort study to appraise.

Article chosen

Nanchen D, Gencer B, Muller O, et al. Prognosis of patients with familial hypercholesterolemia after acute coronary syndromes. Circulation 2016;134(10):698–709. doi:10.1161/CIRCULATIONAHA.116.023007.

Structured abstract (adapted from the above)

Study design: Prospective cohort study.

Setting: Four university hospitals in Switzerland.

Participants: 4,534 patients (mean age 55.1 years, 22.5% female) hospitalised with acute coronary syndrome (ACS), with 20.8% of patients with criteria for familial hypercholesterolaemia (FH).

Outcomes: Coronary events (fatal or non-fatal myocardial infarction) and cardiovascular events (myocardial infarction, ischaemic stroke, transient ischaemic attack, or cerebrovascular or cardiovascular mortality).

Prognostic factors: Age, sex, BMI, smoking, hypertension, diabetes mellitus, existing cardiovascular disease,

Continued

◉ MEDICINE EXAMPLE—cont'd

high-dose statin at discharge, attendance at cardiac reha-bilitation, and the GRACE (Global Registry of Acute Coronary Events) risk score for severity of ACS.

Follow-up period: 1 year.

Main results: During the year after hospitalisation for ACS, 153 patients (3.4%) died, 217 (4.8%) had a fatal or non-fatal myocardial infarction and 275 (6.1%) experienced a cardiovascular event. A further 113 patients (2.5%) experienced non-fatal myocardial infarction. Overall, 79.2% did not meet the criteria for familial hypercholesterolaemia, while its prevalence was 2.5% with the American Heart Association definition, 5.5% with the Simon Broome definition and 1.6% with the Dutch Lipid Clinic definition. The risk of coronary event recurrence after ACS was greater in patients with familial hypercholesterolaemia than without, with an adjusted hazard ratio of 2.46 (95% CI 1.07 to 5.65; $p = 0.034$) for the American Heart Association definition, 2.73 (95% CI 1.46 to 5.11; $p = 0.002$) for the Simon Broome definition and 3.53 (95% CI 1.26 to 9.94; $p = 0.017$) for the Dutch Lipid Clinic definition.

Conclusion: Patients with familial hypercholesterolaemia and ACS have a more than two-fold higher adjusted risk of coronary event recurrence within the first year after discharge than patients without familial hypercholesterolaemia, despite the use of statins.

Is this evidence likely to be biased?

- *Was there a representative and well-defined sample?*
  Yes. The inclusion and exclusion criteria for the sample were clearly defined, and consecutive cases were recruited from four different centres.
- *Were participants recruited at a common point in their disease or condition?*
  Yes. Although it is not clearly reported in this article, the authors provided references for two other articles from the same study that contain further details about the recruitment process. Recruitment was of all consecutive patients who presented within 5 days of pain onset.
- *Was exposure determined accurately?*
  Partially. Although the eligibility and clinical diagnosis of ACS was clearly defined, for familial hypercholesterolaemia, the authors did not assess all the criteria (for example, xanthomas and family history of high LDL cholesterol levels) that could have impacted two of the three scoring systems (Simon Broome and Dutch Lipid Clinic definition). No genetic testing was done to confirm the diagnosis of

familial hypercholesterolaemia, which could have underestimated the risk of cardiovascular events for this group of patients.
- *Were the outcomes measured accurately?*
  Probably. Cardiovascular end points were determined by a panel of three cardiologists who served as independent experts blinded to the diagnosis of familial hypercholesterolaemia. Outcomes were reported as a composite outcome that included both fatal and non-fatal events.
- *Were important confounding factors considered?*
  Yes. Data about a range of factors (including age, sex, BMI, smoking, hypertension, diabetes mellitus, existing cardiovascular disease and severity of ACS) were available from baseline to enable important prognostic factors to be adjusted for with respect to the clinical outcomes. Participants' self-reporting of family history of coronary heart disease may have introduced some recall bias, which might have led to the overestimation of familial hypercholesterolaemia prevalence.
- *Was the follow-up of participants sufficiently long and complete?*
  Yes. The 1 year follow-up is appropriate to capture the post-hospital discharge risk of coronary events, which is the main concern for your patient. However, an extended follow-up would be informative about the risk of cardiovascular events over a longer time.

What are the main results?

In a multivariate analysis, the risk of coronary event recurrence (including fatal or non-fatal myocardial infarction) was higher in patients with familial hypercholesterolaemia than in patients without. This was irrespective of the diagnostic scoring system used: adjusted hazard ratio [HR] 2.46 (95% CI 1.07 to 5.65; $p = 0.034$) for the American Heart Association definition, 2.73 (95% CI 1.46 to 5.11; $p = 0.002$) for the Simon Broome definition and 3.53 (95% CI 1.26 to 9.94; $p = 0.017$) for the Dutch Lipid Clinic definition. For cardiovascular events, statistical significance was reached for the Simon Broome definition only (HR 2.49; 95% CI 1.43 to 4.34; $p = 0.046$).

How might we use this evidence to inform practice?

Although you have some concerns about the study (mostly regarding the exposure measurement), it otherwise appears to be at low risk of bias and you consider the study relevant to your patient. You have a conversation with your patient and explain that similar patients with familial hypercholester-olaemia who have been hospitalised for ACS had more than a two-fold higher risk of coronary event recurrence within the first year after discharge. You remind your patient that it is important for him to maintain a low lipid level by continu-ing to take his medication and by making dietary and other lifestyle changes. You collaborate with him to develop a care plan, including specialist and allied health support.

◎ NURSING EXAMPLE

Clinical scenario
You are an experienced registered nurse working in an adult intensive care unit (ICU). The ICU has a strict regimen of skin assessments being performed regularly by an interdis-ciplinary team and documenting these findings. In addition to these checks, nursing staff perform a complete physical assessment, including of skin integrity, at shift commence-ment. A range of resources are available to use to reduce the risk of pressure injuries, such as alternating pressure mattresses, and yet even with these and regular reposition-ing, some patients still develop pressure injuries. You would like to know if these patients have common clinical or physiological factors and whether it can be predicted which patients are most at risk of developing pressure injuries.

Clinical question
What are the risk factors for critically ill adults (in inten-sive care units) developing pressure injuries?

Search terms and databases used to find the evidence
Database: PubMed—Clinical Queries (with 'prognosis category' and 'narrow scope' selected).
Search terms: (critical illness) AND (pressure injur*) AND (risk factors)

The search returns 55 records. You scan the titles and read the abstracts of several studies that appear relevant. You choose the one that mostly closely matches your clinical question.

Article chosen
Sala J, Mayampurath A, Solmos S, et al. Predictors of pres-sure injury development in critically ill adults: a retrospec-tive cohort study. Intensive Crit Care Nurs 2021;62:102924. https://doi.org/10.1016/j.iccn.2020.102924.

Structured abstract (adapted from the above)
Study design: Retrospective cohort study.
Setting: Five ICUs (medical, surgical, cardiac, neurological and cardiovascular) within an urban academic medical centre.

Participants: 1,587 patients (56% male, mean age 59.6 years) with a documented hospital-acquired pres-sure injury (HAPI) identified through electronic health and quality improvement records.
Outcomes: Presence of a HAPI and staging and location of it.
Prognostic factors: Clinical data considered in the devel-opment of the predictive tool included: demographic data (age, race, gender), mean arterial pressure (MAP), the in-fusion of vasopressors (inotropes), fluid bolus administra-tion, total Glasgow Coma Score (GCS), fraction of inspired oxygen (FiO_2), oxygen saturation, partial pressure of arte-rial oxygen and fraction of inspired oxygen ratio (P/F ratio), total bilirubin, platelet count and creatinine. Total Braden Scale scores were also collected. (Braden scores are an aggregate score with a range from 6 to 23, with lower scores indicating higher risk of developing a pressure in-jury.) Additional clinical data obtained included hospital length of stay, diagnosis of sepsis and comorbid condi-tions (myocardial infarction, congestive heart failure, cerebrovascular accident, chronic pulmonary disease, diabetes mellitus).
Follow-up period: Data were collected throughout par-ticipants' ICU admission. (Median length of stay was 33 days for participants with HAPI and 15 days for partici-pants without HAPI.) The data collection period spanned 2.5 years and included all admissions.
Main results: Nearly half (47%) of the participants had a total Braden Scale score on admission that indicated an increased risk of developing HAPI (≤18). During ICU admission, 81 (5.1%) patients developed a total of 114 HAPI, with 31.8% of the injuries suspected to involve deep tissue. Through logistic regression, individual predic-tors of HAPI were identified as: MAP <60 mmHg (OR 9.88, 95% CI 3.07 to 60.43), administration of vasopres-sors (inotropes) (OR 2.92, 95% CI 1.82 to 4.75), FiO_2 > 50% (OR 3.06, 95% CI 1.58 to 6.67), lowest Braden score (OR 0.71, 95% CI 0.65 to 0.77) and GCS 8 (OR 5.16, 95%

Continued

◎ NURSING EXAMPLE—cont'd

CI 3.05 to 9.23). The association between all risk factors and the development of pressure injuries revealed only MAP <60 mmHg and lowest total Braden score were associated with increased risk of developing HAPI (MAP <60 OR 8.22, 95% CI 1.74 to 147.07, Braden OR 0.79, 95% CI 0.70 to 0.88).

Conclusion: 5% of participants developed a HAPI during their ICU admission, with 31.8% suspected to involve deep tissue injury. Patients that had a low MAP and score ≤18 on the Braden Scale on admission were more likely to develop a HAPI.

Is the evidence likely to be biased?

- *Was there a representative and well-defined sample?*

  Yes. The participants, as defined by the inclusion and exclusion criteria, included all patients admitted to ICU over a 2.5-year period. Participants were evaluated for presence or absence of pressure injury by a skin care team nurse. Two certified wound care nurses independently examined all skin injuries; if the injury was confirmed as a HAPI, the nurses verified its staging using National Pressure Ulcer Advisory Panel recommendations. Patients without a documented pressure injury throughout their ICU stay were included in the comparison group.

- *Were participants recruited at a common point in their disease or condition?*

  Yes, if admission to ICU was considered the common point, although patients varied widely in their reason for admission and health. It should be remembered that this was a retrospective cohort study, and data from all admitted participants were included.

- *Was exposure determined accurately?*

  Yes. Diagnosis, clinical and physiological variables were collated throughout the admission and recorded in the electronic hospital record.

- *Were the outcomes measured accurately?*

  Yes. The primary outcome was the development of a pressure injury during the ICU admission. Assessment of this is as described in response above about whether the sample was representative and well-defined.

- *Were important confounding factors considered?*

  Probably yes. Potential confounding factors (such as age, diagnosis, comorbidities, Braden score) were included as prognostic factors. However, comorbidities were only documented at discharge, so potentially a comorbid condition may have existed at the time

of HAPI development that was not captured in the discharge data coding.

- *Was the follow-up of participants sufficiently long and complete?*

  Yes. Data were available for participants from ICU admission to discharge. As the focus was on the development of a pressure injury during the ICU stay, this is appropriate. There is no report of any participants being lost to follow-up.

What are the main results?

Of the 1,587 participants, 81 (5.1%) developed a pressure injury during their hospital admission. Statistically significant associations were found for some variables between patients with and patients without a HAPI. Patients that developed a HAPI more often had a MAP <60 mmHg, received vasopressor (inotropic) infusions, received larger fluid boluses, required a higher FiO_2 and had a lower P/F ratio compared with patients who did not develop a HAPI. Demographic, physiological and clinical data were combined for a logistic regression model predicting HAPI and only two factors were significant: MAP <60 mmHg (OR 8.22, 95% CI 1.74 to 147.07) and lowest total Braden score up to 2 weeks before HAPI development (OR 0.79, 95% CI 0.70 to 0.88).

How might we use this evidence to guide our practice?

The risk of bias in this study seems low, although you are mindful that it is a retrospective cohort study and is further down the hierarchy of evidence than a prospective cohort study. Pressure injuries are painful for patients and, depending on their severity, they may require surgical intervention which is why they are considered an important patient safety metric. It is well established that they considerably increase hospital length of stay. This study was undertaken in a well-resourced hospital with a specialist skin care team, a hospital-wide education program and specialist equipment available. Even with these resources, 5% of patients developed a HAPI. A key finding of this study is that reduced perfusion and low Braden scores might be able to identify patients at increased risk of developing a HAPI. You next plan to look for research on the sensitivity and specificity of the Braden scale and, if found, to discuss the research and this cohort study at your ward's journal club, with a view to considering if refined or additional strategies to reduce modifiable risk are needed.

HUMAN MOVEMENT EXAMPLE

Clinical scenario

Mrs Williams is 57 years old and has come to you for a fitness assessment. You determine she usually undertakes about 60–90 minutes of physical activity (PA) per week, of at least moderate intensity. This is about half the lower threshold of guideline recommendations of 150 minutes per week. When you ask her what she wants to achieve, she says she hopes that being more active will reduce her cardiovascular disease (CVD) risk. She is concerned about this as her mother had hypertension and a myocardial infarction. However, Mrs Williams is uncertain about the recommendations for duration and intensity in the physical activity guidelines as there is a range in the recommended duration (that is, 150–300 minutes) and both moderate- and vigorous-intensity PA can be included. She is unclear if she should try to increase her duration of PA or her intensity. She currently uses a wearable device (she has a Fitbit), which has an accelerometer to estimate her activity level.

Clinical question

Is greater duration or greater intensity of physical activity, measured with an accelerometer, associated with a greater reduction in risk of cardiovascular disease?

Search terms and databases used to find the evidence

Database: PubMed—Clinical Queries (with 'prognosis category' and 'narrow scope' selected).

Search terms: (physical activity) AND (cardiovascular disease) AND (accelerometer*) AND (duration OR intensity)

This search results in 54 hits. From scanning the titles and abstracts, some are in groups of people with specific conditions, such as diabetes; however, one is a recent study about physical activity measured with an accelerometer in a large cohort, so you start by appraising it.

Article chosen

Ramakrishnan R, Doherty A, Smith-Byrne K, et al. Accelerometer measured physical activity and the incidence of cardiovascular disease: evidence from the UK Biobank cohort study. PLOS Medicine 2021;18(1):e1003487.

Structured abstract (adapted from the above)

Study design: Prospective cohort study (retrospective analysis of data prospectively collected from a sample of a population-based cohort study who wore an accelerometer for 7 days).

Setting: Community-based adults from the United Kingdom.
Participants: 90,211 adults (mean age 62 years; 57.9% female) who agreed to wear an accelerometer over a 7-day period.
Outcome: Cardiovascular incidence (defined as the first hospital admission or death from CVD) obtained from linked health records and a national death index.
Prognostic factors studied: Age, gender, age completed full-time education, social deprivation, ethnicity, smoking status, alcohol consumption, self-rated health, hypertension, BMI, cholesterol, C-reactive protein, glycated haemoglobin (HbA1c), red meat consumption, fresh fruit and cooked vegetable consumption.
Follow-up period: The median follow-up period was 61.9 months (IQR 14.1).
Main results: Higher levels of PA were associated with a lower CVD risk in a linear-dose relationship, which was similar for moderate- and vigorous-intensity PA and overall PA volume status.
Conclusion: Individuals who engage in higher levels of PA had lower risk for CVD, which can be achieved through moderate- and/or vigorous-intensity PA.

Is the evidence likely to be biased?

- *Was there a representative and well-defined sample?*
  Partially. Participant data were obtained from a subsample of the UK Biobank which recruited 500,000 volunteers throughout the UK aged 40 to 69 years from 2006 to 2010 to examine risk factors for diseases of middle and old age. On entry to the Biobank, volunteers provided detailed information and samples for analysis. No further details of the Biobank inclusion criteria are provided; however, the authors note concerns that the UK Biobank is not completely representative of the sampling population (for example, predominantly white and living in higher socio-economically advantaged areas), with 'healthy volunteer' selection bias. The sample used in this study was a sub-sample of the Biobank cohort who participated in a 7-day accelerometer study.[2] This sample consisted of participants who agreed to accelerometer use from random email invitation.[2]

- *Were participants recruited at a common point in their disease or condition?*
  Yes. Data from healthy participants from the Biobank (who were recruited to wear an accelerometer in a previous study and who had high-quality accelerometer data and no CVD prior to the end of their

Continued

◎ HUMAN MOVEMENT EXAMPLE—cont'd

accelerometer wear) were examined, including follow-up data about CVD incident or study end. CVD diagnosis was checked prior to analysis of accelerometer data as shown in a flowchart in a supplementary figure of the article and using criteria defined in the article.

- *Was the exposure measured accurately?*

  Yes. Accelerometers currently provide the best estimates of time spent in varying intensities of PA and remove the subjective bias of self-report. Data were only included if participants met wear time criteria and estimates of moderate and vigorous PA were calculated using published thresholds. (However, it is worth noting that PA guidelines are based on self-reported data, which can make comparability of the PA duration to the guidelines problematic.) Total PA volume was measured as average vector magnitude in milli-gravity (mg) units. Estimated minutes of moderate and vigorous PA per week were calculated from the percentage of time spent in 100–400 mg and >400 mg, respectively. However, accelerometer data in this study were only collected for a 7-day period and that period may not reflect habitual levels of PA.

- *Were the outcomes measured accurately?*

  Yes. CVD incidence was identified from linkages to the national death index and Hospital Episode Statistics.

- *Were important confounding factors considered?*

  Probably. Many known demographic, behavioural and lifestyle factors were included in the analyses. Participants were excluded from analysis if data were missing for age, gender, ethnicity, age completed full-time education, Townsend Deprivation Index, smoking and alcohol consumption.

- *Was the follow-up of participants sufficiently long and complete?*

  Yes. The median follow-up of 5 years provided adequate time for outcome occurrence. However, this varied depending on the geographical location of the participants, with data of surviving participants in England available for 4 years longer than that of participants from Wales and Scotland. There is no reporting of loss to follow up, as this was a retrospective analysis of existing data that met inclusion and exclusion criteria. From an initial sample of 103,687 Biobank participants with accelerometer data, 7,012 were screened out due to low-quality accelerometer data, a further 5,635 were screened out due to CVD diagnosis in health records prior to accelerometer wear, and a further 829 were screened out due to missing data for socio-demographic and health behavioural factors, leaving the analysed sample (90,211).

What are the main results?

The results most relevant to your clinical question are reported as hazard ratios for CVD incidence by quarters of average moderate-intensity and vigorous-intensity physical activities in the participants. The hazard ratios were adjusted for age (stratified by 5-year age-at-risk intervals), sex, ethnicity, education, social deprivation, smoking and alcohol consumption. There was a linear dose–response relationship of PA to risk of incidence of CVD, regardless of whether the PA was moderate intensity, vigorous intensity or as total PA volume. Increasing PA to the next quartile appears to provide greater reduction in risk of CVD incidence. For example, for moderate-intensity PA, compared to the least active people (<524 min/week), the hazard ratios for the increasing quarters of PA were 0.71 (95% CI 0.65 to 0.77) for the quarter of 524–705 min/week, 0.59 (95% CI 0.54 to 0.65) for 705–927 min/week and for the most active quarter (>927 min/week) 0.46 (95% CI 0.41 to 0.51).

How might we use this evidence to inform practice?

The risk of bias of this evidence appears to be quite low and your patient is not dissimilar to the study participants. You advise Mrs Williams that it seems to be that the more PA she does, the better it might be for reducing CVD risk, irrespective of whether this is at a moderate or vigorous intensity (and you bear in mind that these data cannot establish causality). You both discuss a plan and she agrees to start by trying to achieve 150 minutes/week of at least moderate-intensity PA and, where possible, to mix in some vigorous-intensity PA. Over time, she hopes to increase this duration and will aim to incorporate incidental bouts of PA into her daily routine.

PARAMEDICINE EXAMPLE

Clinical scenario
You are a paramedic at the scene of an adult having a cardiac arrest and you have been working through the resuscitation guideline for about 15 minutes. You discuss with your partner whether you should stay at the scene and continue the resuscitation attempt or load the patient into the ambulance and head for the hospital. Your partner thinks it might be better to stay at the scene, but you are not sure what the best option is.

Clinical question
For patients in out-of-hospital cardiac arrest (OHCA), are patient survival outcomes better if you stay at the scene and continue the resuscitation or if you transport the patient to hospital and continue the resuscitation attempt on the way?

Search terms and databases used to find the evidence
Database: PubMed—Clinical Queries (with 'prognosis category' and 'narrow scope' selected).
Search terms: (out-of-hospital cardiac arrest) AND (on-scene resuscitation) and (transport)
The search identified 14 articles, with one article matching the clinical question.

Article chosen
Grunau B, Kime N, Leroux B, et al. Association of intra-arrest transport vs continued on-scene resuscitation with survival to hospital discharge among patients with out-of-hospital cardiac arrest. JAMA 2020;324(11):1058–67.

Structured abstract (adapted from the above)
Study design: Secondary analysis of a cohort study of prospectively collected consecutive non-traumatic adult EMS-treated OHCA data from the Resuscitation Outcomes Consortium Cardiac Epidemiologic Registry.
Setting: Ten study sites in the United States.
Participants: All consecutive patients >18 years of age who had a non-traumatic OHCA between April 2011 and June 2015 and were in the register. OHCA definition: a person found apnoeic and pulseless who received either external defibrillation by bystanders or emergency medical systems (EMS) staff, or chest compressions by EMS staff.
Outcomes: Primary outcome was survival to hospital discharge. Secondary outcome was a good neurological outcome at hospital discharge (a modified Rankin scale <3 [range: 0 = no symptoms or disability to 6 = death]).

Prognostic factors studied: For the time-dependent propensity score analysis, the potential confounders included were: age, gender, location of episode (public or not), witnessed status (bystander vs EMS vs not witnessed), bystander CPR performed or not, interval between emergency phone call and EMS arrival, shockable EMS-recorded rhythm or not, presumed cardiac vs obvious non-cardiac cause, advanced life support (ALS) unit first on scene or not and treatment region.
Follow-up period: Cardiac arrest patients were followed to hospital discharge.
Main results: Of 57,725 consecutive OHCA patients treated by EMS, 43,969 patients (63% male, median age 67 years) had complete data and 27,705 of these were included in a full propensity-matched cohort analysis. Of the full cohort, 11,625 (26%) underwent intra-arrest ambulance transport to hospital and 32,344 (74%) were resuscitated onsite until return of spontaneous circulation (ROSC) or termination of the resuscitation attempt. For those patients who received onsite resuscitation, 12.6% survived to hospital discharge, compared to 3.8% for those patients who underwent intra-arrest ambulance transport to hospital. Using the propensity score analysis, for those OHCA patients surviving to hospital discharge (n = 27,705), survival was higher for those resuscitated onsite (8.5%) compared to those patients who were transported to hospital by ambulance while intra-arrest (4.0%), risk difference 4.6% (95% CI 4.0 to 5.1) and adjusted risk ratio 0.48 (95% CI 0.43 to 0.54). For those patients (15,383) who survived to hospital discharge with good neurological outcomes, the neurological outcome was better for those patients who were resuscitated onsite (7.1%) compared to those patients with intra-arrest ambulance transport to hospital (2.9%), risk difference 4.2% (95% CI 3.5 to 4.9) and adjusted risk ratio 0.60 (95% CI 0.47 to 0.76).
Conclusion: Patients with OHCA who were resuscitated onsite were associated with more likely to survive to hospital discharge and to have a better neurological outcome compared to those patients who received some resuscitation onsite and were then transported to hospital while the resuscitation attempt continued.

Is this evidence likely to be biased?
• *Was there a representative and well-defined sample?*
   Yes. The inclusion criteria were clearly defined for the registry and likely to be representative of the population who experiences OHCA.

Continued

◉ PARAMEDICINE EXAMPLE—cont'd

- *Were participants recruited at a common point in their disease or condition?*
  Yes. Patients were entered into the study if they had a non-traumatic OHCA, were found apnoeic and pulseless on presentation, and received either external defibrillation by bystanders or EMS staff or chest compressions by EMS staff.
- *Was the exposure determined accurately?*
  Yes. Data on whether on-scene resuscitation continued or whether intra-arrest transport occurred prior to any episodes of ROSC came from the registry. Data in this were identified by trained research personnel at individual sites who examined dispatch logs, patient care records, defibrillator files and hospital records.
- *Were the outcomes measured accurately?*
  Yes. Data about survival to hospital discharge and neurological outcome on discharge were collected by the registry from hospital records.
- *Were important confounding factors considered?*
  Mostly. Likely potentially important confounding factors were considered in the time-dependent propensity score analysis and are listed in the abstract in this worked example. However, the authors do acknowledge that some characteristics of patients and responders could not be controlled. For example, confounding by indication may have occurred as EMS personnel might have used certain patient characteristics to estimate who might benefit from intra-arrest transport. Also, in the propensity analysis, not all individual variables were aligned between groups, with intra-arrest patients having more favourable prognostic features (for example, younger, more with initial shockable rhythms in public locations) which may have biased the results towards intra-arrest transport.

- *Was the follow-up of participants sufficiently long and complete?*
  Unclear, but probably not. Patients were only followed to hospital discharge. Other studies involving OHCA have followed patients for up to 5 years post-cardiac arrest or until death. Of the initial 57,725 in the registry, 13,756 (24%) were excluded (many due to missing data) and only 27,705 (48%) were included in the full-propensity matched data analysis.

What are the main results?

For both the full cohort and the propensity-matched cohort, survival to hospital discharge was lower among patients who had intra-arrest transport compared to those who had continued on-scene resuscitation. In the propensity-matched cohort, there was an absolute difference in survival of 4.6% and the risk ratio was 0.48 (95% CI 0.43 to 0.54), which was statistically significant and in favour of those who continued on-scene resuscitation. Table 9.3 contains the main results relevant to the clinical question.

How might we use this evidence to inform practice?

This is a large, well-conducted study that has attempted to minimise risk of bias, although some concerns remain. It is important to remember that it is an observational study and can only provide information about association, not causation, and randomised trials would be needed to examine this before considering change in policy. There is also some uncertainty about the generalisability of the results to other settings, for both EMS and hospital care of OHCA. Even within the study, there was regional variation and result variability among the ten sites (with the point estimates favouring on-scene resuscitation at some sites and intra-arrest transportation at other sites). You decide to discuss this study and its results at the next team meeting.

TABLE 9.3 **Analysis of primary outcome in patients who received on-scene resuscitation and those who had intra-arrest transportation to hospital**

Survival to hospital discharge	Intra-arrest transport *n/N* (%)	On-scene resuscitation *n/N* (%)	Absolute difference (95% CI)	Risk ratio (95% CI)
Full cohort	446/11,625 (3.8%)	4,072/32,344 (12.6%)	8.8% (8.3 to 9.3)	
Propensity-matched cohort*	372/9,406 (3.9%)	1,557/1,829 (8.5%)	4.6% (4.0 to 5.1)	0.48 (0.43 to 0.54)

*primary analysis

PHARMACY EXAMPLE

Clinical scenario

You are a community-based pharmacist. A regular customer (a middle-aged woman) asks your advice about taking vitamin D supplements. She says she was recently diagnosed with vitamin D insufficiency and is concerned following reading a magazine article about how becoming depressed is common among people with low levels of vitamin D. She would like to know if there is any truth to this. You advise her that you will look at the research on this issue and let her know what you find.

Clinical question

Among middle-aged people, is vitamin D level a predictor of new-onset depression?

Search terms and databases used to find the evidence

Database: PubMed—Clinical Queries (with 'prognosis category' and 'narrow scope' selected).

Search terms: (vitamin d) AND (depression)

This search results in 160 articles. You narrow the search by adding '(middle aged)' with an 'and' operator to your search string and this gives 55 articles. You scan the titles and abstract and choose a recent study that most closely matches your clinical question.

Article chosen

Ronaldson A, Arias de laTorre J, Gaughran F, et al. Prospective associations between vitamin D and depression in middle-aged adults: findings from the UK Biobank cohort. Psychol Med 2020;Oct 21:1–9. https://doi.org/10.1017/S0033291720003657.

Structured abstract (adapted from the above)

Study design: Cohort.

Setting: Data were collected from UK Biobank participants from 22 different assessment centres across England, Scotland and Wales.

Participants: Of 502,640 participants aged between 40 and 69 years, 139,128 (28%) (mean age 55.83) completed follow-up.

Outcomes: Vitamin D insufficiency and vitamin D deficiency.

Prognostic factors studied: Socio-demographic variables (age, gender, ethnicity, socio-economic status), social history (alcohol and smoking history) and physical activity (mild, moderate and vigorous).

Follow-up period: 6–10 years.

Main results: Among participants with no depression at baseline ($n = 127,244$), those with vitamin D insufficiency (adjusted odds ratio [aOR] 1.14, 95% CI 1.07 to 1.22) and those with vitamin D deficiency (aOR 1.24, 95% CI 1.13 to 1.36) were more likely to develop new-onset depression at follow-up compared with those with optimal vitamin D levels. Among those with depression at baseline ($n = 11,884$), prospective associations with vitamin D levels and depression were also identified (insufficiency: aOR 1.11, 95% CI 1.00 to 1.23; deficiency: aOR 1.30, 95% CI 1.13 to 1.50).

Conclusion: In middle-aged adults, a prospective association was found between vitamin D status and depression. The findings suggest that vitamin D deficiency and insufficiency might be risk factors for the development of new-onset depression in this population group. Further, vitamin D deficiency might be a predictor of sustained depressive symptoms among middle-aged adults who already have depression.

Is the evidence likely to be biased?

* *Was there a representative and well-defined sample of participants?*

  Partially. Data were extracted from records of participants in the UK Biobank (a large, long-term biobank study of adults aged between 40 and 69 years), who were registered with a general practitioner and living within 25 miles of one of the 22 assessment centres. It is implied, but not explicitly stated, that participants were enrolled consecutively. Inclusion in the UK Biobank database is limited to middle-aged participants, though this is appropriate for the study question. It reportedly differs from the general UK population in terms of demographics (more females, 'less deprived') and health (lower smoking incidence, lower alcohol intake and fewer self-reported health conditions), which could affect the generalisability of findings.

* *Were participants recruited at a common point in the disease or condition?*

  No. Participants in the Biobank database had variable vitamin D levels at the time of recruitment into it (and baseline was the only time that vitamin D levels were measured) and some had depression and some did not (although this was adjusted for in the analyses).

* *Was exposure determined accurately?*

  Yes. Vitamin D levels were measured using a chemiluminescent immunoassay and analysed using thresholds from UK Scientific Advisory Committee on Nutrition for categorising participants to sufficient levels of vitamin D (>50 nmol/L), insufficient levels (20–50 nmol/L) and deficient levels (<20 nmol/L).

Continued

PHARMACY EXAMPLE—cont'd

- *Were the outcomes measured accurately?*
  Unclear. Multiple measures were used to determine depression at baseline, including validated instruments (Patient Health Questionnaire [PHQ]-2) and linked records. At follow-up, depression was only assessed with one self-report measure and it was a different one from that used at baseline—the PHQ-9 (a nine-item questionnaire that scores each of the nine DSM-IV criteria for depression). Neither the PHQ-2 nor the PHQ-9 are measures of clinical depression and are self-administered tools.

- *Were important confounding factors considered?*
  Mostly. This study considered covariates previously demonstrated to impact on depression. Sensitivity analyses were carried out to examine associations with alcohol intake, vitamin D status threshold, continuous PHQ-9 scores using linear regression and baseline depression in the model as a covariate. As the presence of a chronic physical condition could predict new-onset depression, the study adjusted for the number of physical health conditions reported by each participant during baseline assessment, although the authors note that vitamin D might be a marker of chronic non-specific disease, rather than specifically related to depression. Adjustments were also made for the season in which the blood sample was taken, as seasonal variation can impact vitamin D level.

- *Was the follow-up of participants sufficiently long and complete?*
  Yes, for length and no, for completeness. The mental health follow-up questionnaire was sent at 6–10 years after joining the Biobank. However, of the 502,640 Biobank participants, a follow-up mental health questionnaire was only sent to 157,366 participants and data were analysed for the 139,128 participants for whom both baseline vitamin D and follow-up mental health data were available.

What are the main results?
Among participants with no depression at baseline (*n* = 127,244), those with vitamin D insufficiency (aOR 1.14, 95% CI 1.07 to 1.22) and those with vitamin D deficiency (aOR 1.24, 95% CI 1.13 to 1.36) were more likely to develop new-onset depression at follow-up compared with those with optimal vitamin D levels. For every unit (nmol/L) increase in vitamin D, the risk of new-onset depression had a modest decline (aOR 0.996, 95% CI 0.994 to 0.999).

How might we use this evidence to inform practice?
There are some aspects of the study and its risk of bias that concern you, although it appears to be the best available primary study relevant to your clinical question. The study suggests a positive association between low vitamin D level and symptoms of depression, although no causal relationship can be established from this study design. You plan to discuss the findings with your customer when you next see her and suggest that she discuss the study and her concerns with her GP at her next appointment.

OPTOMETRY EXAMPLE

Clinical scenario
You are an optometrist in a suburban practice. A patient, William, is a 35-year-old occasional contact lens wearer who presented with a dendritic corneal ulcer which you diagnosed as a first episode of herpes simplex virus (HSV) keratitis and successfully treated with a 10-day course of topical aciclovir. At his follow-up visit, you confirm that the ulcer has healed and advise him of the known risk of recurrence of epithelial keratitis (14% in the first 12 months based on the seminal Herpetic Eye Disease Study [HEDS][3] results in the United States). William asks you if he can safely resume contact lens wear. You are not aware of contact lenses being an established risk factor for HSV keratitis recurrence but as contact lenses are a known risk for other types of infectious keratitis (for example, bacterial, acanthamoeba), you decide to search for evidence.

Clinical question
In adults with a history of herpes simplex virus keratitis, does contact lens wear increase the risk of recurrence?

Search terms and databases used to find the evidence
Database: PubMed—Clinical Queries (with 'prognosis category' and 'narrow scope' selected).

Search terms: (herpes simplex virus) AND (keratitis) AND (contact lens)

The search returned six records. Three appear to be relevant. Only one focused on contact lens wearers, so you choose it to appraise.

Article chosen

Mucci JJ, Utz VM, Galor A, et al. Recurrence rates of herpes simplex virus keratitis in contact lens and non-contact lens wearers. Eye Contact Lens 2009;35:185–7.

Structured abstract (adapted from the above)

Study design: Retrospective cohort study.

Setting: Hospital eye clinic in one city (Cleveland, Ohio) in the United States.

Participants: 117 patients (65% male); 21 contact lens wearers (median age 40 years) and 96 non-contact lens wearers (median age 53 years), with any previous diagnosis of active HSV keratitis of any type (epithelial, stromal or endothelial disease) in one or both eyes and follow-up time of at least 6 months.

Outcomes: Recurrence rate of HSV keratitis.

Prognostic factors studied: Age, gender, ethnicity, keratitis type, unilaterality/bilaterality, immunosuppression (local and systemic), history of atopy, use of prophylactic antiviral (for example, aciclovir 400 mg twice daily or valaciclovir 500 mg once daily, or famciclovir 500 mg once daily), duration of prophylactic antiviral use, history of previous HSV infection and duration of follow-up.

Follow-up period: Median follow-up was 40 months (range: 8–244 months) for contact lens wearers and 27 months (range: 6–330 months) for non-contact lens wearers.

Main results: 79/117 (68%) patients had a recurrence of HSV keratitis. Among these, a higher proportion of contact lens wearers (95%) than non-contact lens wearers (62%) experienced a recurrence ($p = 0.003$). Contact lens wearers experienced a higher number of recurrences (2 vs 1 mean number of recurrences, $p = 0.002$) and a higher recurrence rate (0.4 vs 0.23 median number of recurrences per year of follow-up, $p = 0.02$) than non-contact lens wearers. In the multivariate analysis, recurrence was associated with contact lens wear, history of previous infection, no prophylactic antiviral use and longer duration of follow-up.

Conclusion: In patients with a history of HSV keratitis, contact lens wear increased the risk of keratitis recurrence.

Is the evidence likely to be biased?

- *Was there a representative and well-defined sample?*

  Yes. The inclusion criteria and exclusion criteria for the sample were clearly defined and cases were obtained from a retrospective chart review of patients who had attended the clinic over a 4-year period and met the criteria. Diagnosis had been confirmed clinically, which is standard practice.

- *Were participants recruited at a common point in their disease or condition?*

  No. Patients were recruited at the time an active infection was recorded in their hospital file. However, about half of the patients had a positive history of previous episodes of HSV keratitis, so this is not an inception cohort study. Contact lens wearers were younger, and more likely to report prophylactic antiviral use (binary variable) and for longer (time on antiviral medication divided by the total follow-up time).

- *Was exposure measured accurately?*

  Unclear. Contact lens wearers were defined as those patients having any record of any type of contact lens use during the follow-up period. This included soft and hard lenses and patients who wore lenses for cosmetic or medical indications. Because of limited chart documentation, the time between recurrence of HSV keratitis and contact lens wear could not be adequately assessed and thus recurrences may have been incorrectly attributed to patients who had stopped wearing contact lenses prior to a recurrence or who wore contact lenses very infrequently.

- *Were the outcomes measured accurately?*

  Probably. Recurrences during follow-up were documented on the hospital eye clinic chart or documented by external ophthalmologists who provided adequate correspondence verifying an episode of recurrence. It is possible, though probably unlikely, that patients could have had undocumented and/or mild recurrences that did not generate correspondence from an outside practitioner or prompt a visit to the hospital clinic.

- *Were important confounding factors considered?*

  Yes. A multivariate analysis that considered many other known risk factors (listed in the abstract) was conducted.

- *Was the follow-up of participants sufficiently long and complete?*

  Yes—for duration; unclear—for completeness. Participants were followed for at least 6 months, which is

Continued

◎ OPTOMETRY EXAMPLE—cont'd

a reasonable duration to monitor for recurrence. Based on HEDS study data,[3] a recurrence rate of at least 9% for the epithelial type and of at least 14% for the stromal type would be expected over 12 months of follow-up. Loss to follow-up was not specified and likely because the study was a retrospective chart review.

What are the main results?

Recurrence of HSV keratitis was observed in almost all (20/21, 95%) of contact lens wearers and the majority (59/96, 62%) of non-contact lens wearers. Table 9.4 lists the relevant prognostic factors that were significantly associated with recurrence from the multivariate analysis, with one of the factors being contact lens wear. Contact lens wearers had a 1.6-fold increased risk (95% CI 1.1 to 2.5) of recurrence per year than non-contact wearers.

How might we use this evidence to inform practice?

You are mindful that this is a retrospective study and while you have some concerns about its risk of bias, it is currently the best available evidence for this clinical question. There is some uncertainty about the generalisability as the cohort consisted of patients who had presented to a hospital eye clinic and thus may have had more severe

TABLE 9.4 Factors significantly associated with increased risk of HSV keratitis recurrence in a multivariate analysis

Risk factor	Odds ratio (95% CI)
Contact lens wear	1.6 (1.1 to 2.5)
History of previous HSV infection	2.0 (1.3 to 2.9)
No history of prophylactic antiviral use	1.6 (1.1 to 2.5)
Longer follow-up time	1.07 (1.0 to 1.1)

disease than those who present to community optometry and general practitioner practices. However, it does appear possible that resumption of contact lens wear may increase the chance of a recurrence of an HSV keratitis in your patient. You will discuss this with him, remind him of the risk of corneal scarring and vision loss in non-epithelial forms of the disease, and recommend he talks with his general practitioner about possible prophylactic oral antiviral use should he wish to resume regular contact lens wear.

REFERENCES

1. Lazzarini PA, Ng V, Kinnear EM, et al. The Queensland high risk foot form (QHRFF)—is it a reliable and valid clinical research tool for foot disease? J Foot Ankle Res 2014;7:7.

2. Doherty A, Jackson D, Hammerla N, et al. Large scale population assessment of physical activity using wrist worn accelerometers: the UK Biobank Study. PLOS ONE 2017;12(2): e0169649.

3. Herpetic Eye Disease Study Group. Predictors of recurrent herpes simplex virus keratitis. Cornea 2001;20:123–8.

Understanding Evidence from Qualitative Research

Karin Hannes and Sally Bennett

LEARNING OBJECTIVES

After reading this chapter, you should be able to:

- Appreciate the role of qualitative research in providing information about people's experiences, beliefs, values and concerns
- Describe the basic assumptions that underpin commonly used qualitative research methodologies and the basic considerations for undertaking qualitative research
- Develop a qualitative clinical question

- Have a basic understanding of how to search for qualitative research
- Assess the quality (critical appraisal) of qualitative research articles
- Have a basic understanding of how to interpret the findings of qualitative research articles
- Discuss how the findings of qualitative research may be used in practice

This chapter primarily focuses on questions that relate to the experiences of patients and health professionals and the meaning they associate with these experiences. Qualitative researchers seek to understand human experiences and behaviour in a particular healthcare context. They may also be interested in the question of how relationships with other people, health professionals, environments and systems are negotiated, established, strengthened or restored. As we have seen in earlier chapters, evidence-based health care encourages us to find and use the best available evidence in practice. Health professionals seek evidence to substantiate the worth of a wide range of activities and interventions, and therefore the type of evidence needed depends on the nature of the activity and its purpose. Sometimes, evidence that arises from qualitative research is sought and utilised.[1] Qualitative research seeks to make sense of phenomena in terms of the meanings that people bring to them.[2] Evidence from qualitative studies that explore the experience of patients and health professionals has an important role in helping us to understand the particularities associated with individuals, families and communities.

Qualitative research attempts to increase our understanding of:

- how individuals and communities perceive health, manage their own health and make decisions related to health service usage
- the culture of communities and organisations in relation to implementing change and overcoming barriers to the use of new knowledge and techniques
- how patients experience health, illness and the health system
- the usefulness, or otherwise, of components and activities of health services that cannot be measured in quantitative outcomes (such as health promotion and community development)
- the behaviours/experiences of health professionals, the contexts of health care, and why we behave/experience things in certain ways.

The following scenario provides an example of questions that qualitative research can help to inform.

◎ CLINICAL SCENARIO

You are a nursing manager who is planning to move from working in an acute general ward to managing a cancer care ward and related outpatient facility. Before making this move, you wish to understand more about the cancer care system and, in particular, the environment in which patients are treated, how this is experienced by nursing staff and patients, and how it may affect patients' sense of wellbeing. You decide to do some reading on these various issues.

As you can see, this scenario suggests that the nursing manager wants information about how patients receiving treatment for cancer experience the cancer care facilities and its environment. In addition, you could add the perspectives of family members and carers to those of the patients. For example, *How do patients feel about their physical and social environments, and their interactions with those who care for them? What do patients, family members and staff think could be improved or changed in the cancer care facility environment?* These questions could be explored through qualitative research.

Qualitative research can generate evidence that informs us when making clinical decisions on matters related to the feasibility, appropriateness or meaningfulness of a certain intervention or activity. We will look at each of these in turn. Feasibility can be described as the extent to which an activity is practical and practicable. *Clinical feasibility* is about whether an activity or intervention is physically, culturally or financially practical or possible within a given context. *Appropriateness* is the extent to which an intervention or activity fits with or is apt in a situation. *Clinical appropriateness* is about how an activity or intervention relates to the context in which care is given. *Meaningfulness* refers to how an intervention or activity is experienced by the people receiving it. It relates to the personal experience, opinions, values, thoughts, beliefs and interpretations of individuals. Qualitative research does not always involve the evaluation of an intervention. It may also seek to understand how patients try to cope with their disease or how they experience illness in a broader social–cultural context. Apart from focusing on an intervention, qualitative research can also focus on a certain phenomenon of interest.

This chapter introduces different qualitative methodologies that can be used in qualitative research to help us explore patients' experiences, behaviours and concerns. It also presents a stepwise approach to developing qualitative clinical questions and searching for, appraising and applying qualitative evidence.

QUALITATIVE RESEARCH: THE VALUE OF DIFFERENT PHILOSOPHICAL PERSPECTIVES AND METHODOLOGIES IN RESEARCHING PEOPLE'S EXPERIENCES AND BEHAVIOURS

Qualitative research that focuses on patients' (and health professionals') experiences, behaviours and concerns assists people to tell their stories about what it is like to be a certain person, living in a particular time and place, in relation to a set of circumstances, and analyses the data generated to describe human experience and meaning. Qualitative researchers collect and analyse words, pictures, drawings, photos, videos, information from virtual reality and the internet, and other non-numerical data, because these are the media through which people express themselves and their relationships to other people and their world. This means that if researchers want to know what the experience of care is like, they may want to ask the people receiving that care to describe or visualise their experience to capture the rich meaning. Through these approaches, the enduring realities of people's experiences are not oversimplified and subsumed into a number or a statistic.

All research has underlying philosophical positions or assumptions that represent a researcher's worldview (ontology) or ideas about the nature of the reality we study. Quantitative research is mainly driven by a positivistic research position subscribing to the idea that information derived from sensory experience (what we can see, hear, smell, taste or feel), interpreted through reason and logic, forms the source of scientifically based knowledge.[3] It holds that society, systems, structures and cultures, like the physical world, operate according to general laws that can be detected through research.

In qualitative research, two common philosophical perspectives that are helpful for us to understand are the *interpretive* and *critical* perspectives. Interpretive research is undertaken with the assumption that reality is socially constructed through the use of language and shared meanings. They acknowledge the existence of multiple versions of 'the truth', depending on the perspective or disciplinary lens we use to interpret our complex reality. This is considered the basis for further debate and understanding. From the critical perspective, knowledge is considered to be value-laden and shaped by historical, social, political, gender and economic conditions. Critical researchers acknowledge the capacity of humans to influence and construct their reality. However, they are sensitive to external conditions that interfere in such processes and are beyond the control of the individual or may even be invisible for them. If these conditions remain unquestioned, they may serve to oppress particular groups.[4]

Critical approaches in qualitative research ask not just what is happening, but why, and seek to generate theory and knowledge to help raise our awareness and assist people to bring about *change*. In the last decade, healthcare researchers have also started to engage with post-human perspectives on research, 'making visible the more than human forces and power relations that constitute subjectivity and health practices'.[5] Such perspectives challenge the human-centred division and conceptualisation of care and clinical practice in the sense that they assign a form of agency to material things, which means that things can influence humans as much as the other way around.

Researchers' worldviews have implications for how they study the world or generate knowledge. Positivists will try to *measure* things as they are (where possible, using a standard, validated set of instruments), controlling contextual factors that may influence causal chains or correlations between particular variables. Interpretive researchers, on the other hand, attempt to *understand* phenomena through listening to people or watching what they do to interpret meaning.[6] Instead of using measurement instruments, they consider themselves an instrument through which reality is understood. Critical researchers take a different approach again. They will try to *influence* the situations or living conditions of the people they work with. Their role in the research process is often of a more facilitating nature, guiding their target group towards a consciousness level that allows them to transform their situation.

Different qualitative methodologies may be used depending on the underlying philosophical perspective. For example, phenomenology, grounded theory and ethnography are commonly used 'interpretive' methodological approaches to research because they all aim to describe and understand phenomena; whereas researchers who seek to generate change by bringing problems or injustices forward for conscious debate and consideration may choose methodological approaches such as action research or discourse analysis. Although these and other methodologies are discussed separately in this chapter, qualitative researchers often combine elements from different methodologies when undertaking their research. Each qualitative research approach aims to achieve different things; and when differing perspectives are put together, they provide a multifaceted view of the subject of inquiry that deepens our understanding of it. In this sense, they are not substitutes for each other due to some essential superiority of one method over another; rather, they represent a theoretical 'toolkit' of devices. Depending on the task at hand, one methodology on one occasion may be a more useful tool than another. We will describe commonly used methodologies in this chapter.

QUALITATIVE METHODOLOGIES USED IN HEALTH RESEARCH

Phenomenology

A phenomenological research approach values human perception and subjectivity and seeks to explore what an experience is like for the individual concerned.[7] The basis of this approach is a concept called 'lived experience'. This means that people who are living presently, or have lived an experience previously, are in the best position to speak of it, to inform others of what the experience is like or what it means to them. Phenomenology is concerned with discovering the 'essence' of experience. It usually draws on a very small sample of research participants (between three and ten), and asks the question: '*What was it like to have that experience?*' Large sample sizes such as those needed in quantitative research are not required, as the aim is to gather detailed information to understand the depth and nature of experiences. Data are collected using a focused, but non-structured, interview technique to elicit descriptions of the participant's experiences. This style of interview supports the role of the researcher as one who does not presume to know what the important aspects of the experience to be revealed are. Interviews may be undertaken as one-to-one interviews or as focus groups. Several steps are involved in thematic data analysis.[7] The interviews are transcribed verbatim and read by researchers who attempt to totally submerge themselves in the text to identify the implicit or essential themes of the experience, thus seeking its fundamental meaning.

The strength of this method is that it seeks to derive meaning and knowledge from the phenomena themselves and, although it is generally conceded that unmediated access to a phenomenon is never possible (that is, the exclusion of all prior perceptions and research bias), the emphasis on the experience of the participants ensures that this model represents as closely as possible the participants' perspective.[8,9] The perspectives that arise help to shape the categories of concern in terms of the issues the participants themselves identify. Through the phenomenological method, participants contribute substantially to informing and describing the field of inquiry that future policy needs to address.

◎ **CLINICAL SCENARIO (CONTINUED)**

Potential contribution of evidence from phenomenological research

The findings of phenomenological research studies could usefully provide evidence to the nurse manager related to the lived experience of being a patient engaged in a cancer care facility and the meanings that patients associate with this experience.

Grounded theory

Grounded theory is a methodology developed by sociologists Glaser and Strauss[10] to express their ideas of generating theory from the 'ground' to explain data collected during the study, using an 'iterative' (or cyclical/circular) approach whereby data are gathered using an ongoing collection process from a variety of sources. Grounded theorists use a theoretical sample of people that are most likely to be the best informants to deliver the building blocks for the theory to be developed. Theoretical samples work towards a saturation point. That is, the point in which no new themes or issues emerge from the data. Glaser and Strauss developed this approach in their ground-breaking work on death and dying in hospitals.[10] Strauss and Corbin[11] have developed an approach that begins with open coding of data and requires the researcher to take the data apart. The approach distinguishes itself from phenomenology in putting a heavy emphasis on understanding the parts from a text to construct the overall picture of *'What is going on here?'*.

 CLINICAL SCENARIO (CONTINUED)

Potential contribution of evidence from grounded theory research

The findings of grounded theory research studies could usefully provide evidence to the nurse manager related to the development of a new, theoretical understanding of what being a patient in a cancer care facility means, grounded or based on the experience of patients.

Ethnography

The term 'ethnography' was used originally to describe a research technique that studied groups of people who: shared social and cultural characteristics; thought of themselves as a group; and shared common language, geographical locale and identity. Classic ethnographies portray cultures, providing 'a portrait of the people' (the literal meaning of the term 'ethnography'), and move beyond descriptions of what is said and done to understand 'shared systems of meanings that we call culture'.[12] An ethnographer comes to understand the social world of the group to develop an inside view, while recognising that it will emerge from an outside perspective. In this sense, the researcher attempts to experience the world of the 'other' (euphemistically referred to as 'going native'), while appreciating that the experience emerges through the 'self' of the researcher. Ethnography involves participant observation, the recording of field notes and interviewing key informants. The identifying feature of participant observation is the attempt

to reconstruct a representation of a culture that closely reflects 'the native's point of view'.

 CLINICAL SCENARIO (CONTINUED)

Potential contribution of evidence from ethnography

The findings of ethnographic research studies could usefully provide evidence to the nurse manager related to the norms, patterns and group meanings of patients receiving treatment in a cancer care facility. Through observation and the accounts of members of the group, researchers can study how people respond to their care environment.

Action research

Action research is the pursuit of knowledge through working collaboratively on describing the social world and acting on it to change it. Through this, critical theory and understandings are generated. Action research asks the question, *'What is happening here, and how could it be different?'* It involves reflecting on the world and then entering into a cyclical process of reflection, change and evaluation. Data collected in action research include transcripts of group discussions, as well as quantitative and qualitative data suggested by the participative group. Both types of data are analysed concurrently. Themes, issues and concerns are extracted and discussed by both the research team and the participative group. Action research provides a potential means for overcoming the frequent failure of externally generated research to be embraced by research consumers, who often regard this form of research as unrelated to and not associated with their practice.

 CLINICAL SCENARIO (CONTINUED)

Potential contribution of evidence from action research studies

The findings of action research studies could usefully provide evidence to the nurse manager related to outcomes by involving people being treated for cancer in critiquing the care they receive and in developing and implementing action to change those things they identify as challenging in the cancer care environment.

Discourse analysis

Discourse analysis has its roots in postmodern thinking and emerged in several academic disciplines in the last few decades of the 20th century. It has played an important role in creating new ways of developing ideas in the arts, science and culture. At its simplest (and it is far from simple!), postmodernism is a response to modernity—the period when science was trusted and represented progress—and essentially focuses on questioning the centrality of both science and established principles, disciplines and institutions to achieving progress. The nature of 'truth' is a recurring concern to postmodernists, who generally claim that there are no truths but instead there are multiple realities and that understanding of the human condition is dynamic and diverse. The notion that no one view, theory or understanding should be privileged over another is a belief of postmodernist critique and analysis. The scrutiny and breakdown of ideas that are associated with postmodernism are most frequently applied through the discursive analysis of texts. Discourse is defined as to 'talk, converse; hold forth in speech or writing on a subject; give forth'.[13] Thus, 'discourse analysis' essentially refers to the capturing of public, professional, political and even private discourses, and to deconstructing these 'messages'. Discursive analysis aims at revealing what is being said, thought and done in relation to a specific topic or issue.

 CLINICAL SCENARIO (CONTINUED)

Potential contribution of evidence from discursive studies

The findings of discursive studies could usefully provide evidence to the nurse manager that arises out of deconstructing what patients and health professionals say; the origins of existing, dominant views; and the way in which strongly held, powerful discourses may 'silence' or 'marginalise' the voices of patients particularly with respect to what would support them in their treatment environment.

Within and cross-case studies

Case studies provide an in-depth perspective on a particular unit of analysis; a patient, a care facility, a group of health professionals, a hospital ward, etc. In some studies, one unit is analysed as a single, stand-alone entity. More often, though, multiple cases are compared with each other to generate a better understanding of how processes and patterns revealed in one particular case translate into another.[14,15] From a data-analytical perspective, it makes sense to first engage in a descriptive within-case analysis and extend it with cross-case analysis.[16] When researchers analyse cases independently for key content, they generate an initial understanding of what is at stake in each unit of

analysis. In a second step, researchers may wish to evaluate how key aspects related to their topic of investigation may vary across different units of analysis to detect patterns and commonalities relevant to the research question. From here, a synthesis is developed that captures the essence or variation between cases and, where possible, detects patterns and commonalities.

 CLINICAL SCENARIO (CONTINUED)

Potential contribution of evidence from within and cross-case research

A single case study may look at how one particular hospital cancer care facility succeeds in creating a stimulating environment that facilitates the wellbeing of patients. Cross-comparing different cancer care facilities in a multiple case study will enable researchers to identify key factors that contribute to people's sense of satisfaction with care or hamper it.

Artistic and design-based methods

Aside from these core methodologies, other more creative approaches have been developed to generate evidence, most notably within the field of artistically inspired and design-based research. Design-based research informs best practice decisions in building processes. Evidence-based design methodologies can be applied to any type of environmental intervention. However, in health, they are most often used to design and evaluate care facilities.[17] Design researchers investigate the physical, psychological and social effects of the built environment on its users. Design studies inspired by qualitative methods usually include a strong visual research component in combining characteristics of build environments with narrative storylines. In arts-based research, an art form is used as a medium to convey meaning.[18] In arts-informed research, approaches are embedded in a qualitative research design, mostly as a data collection or dissemination technique. In arts-based research, however, the epistemology of art making is prioritised over conventional qualitative research methods. It is the artistic process that is used as a primary way of understanding, exploring, investigating or examining patients' experiences, social welfare and health-related phenomena of interest.[19]

Qualitative research evidence is an important source of knowledge. Its value lies in its ability to systematically examine questions about issues such as experiences, opinions, reasons for behaviours and complex relationships that are unable to be answered by quantitative research.

CONSIDERATIONS WHEN UNDERTAKING QUALITATIVE RESEARCH

The methods used in qualitative research differ in several ways from quantitative research. We will look very briefly at some issues that researchers consider when undertaking qualitative research so that, when you are reading this type of research, you can better appreciate how the research quality can be appraised.

Selecting participants

Compared to quantitative research, qualitative research uses much smaller sample sizes because the goal of this research is to understand something in detail. It is not uncommon to see sample sizes of between five and 25, or even smaller, depending on the study design used. Participants (or documents in the case of discourse analysis) are often sampled using approaches such as convenience, purposive or theoretical sampling, and researchers may opt to continue to invite participants until data saturation is reached (the point at which no new themes or issues emerge from the data). Expectations about the richness of data that particular stakeholders can bring to the study largely determine the specific selection of participants.

Data collection approaches

Questionnaires are rarely used to gather qualitative data (although some researchers gather data this way using open-ended questions within a questionnaire). Data are most often collected by interviews with individuals or focus groups, observation and field notes, or by creative approaches such as photography or drawings. Interviewers often have an interview guide of the types of questions they need to ask, but this can be used flexibly during the interviews. Factors of importance that can affect the data being gathered include who does the interviewing or is present, the power relationships between the interviewer and participants or between the observer and those being observed, as well as *where* the interviews or observations are conducted. For example, people are likely to provide different information if an interview is held next to a person's bedside in a hospital than if it is undertaken at the person's home. Similarly, *when* the interview is undertaken within the context of the person's health trajectory can be important.

Data analysis

The data being analysed in qualitative research are the words from interviews, or information from observations, documents or creative sources, rather than numbers. The approach to data analysis looks different depending on what overall qualitative research method is being used.

Analysis is the systematic search for meaning. In many cases, this means breaking up the data into smaller chunks of information and reconfiguring them again into a consistent whole, as in thematic types of analysis. But it can equally refer to a thorough exploration of content based on keyword analysis or constant comparative analysis promoted in grounded theory. Depending on the type of data that goes into the study—texts, objects or field notes—the analytical focus might be on events or happenings, use of words, symbols and semiotics (for example, in the case of images), narrative structures and content or discourse. Researchers that adopt a theoretical framework in their study are likely to return to its core concepts in the analytical phase to make sense of the data. For inductive designs, the 'end product', independently of whether it is a new theory or a detailed narrative, should be more than the sum of its parts and more than a simple cut-and-paste exercise. It is the researchers' job to create this extra value through a structured account and by linking the insights generated to broader debates and discussions in health care.

One commonly used approach to analysis of data, particularly from interviews, is *thematic analysis* and this is now described in more detail. However, keep in mind that it is by no means the only type of analysis used in qualitative research. Thematic analysis is relatively easy to understand compared to more interpretive approaches, but an interpretive slant can also be brought into thematic analysis if needed. It is well suited to investigation of clinical phenomena for the purpose of capturing themes and patterns in a data set that can inform clinical understanding.[20] It summarises large amounts of data by offering themes that bring the data together.

The process of carrying out a thematic analysis consists of six core steps.[21] In a first step, the researchers familiarise themselves with the data (often in the form of words) to inform initial ideas about what is happening in the data with a focus on what was said. Second, researchers engage in line-by-line coding to indicate the parts that are interesting or important in the snippets of text analysed. In a third step, researchers start looking for patterns among the coded fragments to develop themes. The analytical effort moves towards a more abstract conceptualisation of study content. In a fourth step, these preliminary themes are examined against the original data. All evidence in support of a particular theme is clustered. Step five is concerned with theme definition and labelling. Themes, sub-themes and original research fragments that were originally difficult to code become clear. This is also the phase in which researchers might ask the original people interviewed to comment on summaries of data generated (referred to as 'member checking'), and/or the researchers' interpretation of the data to invite feedback. The report developed in step six is usually quite detailed, reflects the researchers' final ideas, and presents short quotes from the interview data to illustrate the themes generated.

USING QUALITATIVE EVIDENCE: A STEPWISE APPROACH

Structuring a qualitative question

The nurse manager described in the clinical scenario at the beginning of this chapter wants to find out how the experience of the environment of cancer care facilities impacts on the wellbeing of people receiving treatment for cancer. The PICO format described in Chapter 2 does not do full justice to the variety of qualitative questions that can emerge within different methodologies; however, it is a helpful tool for structuring qualitative questions. Generally, there is no 'comparison' in a qualitative question, and the 'I' refers to 'interest' or 'issue' rather than intervention. And sometimes you may wish to add the term 'evaluation' (that is, *what is it that we are wanting to see evaluated?*), as this may be more appropriate than 'Outcome'.

> ### ◎ CLINICAL SCENARIO (CONTINUED)
>
> **Structuring the question**
> From this scenario, a suitable qualitative question could be:
> - How does the perceived experience of the cancer care facility environment (*Phenomenon of Interest*) affect the wellbeing (*Evaluation*) of patients who are receiving cancer treatment (*Population/Perspective*)?

Searching for qualitative evidence

Using the term 'qualitative research' can be problematic. The word 'qualitative' is frequently used to describe a singular, specific methodology (for example, 'in this study, a qualitative methodology was pursued'), when—in its broadest sense—it is an umbrella term that encompasses a wide range of methodologies stemming from many diverse traditions.

In Chapter 3, we provided you with some search strategies for locating qualitative research in MEDLINE, CINAHL, Embase and PsycINFO. Qualitative researchers tend to privilege specificity over sensitivity in searching for information to avoid irrelevant hits. They usually feel comfortable using initially retrieved items as a starting point for applying supplementary search techniques such as related article searches, reference lists and hand searching less conventional databases,[22] including those containing evidence beyond the written word, such as prototypes, designs and arts-based

research data.[23] You may wish to opt for a multiple-term strategy that minimises the difference between a sensitive and a specific search—for instance, by combining the content terms with the following methodological terms: interview:.mp. OR experience:.mp. OR qualitative.tw.[24] However, if you wish to look for a particular method, relevant terms such as *phenomenology* or *grounded theory* or *arts-based* will need to be used.

> ### ◎ CLINICAL SCENARIO (CONTINUED)
>
> **Finding the evidence to answer the question**
> The topic is about patients' experience of the cancer care facility *environment*. The nurse manager searches in PubMed, CINAHL and EMBASE, but does not find any relevant articles. She considers that if any research had been done on this topic it might not have been published in a health journal, so decides to search Scopus, a database that includes a range of disciplines as well as health sciences. One possible search strategy is:
> "Cancer care facilit*" AND environment AND wellbeing AND (interview OR experience OR qualitative)
> Using the broad search scope, one article[25] looks relevant because it considers environmental design and spaces within cancer care facilities.

> ### ◎ CLINICAL SCENARIO (CONTINUED)
>
> **Structured abstract of the chosen article**
> **Citation:** Jellema P, Annemans M, Heylighen A. The roles of cancer care facilities in users' well-being. Building Res Info 2020;48(3):254–68.
> **Study design:** This qualitative study combined a thematic analysis loosely inspired by grounded theory with a photovoice approach.
> **Study question:** The study aimed to 'describe the role(s) cancer care facilities play in the users' wellbeing and to identify spatial aspects contributing to these roles'.
> **Context:** People receiving cancer treatment (from four different hospitals), their relatives, and care professionals. The primary interest lay in patients' experiences in their social and spatial context.
> **Participants:** 15 adults: five who were receiving cancer care, five of their relatives and five care professionals.
> **Data collection method:** A combined approach that included interviews, photographs, building plans and walking around the environment while interviewing.

Continued

⊚ CLINICAL SCENARIO (CONTINUED)—cont'd

Analysis: A qualitative analysis was conducted through an iterative process of memo-writing, coding and categorising research data from field notes, interview transcripts and photographs, and discussions within the research team.

Key findings: Three main themes were identified: (1) 'containing and mediating the confrontation with cancer', which was about confronting experiences of facilities that were stressful, especially sensory qualities such as smells and sounds; people's first encounter with the care facility; and the facility's spatial organisation, including routes and transitions outside and within the building, ease of access and places for privacy; (2) 'coping with limitations and opportunities', which referred to routine practices, flexibility and adaptability of spaces, and creating different atmospheres; and (3) 'changeability', which was about changing corporeality and identity and changes in the care environments and their effects.

Conclusion: Recommendations include aiming to improve patients' first encounters with a facility, the spatial organisation and atmosphere of the facility such as offering 'homelike' spaces and qualities in designated spaces and using spaces flexibly while ensuring spatial stability. More attention should be given to the specific design challenges of entrances, routes and transitional spaces to improve the experience of patients and their relatives and to support care professionals in utilising their work environment more flexibly.

Critically appraising qualitative evidence

Qualitative approaches are located in diverse understandings of knowledge; they do not distance the researcher from the researched; and the data analysis is legitimately influenced by the researcher when they interpret the data. This poses considerable challenges in appraising or assessing the quality of qualitative research. Quality assessment assists users to evaluate whether a primary research study has been conducted properly and whether the evidence it produced can be trusted. In a recent review, 102 critical appraisal instruments were identified in which 22 different themes were discussed.[26] Criteria that appear in most instruments were related to clear statements of findings, rigorous processes of data collection, sampling and analysis. Other criteria such as involvement of stakeholders and spelling out the practicalities of a research project appeared in fewer than three instruments. This suggests that not all criteria are considered equally valid by all developers.

Given the variety of views of qualitative researchers, it seems unlikely that the international research community will come to an agreement on a particular instrument as the standard for appraisal of qualitative research, at least in the near future. In the absence of a clear consensus on the criteria that should be used, users need to position themselves in these debates. Important questions to ask yourself when engaging in an assessment of quality include, for example: Has the study been conducted according to the methodological state of the art? Is it 'good enough'? In other words, does it move beyond basic methodological requirements, such as providing participants' quotes to demonstrate the credibility of the author's statement, into an in-depth interpretation that has broader relevance to the reader and is grounded in the data? Each instrument has its strengths and weaknesses. This is also the outcome of a comparison of two popular critical appraisal instruments: QARI (Qualitative Assessment and Review Instrument)[27] and CASP (Critical Appraisal Skills Programme).[28]

We cross-compared the quality criteria from both instruments. They each contain ten quality criteria.[27,28] In the comparison, we emphasise the extent to which both instruments facilitate the assessment of trustworthiness in qualitative research. In earlier chapters, you learnt that assessing the risk of bias of a study is a major aim when critically appraising quantitative data. Internal validity in quantitative research is assessed by establishing the extent to which the design and conduct of a study address potential sources of bias. This focus on limiting bias to establish internal validity does not fit with the philosophical foundations of qualitative approaches to inquiry. In qualitative research, the focus can be on the *rigour* of the research design, as well as on the quality of reporting. Others argue that quality of reporting is only a facilitator of appraising qualitative research papers and that the focus should be on evaluating validity in terms of trustworthiness or 'believability', referring to the kinds of understanding we have of the phenomena under study (accounts identified by researchers) and whether these are subject to potential flaws. Potential flaws can occur, for example, in the translation from statements of study participants into researcher statements or from study findings into a conclusion.

We tend to adopt the latter approach, emphasising that statements need to be grounded in research evidence, that we need to know whether statements from a researcher accurately reflect the ideas participants intended to reveal, and that the set of arguments or the conclusion derived from a study necessarily follows from the premises. To facilitate comparison between the QARI and the CASP, we took the 11 main headings (left column of Table 10.1) reported in Hannes and colleagues[29] and adapted the original table for this comparison.

TABLE 10.1 **Comparison of appraisal criteria in the QARI instrument and the CASP checklist**

Main heading	QARI instrument appraisal criteria (original criterion numbering)	CASP checklist instrument appraisal criteria (original criterion numbering)
	There is congruity between:	Screening questions: (1) Was there a clear statement of the aims of the research? *Consider what the goal of the research was, why it is important, and its relevance.* (2) Is a qualitative methodology appropriate? *Consider whether the research seeks to interpret or illuminate the actions and/or subjective experiences of research participants.*
Theoretical framework	(1) The stated philosophical perspective and the research methodology. *Consider whether the article clearly states the philosophical or theoretical premises on which the study is based. Does the article clearly state the methodological approach on which the study is based? Is there congruence between the two? For example:* • *An article may state that the study adopted a critical perspective and a participatory action research methodology was followed. There is congruence between a critical view (focusing on knowledge arising out of critique, action and reflection) and action research (an approach that focuses on working with groups to reflect on issues or practices and to consider how they could be different, on acting to change and on identifying new knowledge arising out of the action taken).* • *An article states that the study adopted an interpretive perspective and that a survey methodology was followed. In this example, there is incongruence between an interpretive view (focusing on knowledge arising out of studying what phenomena mean to individuals or groups) and surveys (an approach that focuses on asking standard questions to a defined study population).* • *An article may state that the study was qualitative or used qualitative methodology (such statements do not demonstrate rigour in design) or make no statement about the philosophical orientation or methodology.*	

Continued

TABLE 10.1   Comparison of appraisal criteria in the QARI instrument and the CASP checklist—cont'd

Main heading	QARI instrument appraisal criteria (original criterion numbering)	CASP checklist instrument appraisal criteria (original criterion numbering)
Appropriate-ness of research design	(2) The research methodology and the research question or objectives. *This question seeks to establish whether the study methodology is appropriate for addressing the research question. For example:* • *A report may state that the research question was to seek understandings of the meaning of pain in a group of people with rheumatoid arthritis and that a phenomenological approach was taken. Here, there is congruity between this question and the methodology. However, a report which states that the research question was designed to establish the effects of counselling on the severity of pain experience and that an ethnographic approach was pursued lacks congruity. This is because cause-and-effect cannot be addressed using an ethnographic approach.*	(3) Was the research design appropriate to address the aims of the research? *Consider whether the researcher has justified the research design. (For example, have they discussed how they decided which methods to use?)*
Data collection	(3) The research methodology and the methods used to collect data. *This question guides reviewers to consider whether the data collection methods are appropriate to the stated methodology. For example:* • *An article may state that the study pursued a phenomenological approach and that data were collected through phenomenological interviews. In this instance, there is congruence between the methodology and data collection.* • *An article stated that the study pursued a phenomenological approach and that data were collected through a postal questionnaire. This would indicate incongruence between the methodology and data collection. This is because phenomenology seeks to elicit rich descriptions of the experience of a phenomenon that cannot be achieved through seeking written responses to standardised questions.*	(4) Was the recruitment strategy appropriate to the aims of the research? *Consider whether the researcher has explained how the participants were selected, why the participants they selected were the most appropriate to provide access to the type of knowledge sought by the study, and whether there are any discussions around recruitment (e.g. why some people chose not to take part).* (5) Were the data collected in a way that addressed the research issue? *Consider whether the setting for data collection was justified, it is clear how data were collected (e.g. focus group, semi-structured interview, etc.), the researcher has justified the methods chosen, the researcher has made the methods explicit (e.g. for interview method, is there an indication of how interviews were conducted, and did they use a topic guide?), methods were modified during the study (if so, has the researcher explained how and why?), the form of data is clear (e.g. tape recordings, video material, notes, etc.), the researcher has discussed saturation of data.*

TABLE 10.1   Comparison of appraisal criteria in the QARI instrument and the CASP checklist—cont'd

Main heading	QARI instrument appraisal criteria (original criterion numbering)	CASP checklist instrument appraisal criteria (original criterion numbering)
Data analysis	(4) The research methodology and the representation and analysis of data. *Are the data analysed and represented in ways that are congruent with the stated methodological position?* *For example:* • *An article may state that the study pursued a phenomenological approach to explore people's experience of grief by asking participants to describe their experiences of grief. If the text generated from asking these questions is searched to establish the meaning of grief to participants and the meanings of all participants are included in the report findings, then this represents congruity.* • *An article might focus only on the meanings that were common to all participants and discard single reported meanings, which would not be appropriate in phenomenological work.*	(8) Was the data analysis sufficiently rigorous? *Consider whether there is an in-depth description of the analysis process, thematic analysis is used (if so, is it clear how the categories/themes were derived from the data?), whether the researcher explains how the data presented were selected from the original sample to demonstrate the analysis process, whether sufficient data are presented to support the findings, to what extent contradictory data are taken into account, and whether the researcher critically examined their own role, potential bias and influence during analysis and selection of data for presentation.*
Findings	(5) The research methodology and the interpretation of results. *Are the results interpreted in ways that are appropriate to the methodology?* *For example:* • *An article may state that a study pursued a phenomenological approach to explore people's experience of facial disfigurement and these results are used to inform health professionals about accommodating individual differences in care. In this example, there is congruence between the methodology and this approach to interpretation.* • *An article states that the study pursued a phenomenological approach to explore people's experience of facial disfigurement and the results are used to generate practice checklists for assessment. In this case, there is incongruence between the methodology and this approach to interpretation, as phenomenology seeks to understand the meaning of a phenomenon for the study participants and cannot be interpreted to suggest that this can be generalised to total populations to a degree where standardised assessments will have relevance across a population.*	(9) Is there a clear statement of findings? *Consider whether the findings are explicit, there is adequate discussion of the evidence both for and against the researcher's arguments, the researcher has discussed the credibility of their findings (e.g. triangulation, respondent validation, more than one analyst) and whether the findings are discussed in relation to the original research questions.*

Continued

TABLE 10.1   **Comparison of appraisal criteria in the QARI instrument and the CASP checklist—cont'd**

Main heading	QARI instrument appraisal criteria (original criterion numbering)	CASP checklist instrument appraisal criteria (original criterion numbering)
Context	**(6)** There is a statement locating the researcher culturally. *Are the beliefs and values and their potential influences on the study declared? The researcher plays a substantial role in the qualitative research process, and it is important when appraising evidence that is generated in this way to know the researcher's cultural and theoretical orientation. A high-quality report will include a statement that clarifies this.*	
Impact of investigator	**(7)** The influence of the researcher on the research, and vice versa, is clear. *Are the potential for the researcher to influence the study and the potential of the research process itself to influence the researcher and the interpretations acknowledged and addressed? For example: Is the relationship between the researcher and the study participants addressed? Does the researcher critically examine their own role and potential influence during data collection? Is it reported how the researcher responded to events that arose during the study?*	**(6)** Has the relationship between researchers and participants been adequately considered? *Consider whether it is clear that the researcher critically examined their own role, potential bias and influence during formulation of research questions, data collection, including sample recruitment and choice of location, how the researcher responded to events during the study and whether they considered the implications of any changes in the research design.*
Believability	**(8)** Participants, and their voices, are heard. *Generally, articles should provide illustrations from the data (such as quotes from participants) to show the basis of their conclusions and to ensure that participants are represented in the article.*	
Ethics	**(9)** The research is ethical according to current criteria or, for recent studies, there is evidence of ethical approval by an appropriate body. *An ethics committee approved the project proposal.*	**(7)** Have ethical issues been taken into consideration? *Consider whether there are sufficient details of how the research was explained to participants for the reader to assess whether ethical standards were maintained, and whether the researcher has discussed issues raised by the study (e.g. issues around informed consent or confidentiality, or how they have handled the effects of the study on the participants during and after the study).*

TABLE 10.1 Comparison of appraisal criteria in the QARI instrument and the CASP checklist—cont'd

Main heading	QARI instrument appraisal criteria (original criterion numbering)	CASP checklist instrument appraisal criteria (original criterion numbering)
Evaluation/ Outcome	**(10)** Conclusions drawn in the research report do appear to flow from the analysis, or interpretation, of the data. *This criterion concerns the relationship between the findings reported and the views or words of study participants. In appraising an article, appraisers seek to satisfy themselves that the conclusions drawn by the research are based on the data collected—the data being the text that is generated through observation, interviews or other processes.*	
Value and implications of research		**(10)** How valuable is the research? *Consider whether the researcher discusses the contribution the study makes to existing knowledge or understanding (e.g. do they consider the findings in relation to current practice or policy, or relevant research-based literature?), identifies new areas where research is necessary, and discusses whether or how the findings can be transferred to other populations, or other ways the research may be used.*

There is a lot of common ground in what both instruments cover. One feature of the QARI tool that is not present in the CASP tool is the ability it provides to check the congruence between these aspects of a study. QARI also focuses on the extent to which the influence of the researcher is acknowledged, and that what participants said is represented in the findings and forms the basis of any conclusions drawn. There are some other interesting differences between the instruments compared.[29] The QARI tool does not include an item about relevance or transferability of findings. Whether 'relevance' is an issue that needs to be evaluated in the context of a critical appraisal exercise is debatable. Like ethics, the 'relevance' criterion most likely has its roots in the idea that research should address the concerns of health professionals, rather than be the product of individual academic interest.

The CASP checklist, with its pragmatic focus on the different phases in a research project, does not engage substantially with the theoretical and paradigmatic level for which one needs to be an experienced qualitative researcher. It is more user-friendly to novice researchers.

Overall, CASP does a better job than QARI in capturing the audit trail of individual studies and, as such, enables reviewers to evaluate whether a study has been conducted according to the 'state of the art' for a particular method. The questions posed by the CASP tool remind the reader to think about the idea of *rigour* (whether thorough and appropriate approaches have been applied to key research methods in the study); *credibility* (whether the findings are well presented and meaningful); and *relevance* (how useful the findings are to you and your organisation). Within the qualitative research tradition, there are specific strategies that the researcher can use to improve the credibility of the research, and these are indicated in the CASP tool as a prompt for the reader to consider them. For example, the researcher may make use of triangulation and respondent validation. To explain further: *triangulation* occurs when data are collected and considered from several different sources, which may help to confirm the findings or to increase the completeness of data collected.[30] *Respondent validation* (also known as 'member checking') is where the researcher seeks confirmation and clarification from the participants that the data accurately reflect what they meant or wanted to say.

Another important feature of qualitative research is that the researcher is integral to the research process. It is important, therefore, that their role is considered and explained in the research report. The CASP tool prompts the reader to ask whether the researcher critically examined their own role, potential bias and influence during analysis and selection of data for presentation. One of the strengths of the QARI tool is that it suggests that the reader evaluate whether the researchers have reflected on their cultural and theoretical background and provided a rationale for the methodological choices made to control

their impact on the research. It also evaluates whether researchers have reflected on how their choice of method might have influenced the findings, which is equally as important as thinking about what the potential impact of the researcher has been. Both instruments can assist us in evaluating the methodological quality of studies; however, their approach to appraising qualitative research is somewhat different.

To illustrate the assessment of quality (or critical appraisal) process, we will evaluate the clinical scenario using the ten QARI criteria. Additional insights generated by using the CASP tool are added at the end of each of the QARI comments.

◎ CLINICAL SCENARIO (CONTINUED)

Assessment of quality of the chosen article

1. **Congruity between the stated philosophical perspective and the research methodology**

   In this study, the researchers wanted to provide insight into the roles that cancer care facilities play in the well-being of people receiving treatment. The authors state that their approach was informed by a constructionist paradigm, that they assumed a pluralist position and 'an understanding that knowledge is constructed in the interchanges between people, objects and activities'. The authors indicate that they adopted a more integrative onto-epistemological approach as a point of departure that emphasises the intersubjective nature of the research activities. They pay particular attention to bridging the gap between the researcher and the person with cancer and with inclusion of human and non-human components in the research environment. They also indicate that they used a polylogic research approach that, alongside the researcher and the researched, explicitly incorporates place into the methodology through the combined use of photovoice methodology and more conventional qualitative descriptive methods. Participants were asked to objectify their perspectives by adopting the position of a researcher themselves. This methodological approach is in line with the constructionist position that guides their research.

   The CASP checklist does not evaluate this criterion.

2. **Congruity between the research methodology and the research question or objectives**

   Given that the aim was to understand cancer patients' experiences and a combination of photovoice methodology with a more descriptive qualitative approach to analysis was used, this criterion appears to be met.

Additional comment from the CASP checklist: The mixed research design was justified and is appropriate to address the aims of the research.

3. **Congruity between the research methodology and the methods used to collect data**

   The researchers used a combined approach to data collection that included interviews (at home or at a preferred location and while walking in and around the facility), participant photographs and collecting building plans. This method is consistent with the overall mixed design of the study that pays attention to both visual markers of the environment and textual accounts of how the environment is experienced by patients as well as family.

Additional comments from the CASP checklist: The settings for the recruitment of participants and the sites where the research was conducted are clearly described, as is the number of participants involved in each group (patients, relatives, carers). While there were clear criteria for patients, these were absent for the other groups, and relatives and carers were selected based on referral of the patient. Patient recruitment was largely based on convenience sampling. However, the variety in participant demographic characteristics was monitored via a sequential enrolment procedure of involved people. The authors further provided relevant information about reasons for the drop-out of one participant. Less is known about how potential participants were approached and whether some declined involvement. Data saturation was not the aim. Rather, sampling was guided by involving patients from 'contrasting spatial situations' to provide insight to a variety of facilities.

4. Congruity between the research methodology and the analysis and representation of data

The authors explained that field notes, interview transcriptions and photographs were collected and sorted in NVivo. A qualitative analysis was conducted, based roughly on the QUAGOL guide (Qualitative Analysis Guide of Leuven) through an iterative process of memo-writing, code and category development, and discussions with the research team. QUAGOL offers a comprehensive method to guide the process of qualitative data analysis, loosely connected to the principles of grounded theory, but the different steps were not outlined. This method of analysis is congruous with the overall descriptive analytical approach used. There was representation of data through the quotes provided in the results as well as photos of interest to the participants. This does justice to the integrative methodological approach opted for.

Additional comment from the CASP checklist: A fairly general description of the data analysis process was provided and it is not explained how the data presented were selected from the original QUAGOL guide to demonstrate the analysis process. There are sufficient quotes and photos used to illustrate the results, and contradictory data are clearly indicated, with respect to the opinions of different target groups involved. The researchers' relationship with the participants was clearly described, but not their own role during data selection and analysis.

5. Congruence between the research methodology and the interpretation of results

The results were interpreted as three main themes, which are reported in the abstract earlier in this worked example. The authors highlight that for patients, the experience of transitions between different spaces is strongly linked to their corporeality before suggesting some more specific recommendations in relation to barriers and opportunities identified in the study. Similarly, the experiences of relatives and care providers are also discussed and recommendations provided. The findings and their interpretation are congruent with the multiple method strategy proposed in that you can clearly see the patients' perspectives and the socio-spatial meanings they were making of their treatment environment.

Additional comment from the CASP checklist: The findings were explicit, and the data clearly illustrated the themes. The findings were discussed in relation to the original research question. Negative and positive experiences are highlighted, which brings balance in the interpretation.

6. Locating the researchers culturally or theoretically

The beliefs and values of the researchers, and where they were located culturally, is not explicitly stated. Based on their affiliations, the team are based at a western European university. They include an explicit statement about their disciplinary backgrounds and the complementarity this brings. It suggests that the data have been read from multiple perspectives and this may have corrected for a potential over- or under-interpretation. The authors bring richness in spelling out their theoretical framing, both on the level of philosophical underpinnings of the study design and on the level of concepts guiding the analysis and interpretation of the content.

Additional comment from the CASP checklist: The CASP checklist does not specifically address whether the researchers have declared their cultural or theoretical position.

7. Influence of the researchers on the research, and vice versa, is addressed

The researchers describe several strategies related to how they personally related to the study topic, such as peer debriefing strategies, expert consultation and memo-writing. Other techniques to improve credibility of the results were pilot studies and follow-up interviews to gain further insight into experiences.

Additional comment from the CASP checklist: There are different traces of a critical examination of the researchers' role, potential bias and influence in this study, most notably member checking with participants. While this has mainly been done for the purpose of checking the translation from one language to another, it would perhaps have been more useful to check the researchers' initial interpretation of data collected. The researchers also engaged in retrospective reflection based on a triangulation strategy in which they gathered different types of data at different points in time and presented emerging insights to an

Continued

expert panel (of former cancer patients, a relative, a nurse and a director of a care facility) to enhance trust-worthiness and confirmability.

8. **Representation of participants and their voices**
   The article illustrates each of the themes by presenting excerpts from the interviews with participants and therefore demonstrates compliance with this criterion. It also presents visual evidence of material dimensions of the hospital environment to support certain claims made by participants or researchers.

   Additional comment from the CASP checklist: This item is addressed as part of the representation of the findings (item 4).

9. **Ethical approval by an appropriate body**
   An ethics committee approved the project proposal.

Additional comment from the CASP checklist: The authors state that all participants gave written, informed consent to participate in the study. They provide a very detailed account of how they dealt with ethical challenges for the visual component of the study.

10. **Relationship of conclusions to analysis or interpretation of the data**
    The study concludes with a set of recommendations. The conclusions are well supported by the participants' responses and photos and appear to have clearly flowed from the analysis and interpretation of data.

    Additional comment from the CASP checklist: The CASP checklist does not specifically look at the relationship between the analysis and the conclusions.

Further comments related to critical appraisal

A useful resource to further understand assessing methodological limitations of qualitative research is a guidance series written by the Cochrane Qualitative and Implementation Methods Group.[31–36] The guidance is intended for use in conjunction with the current edition of the Cochrane Handbook of Systematic Reviews of Interventions, particularly the chapter on qualitative evidence.[37] Although that guidance focuses on qualitative evidence appraisal in the context of systematic reviews, it lists the key domains that need to be considered when assessing the methodological strengths and limitations of qualitative studies and provides guidance on considerations when choosing a tool for assessment of qualitative studies. It also provides guidance on how to deal with the outcome of the quality assessment exercise,[37] which is important to think about. Should you judge certain studies as methodologically flawed when particular criteria are not met? What is the minimum number of criteria that should be met? Should you prefer to work with findings of studies that obtain a higher score on the appraisal exercise, or should you focus on the content of those that align well with your particular needs? Is there merit in describing the limitations of a study that we have observed from reading the research report, without excluding any of them, and what are the potential risks in doing so?

The study that we evaluated scores relatively well on most criteria. It also illustrates how the philosophical position of the researchers towards the research project determined not only the choice of an appropriate method,

but also the window through which they examined the data. It had a direct impact on the way the findings were interpreted and presented, such as inclusion of building plans and participants' photos as well as quotations in the results.

This section ends with some guidance on how to make sense of the appraisal as a whole. Pearson[27] offers the following categorisation of judgment about the content of a qualitative article. Overall, the content of the article may be considered:

- *Unequivocal:* the evidence is beyond reasonable doubt and includes findings that are factual, directly reported/observed and not open to challenge.
- *Credible:* the evidence, while interpretative, is plausible in light of the data and theoretical framework. Conclusions can be logically inferred from the data; but because the findings are essentially interpretative, these conclusions are open to challenge.
- *Unsupported:* findings are not supported by the data and none of the other level descriptors apply.

The next issue to consider is how we might use the findings in practice.

Applying qualitative evidence

Research from qualitative studies can inform health professionals' thinking about similar situations/populations that they are working with. However, the way in which findings from qualitative evidence might be used in practice differs from quantitative research. Quantitative research findings are reported in terms of the probability (for example) of an outcome occurring when a particular intervention is implemented, in the same way, for a defined patient group. This therefore requires health professionals to accept a generalisation that the research findings can be applied to patients similar to those in the study. In quantitative research, this concept is referred to as *generalisability*. There are objections to the application of qualitative findings in practice because of the theoretical underpinnings of many qualitative methodologies. Principally, this relates to the idea that 'truth' is contextual, or for certain methodologies 'in the moment', and therefore only representative of a particular person or group at *that* time and within *that* context. Therefore, it is argued that the findings of a qualitative study of one group of people in a single study cannot be extrapolated to other people, groups or contexts. Researchers who follow this line of argument claim that the pooling and/or application of qualitative findings is, in effect, an attempt to formulate a result that can be generalised across a population and, as such, is an inappropriate use of qualitative findings.

Other researchers have developed a strong opposing view and suggest that the term 'generalisability' is being misinterpreted. Sandelowski and colleagues[38] have put forward that the argument against the pooling or application of qualitative findings is founded on a 'narrowly conceived' view of what constitutes generalisability—that is, a view that sees it in relation to the representativeness (in terms of size and randomisation) of a sample and of statistical significance. They argue that qualitative research has the capacity to produce generalisations—but they are suggestive or naturalistic (or realistic) in nature rather than generalisations that are predictive, as is the case in quantitative research.[38] The CASP checklist adds the criterion of relevance or transferability of findings as an important issue to be evaluated when reading a research paper and, depending on the type of qualitative design used, it seems reasonable to do so. There is little reason to believe that a theoretical or conceptual model that is based on a theoretical sample that used a maximum variation strategy (sampling to maximise diversity of participants represented), reached a point of saturation, and was tested in different settings (for example, as grounded theory approaches do) could not be considered transferable or relevant to other settings. However, bear in mind that many qualitative researchers aim just to understand a phenomenon, rather than intend for the findings to be generalised to other settings.

◎ CLINICAL SCENARIO (CONTINUED)

Applying qualitative evidence in the clinical scenario

The results of this study have increased your understanding of the perceived impact of the environment of a cancer care facility on patients' wellbeing. Once you are working in the cancer care facility, you plan to use this information to:

- raise awareness of patients' experiences of their care environment among the staff who work there
- involve the multidisciplinary team to review the way in which cancer care wards and facilities can be built or adapted to:
  - encourage social interaction between patients, family members and health professionals
  - encourage managers to invest in the material dimension and architectural feel of their hospital wards and cancer care facilities
  - increase patients' and families' sense of calm, comfort and orientation and reduce environmental stresses experienced by patients and by staff.
- Provide a system for patients and their families to provide feedback about the facility environment, the processes used and their experiences.

SUMMARY

- The experiences of patients (and of health professionals, for that matter) are a rich source of evidence for practice and policy. Investigating them can increase our understanding of how individuals and communities perceive health, manage their own health and make decisions related to health service usage.
- High-quality qualitative research uses rigorous processes to elicit and analyse data related to patients' experiences, perceptions and types of relationships with human and non-human agencies in the clinical environment.
- There are a number of well-established descriptive and interpretive qualitative research methodologies, including (but not limited to) phenomenology, grounded theory,

ethnography, action research, discourse analysis, within and cross-case analysis, and design and arts-based research. These methods are adaptable and may be used in conjunction with each other.
- Appraising qualitative evidence requires an assessment of the quality of the research in relation to the research methodology, methods and analyses used, and the interpretation of data. Critical appraisal instruments may help us in evaluating whether studies are conducted according to the methodological state of the art. However, as with appraisal instruments for quantitative research, appraisal checklists only capture what has been reported.

REFERENCES

1. Pearson A, Wiechula R, Court A, et al. The JBI model of evidence-based healthcare. Int J Evidence-based Healthcare 2005;3:207–15.
2. Denzin NK. The art and politics of interpretation. In: Denzin N, Lincoln Y, editors. Handbook of qualitative research. Thousand Oaks, CA: Sage; 1994. pp. 500–15.
3. Macionis JJ, Gerber LM. Sociology. 7th ed. Don Mills, Ontario: Pearson Education Canada; 2011.
4. Berman H, Ford-Gilboe M, Campbell JC. Combining stories and numbers: a methodologic approach for a critical nursing science. Adv Nurs Sci 1998;21(1):1–15.
5. McLeod K, Fullagar S. Remaking the post 'human': a productive problem for health sociology. Health Sociol Rev 2021;30(3):219–28.
6. Lockwood C, Porrit K, Munn Z, et al. Chapter 2: Systematic reviews of qualitative evidence. In: Aromataris E, Munn Z, editors. JBI Manual for Evidence Synthesis. JBI; 2020. Online. Available from https://synthesismanual.jbi.global (accessed 15 March 2022).
7. Manen M. Researching lived experience: human science for an action sensitive pedagogy. Toronto: Althouse Press; 1997.
8. Koch T. Establishing rigour in qualitative research: the decision trail. J Adv Nurs 1993;19:976–86.
9. Koch T. Implementation of a hermeneutic inquiry in nursing: philosophy, rigour and representation. J Adv Nurs 1996;24:174–84.
10. Glaser B, Strauss A. The discovery of grounded theory: strategies for qualitative research. New York: Aldine de Gruyter; 1967.
11. Strauss A, Corbin J. Basics of qualitative research: grounded theory procedures and techniques. London: Sage; 1990.
12. Boyle J. Styles of ethnography. In: Morse J, editor. Critical issues in qualitative research methods. Thousand Oaks, CA: Sage; 1994. pp. 159–85.
13. Concise Oxford English Dictionary. Oxford: Oxford University Press; 1964.
14. Patton MQ. Qualitative research and evaluation methods. 4th ed. Thousand Oaks, CA: Sage; 2015.
15. Yin RK. Designing single- and multiple-case studies. In: Bennett N, Glatter R, Levacic R. Improving educational management through research and consultancy. London: Sage; 1994. pp. 135–55.
16. Miles MB, Huberman M, Saldana J. Qualitative data analysis: a methods sourcebook. 4th ed. Thousand Oaks, CA: Sage; 2020.
17. Alfonsi E, Capolongo S, Buffoli M. Evidence Based Design and healthcare: an unconventional approach to hospital design. Ann Ig 2014;26(2):137–43.
18. Barone T, Eisner EW. Arts based research. Thousand Oaks, CA: Sage Publications; 2012.
19. Gerber N, Biffi E, Biondo J, et al. Arts-based research in the social and health sciences: pushing for change with an interdisciplinary global arts-based research initiative. Forum Qual Soc Res 2020;21(2):15.
20. Thorne S, Kirkham SR, O'Flynn-Magee K. The analytic challenge in interpretive description. Int J Qual Methods 2004;3(1):1–11.
21. Braun V, Clarke V. Using thematic analysis in psychology. Qual Res Psych 2006:3(2):77–101.
22. Harris JL, Booth A, Cargo M, et al. Cochrane Qualitative and Implementation Methods Group guidance series-paper 2: methods for question formulation, searching, and protocol development for qualitative evidence synthesis. J Clin Epidemiol 2018;97:39–48.
23. Hannes K, Coemans S. 2016. The (app)sense of numbers and narratives in social science research. In: 'A Truly Golden Handbook': the scholarly quest for utopia. Leuven, BE: Leuven University Press; 2016. pp. 480–93.
24. Wong S, Wilczynski N, Haynes RB, et al. Developing optimal search strategies for detecting clinically relevant qualitative studies in MEDLINE. Medinfo 2004;11:311–16.
25. Jellema P, Annemans M, Heylighen A. The roles of cancer care facilities in users' well-being. Building Res Info 2020;48(3): 254–68.
26. Munthe-Kaas HM, Glenton C, Booth A, et al. Systematic mapping of existing tools to appraise methodological strengths and limitations of qualitative research: first stage in the development of the CAMELOT tool. BMC Med Res Methodol 2019;19(1):113.
27. Pearson A. Balancing the evidence: incorporating the synthesis of qualitative data into systematic reviews. JBI Reports 2004;2:45–64.
28. Critical Appraisal Skills Programme (CASP). 10 questions to help you make sense of qualitative research. England: Public Health Resource Unit; 2013. Online. Available: www.casp-uk.net/casp-tools-checklists (accessed 14 March 2022).
29. Hannes K, Lockwood C, Pearson A. A comparative analysis of three online appraisal instruments' ability to assess validity in qualitative research. Qual Health Research 2010;20:1736–43.
30. Shih F. Triangulation in nursing research: issues of conceptual clarity and purpose. J Adv Nurs 1998;28(3):631–41.
31. Noyes J, Booth A, Cargo M, et al. Cochrane Qualitative and Implementation Methods Group guidance series-paper 1: introduction. J Clin Epidemiol 2018;97:35–8.
32. Harris JL, Booth A, Cargo M, et al. Cochrane Qualitative and Implementation Methods Group guidance series-paper 2: methods for question formulation, searching, and protocol development for qualitative evidence synthesis. J Clin Epidemiol 2018;97:39–48.
33. Noyes J, Booth A, Flemming K, et al. Cochrane Qualitative and Implementation Methods Group guidance series—paper 3: methods for assessing methodological limitations, data extraction and synthesis, and confidence in synthesized qualitative findings. J Clin Epidemiol 2018;97:49–58.
34. Cargo M, Harris J, Pantoja T, et al. Cochrane Qualitative and Implementation Methods Group guidance series—paper 4: methods for assessing evidence on intervention implementation. J Clin Epidemiol 2018;97:59–69.

35. Harden A, Thomas J, Cargo M, et al. Cochrane Qualitative and Implementation Methods Group guidance series—paper 5: methods for integrating qualitative and implementation evidence within intervention effectiveness reviews. J Clin Epidemiol 2018;97:70–8.

36. Flemming K, Booth A, Hannes K, et al. Cochrane Qualitative and Implementation Methods Group guidance series—paper 6: reporting guidelines for qualitative, implementation, and process evaluation evidence syntheses. J Clin Epidemiol 2018;97:79–85.

37. Noyes J, Booth A, Cargo M, et al. Chapter 21: Qualitative evidence. In: Higgins JPT, Thomas J, Chandler J, et al., editors. Cochrane handbook for systematic reviews of interventions. Version 6.3 (updated February 2022). The Cochrane Collaboration; 2022. Online. Available from www.training.cochrane.org/handbook/ (accessed 15 March 2022).

38. Sandelowski M, Docherty S, Emden C. Focus on qualitative methods. Qualitative metasynthesis: issues and techniques. Res Nurs Health 1997;20:365–71.

11

Understanding Evidence from Qualitative Research
Examples of Assessment of Quality (Critical Appraisal) from Different Health Professions

Romi Haas, Sally Bennett, Bridget Abell, John Bennett, Fiona Bogossian, Ryan Causby, Anthony Scott Devenish, Carolyn Ee, Roma Forbes, Rebecca Packer and Shelly Wilkinson

This chapter is an accompaniment to the previous chapter (Chapter 10), where the steps involved in answering a clinical question about patients' experiences and concerns were explained. To further help you learn how to assess the quality (critically appraise) the evidence for this type of question, this chapter contains worked examples of questions about patients' experiences and concerns.

The Critical Appraisal Skills Program (CASP) qualitative checklist[1] for assessing the quality of qualitative research has been used as a guide in each of the examples that follow. The CASP checklist is lengthy, and so for the purpose of brevity we have omitted the two screening items at the beginning of the checklist that ask: '*Was there a clear statement of the aims?*' and '*Is a qualitative methodology appropriate?*' The authors who contributed examples to this chapter had already screened their chosen articles, and therefore we have not provided comments on these two items and you will see that each assessment of quality (appraisal) begins with item 3 of the checklist.

It is important to understand that the CASP checklist for qualitative research provides a technical/pragmatic assessment of quality. The CASP tools were developed from guides produced by the Evidence-Based Medicine Working Group and published in the *Journal of the American Medical Association*.[2] One of the guides addresses qualitative research[3] but does not consider the philosophical or theoretical perspectives of qualitative research or philosophical perspectives of the researcher, as you will have seen in the QARI tool in Chapter 10. An explanation and comparison of the features of the QARI tool and the CASP checklist was provided in Chapter 10.

You will also see that the third item in the CASP checklist asks about *research design*, and this needs clarification as it is subject to interpretation. Specifically, it asks: '*Was the research design appropriate to address the aims of the research?*' It also prompts the reader to consider '*Whether the researcher has justified the research design. (For example, have they discussed how they decided which methods to use?)*' There are no specific guidelines about what the CASP tool means by 'research design' or 'methods to use'. In the examples that follow, we have taken the position that 'research design' refers to 'research methodology' (that is, phenomenology, grounded theory, ethnography, etc.), where relevant information was reported.

The CASP tool is just one example of a checklist for assessing the quality of qualitative evidence, and there are others that have a slightly different focus, with no consensus about the ideal approach that should be used. The following worked examples illustrate the use of the CASP checklist for appraising the quality of qualitative research in a range of different disciplines.

◎ OCCUPATIONAL THERAPY EXAMPLE

Clinical scenario

As an occupational therapist, you work in a large private practice in a metropolitan area of Australia which offers services for children, a large number of whom have autism spectrum disorder. You work mainly with young children. Many of your clients with autism also have high levels of anxiety, which contributes to their difficulty with engaging in therapy sessions. You want to meet with the owner of the private practice to discuss the possibility of using therapy dogs in some of your occupational therapy sessions, as you have additional training in animal-assisted therapy and have a dog (a female Labrador called Jaffer) who you have had trained during the last year in the hope she could be used in some form of animal-assisted therapy in future. However, before meeting with the owner of the practice, you decide to look at the literature to understand the evidence for animal-assisted therapy with children with autism (which appears to have some benefit). In particular, you want to understand how the use of therapy dogs in occupational therapy might be perceived by clients' parents. You decide to do a search on this topic.

Clinical question

How do parents of children with autism perceive the use of therapy dogs in occupational therapy sessions?

Search terms and databases used to find the evidence

Database: PubMed—Health Services Research Queries (with 'qualitative research category' and 'narrow scope' selected), which is accessed through https://www.nlm.nih.gov/nichsr/hedges/search.html.

Search terms: (dog OR canine) AND occupational therapy AND autism AND parents

This search retrieved three results. Two studies look highly relevant and you decide to read both in detail; however, the following article focused on parents of younger children, so you decide to appraise this one first.

Article chosen

Hill JR, Ziviani J, Driscoll C. Canine-assisted occupational therapy for children on the autism spectrum: parents' perspectives. Austr Occup Ther J 2020;67(5):427–36. doi: 10.1111/1440-1630.12659.

Structured abstract (adapted from the above)

Study design: An interpretive descriptive design, within the context of a pilot randomised controlled trial (RCT) on the effect of canine-assisted therapy with children who had an autism spectrum disorder.

Study question: Authors sought to better understand the engagement of children on the autism spectrum participating in canine-assisted occupational therapy sessions from the perceptions of their parents.

Setting: Telephone interviews with parents of children following their participation in a RCT of canine-assisted occupational therapy in Brisbane, Australia.

Participants: Ten participants (nine mothers, one father) of children between the age of 4 years and 6 years 11 months, diagnosed with autism spectrum disorder who had participated in an occupational therapy program (seven × 1-hour sessions) incorporating canine-assisted therapy and, as parents, had observed and participated in the sessions.

Data collection method: A researcher not involved in the delivery of the intervention undertook semi-structured interviews with each parent, via telephone, to understand their experience of canine-assisted occupational therapy with their child.

Analysis: Interviews were recorded, transcribed verbatim and checked for accuracy. Inductive thematic analysis was undertaken by two researchers to generate a coding system, which was then used by both researchers to code all transcripts. Themes emerged from the coding, with the two researchers meeting regularly to ensure consensus.

Key findings: Four themes were identified describing parents' experiences: 'therapist qualities', 'goal-directed (canine-assisted) therapy', 'emotional safety' and 'therapy engagement'. Parents expressed that the presence of the dog appeared to provide emotional safety within the sessions and this seemed to help build child–therapist rapport. However, parents felt that the skills and qualities of the therapist and the use of goal-directed therapy were essential for children's engagement, in addition to the presence of the therapy dog.

Conclusion: The authors concluded that while the therapy dog enabled children's engagement in therapy, this study highlighted that the skill of the occupational therapist was essential for harnessing the motivational aspects of this intervention, and was critical for supporting children's sense of control, security and competence.

Continued

◎ OCCUPATIONAL THERAPY EXAMPLE—cont'd

Is the evidence rigorous and sufficiently reported?
Detailed questions from CASP

1. **Was the research design appropriate to address the aims of the research?**
   Consider:
   - *Whether the researcher has justified the research design (that is, type of qualitative research). (For example, have they discussed how they decided which method to use?)*
     The researchers reported using an interpretive descriptive methodology undertaken within the context of a pilot RCT and very briefly justified this choice by indicating it was well suited to 'inform clinical understanding of interventions experienced by participants'. This approach and justification fit with the aims of the research.

2. **Was the recruitment strategy appropriate to the aims of the research?**
   Consider:
   - *Whether the researcher has explained how the participants were selected.*
     Parents who were interviewed had to have participated in the pilot RCT (by observing and participating in canine-assisted occupational therapy sessions) and thus purposeful sampling was used. Eligibility to be in the trial included that the child was between the age of 4 years and 6 years 11 months; had a diagnosis of autism spectrum disorder; and had to have had previous positive experiences with dogs. For the current qualitative study, parents needed to have participated in the therapy sessions and be available to undertake a telephone interview. Twenty-two children had participated in the trial; however, no specific details are provided as to why only ten of the parents participated in the interviews for this study—that is, whether this number had been planned, or if the plan had been to interview all of them if they had been interested and available to interview.
   - *Whether they explained why the participants they selected were the most appropriate to provide access to the type of knowledge sought by the study.*
     The researchers explained that participants were eligible to participate if they and their children had participated in the intervention in the RCT. This meant that participants would have knowledge appropriate for the study, although more information

   about the representativeness of the parent's gender in relation to the gender of those in the RCT would have been informative, given that 90% of the parents interviewed were female.
   - *Whether there are any discussions around recruitment (for example, why some people chose not to take part).*
     This is not specifically reported in the article.

3. **Were the data collected in a way that addressed the research issue?**
   Consider:
   - *Whether the setting for data collection was justified.*
     The interviews were conducted via telephone after the completion of the therapy session, but the reason for this was not explained. There may be advantages and disadvantages to telephone versus face-to-face interviews that would be helpful for the reader of this study to take into consideration.
   - *Whether it is clear how data were collected (for example, focus group, semi-structured interview, etc.).*
     Semi-structured interviews were conducted at the conclusion of the canine-assisted occupational therapy sessions by a researcher who was an experienced occupational therapist and had not provided the intervention.
   - *Whether the researcher has justified the methods chosen.*
     The authors do not specifically provide justification for use of individual interviews, but it is somewhat self-evident that the therapy sessions had been individual and thus individual interviews would be appropriate for this study.
   - *Whether the researcher has made the methods explicit. (For example, for interview method, is there an indication of how interviews were conducted, or did they use a topic guide?)*
     The interview process is well described, including that the interviewer had not been involved in the delivery of the intervention, that the interviews occurred by telephone, and that a copy of the interview guide was provided. Some of the interviews were very short (5 min 43 s and 16 min 58 s), compared to many qualitative interviews. The researchers do not comment on the reason for this, and whether this was sufficient time to hear fully from the participants.

- *Whether methods were modified during the study. If so, has the researcher explained how and why?*
  The researchers do not mention any changes to the research methods during the study.
- *Whether the form of data is clear (for example, tape-recordings, video material, notes, etc.).*
  It is clearly stated that interviews were audio-recorded and transcribed verbatim.
- *Whether the researcher has discussed saturation of data.*
  No mention of data saturation was made, and it would have been helpful to know whether the researchers felt data saturation may have been reached by interviewing only ten parents of the 22 participants, particularly given that some of the interviews were quite brief.

4. **Has the relationship between researcher and participants been adequately considered?**
  Consider:
  - *Whether the researcher critically examined their own role, potential bias and influence during:*
    - *Formulation of the research questions.*
      The researchers had previously undertaken a systematic review and RCT about the effect of canine-assisted therapy and indicated the need to gain a better understanding of child engagement in therapy, which they sought to do through this qualitative study. In addition, the lead author had training in the use of canine-assisted therapy and ownership of a therapy dog which would have played a role in formation of the research question. Their role in the RCT and experience in canine-assisted therapy was acknowledged by the author, and some limited discussion about how they managed potential bias was discussed.
    - *Data collection, including sample recruitment and choice of location.*
      No specific mention is made about the role of the researchers or potential biases in recruitment. The researchers indicate that the interviews were carried out by an occupational therapist who was a researcher in the study but who did not provide the intervention.
  - *How the researcher responded to events during the study and whether they considered the implications of any changes in the research design.*
    No changes are reported.

5. **Have ethical issues been taken into consideration?**
  Consider:
  - *Whether there are sufficient details of how the research was explained to participants for the reader to assess whether ethical standards were maintained.*
    The paper indicates that all participants provided written consent to participate in this study, but no further details are provided.
  - *Whether the researcher has discussed issues raised by the study (for example, issues around informed consent or confidentiality or how they have handled the effects of the study on the participants during and after the study).*
    The researchers gave parents and children a pseudonym and personal information was removed from transcripts to ensure confidentiality. It would have been interesting to have had information about how they handled any effects of the interviews, but this was not reported. It is assumed that the interviews would have allowed for a 'debriefing' for the parents following the intervention with an experienced therapist which may have been helpful for participants, but this is not stated per se.
  - *Whether approval has been sought from the ethics committee.*
    Approval from appropriate ethics committees were obtained.

6. **Was the data analysis sufficiently rigorous?**
  Consider:
  - *Whether there is an in-depth description of the analysis process. Whether thematic analysis is used. If so, is it clear how the categories/themes were derived from the data?*
    A detailed description of the analysis is provided. The authors employed inductive thematic analysis as per interpretive description. The authors describe how coding, categories and themes were derived.
  - *Whether the researcher explains how the data presented were selected from the original sample, to demonstrate the analysis process.*
    Examples of quotes from participants are provided to illustrate some of the themes, but it is not clear how these were selected.
  - *Whether sufficient data are presented to support the findings. To what extent are contradictory data taken into account?*
    Many examples of participant quotes are provided; however, no mention was made about whether or not there were any contradictory data.

Continued

◉ OCCUPATIONAL THERAPY EXAMPLE—cont'd

- *Whether the researcher critically examined their own role, potential bias and influence during analysis and selection of data for presentation.*

  The authors acknowledged that the first author conducted the occupational therapy intervention sessions and was also one of the researchers who undertook the qualitative data analysis. The other authors provided independent analysis and interpretation of findings to mitigate the risk of potential bias. For example, two authors undertook the analysis and also met on multiple occasions to consider broad questions about the parents' experience of participating and how that related to occupational therapy practice and facilitating therapy engagement with children on the autism spectrum.

7. Is there a clear statement of findings?
Consider:

- *Whether the findings are explicit. Whether there is adequate discussion of the evidence both for and against the researcher's arguments.*

  The findings are very clearly presented. Although the parents' comments were overwhelmingly positive about the use of a therapy dog, the authors were careful to note that parents also recognised the role of the therapist and that the presence of the dog alone was not considered sufficient to engage the children. Authors went on to consider the literature around the therapist and dog as a team, and the need to better understand the mechanisms at play, and cautioned about the need for therapists to have appropriate training prior to incorporating therapy dogs into therapy.

- *Whether the researcher has discussed the credibility of their findings (for example, triangulation, respondent validation, more than one analyst).*

  The researchers present some discussion of credibility, including: the use of two researchers to develop codes and themes; the inclusion of substantive quotes from participants; and the use of respondent validation/member checking. A stronger reflexivity statement would have been valuable given the first author's interest in and experience of the topic.

- *Whether the findings are discussed in relation to the original research question.*

  The findings are clearly discussed in relation to the original objective of the research.

8. How valuable is the research?
Consider:

- *Whether the researcher discusses the contribution the study makes to existing knowledge or understanding. (For example, do they consider the findings in relation to current practice or policy, or relevant research-based literature?)*

  The article discusses the findings from this study in relation to research about the motivational framework of social determination theory for fostering a child's engagement in therapy. The researchers suggest that the findings from this study highlight how the therapist's skill in using therapy dogs may accelerate the therapeutic relationship and contribute to the child's engagement in therapy. The article also discussed a range of clinical implications, including the need for the therapist to be adequately trained to use dogs in therapy.

- *Whether they identify new areas where research is necessary.*

  The authors note the need for further RCTs to establish the effectiveness of canine-assisted therapy as part of occupational therapy with children with autism, as well as research to better understand the mechanisms through which beneficial effects of the therapist–canine team might be experienced.

- *Whether the researchers have discussed whether or how the findings can be transferred to other populations or considered other ways the research may be used.*

  The authors briefly indicate that the research focused on children with autism spectrum disorder between the age of 4 years and 6 years 11 months, and that the findings needed to be interpreted accordingly. For children to be eligible to participate in the trial, they had to have previous positive experience with dogs and thus the observations made by their parents may not apply to children who do not meet this criterion. Experienced therapists are unlikely to choose to use therapy dogs in clinical practice unless children are comfortable with them, but this issue is not discussed.

What are the main findings?

Four themes were identified in this paper which highlighted parents' perceptions about their children's engagement in canine-assisted occupational therapy. The theme *'therapist qualities'* described parents' perspectives about the relationship between the child and the therapist as being essential to successful therapy (regardless of whether the therapist worked with or without a dog), and that they valued the therapist being calm, patient and responsive to the child and accepting of both child and parent. The theme 'goal-directed (canine-assisted) therapy' described parents' perceptions of the way in which the therapist incorporated the dog in therapy while remaining goal focused. The theme 'emotional safety' captured parents' views that the dog contributed to a calm and relaxed therapy session, and that patting the dog contributed to the child's emotional regulation and provided something similar to a friendship experience between their child and the therapy dog. Finally, the theme 'therapy engagement' was about parents' perception of the therapy dog accelerating the connection between their child and the therapist, the increased motivation and engagement their child seemed to show in therapy with a dog present, as well as their ability to maintain attention and persistence in therapy.

How might we use this evidence to inform practice?
This appears to be a fairly well-designed and conducted study which took place within the context of an RCT testing the effect of the intervention. Although the small pilot RCT showed no difference between groups (and the papers describing the RCT should be read in concert with

this study), this study provides additional useful information about parents' perspectives on the use of therapy dogs. The results were overwhelmingly positive, and participants provided many examples of how the skill of the occupational therapist and therapy dog contributed to the child's engagement in the intervention. The fact that the associated trial did not find any difference between the intervention group and the control group does not take away from the importance of this study with respect to the experience of parents—what they had observed, the benefits they had perceived and the insights they provided—all of which can inform both the use of therapy dogs in practice as well as design of future research into the effects of therapy dogs.

Returning to the case scenario, as a therapist who is interested in incorporating therapy dogs in your practice the article provides very useful information for you to consider and the various issues to raise with the owner of the practice. You decide to read the other papers on this topic to better understand how to choose which children are suitable to use therapy dogs with, and to look at the available systematic reviews about the effects of canine-assisted therapy for children with autism more generally in preparation for your meeting with the practice owner.

◎ PHYSIOTHERAPY EXAMPLE

Clinical scenario
You are a physiotherapist who works in a private practice that specialises in non-operative management of patients with persistent musculoskeletal conditions. In recent meetings with colleagues, you have noticed there have been shared experiences of managing patients with persistent hip pain who present with unhelpful beliefs surrounding their condition which is impacting their subsequent engagement in physiotherapy management. You decide to explore this further to better understand why this may be occurring so that you can share this with your colleagues in an upcoming clinic in-service with the goal of better managing patients with this complaint.

Clinical question
What are the beliefs of people living with persistent hip pain about their condition?

Search terms and databases used to find the evidence
Database: PubMed (with 'qualitative research category' and 'narrow scope' selected), which is accessed through https://www.nlm.nih.gov/nichsr/hedges/search.html.

Search terms: hip pain AND (persistent OR chronic) AND beliefs.

Your search strategy retrieves 8 articles. You choose a study that is relevant to your research question and focuses on people with hip pain who were candidates for surgery but agreed to participate in a physiotherapy intervention.

Article chosen
de Oliveira B, Smith A, O'Sullivan P, et al. 'My hip is damaged': a qualitative investigation of people seeking care for persistent hip pain. Br J Sports Med 2020; Jul. doi: 10.1136/bjsports-2019-101281.

Structured abstract (adapted from the above)
Study design: Cross-sectional general qualitative study using interviews based on the 'Common Sense Model'.
Study question: The aim of this study was to explore how people seeking care for persistent hip pain and disability make sense of their symptoms, their strategies to cope with pain and their experiences in seeking health care.

Continued

◎ PHYSIOTHERAPY EXAMPLE—cont'd

Setting: A private orthopaedic clinic in Perth, Western Australia.

Participants: 16 adults who were consulting an orthopaedic surgeon for persistent hip pain and were candidates for surgery but had agreed to participate in a physiotherapy-directed cognitive functional intervention.

Data collection method: Individual interviews were conducted by the lead author in a consultation room of the participating clinic ($n = 15$) or over the phone ($n = 1$) one week prior to commencing the intervention. Interviews based on the Common Sense Model explored patients' beliefs about the identity (diagnosis), causes, consequences, timeline and controllability of their symptoms, their strategies to cope with pain and their experiences in seeking health care. Interviews were recorded and then transcribed.

Analysis: Data were analysed thematically using a framework approach. Two authors classified interview responses into *a priori* categories. Data classified under each category were then analysed using inductive coding methods. The two authors then independently performed inductive coding on four transcripts to develop an index of codes which was then applied to all transcripts by one author. Themes were developed by the wider research team based on the coding.

Key findings: Four key themes were identified: (1) 'lay' versus 'informed' perceptions of cause; (2) 'fissures and tears': the use of the diagnostic jargon; (3) 'fixing damage' and 'controlling symptoms'; and (4) exercise, sleep and the threat to mental health.

Conclusion: The authors concluded that the negative beliefs relating to 'damaged' hip structures held by people with persistent hip pain and disability contributed to them avoiding physical activity, which then impaired their sleep, emotional wellbeing and physical health. Targeting pain beliefs and coping strategies may provide opportunities for more effective management of persistent hip pain.

Is the evidence rigorous and sufficiently reported?
Detailed questions from CASP

1. **Was the research design appropriate to address the aims of the research?**
   Consider:
   - *Whether the researcher has justified the research design. (For example, have they discussed how they decided which method to use?)*
     The use of qualitative research is appropriate to explore how people seeking care for persistent hip pain make sense of their symptoms, their strate-gies to cope with pain and their experiences in seeking health care. The authors used the 'Common Sense Model' as a validated framework to explore how people make sense of their musculo-skeletal symptoms. However, the authors did not clearly state which qualitative research method was used, only that a 'qualitative interview study' was conducted.

2. **Was the recruitment strategy appropriate to the aims of the research?**
   Consider:
   - *Whether the researcher has explained how the participants were selected.*
     Potential participants were recruited by two private orthopaedic surgeons within one private clinic. All eligible patients were invited to participate. Of the 28 people who met criteria, 11 declined or were unable to be contacted. One further individual was excluded from analysis due to being pregnant.
   - *Whether they explained why the participants they selected were the most appropriate to provide access to the type of knowledge sought by the study.*
     The authors clearly outline eligibility criteria. Patients were eligible to participate if they were aged 18 years and over, were consulting an orthopaedic surgeon for persistent hip pain and were candidates for surgery but had agreed to participate in a physiotherapy-directed cognitive functional intervention. It is inferred that these participants were deemed appropriate because they are seeking care for persistent hip pain. However, there were no eligibility criteria regarding the pain duration, and it is unclear why participants who were not candidates for surgery were excluded.
   - *Whether there are any discussions around recruitment (for example, why some people chose not to take part).*
     The authors state that 16 of the 28 eligible participants were interviewed. It is not clear how many eligible patients declined versus were unable to be contacted, and the reasons for declining are also unclear. The authors did not collect demographic data on the 11 people who were referred to the intervention but declined to participate.

3. **Were the data collected in a way that addressed the research issue?**
Consider:
- *Whether the setting for data collection was justified.*
Individual interviews were conducted in a consultation room of the participating clinical site ($n = 15$) or over the phone ($n = 1$). The choice of data collection site was not explained. Interviews were scheduled before participants began the intervention. Therefore, we can assume that the physiotherapists conducting the intervention would not have influenced patient beliefs.
- *Whether it is clear how data were collected (for example, focus group, semi-structured interview, etc.).*
Data were collected using interviews. The authors do not explicitly state the structure of these interviews, although they outline that 'the interview schedule was structured on the Common Sense Model' which implies that interviews were likely to have been structured to some extent.
- *Whether the researcher has justified the methods chosen.*
The authors do not directly justify the methods chosen for collection of data; however, the approach appears to be congruent with the aim of the study.
- *Whether the researcher has made the methods explicit. (For example, for interview method, is there an indication of how interviews were conducted, or did they use a topic guide?)*
The authors indicate 'the interview schedule was structured on the Common Sense Model'. The questions used in the interviews are described in the section on data collection and are consistent with the use of this model.
- *Whether methods were modified during the study. If so, has the researcher explained how and why?*
There is no explanation as to whether any of the methods were modified during the study. However, one participant was interviewed over the phone rather than in person. It is unclear as to whether this was a planned or a pragmatic change to the methods.
- *Whether the form of data is clear (for example, tape-recordings, video material, notes, etc.).*
It is clearly stated that interviews were audio-recorded and transcribed prior to analysis.
- *Whether the researcher has discussed saturation of data.*
No explanation of data saturation methods is provided. Although the authors state 'the patterns we identified among the 16 participants were sufficient to answer our research question', they also acknowledge this was a 'small convenience sample'.

4. **Has the relationship between researcher and participants been adequately considered?**
Consider:
- *Whether the researcher critically examined their own role, potential bias and influence during:*
  - *Formulation of the research questions.*
  The authors outline that they have a shared interest in cognitive behavioural interventions for musculoskeletal pain; and therefore their shared worldview, or 'lens', may have influenced both the design and conduct of the study.
  - *Data collection, including sample recruitment and choice of location.*
  The authors outline that eligible participants were identified by two orthopaedic surgeons; however, they do not state who approached these candidates to participate nor who contacted the participants to organise interviews. It is also unclear why one interview was conducted by telephone.
- *How the researcher responded to events during the study and whether they considered the implications of any changes in the research design.*
One individual was excluded from analysis due to being pregnant. This is stated as an exclusion criterion, but it is unclear whether this individual was interviewed. Otherwise, the methods do not appear to have changed in the study.

5. **Have ethical issues been taken into consideration?**
Consider:
- *Whether there are sufficient details of how the research was explained to participants for the reader to assess whether ethical standards were maintained.*
The authors do not provide details of how the research was explained to participants and state that patient consent for publication was not required, but the study was cleared by a Human Ethics Research Committee. Pseudonyms are used in the reporting of supporting quotes and demographic and clinical data.

Continued

⊚ **PHYSIOTHERAPY EXAMPLE—cont'd**

- *Whether the researcher has discussed issues raised by the study (for example, issues around informed consent or confidentiality or how they have handled the effects of the study on the participants during and after the study).*

  It is unclear if, and to what extent, informed patient consent was obtained given that it states that patient consent for publication was not required. It is therefore unclear whether the participants were adequately informed prior to partaking in the interviews. The authors also did not report if any issues arose as a result of this study or how such issues may have been handled.

- *Whether approval has been sought from the ethics committee.*

  The study was approved by both the Hollywood Private Hospital Research Ethics Committee and the Curtin University Human Research Ethics Committee.

6. **Was the data analysis sufficiently rigorous?**

  Consider:

- *Whether there is an in-depth description of the analysis process. Whether thematic analysis is used. If so, is it clear how the categories/themes were derived from the data?*

  The data analysis processes are clearly outlined. A framework approach was used for data analysis. Two authors classified interview responses into *a priori* categories and then independently performed inductive coding on four transcripts to classify data under each category and develop an index of codes. One author then applied the index to all transcripts. Reoccurring codes were identified and emerging interpretations were discussed and challenged among the study researchers. NVivo was used to facilitate analysis. The manuscript depicts the *a priori* categories, index of codes and themes.

- *Whether the researcher explains how the data presented were selected from the original sample to demonstrate the analysis process.*

  There is no explanation as to how the data presented were selected from the original sample.

- *Whether sufficient data are presented to support the findings. To what extent are contradictory data taken into account?*

  Sufficient data are presented to support the findings, with data presented within the text and a table of supporting quotes from the article for each theme. Contradictory data appear to be taken into account. For example, the authors describe cases when 'lay'

perceptions of cause were favoured by participants over 'informed' perceptions and where these perceptions were reversed.

- *Whether the researcher critically examined their own role, potential bias and influence during analysis and selection of data for presentation.*

  Emerging interpretations of the data were discussed and challenged among the researchers in this study, acknowledging their different professional backgrounds as clinical physiotherapists, orthopaedic surgeons and physiotherapists with expertise in qualitative research. The authors also acknowledge that their lens (worldview) may have influenced the study and that alternative interpretations of data are possible. The authors claim to address this by acknowledging their lens, and providing the interview schedule, code book and supporting quotes to leave an 'audit trail'.

7. **Is there a clear statement of findings?**

  Consider:

- *Whether the findings are explicit. Whether there is adequate discussion of the evidence both for and against the researcher's arguments.*

  The authors have provided data that reflect views that both support and refute the prevailing interpretations.

- *Whether the researcher has discussed the credibility of their findings (for example, triangulation, respondent validation, more than one analyst).*

  The data were provided by patients as the only participant group and more than one researcher undertook analysis. Validation of data from participants is not outlined.

- *Whether the findings are discussed in relation to the original research question.*

  The findings are discussed with clear links to the original research question and aims.

8. **How valuable is the research?**

  Consider:

- *Whether the researcher discusses the contribution the study makes to existing knowledge or understanding. (For example, do they consider the findings in relation to current practice or policy, or relevant research-based literature?)*

  The authors discuss how these study findings relate to existing research and the clinical implications of their findings in relation to imaging reports, patient education and self-management. The authors argue that by illustrating the role of biopsychosocial factors influencing a person's hip pain and disability, these findings strengthen calls to action to change the prevailing biomedical paradigm and reduce reliance on imaging as a sole explanation of a person's pain experience. They also suggest alternative evidence-based health messages when communicating with people with persistent hip pain.

- *Whether they identify new areas where research is necessary.*

  The authors acknowledge that although the current findings reinforce existing literature relating to patient beliefs, there is a need for future research that includes larger, more generalisable samples. They also suggest future research to address the question, 'What is the ideal message for patients with hip pain?'

- *Whether the researchers have discussed whether or how the findings can be transferred to other populations or considered other ways the research may be used.*

  The authors acknowledge that the insights gained from the small convenience sample are of 'limited generalisability'. They argue, however, that their 'rich description' of the demographic and clinical characteristics of this sample will assist readers in making judgments about the transferability of the study findings to their own clinical settings.

What are the main findings?

Four key themes were identified: (1) 'Lay' versus 'informed' perceptions of cause. This related to strong beliefs that hip pain was caused by largely structural and biomechanical factors, and often attributed to physical activity experienced earlier in life. Participants often experienced conflict between their own perceptions of the cause of their hip pain and explanations provided by their healthcare provider. (2) 'Fissures and tears': the use of the diagnostic jargon. This theme related to many participants who perceived that the imaging findings could explain the symptoms they were experiencing. (3) 'Fixing damage' and 'controlling symptoms' related to the optimism towards various treatments (for example, exercise, stem cell injections or surgery) that participants believed would 'fix' their condition. This also reflected the experiences of 'failed treatments' that took a psychological toll on participants. Lastly, (4) exercise, sleep and the threat to mental health reflected the perceived consequences of being unable to exercise or sleep, including worry about one's overall health, and disruption to paid work and relationships.

How might we use this evidence to inform practice?

These study findings have provided an ideal impetus for discussion at the upcoming clinic in-service you have planned. The key clinical recommendations include: (1) adoption of minimally threatening language and the provision of normative age-related data when interpreting imaging findings and an explanation that imaging findings should be considered in conjunction with clinical features; (2) patient education regarding the multidimensional complexity of musculoskeletal pain and opportunities for self-management focused on modifiable risk factors such as beliefs, physical activity, sleep and weight management; and (3) the use of alternative evidence-based health messages that aim to promote positive health behaviours for people with persistent hip pain. It is hoped that the clinical application of these findings by physiotherapists at your practice will improve the management of patients presenting with persistent hip pain.

◎ MEDICINE EXAMPLE

Clinical scenario

You work as a general practitioner (GP) in a practice with seven other GPs. You frequently see people who have depression and prescribe anti-depressants if needed. A visiting psychiatrist has been invited to a meeting being held in your practice about managing people with depression. You have a number of patients who have been on anti-depressants for a long time and you plan to raise this as a management issue at the meeting. You decide to look at the literature around long-term anti-depressant use, including patients' viewpoints.

Clinical question

What are patients' views and experiences of long-term anti-depressant use?

Search terms and databases used to find the evidence

Database: PubMed—Health Services Research Queries (with 'qualitative research category' and 'narrow scope' selected), which is accessed through https://www.nlm.nih.gov/nichsr/hedges/search.html.

Search terms: long-term AND antidepressant AND (primary care OR general practice)

Continued

◎ MEDICINE EXAMPLE—cont'd

This search strategy retrieved 28 articles. Many are about discontinuation of anti-depressants, but you select one that appears particularly relevant that provides information about patients' and GPs' perspectives on long-term use.

Article chosen

Bosman R, Huijbregts K, Verhaak P, et al. Long-term anti-depressant use: a qualitative study on perspectives of patients and GPs in primary care. Br J Gen Pract 2016;66(651): e708–e719.

Structured abstract (adapted from the above)

Study design: A 'qualitative study' using semi-structured, in-depth interviews.

Study question: To understand the motivations of patients and GPs contributing to long-term anti-depressant use and to gain insight into possibilities to prevent unnecessary long-term use.

Setting: Primary care in the Netherlands.

Participants: 38 patients (age range 30–68 years, 74% female) on anti-depressants for anxiety or depressive disorders, with 20 patient–GP dyads that could be analysed.

Data collection method: In-depth, semi-structured interviews with patients were mostly carried out in the patients' homes. Patients were never present during the GP interviews, and vice versa. A lengthy topic list used to guide the interviews is available in the article appendix. Interviews were recorded and then transcribed.

Analysis: Analysis was based on the constant comparative method, with an iterative process of data analysis and interviews. This allowed for updating the topic list to consider emerging themes. New topics were identified and predetermined topics checked so that both inductive and deductive approaches to analysis were used.

Key findings: The motives and barriers of patients and GPs to continue or discontinue anti-depressants were influenced by access to supportive guidance during discontinuation, the personal circumstances of the patient, and considerations of the patient or GP. Information suggested a large variation in policies of general practices around long-term use and continuation or discontinuation of anti-depressants. Patients and GPs seemed unaware of the mismatch between each other's expectations about who should initiate discussions about discontinuation and the amount of support needed for it.

Conclusion: Although themes about the motives and barriers to anti-depressant continuation or discontinuation were the same for patients and GPs, discrepancies between the patient and their GP were also evident. A more definite treatment plan discussed by both patient and GP may prevent unnecessary long-term use of anti-depressants.

Is the evidence rigorous and sufficiently reported?

Detailed questions from CASP

1. **Was the research design appropriate to address the aims of the research?**

   Consider:
   - *Whether the researcher has justified the research design. (For example, have they discussed how they decided which method to use?)*

     The use of qualitative research is appropriate for investigating the motivations of patients and GPs contributing to long-term anti-depressant use. However, the authors did not state clearly which qualitative research methodology (design) was used to inform the methods of the study. They did, however, note that their approach to analysis fits with an instrumental–pragmatic approach.

2. **Was the recruitment strategy appropriate to the aims of the research?**

   Consider:
   - *Whether the researcher has explained how the participants were selected.*

     A two-way snowballing recruitment approach was used, whereby either GPs were recruited and then asked to recruit patients, or patients were recruited and asked to recruit their GP. The methods for recruitment are clearly explained.
   - *Whether they explained why the participants they selected were the most appropriate to provide access to the type of knowledge sought by the study.*

     Some information is available from the study eligibility criteria.
   - *Whether there are any discussions around recruitment (for example, why some people chose not to take part).*

     Although 30 GP–patient dyads were recruited, only 20 of these could be analysed because 'either the patient or the GP did not mention the other person'. This was not discussed in more detail.

3. **Were the data collected in a way that addressed the research issue?**

Consider:

- *Whether the setting for data collection was justified.*
  The setting was not justified. Patient participants were mostly interviewed at home. Where GPs were interviewed was not stated but is likely to have been in their practice. Patients were never present during the GP interviews, and vice versa. Dyads were discussed depending on the focus of the interview and available time.
- *Whether it is clear how data were collected (for example, focus group, semi-structured interview, etc.).*
  Semi-structured interviews were used.
- *Whether the researcher has justified the methods chosen.*
  The methods chosen (semi-structured interviews) are not explicitly justified but are congruent with the aim of the study.
- *Whether the researcher has made the methods explicit. (For example, for interview method, is there an indication of how interviews were conducted, or did they use a topic guide?)*
  The interviews used a topic guide (which is provided) and the authors explain how it was generated.
- *Whether methods were modified during the study. If so, has the researcher explained how and why?*
  The methods do not appear to have changed during the study.
- *Whether the form of data is clear (for example, tape-recordings, video material, notes, etc.).*
  It is stated that interviews were recorded and then transcribed.
- *Whether the researcher has discussed saturation of data.*
  The authors state: 'Data collection ended when data were saturated; that is, the information was repeating itself and no new information was added based on four new interviews.'

4. **Has the relationship between researcher and participants been adequately considered?**

Consider:

- *Whether the researcher critically examined their own role, potential bias and influence during:*
  - *Formulation of the research questions.*
    There is no comment about this in the article.

- *Data collection, including sample recruitment and choice of location.*
  Four master students unrelated to the participants conducted the interviews. Authors do not consider their role or potential for bias or influence.
- *How the researcher responded to events during the study and whether they considered the implications of any changes in the research design.*
  The methods do not appear to have changed during the study.

5. **Have ethical issues been taken into consideration?**

Consider:

- *Whether there are sufficient details of how the research was explained to participants for the reader to assess whether ethical standards were maintained.*
  Details of how the research was explained to participants are not clear. The authors simply state: 'The research team contacted interested patients and GPs, and provided them with additional information.'
  It is not clear if/how ethical standards were maintained.
- *Whether the researcher has discussed issues raised by the study (for example, issues around informed consent or confidentiality or how they have handled the effects of the study on the participants during and after the study).*
  The authors do not discuss issues raised by the study.
- *Whether approval has been sought from the ethics committee.*
  The study was approved by a university ethics committee.

6. **Was the data analysis sufficiently rigorous?**

Consider:

- *Whether there is an in-depth description of the analysis process. Whether thematic analysis is used. If so, is it clear how the categories/themes were derived from the data?*
  Analysis is clearly described. It was based on the constant comparative method, allowing the topic list to be updated in the light of emerging themes. The authors state that this fits with an instrumental–pragmatic approach. The authors describe how themes were derived: 'Two interviewers coded the first two interviews independently, codes were then compared, and consensus was reached about an initial framework. Analysis was continued

Continued

by updating the coding framework after every two interviews and at research group meetings.' To analyse dyads, interview parts in which the patient spoke about their GP and vice versa were coded separately.

- *Whether the researcher explains how the data presented were selected from the original sample, to demonstrate the analysis process.*
  This is not clearly explained.
- *Whether sufficient data are presented to support the findings. To what extent contradictory data are taken into account.*
  Sufficient data are presented, and both positive and negative perspectives are reported.
- *Whether the researcher critically examined their own role, potential bias and influence during analysis and selection of data for presentation.*
  The researcher did not critically examine their own role or potential biases and influence during analysis and selection of data.

7. **Is there a clear statement of findings?**
   Consider:
   - *Whether the findings are explicit. Whether there is adequate discussion of the evidence both for and against the researcher's arguments.*
     The authors presented a balanced discussion of the issues derived from participants' statements, reflecting their positive and negative perceptions.
   - *Whether the researcher has discussed the credibility of their findings (for example, triangulation, respondent validation, more than one analyst).*
     The data were provided by both GPs and patients, and more than one analyst was involved in data analysis. No respondent validation was used.
   - *Whether the findings are discussed in relation to the original research question.*
     The findings are clearly discussed in relation to the original objective.

8. **How valuable is the research?**
   Consider:
   - *Whether the researcher discusses the contribution the study makes to existing knowledge or understanding. (For example, do they consider the findings in relation to current practice or policy, or relevant research-based literature?)*
     The authors discuss whether 'a more definite treatment plan discussed by both patient and GP may prevent unnecessary long-term use. This long-term plan should include agreements about who

initiates future contact, and the frequency and method of this contact.'

- *Whether they identify new areas where research is necessary.*
  The authors indicate that further research is needed to determine how widespread the expressed opinions are. They also note the need for evidence regarding relapse risk for individual patients.
- *Whether the researchers have discussed whether or how the findings can be transferred to other populations or considered other ways the research may be used.*
  No statements are made about transferability of findings, but practical recommendations are made as to how the results might be used. For example, the authors recommend that GPs and patients discuss a more definite treatment plan to prevent unnecessary long-term use of anti-depressants, including who initiates future contact, and the frequency and method of this contact.

What are the main findings?

The reasons that patients wanted to discontinue anti-depressants included the possibility of physical dependency, a negative perception of anti-depressants and concerns about side effects. Patients did not necessarily agree that GPs were suitable to provide supportive guidance during discontinuation. For example, patients thought GPs did not have enough time or sufficient knowledge about discontinuation. Patients wanted to receive more support (such as 1 hour per week) than what GPs thought was needed (such as 10–20 minutes per week or fortnight). Information from dyads suggested a large variation in long-term use or discontinuation policies and practices of different GPs. There were also differences between patients and GPs about who should be initiating discussions about discontinuation.

How might we use this evidence to inform practice?

This study provides some useful information for your general practice to consider which you plan to raise at the next practice meeting. First, your practice could consider a standard approach to consultations involving the prescription of anti-depressants whereby a treatment plan is formulated between the GP and the patient regarding who initiates future contact, and the frequency and method of this contact. A practice nurse could possibly have a role in monitoring patients using anti-depressants, and reminders provided via the practice prescription system to bring repeat prescriptions to the GP's attention.

◎ NURSING EXAMPLE

Clinical scenario

You are an experienced paediatric nurse who after 20 years of work in an acute hospital is about to take up a new role in a paediatric hospice. The hospice provides palliative care for children with life-limiting conditions, with a focus on enhancement of quality of life for the children and their families. In preparation for your new role, you want to understand strategies that can enhance end-of-life care and how you can sensitively offer these to families. A colleague who has suffered the loss of a child tells you how valuable legacy or memory making was for them.

Clinical question

How do parents of children who are in palliative care experience memory making?

Search terms and databases used to find the evidence

Database: PubMed—Advanced search.
Search terms: parent AND experience AND child AND palliat* AND memory
Search results: The search yielded a total of 11 studies, only two of which closely matched the question. The remainder addressed: other populations (mothers only); in settings other than palliative care; with varied interventions (birth planning, bereavement support, funeral services); and other outcomes such as death from cancer. The selected study was primary research, recently published and conducted in Ireland, a country where healthcare systems and the provision of hospice care is similar to the setting where the findings might be applied.

Article chosen

Clarke T, Connolly M. Parent's lived experience of memory making with their child at or near end of life. Am J Hosp Palliat Care 2022 Jul;39(7):798–805. doi: 10.1177/10499091211047838. Epub 2021 Sept 16.

Structured abstract (adapted from the above)

Study design: Qualitative study with individual interviews.
Study question: To explore the lived experience a memory-making process had on parents of children who were at or near end of life.
Context: Parents whose child had received care from a children's hospice in Ireland.
Participants: Six parents (all mothers) whose child had died and who had engaged in memory making.
Data collection method: Sampling was purposive and potential participants were identified from a bereavement database of the hospice. A gatekeeper sent the invitations to participate and parents whose child had died in the last 12 months were not contacted. The interview questions were based on topics of relevance to the study aim. Interviews were conducted in a quiet, private environment and participants were given a choice of location for the interview. Data was audio-recorded using a digital recorder. Reflective journal notes were made after each interview and field notes were taken during the interviews.

Analysis: Verbatim transcripts were thematically analysed using a phenomenological approach (Van Manen's three stages). Transcripts were read while listening to the recordings. Reflective journal notes and field notes were included in the analysis.

Key findings: Three main themes emerged from the data: (1) *making the memories*; (2) *the impact now of memory making*; and (3) *the end-of-life care journey*. The findings provide insight into this activity in children's palliative care and the benefits to and satisfaction of parents during a time of great distress for families.

Is this evidence rigorous and sufficiently reported?

Detailed questions from CASP

1. **Was the research design appropriate to address the aims of the research?**
   Consider:
   - *Whether the researcher has justified the research design.*
     A hermeneutic phenomenological design was justified on the basis that it provides a philosophical and methodological approach that can be applied to a broad range of clinical research investigations in nursing.

2. **Was the recruitment strategy appropriate to the aims of the research?**
   Consider:
   - *If the researcher has explained how the participants were selected.*
     The article provides a clear description of the purposive sampling strategy used to select participants.
   - *If they explained why the participants they selected were the most appropriate to provide access to the type of knowledge sought by the study.*
     The participants selected appear to be appropriate to meet the study's aims, although this was not explicitly justified. To obtain a purposive sample, the bereavement database of the hospice was used to identify individuals suitable to recruit as

Continued

◎ NURSING EXAMPLE—cont'd

participants. Participants were parents of children who had been cared for in the hospice and who had participated in memory making at or near the child's death.

- *If there are any discussions around recruitment (for example, why some people chose not to take part).*
  Based on permission from the ethics committee, parents whose child had died in the last 12 months were not contacted. There is no information provided regarding the number of invitations that were issued; only that six bereaved parents responded to the invitation. Although mothers and fathers were invited to take part, only mothers took part in the interviews.

3. **Was the data collected in a way that addressed the research issue?**
   Consider:
   - *Whether the setting for data collection was justified.*
     The interviews were conducted in a quiet, private environment without interruption. This was justified as enabling participants to talk freely about their very personal experiences regarding the death of their child and the subsequent memory-making process. Although participants were given a choice of location, only one participant chose to have the interview conducted at the hospice. No reason is provided for this decision. The remaining participants chose to be interviewed in their own homes.
   - *Whether it is clear how data were collected (for example, focus group, semi-structured interview etc.).*
     The collection of data by individual interview has been made explicit. The interview schedule has been provided and suggests that these were semi-structured interviews.
   - *Whether the researcher has justified the methods chosen.*
     No specific justification has been given for individual interviews as a data collection method. However, this appears to be appropriate given the sensitive nature of the topic.
   - *Whether the researcher has made the methods explicit. (For example, for interview method is there an indication of how interviews were conducted, or did they use a topic guide?)*
     The interview schedule was used to facilitate an exploration of the topics of relevance and includes questions relating to experiences, feelings, participation

by family members, support and suggestions for development of the service.

- *Whether methods were modified during the study. If so, has the researcher explained why?*
  There is no indication that the methods were altered during this study.
- *Whether the form of the data is clear (for example, tape-recordings, video material, notes, etc.).*
  The researchers have indicated that interviews were audio-recorded using a digital recorder and transcribed prior to analysis.
- *Whether the researcher has discussed saturation of the data.*
  The researchers have not discussed data saturation, and as there is no indication that the number of participants was open-ended it is unlikely that data saturation informed sampling.

4. **Has the relationship between research and participants been adequately considered?**
   Consider:
   - *Whether the researcher critically examined their own role, potential bias and influence during:*
     - *Formulation of the research questions.*
       The authors'/researchers' affiliations and qualifications suggest that they may have some deeper experience or engagement in palliative care and nursing; however, this has not been acknowledged in the formulation of research questions.
     - *Data collection, including sample recruitment and choice of location.*
       The authors'/researchers' affiliations suggest that they may have some connection with the hospice, as all are in Dublin. The 'principal researcher' (although not specified) knew all the participants in a professional capacity and was involved in their care either during end of life, memory making, or the post-bereavement visit to bring the finished memory-making creations to the family. The authors acknowledge the potential influence of this lack of independence on participants' decisions to participate, the interview process and findings. They counter that the previous relationship may have enabled the participants to be comfortable, open and honest in recounting their experiences. The researchers do not specifically identify who conducted the interviews; they simply refer to 'the interviewer'.

- *How the researcher responded to events during the study and whether they considered the implications of any changes in the research design.*

  There were no events reported during the study that would have implications for changes in the research design.

5. **Have ethical issues been taken into consideration?**

  Consider:

  - *Whether there are sufficient details of how the research was explained to participants for the reader to assess whether ethical standards were maintained.*

    The researchers have provided details regarding ethical permission to conduct the study. The authors report that the interviewer gave opportunity for each participant to seek clarification before commencing the interview and any questions or concerns were addressed.

  - *Whether the researcher has discussed issues raised by the study (for example, issues around informed consent or confidentiality, or how they handled the effects of the study on participants during and after the study).*

    Participants gave written consent to participate. Although confidentiality was not explicitly mentioned, it would likely have been attended to as part of ethical clearance requirements. It is reasonable to expect that this type of study may impact participants who are mothers whose children have died and may be potentially vulnerable. Although this has been acknowledged tangentially through the exclusion of parents whose child had died in the last 12 months, it is unclear how the researchers may have handled these effects.

  - *Whether approval has been sought from the ethics committee.*

    The researchers have reported ethical approval from the hospice ethics committees, and that an exemption was granted by another university school committee.

6. **Was the data analysis sufficiently rigorous?**

  Consider:

  - *Whether there is an in-depth description of the analysis process. Whether thematic analysis is used. If so, is it clear how the categories/themes were derived from the data?*

    The thematic analysis was undertaken following Van Manen's approach in three analytic steps: (1) turning to a phenomenon of interest; (2) conducting an investigation of the phenomenon; and (3) reflecting on the essential themes. Each step was described, and its interpretation outlined. The process of analysis was further described as a selective data analysis technique in which verbatim transcripts were read several times, while listening to the recording of the interviews, as well as consideration of reflective journal notes and field notes. Although categories included within each theme are presented in Table 4 of the article, it is unclear how the categories were selected from the data.

  - *Whether the researcher explains how the data presented were selected from the original sample, to demonstrate the analysis process.*

    There is no detail reported on how data were selected for presentation.

  - *Whether sufficient data are presented to support the findings. To what extent contradictory data are taken into account.*

    For each of the organising themes, there are several rich quotes used to support and illustrate, and these seem to follow the identified categories in each theme. There was no contradictory data presented, although it is foreseeable that there was limited variation in the data within the small sample size ($n = 6$).

  - *Whether the researcher critically examined their own role, potential bias and influence during analysis and selection of data for presentation.*

    There has been no critical examination of the role of the researchers with respect to influence on the analysis and presentation of data.

7. **Is there a clear statement of findings?**

  Consider:

  - *Whether the findings are explicit. Whether there is adequate discussion of the evidence both for and against the researcher's arguments.*

    The discussion reflects on the findings in relation to the literature on memory making and the value it holds for parents. There is one section of the discussion that refers to the skill, sensitivity and timing of the professional conducting the memory-making activities which is not strongly represented as a category or theme or in quotes and is not supported with existing literature.

Continued

⊚ NURSING EXAMPLE—cont'd

- *Whether the researcher has discussed the credibility of their findings (for example, triangulation, respondent validation, more than one analysis).*

   All verbatim transcripts of interviews were checked for accuracy by both researchers. Although the authors indicate '**we** (emphasis added) aimed to capture the meaning ...', it is unclear whether the two researchers conducted the analysis and if, or how, consensus was reached. There was no mention of the participants being shown the transcripts, or that clarification was sought from participants as to the intention of their statements. One could suppose that inclusion of the reflective journal of notes after each interview and of the field notes from each interview was a means of strengthening the credibility of their findings.

- *Whether the findings are discussed in relation to the original research question.*

   The researchers set out to explore the lived experiences of parents who had engaged in a memory-making process at or near the point of their child's death. To that extent, they have provided a rich and well-structured description of those experiences.

8. How valuable is the research?

Consider:

- *Whether the researcher discusses the contribution the study makes to existing knowledge or understanding. (For example, do they consider the findings in relation to current practice or policy, or relevant research-based literature?)*

   This study contributes to knowledge about parental experiences of memory making. Although this is largely a descriptive study, it does illustrate that the experiences of parents are consistent with the purpose of memory making. In their conclusion, the authors indicate that this research highlighted the skills required to provide this service in a compassionate and sensitive manner.

- *Whether they identify new areas where research is necessary.*

   The researchers identify that more research is required to enhance and confirm the importance of memory-making activity as an essential component in children's palliative care and that further investigation will lead to improvements in the service provided and outcomes.

- *Whether the researchers have discussed whether or how the finding can be transferred to other populations or considered other ways the research can be used.*

   The researchers acknowledge the limitations of the small sample and single-site recruitment—which is perhaps less pertinent than that of data saturation. The findings are similar to those undertaken in other geographic locations, suggesting some transferability between settings and populations.

What are the main findings?

Mothers identified the benefits of and satisfaction with the provision of a memory-making service in a children's hospice. Three main themes emerged: (1) *making the memories*, which relates to all participants wanting to make the most of precious time and create cherished memories and keepsakes; (2) *the impact of memory making*, which relates to how parents were underprepared for the overwhelming experience of receiving the creations but also overjoyed; and (3) *the end-of-life care journey*, which relates to the importance of being able to choose the location for end-of-life care where possible.

How might we use this evidence to inform practice?

This research highlighted the value of memory making to bereaved parents. Palliative care discussions with parents and families should include information about memory making, and perceptions of parents in this research might be communicated in these discussions. You hope to be able to offer this experience to families in your new role within a paediatric hospice and decide to read other research in this area in preparation.

⊚ SPEECH PATHOLOGY EXAMPLE

Clinical scenario

You are part of a multidisciplinary in-patient rehabilitation team providing speech pathology services to people with dysphagia (swallowing disorders). Part of your role is to provide education to caregivers about the transition home and what to expect regarding any adjustments that might need to be made for patients with dysphagia. You want to provide caregivers with real-life examples, so you decide to look for research published in this area to inform your discussions.

Clinical question

What are the experiences of caregivers of people with dysphagia living at home?

Search terms and databases used to find the evidence

Database: PubMed—Health Services Research Queries (with 'qualitative research category' and 'narrow scope' selected), which is accessed through https://www.nlm.nih.gov/nichsr/hedges/search.html.

Search terms: dysphagia AND caregivers AND community
The search retrieves eight articles. The first study matches your research question and focuses on the lived experiences of caregivers supporting people with dysphagia living at home in Queensland, Australia.

Article chosen

Howells SR, Cornwell PL, Ward EC, et al. Living with dysphagia in the community: caregivers 'do whatever it takes'. Dysphagia 2021. doi: 10.1007/s00455-020-10117-y.

Structured abstract (adapted from the above)

Study design: Qualitative descriptive study grounded in phenomenology.
Study question: To understand the experience of supporting a person with dysphagia of various aetiologies living in the community from the caregiver perspective.
Setting: Community within Queensland, Australia.
Participants: 15 caregivers (mean age 72.8 years, 13 female) of 14 unique people with dysphagia. Caregivers were either a partner, child or friend living with a person with dysphagia.
Data collection method: Convenience sampling was used to recruit participants caring for an adult with dysphagia from a government health service, speech-language pathology private practice clinics and media coverage. Individual, face-to-face semi-structured interviews were conducted by one researcher in the participant's home. Topics included caregiver perspectives on supporting someone with dysphagia at home, how they had adjusted and perceived barriers, and enablers and key issues in supporting a person with dysphagia at home. All interviews were audio-recorded, and the primary researcher kept a reflective journal.
Analysis: Data were analysed using thematic analysis. Two transcripts were independently coded using an inductive, semantic approach to generate a code list which was then refined and applied to all transcripts. Codes were collapsed into themes, sub-themes and categories. Respondent validation was requested on the main findings of the study and eight participants confirmed the authors' interpretation of their experiences.

Key findings: The overarching theme of 'You do whatever it takes' reflected the experience of supporting a family member or friend with dysphagia at home. This theme was underpinned by three sub-themes where caregivers described *being a caregiver, support networks* and *practicalities of living with dysphagia*. In order to live successfully with dysphagia, caregivers provided practical and emotional support to people with dysphagia.

Conclusion: The authors concluded that through understanding the caregiver perspective, health professionals will be better placed to involve and support caregivers in their role of caring for those living with dysphagia in the community.

Is the evidence rigorous and sufficiently reported?

Detailed questions from CASP

1. **Was the research design appropriate to address the aims of the research?**
   Consider:
   - *Whether the researcher has justified the research design. (For example, have they discussed how they decided which method to use?)*
     The study design used a qualitative descriptive approach grounded in phenomenology. Although this approach was not explicitly justified, it is considered appropriate to understand the caregiver experience of supporting a person with dysphagia living in the community.

2. **Was the recruitment strategy appropriate to the aims of the research?**
   Consider:
   - *Whether the researcher has explained how the participants were selected.*
     The authors provide a clear description of the convenience sampling strategy used to select participants. However, it is unclear whether participants were recruited from one or multiple health services.
   - *Whether they explained why the participants they selected were the most appropriate to provide access to the type of knowledge sought by the study.*
     The eligibility criteria appear to be appropriate to meet the study's aims, although this was not explicitly justified. It is also unclear how a 'known diagnosis' of dysphagia was confirmed, particularly for participants recruited through media coverage.

Continued

⊚ SPEECH PATHOLOGY EXAMPLE—cont'd

This potentially raises uncertainty regarding the appropriateness of the study participants. However, the diet and fluid recommendations presented in Table 1 in the article support the diagnosis of dysphagia.

- *Whether there are any discussions around recruitment (for example, why some people chose not to take part).*

  There is no discussion in the article regarding the number of eligible participants who were invited to participate in the study or reasons why some people chose not to take part.

3. **Were the data collected in a way that addressed the research issue?**

  Consider:

  - *Whether the setting for data collection was justified.*
    Participants were interviewed in their home. This appears to be appropriate but is not explicitly justified by the authors.
  - *Whether it is clear how data were collected (for example, focus group, semi-structured interview, etc.).*
    The collection of data by individual, face-to-face semi-structured interviews has been made explicit.
  - *Whether the researcher has justified the methods chosen.*
    No specific justification has been provided for individual, semi-structured interviews as a data collection method, although this appears to be appropriate.
  - *Whether the researcher has made the methods explicit. (For example, for interview method, is there an indication of how interviews were conducted, or did they use a topic guide?)*
    The interview topic guide was provided in an appendix and gives a clear indication of how the interviews were conducted.
  - *Whether methods were modified during the study. If so, has the researcher explained how and why?*
    The methods do not appear to have been modified during the study; however, questions were adapted or not asked depending on the issues raised by each participant 'to maintain conversational flow during the interview'.
  - *Whether the form of data is clear (for example, tape-recordings, video material, notes, etc.).*
    The authors have indicated that interviews were audio-recorded and transcribed verbatim for analysis. The primary researcher also kept a reflective journal and completed an entry after each interview.

- *Whether the researcher has discussed saturation of data.*

  The authors indicate that a reflective journal assisted in identifying when data saturation was considered to have been reached and that this was determined to occur in the last three to four interviews, when no new information was generated. However, it is unclear how new data were incorporated within the code list, which was initially developed after coding two transcripts, and there is no mention that data collection and analysis occurred iteratively.

4. **Has the relationship between researcher and participants been adequately considered?**

  Consider:

  - *Whether the researcher critically examined their own role, potential bias and influence during:*
    - *Formulation of the research questions.*
      The authors' affiliations and qualifications suggest they may have some experience in speech pathology; however, this has not been acknowledged in the formulation of the research questions.
    - *Data collection, including sample recruitment and choice of location.*
      There does not appear to be a pre-existing relationship between the primary researcher and the participants since eligible participants were identified by their healthcare provider and invitations were then forwarded to the primary researcher.
  - *How the researcher responded to events during the study and whether they considered the implications of any changes in the research design.*
    There were no events reported during the study that would have implications for changes in the research design.

5. **Have ethical issues been taken into consideration?**
  Consider:

  - *Whether there are sufficient details of how the research was explained to participants for the reader to assess whether ethical standards were maintained.*
    There is no explicit explanation of how the details of the research were explained to participants. However, the authors have provided details regarding ethical approval to conduct the study and indicate that all participants provided written informed consent.
  - *Whether the researcher has discussed issues raised by the study (for example, issues around informed consent or confidentiality or how they have handled*

the effects of the study on the participants during and after the study).

The authors indicate that all participants provided written informed consent. Participants were de-identified in the reporting of results. The authors did not report if any issues arose as a result of this study or how such issues may have been handled.

- *Whether approval has been sought from the ethics committee.*

The authors explicitly state that ethical approval was granted through the relevant health service and university human research ethics committees.

6. **Was the data analysis sufficiently rigorous?**

Consider:

- *Whether there is an in-depth description of the analysis process. Whether thematic analysis is used. If so, is it clear how the categories/themes were derived from the data?*

There is a clear description of the analysis process. Thematic analysis, as described by Braun and Clarke, was utilised. Two authors independently coded the first two transcripts. This was followed by a meeting to discuss the coding and generate a final list of codes. The remaining transcripts were then coded using this list. Codes were then collapsed into themes, sub-themes and categories. The themes, sub-themes and categories appear to be coherent, and quotes are provided to support each category.

- *Whether the researcher explains how the data presented were selected from the original sample, to demonstrate the analysis process.*

The authors indicate that quotes by participants that resonated with the overarching themes were noted and attributed to the participant's identifier. However, there is no detail reported about how the quotes presented were selected.

- *Whether sufficient data are presented to support the findings. To what extent are contradictory data taken into account?*

Sufficient data in the form of several rich participant quotes are used to support the findings, and contradictory viewpoints are presented.

- *Whether the researcher critically examined their own role, potential bias and influence during analysis and selection of data for presentation.*

A critical examination of the author's role, potential bias and influence is not reported.

7. **Is there a clear statement of findings?**

Consider:

- *Whether the findings are explicit. Whether there is adequate discussion of the evidence both for and against the researcher's arguments.*

A balanced discussion regarding the role of the caregiver in supporting people with dysphagia is presented. Differing viewpoints are highlighted by the authors.

- *Whether the researcher has discussed the credibility of their findings (for example, triangulation, respondent validation, more than one analyst).*

Credibility of findings is evident. Participants were given an opportunity to validate the author's interpretation, and eight out of 15 participants confirmed the findings. A reflective journal was kept 'to encourage transparency in the research process'. Although the authors state that two researchers completed the initial coding independently, coded two transcripts to ensure consistency in coding and a meeting was held to generate a final list of codes, it is unclear if the themes, sub-themes and categories were discussed, challenged and accepted by the wider research team.

- *Whether the findings are discussed in relation to the original research question.*

The findings are clearly presented in relation to the original research question and provide a rich description of the experience of supporting a person with dysphagia in the community from a caregiver perspective.

8. **How valuable is the research?**

Consider:

- *Whether the researcher discusses the contribution the study makes to existing knowledge or understanding. (For example, do they consider the findings in relation to current practice or policy, or relevant research-based literature?)*

Findings are presented and discussed in relation to the current research literature. Clinical implications of the findings are clearly presented. The authors argue that speech-language pathologists must incorporate caregivers as a direct recipient of dysphagia services and ensure that practices cater for the practical and psychosocial needs of supporting a person with dysphagia at home.

Continued

◎ SPEECH PATHOLOGY EXAMPLE—cont'd

- *Whether they identify new areas where research is necessary.*

  Limited discussion on further research is presented, although the authors state that future research should seek greater participant diversity and consider engaging with caregivers about their experiences at multiple time points to better understand the process of adjustment to supporting an individual with dysphagia.

- *Whether the researchers have discussed whether or how the findings can be transferred to other populations or considered other ways the research may be used.*

  The authors acknowledge 'the viewpoints of caregivers in the study may not reflect experiences of caregivers supporting those with more severe dysphagia'. However, they hypothesise that the issues described would be exacerbated for caregivers supporting people with more severe dysphagia. The authors also acknowledge that caregiver experiences from a range of demographics are difficult to infer due to the homogenous demographics of the caregivers recruited (predominantly female, over 65 years old and retired). The research aim was to understand the experience of supporting a person with dysphagia of varying aetiologies, including neurological conditions of stroke and Parkinson's disease, but the authors do not acknowledge that only three out of 14 individuals with dysphagia had a dysphagia aetiology other than Parkinson's disease or stroke.

What are the main findings?

This study revealed an overarching theme of 'You do whatever it takes', describing the caregiver experience of supporting a family member or friend with dysphagia at home. This was underpinned by three sub-themes,

where caregivers described: (1) being a caregiver, which was reflected across the complexity of caring, caregiver capacity and capability, the person with the health condition, and caregiver response to dysphagia and caring; (2) support networks, which reflected receiving support from family and friends and the potential value of speech language pathology input; and (3) practicalities of living with dysphagia, which reflected a range of practical strategies utilised during mealtimes and challenges to going out.

Caregivers described taking on new roles and making adaptations to ensure that people with dysphagia receive adequate support and care. Dysphagia was considered in the context of the overarching health condition, as managing other issues associated with the health condition may be a higher priority for caregivers. While caregivers felt capable to manage dysphagia, support from speech language pathologists was valuable in terms of the education and practical strategies provided.

How might we use this evidence to inform practice?

Through understanding the caregiver experience, you feel better prepared to involve and support caregivers who are supporting a person with dysphagia at home. In your discussion with caregivers of people with dysphagia, you will need to consider dysphagia in relation to the health condition of each patient and the priorities of the patient and their caregiver. You will need to discuss the medical complications associated with dysphagia, as well as the psychosocial impacts and practical strategies that can be used to mediate those impacts on both the patient and the caregiver. Strategies suggested by caregivers in the article could be used as a starting point to facilitate a discussion on supporting dysphagia in the home. It will be important to provide caregivers information on where they can receive support at a later time if dysphagia management is not currently a priority.

◎ HUMAN MOVEMENT STUDIES EXAMPLE

Clinical scenario

You are an exercise physiologist who owns and runs a successful private exercise physiology clinic offering a range of services, including group exercise sessions in your gym. One of your new clients is the owner of a small business who runs regular mothers' groups for local

women. She tells you that the mothers in her groups are always struggling to get back into exercise and physical activity after birth. You mention that group exercise classes are often a good way to begin. After chatting for a while, you both realise that there are no suitable postnatal exercise groups in the area, and you feel there may be an opportunity to partner to provide classes for these women. While you are experienced at providing exercise classes, you know that there are significant challenges to exercise participation in postpartum women. You wonder if there are specific ways to design your new program to ensure it best meets their needs and has the best chance of success.

Clinical question
What are the perceptions about characteristics of effective group-based exercise programs for postnatal women?

Search terms and databases used to find the evidence
Database: PubMed—Health Services Research Queries (with 'qualitative research category' and 'narrow scope' selected), which is accessed through https://www.nlm.nih.gov/nichsr/hedges/search.html.
Search terms: postpartum AND (group physical activity program)

This search retrieved 27 results. By reading the titles and abstracts, it could be seen that several focused on general barriers and enablers to physical activity postpartum, while others considered influences on postpartum physical activity for specific diseases or conditions (gestational diabetes, obesity, depression). Several others provided interventions/programs to increase physical activity which were not group based. Two appeared useful but had more focus on characteristics of health promotion/public health programs. One remaining study focused on perceptions of the characteristics of key stakeholders and community organisations that support women to sustain their engagement with physical activity programs after birth in the Australian context, and you retrieve the full text of this one.

Article chosen
Peralta LR, Yager Z, Prichard I. Practice-based evidence: perspectives of effective characteristics of Australian group-based physical activity programs for postpartum women. Health Prom J of Austr 2021; Nov 28. doi: 10.1002/hpja.561.

Structured abstract (adapted from the above)
Study design: A constructivist qualitative research study using semi-structured interviews.
Study question: To explore perceptions about the design and delivery of group-based community physical activity (PA) programs for women after pregnancy, including effective characteristics and contextual barriers.

Setting: The surrounding regions of Sydney (including Newcastle and Wollongong) and Wagga Wagga, Australia.
Participants: Ten participants (mean age 39 years, nine females, eight small business owners, nine different organisations) who were locally designing and implementing group-based community PA programs for postpartum women. They were identified to take part by using recommendations from physically active women in a previous study conducted by the authors, and via professional networks.
Data collection method: The lead researcher collected all data using virtual (Zoom®) ($n = 8$) and face-to-face ($n = 2$) semi-structured interviews. The interview guide was based on literature, the PRACTIS framework for informing program implementation and scale-up of PA programs, and expertise within the research team. Questions were applied consistently across all interviews using a flexible approach to probe and lasted on average 31 minutes. Data collection ceased after one round of recruitment as key themes were repeated and no new information emerged (data saturation).
Analysis: Interviews were recorded, transcribed verbatim and checked for accuracy. Thematic analysis was undertaken inductively by two researchers on a sample of transcripts ($n = 3$) to generate a coding framework. This was then used by one researcher to inductively code all other transcripts. Some deductive codes were also applied from existing literature and theory. Codes were grouped into themes, which were discussed by all researchers.
Key findings: Four main themes and 12 sub-themes emerged for the design and implementation of community-based group PA programs for postpartum women. The main themes were: (1) effective practitioners have a history of, and passion for women's health and PA; (2) low-cost, connected approaches attract women into community group-based PA programs; (3) inclusive, flexible, varied and holistic approaches sustain participation; (4) connections should be utilised to overcome barriers to community group-based PA programs.
Conclusion: The authors concluded that practice-based evidence from existing programs should be used to inform the development and implementation of future group PA programs in the community. Specifically, new programs should be designed and implemented by providers with a history and passion for women's health/PA, be low in cost, and use connected approaches that are inclusive, flexible, varied and holistic that prioritise physical, emotional and social wellbeing.

Continued

◎ HUMAN MOVEMENT STUDIES EXAMPLE—cont'd

Is the evidence rigorous and sufficiently reported?
Detailed questions from CASP

1. **Was the research design appropriate to address the aims of the research?**

   Consider:

   • *Whether the researcher has justified the research design (that is, type of qualitative research). (For example, have they discussed how they decided which method to use?)*

   The researchers reported using a qualitative research design, taking a constructivist philosophical view, but did not state the specific qualitative research methodology they employed. They clearly justified their choice of a constructivist approach as being able to explore 'stakeholder perspectives of the development of social processes and the interpretation of the social world that they have created for postpartum women'.

2. **Was the recruitment strategy appropriate to the aims of the research?**

   Consider:

   • *Whether the researcher has explained how the participants were selected.*

   The authors provide a clear description of the purposive sampling strategy used to select participants. They asked postpartum women from another study to recommend stakeholders involved in the design and implementation of group-based PA programs who they had utilised to be active in the early postpartum period. They also recruited some participants via their own professional networks.

   • *Whether they explained why the participants they selected were the most appropriate to provide access to the type of knowledge sought by the study.*

   The researchers were interested in understanding the design and delivery of group-based community PA programs for postpartum women, so they sought to select stakeholders who had direct experience in this field. It is clear that those selected were appropriate for providing knowledge for the study.

   • *Whether there are any discussions around recruitment (for example, why some people chose not to take part).*

   There is no information provided regarding the number of invitations for recruitment that were issued and how many chose not to participate; only that

   seven participants were identified through postpartum women from another research study and that three participants were identified through the first author's professional networks.

3. **Were the data collected in a way that addressed the research issue?**

   Consider:

   • *Whether the setting for data collection was justified.*

   Eight interviews were conducted via videoconference, which was justified given COVID-19 restrictions at the time and because videoconference was considered less burdensome for participants who may have found it hard to find the time to travel to a face-to-face interview. Two face-to-face interviews were conducted in a convenient location for both parties; however, the reasoning behind the face-to-face interviews is unclear.

   • *Whether it is clear how data were collected (for example, focus group, semi-structured interview, etc.).*

   The collection of data by individual semi-structured interviews is clear.

   • *Whether the researcher has justified the methods chosen.*

   The authors clearly justify their chosen methods, interview guide and underlying framework. The authors justify the use of semi-structured interviews to provide a detailed and wide-reaching examination of the physical, mental and social aspects of the design and implementation of their community group-based PA programs during the postpartum period.

   • *Whether the researcher has made the methods explicit. (For example, for interview method, is there an indication of how interviews were conducted, or did they use a topic guide?)*

   The interview guide is provided along with the related PRACTIS contructs on which each question is based.

   • *Whether methods were modified during the study. If so, has the researcher explained how and why?*

   There is no indication that methods were modified during the study. However, the authors state that questions were applied consistently across all interviews and that the interviewer took a flexible and responsive approach to probe and explore 'in order to enhance the authenticity of each participant's response'.

- *Whether the form of data is clear (for example, tape-recordings, video material, notes, etc.).*

  The authors clearly state that interviews were recorded and transcribed verbatim by an online transcription service.

- *Whether the researcher has discussed saturation of data.*

  The authors clearly discuss how saturation was considered and applied to data collection/recruitment. They outline that data saturation was gauged by 'a comprehensive coverage of issues, repeated references to key themes, and an absence of new perspectives', and that saturation was reached with the first round of invited participants.

4. **Has the relationship between researcher and participants been adequately considered?**

   Consider:

   - *Whether the researcher critically examined their own role, potential bias and influence during:*

     - *Formulation of the research questions.*

       The lead author conceptualised the study after experiencing the benefits of participation in a community group-based PA program for postpartum women.

     - *Data collection, including sample recruitment and choice of location.*

       The researchers clearly outlined how their own demographics (as women with children) and experiences may have impacted on the study. While this may have introduced some bias, they also felt it gave them greater connection with the study participants. The authors provide examples of how they tried to account for any biases, such as checking with the literature and researchers with other experiences, and reflecting on potential biases and interpretations during the data analysis process.

   - *How the researcher responded to events during the study and whether they considered the implications of any changes in the research design.*

     There were no events reported during the study that would have implications for changes in the research design.

5. **Have ethical issues been taken into consideration?**

   Consider:

   - *Whether there are sufficient details of how the research was explained to participants for the reader to assess whether ethical standards were maintained.*

     The researchers have outlined that participants were emailed a description of the research project prior to consenting.

   - *Whether the researcher has discussed issues raised by the study (for example, issues around informed consent or confidentiality or how they have handled the effects of the study on the participants during and after the study).*

     Informed consent was obtained in writing before the interview and confirmed again verbally at the start of each interview. Quotes from participants were de-identified in the manuscript. Although the topic is not expected to be sensitive, the authors did not report if any issues arose as a result of participating in this study.

   - *Whether approval has been sought from the ethics committee.*

     Approval from the institutional research ethics committee was obtained.

6. **Was the data analysis sufficiently rigorous?**

   Consider:

   - *Whether there is an in-depth description of the analysis process. Whether thematic analysis is used. If so, is it clear how the categories/themes were derived from the data?*

     A detailed description of the analysis process is provided. The authors employed thematic analysis in six stages. Two researchers individually coded the transcripts of three interviews inductively, then compared these and jointly agreed on a coding framework. A single researcher then immersed themselves in the remaining transcripts and coded these using both inductive and deductive approaches. Multi-coding of the same text was allowed. All researchers then mapped codes together to identify higher level themes that emerged from the interview data. The relationship between the codes, sub-themes and themes are clearly displayed in Table 3 of the article.

   - *Whether the researcher explains how the data presented were selected from the original sample, to demonstrate the analysis process.*

     Examples of quotes from participants are provided to illustrate the themes and sub-themes, but it is not clear how these particular quotes were selected through the process of data analysis.

Continued

◎ HUMAN MOVEMENT STUDIES EXAMPLE—cont'd

- *Whether sufficient data are presented to support the findings. To what extent are contradictory data taken into account?*

  Rich data are presented with extensive examples of participant quotes. The research question does not particularly lend itself to considering contradictory data. There were multiple recommendations provided for designing and delivering these types of PA programs, but they could generally be grouped into four themes.

- *Whether the researcher critically examined their own role, potential bias and influence during analysis and selection of data for presentation.*

  It is acknowledged that inductive analysis may lead to the emergence of themes influenced by the researcher's prior knowledge and understanding. However, the researchers provide a detailed critique of their own perspectives, and the use of some deductive codes based on theoretical and research literature and multiple coders helped to minimise this interpretation bias.

7. Is there a clear statement of findings?

Consider:

- *Whether the findings are explicit. Whether there is adequate discussion of the evidence both for and against the researcher's arguments.*

  The findings are very clearly presented. The authors did not have a particular position at the start of the study, so conclusions and recommendations are drawn from themes that emerged. The authors provided an adequate discussion of the range of issues involved.

- *Whether the researcher has discussed the credibility of their findings (for example, triangulation, respondent validation, more than one analyst).*

  The researchers present some discussion of credibility, including: the use of multiple researchers to develop codes and classify themes; the inclusion of substantive quotes from participants; and use of an established framework. They acknowledge they did not use respondent validation/member checking in an effort to reduce participant burden.

- *Whether the findings are discussed in relation to the original research question.*

  The findings are clearly discussed in relation to the original objective of the research.

8. How valuable is the research?

Consider:

- *Whether the researcher discusses the contribution the study makes to existing knowledge or understanding. (For example, do they consider the findings in relation to current practice or policy, or relevant research-based literature?)*

  The article discusses the congruency of several themes with previous research relating to group-based PA programs for postpartum women. Implications for the design and implementation of community group-based PA programs for postpartum women are clearly articulated, including strategies to engage and sustain the participation of postpartum women.

- *Whether they identify new areas where research is necessary.*

  The researchers identify that further research should investigate the feasibility, acceptability and effectiveness of using digital technology to supplement community PA programs.

- *Whether the researchers have discussed whether or how the findings can be transferred to other populations or considered other ways the research may be used.*

  The authors do not explicitly state ways the findings may be transferable to other settings and participants but acknowledge that perspectives may be limited due to the small sample size. They do suggest, though, that gathering information about existing community programs (including cost, reach, acceptability and fit) can be effectively applied to help inform decisions about the design and implementation of new programs, and to scale up of existing ones.

What are the main findings?

Stakeholder perspectives about the design and implementation of community-based group PA programs for postpartum women were grouped into four broad themes which were presented as recommendations for future programs. These were: (1) effective practitioners have a history of, and passion for, women's health and PA; (2) low-cost, connected approaches attract women into community group-based PA programs; (3) inclusive, flexible, varied and holistic approaches sustain participation; and (4) connections should be utilised to overcome barriers to community group-based PA programs. The practitioners interviewed were able to locate gaps in current community PA programs, either through occupational or motherhood experiences. Interestingly, they were able to intuitively design and implement strategies that enhanced postpartum women's physical, social and emotional wellbeing to overcome barriers to PA.

How might we use this evidence to inform practice?

This appears to be a well-designed and conducted study which took place within the Australian context. It provides some useful information for you to consider as an exercise physiologist trying to establish a group exercise program for postpartum women. Importantly, the findings reinforce the importance of doing this in partnership with the mothers' groups as a way of attracting women to the classes and establishing community connection. You may, however, need to consider running these classes outside of your clinic environment to make them more inclusive, accessible and child-friendly. You can also use your connections with other women's health professionals to deliver educational sessions at the classes and during mothers' groups. This will ensure your program has a focus on the physical, emotional and social wellbeing required. Initially, you should also offer these classes at a reduced rate, with trial sessions and no lock-in memberships. You take this information to your client and together decide to work on establishing a group exercise program for postnatal women.

◎ NUTRITION AND DIETETICS EXAMPLE

Clinical scenario

You are a new dietitian providing outpatient services to patients with chronic diseases, such as type 2 diabetes, cardiovascular disease and obesity, that require multiple visits to facilitate behaviour change. You have heard that developing a meaningful 'therapeutic relationship' can enhance patient outcomes. You want to understand how to best support patients in achieving their goals through improving your counselling and rapport-building skills to maximise the relationship between you and your clients.

Clinical question

How can dietitians develop meaningful relationships with clients to enhance their management of lifestyle-related chronic diseases?

Search terms and databases used to find the evidence

Database: PubMed—Health Services Research Queries (with 'qualitative research category' and 'narrow scope' selected), which is accessed through https://www.nlm.nih.gov/nichsr/hedges/search.html.
Search terms: dietitian AND (client OR patient) AND relationship AND "chronic disease"

This search strategy retrieved seven articles. You choose a study that matches your question and focuses on development of the therapeutic relationship between dietitians and their clients with chronic disease.

Article chosen

Nagy A, McMahon A, Tapsell L, et al. Developing meaningful client–dietitian relationships in the chronic disease context: an exploration of dietitians' perspectives. Nutri Diet 2020;77:529–41. https://doi.org/10. 1111/1747-0080. 12588.

Structured abstract (adapted from above)

Study design: Qualitative study design guided by Charmaz's constructivist grounded theory.
Study question: How do dietitians perceive their process of developing meaningful relationships with clients managing lifestyle-related chronic diseases?
Setting: Dietitians in Australia consulting with clients individually within the free-living environment (that is, not in hospital).
Participants: 22 qualified dietitians (19 female, 16 aged 20–39) working in Australia, who were currently managing, or had recent experience of managing, adult clients regarding lifestyle-related chronic diseases (overweight and obesity, type 2 diabetes, cardiovascular disease).
Data collection method: Purposive sampling occurred in three stages. Dietitians were recruited through initial, snowball and theoretical sampling. Online videoconference and telephone semi-structured interviews were conducted by the lead author. Participant demographic information was collected through an online survey and field notes were documented during and after each interview.

Continued

◎ NUTRITION AND DIETETICS EXAMPLE—cont'd

Analysis: Recorded interview transcripts were analysed using grounded theory methods. The lead author/researcher undertook initial coding, followed by focused coding to categorise significant and similar initial codes at a more abstract level. Finally, theoretical coding was conducted where comparisons were analysed between focused codes to produce more abstract and advanced theoretical codes. Detailed memos documented relationships between codes. These memos were used in conjunction with discussions with the research team to construct the final conceptual model. A constant comparison technique was applied. Data collection and analysis ceased when data saturation was reached.

Key findings: A conceptual model developed from the data that showed the dietitian's role in developing the client–dietitian relationship is complex. Key elements identified and described were 'sensing a professional chemistry', and the dietitian's skills in 'balancing professional and social relationships' and 'managing tension with competing influences'. Influences were categorised as relating to the client and dietitian as individuals (for example, their values), their support network and external contextual factors (for example, working with interpreters).

Conclusion: The authors concluded that developing relationships with clients in the chronic disease context appears complex due to the dietitian's role of managing multiple interrelated elements and influential factors simultaneously. The appropriate management depends on the dietitian as both a person and a professional, and the individual client. It was felt that further research should explore: (1) clients' perspectives of relationship development; and (2) how knowledge of practitioner–client relationships in other disciplines may be utilised to enhance dietetic service delivery.

Is the evidence rigorous and sufficiently reported?
Detailed questions from CASP

1. **Was the research design appropriate to address the aims of the research?**
   Consider:
   - *Whether the researcher has justified the research design (that is, type of qualitative research). (For example, have they discussed how they decided which method to use?)*
     The use of a qualitative approach, particularly the use of grounded theory, was explicitly justified by the authors of the paper. They outlined the benefit of the approach as providing 'complex and detailed

understanding' of an area, as they needed a 'deeper and more comprehensive understanding of client–dietitian relationship development'. Grounded theory was justified for the purpose of 'generating a theory for a process or an action'. They further explained that grounded theory guided the study design, including sampling and data collection and analysis, through a constructivist view, where findings are recognised as a subjective interpretation of the researcher.

2. **Was the recruitment strategy appropriate to the aims of the research?**
   Consider:
   - *Whether the researcher has explained how the participants were selected.*
     The authors clearly articulate the three-staged process of purposive sampling for the study. They build from using a professional association membership (Dietitians Australia) to identify participants, to using snowball sampling through professional network connections, and finally a 'theory-informed' approach (aligned with grounded theory), using targeted sampling of dietitians to meet the needs generated within the data.
   - *Whether they explained why the participants they selected were the most appropriate to provide access to the type of knowledge sought by the study.*
     The justification for the selection of dietitians working within lifestyle-related chronic disease management was clearly articulated. This was because the dietitian and client generally have multiple interactions over an extended period of time in this setting.
   - *Whether there are any discussions around recruitment (for example, why some people chose not to take part).*
     The authors explained that, although a total of 47 dietitians were contacted or expressed an interest in participating, only 22 participated in the study. Reasons for declining included: time constraints ($n = 4$), health reasons ($n = 1$), because they did not meet the inclusion criteria ($n = 2$), or lack of response to the invitation email ($n = 18$).

3. **Were the data collected in a way that addressed the research issue?**
   Consider:
   - *Whether the setting for data collection was justified.*
     The setting for data collection was clearly justified. Online videoconference or telephone interviews

were offered to account for distances between geographic locations as participants were dietitians across Australia. Telephone interviews were conducted at a participant's request or when technical problems occurred with the videoconferencing software.

- *Whether it is clear how data were collected (for example, focus group, semi-structured interview, etc.).*
  The collection of data by individual semi-structured interview has been made explicit.
- *Whether the researcher has justified the methods chosen.*
  The researchers justify the use of semi-structured interviews to ensure that 'key questions were addressed while allowing flexibility in following participants' leads'.
- *Whether the researcher has made the methods explicit. (For example, for interview method, is there an indication of how interviews were conducted, or did they use a topic guide?)*
  Although the actual interview guide is not provided, the authors outline that an interview guide was collaboratively developed, with probes identified from empirical literature. It was clearly articulated that interview questions were open-ended and included asking participants to identify key elements of successful interactions with clients. To support the collection of rich data, participants were provided with the interview questions via email before their interview to ensure ample time to reflect on their responses.
- *Whether methods were modified during the study. If so, has the researcher explained how and why?*
  The only modification noted by the authors was the offer of telephone interview if technological problems occurred with the videoconferencing software.
- *Whether the form of data is clear (for example, tape-recordings, video material, notes, etc.).*
  The authors state that interviews were recorded using a digital audio-recorder and transcribed verbatim. Field notes were also kept by the interviewer/lead researcher during and after each interview, which included details such as how the interview was conducted (including any technical problems).

- *Whether the researcher has discussed saturation of data.*
  The authors clearly outline that data collection and analysis occurred simultaneously and ceased when data saturation was reached. They noted that this was when no new codes emerged, as per grounded theory methods, and outlined that data saturation recognition was enabled through continuous data interrogation using cross-comparison techniques, recording detailed analytical memos and discussing the analysis with the research team throughout the study.

4. **Has the relationship between researcher and participants been adequately considered?**
Consider:
- *Whether the researcher critically examined their own role, potential bias and influence during:*
  - *Formulation of the research questions*
    The authors explicitly discuss their biases and their management in the context of the grounded theory methodology, with the researcher being actively involved in the research process. Although the lead author's biases as a novice researcher and qualified female dietitian prior to and during the study were acknowledged and reflected upon, the nature of these preconceptions and the potential influence of these on the formulation of the research questions were not explicitly documented.
  - *Data collection, including sample recruitment and choice of location*
    The authors acknowledged that a relationship between some participants and the primary researcher existed prior to the study commencing but did not examine how this may have influenced data collection. The authors also outlined that the emerging analysis was challenged in light of the lead author's reflections on her biases as a novice researcher and qualified female dietitian, both throughout coding and in discussion with the research team.
- *How the researcher responded to events during the study and whether they considered the implications of any changes in the research design.*
  This was not relevant, as there were no events reported during the study that would have implications for changes in the research design.

Continued

◎ NUTRITION AND DIETETICS EXAMPLE—cont'd

5. **Have ethical issues been taken into consideration?**
   Consider:
   - *Whether there are sufficient details of how the research was explained to participants for the reader to assess whether ethical standards were maintained.*
     The researchers have provided details regarding ethical permission to conduct the study and clearly state that 'all participants gave informed consent prior to participating'. The nature of how the research was explained to participants was not explicit, only that 'dietitians who confirmed they met the inclusion criteria were sent an information sheet and consent form to sign and return'.
   - *Whether the researcher has discussed issues raised by the study (for example, issues around informed consent or confidentiality or how they have handled the effects of the study on the participants during and after the study).*
     Participants were assigned numerical codes during the transcription process. The authors did not explicitly note if any issues arose as a result of this study or how they handled any such issues during or after the study.
   - *Whether approval has been sought from the ethics committee.*
     The authors state: 'This study was approved by the University of Wollongong Health and Medical Human Research Ethics Committee (2017/575).'

6. **Was the data analysis sufficiently rigorous?**
   Consider:
   - *Whether there is an in-depth description of the analysis process. Whether thematic analysis is used. If so, is it clear how the categories/themes were derived from the data?*
     The authors provide a clear and detailed outline of the steps taken in the analysis according to grounded theory methods. The lead author/researcher undertook initial coding where each line or segment of data was coded. Focused coding was then used to categorise significant and similar initial codes at a more abstract level. Finally, theoretical coding was conducted where comparisons were analysed between focused codes to produce more abstract and advanced theoretical codes. The authors outlined that detailed memos were written throughout the process to document relationships between codes. These memos were used in conjunction with discussions with the research team to construct the final conceptual model. Data collection and analysis ceased when data saturation was reached (when no new codes emerged as per grounded theory methods). The authors stated the use of cross-comparison techniques, recording detailed analytical memos and discussing the analysis with the research team throughout the study allowed for continuous interrogation of the data and recognition of data saturation. Further, this constant comparison technique was applied to the interviews as a whole to distinguish similarities and differences between codes, and memos regarding this were documented. This technique was also used once the conceptual model was finalised to ensure the analysis reflected transcripts and memos, and to enhance study rigour. Other memos were kept to document code definitions, possible analytical avenues and further questions of the data. Findings were presented during regular meetings with authors where raw data were discussed, the emerging analysis was critiqued and potential analytical avenues were raised.
   - *Whether the researcher explains how the data presented were selected from the original sample, to demonstrate the analysis process.*
     There is no detail reported about how the data presented were selected from the original sample.
   - *Whether sufficient data are presented to support the findings. To what extent are contradictory data taken into account?*
     Sufficient data are presented in the form of rich quotes illustrating each category and subcategory and both positive and negative perspectives are reported.
   - *Whether the researcher critically examined their own role, potential bias and influence during analysis and selection of data for presentation.*
     The primary researcher critically examined their role with respect to influence on analysis but not on the presentation of data. Reflections were documented within written memos regarding emerging codes which were embedded within the analysis. It was noted that this process enabled the lead researcher to be aware of preconceptions held. This was felt to facilitate a more critical approach

to data analysis, where the emerging analysis was challenged in light of these reflections both throughout coding and in discussions with the research team.

7. **Is there a clear statement of findings?**
Consider:

- *Whether the findings are explicit. Whether there is adequate discussion of the evidence both for and against the researcher's arguments.*

   The findings are clearly presented, including a novel model of relationship development in chronic disease management offering a more in-depth and comprehensive representation than currently understood in dietetics.

- *Whether the researcher has discussed the credibility of their findings (for example, triangulation, respondent validation, more than one analyst).*

   The researchers present some discussion of the credibility of their findings, including: the use of two researchers to check the accuracy of transcript recordings; the inclusion of substantive quotes from participants; the reflexive processes employed by the lead author; and regular meetings among the authors to discuss the raw data, critique the emerging analysis and raise potential analytical themes. Although participants were invited to check their transcript, it was noted that only one participant elected to do so.

- *Whether the findings are discussed in relation to the original research question.*

   The findings are clearly discussed in relation to the original objective of the research, being to explore dietitians' perspectives of how they develop meaningful relationships with clients managing lifestyle-related chronic diseases.

8. **How valuable is the research?**
Consider:

- *Whether the researcher discusses the contribution the study makes to existing knowledge or understanding. (For example, do they consider the findings in relation to current practice or policy, or relevant research-based literature?)*

   This study extends knowledge of the development of the therapeutic relationship between client and dietitian in the management of chronic diseases in an outpatient setting. The findings are not only presented through a dietetics lens, but are positioned within the wider medical and psychology-based literature about the multidimensional nature of establishing therapeutic relationships.

- *Whether they identify new areas where research is necessary.*

   The authors identify that further research is needed to advance the dietitian profession's understanding of meaningful relationships, particularly from the client's perspective, and how knowledge of practitioner–client relationships in other health disciplines may be utilised to enhance dietetic service delivery. In particular, the authors highlight that further research is needed in understanding how dietitians (can) balance professional and social relationships.

- *Whether the researchers have discussed whether or how the findings can be transferred to other populations or considered other ways the research may be used.*

   The applicability to other populations is not explicitly discussed. Although the researchers acknowledge that perspectives of dietitians not interviewed may have differed from those in the present study, they also suggest the sample appears to reflect the mostly female-dominated dietetic profession in Australia that primarily works in New South Wales, Queensland and Victoria.

What are the main findings?

This study has produced a novel model of relationship development in chronic disease management from the dietitian's perspective which offers a more in-depth and comprehensive representation than is currently understood in dietetics. This has been achieved by building on the knowledge of individual qualities important for client–dietitian relationships within the literature ('sensing a professional chemistry' and 'balancing professional and social relationships'), and by identifying meaningful processes underlying those qualities and how they might interact with each other ('managing tension with competing influences'). Dietitians are called on to add to their repertoire by developing personal/professional skills to manage the tension between this direct interaction and factors that may influence it to better establish meaningful relationships with clients in a chronic disease context.

How might we use this evidence to inform practice?

The findings from this study have implications for personal practice of new dietitians, their training and

Continued

◎ NUTRITION AND DIETETICS EXAMPLE—cont'd

practice-directed research. Personally, practising dietitians should explore the concept of 'professional chemistry' in dietetics, and how it might compare to dimensions of therapeutic relationships explicitly identified in other disciplines, particularly in psychology-based literature. This would allow a deeper understanding of how to appropriately balance professional and social relationships when interacting with clients and may further support dietitians to deliver optimal dietetic care. Additionally, this highlights the importance of professional self-awareness and accentuates the importance of dietitians engaging in regular and critical reflective practice. In training of dietitians-to-be, greater interdisciplinary collaboration between dietetics and psychology may benefit dietitians in better understanding therapeutic relationships.

◎ PARAMEDICINE EXAMPLE

Clinical scenario

You are a paramedic supervisor and have heard that a number of your front-line workers are becoming increasingly dissatisfied because of repeated attacks of aggression from patients and hospital staff alike. You arrange a department meeting to discuss what strategies can be put in place to reduce the frequency of these occurrences and the impacts of these attacks. You decide to consult the recent literature to find studies that have specifically sought paramedics' experiences of aggression in the workplace.

Clinical question

What are the experiences of paramedics who encounter aggression in the workplace, and what is the impact of these experiences?

Search terms and databases used to find the evidence
Database: PubMed
Search terms: (paramedic OR paramedicine OR prehospital OR ambulance) AND (rudeness OR incivility OR "workplace violence") AND (qualitative OR interview* OR themes)

This search strategy retrieved 28 articles. You choose an article that appears to match your study question and focuses on front-line paramedics working for one NHS Ambulance Trust in England.

Article chosen

Credland NJ, Whitfield C. Incidence and impact of incivility in paramedicine: a qualitative analysis. Emerg Med J 2021; May 26. doi: 10.1136/emermed-2020-209961.

Structured abstract (adapted from the above)
Study design: A qualitative study with an interpretivist perspective.

Study question: To explore experiences of incivility among front-line paramedics, who were encouraged to consider their experiences and identify what impact these experiences had.

Setting: One NHS Ambulance Trust in England between June and December 2019.

Participants: 14 front-line paramedics (25–45 years of age, four females).

Data collection method: Purposive sampling was used to recruit paramedics through the Trust newsletter and Twitter feeds. Participants underwent in-depth semi-structured interviews conducted by a non-paramedic researcher to reduce bias. The interview schedule was based on experiences and impacts of incivility, including suggestions about reducing incivility and coping strategies. Interviews were conducted at the participant's convenience and were audio-recorded and then professionally transcribed. Reflexive field notes were also taken.

Analysis: Transcripts were analysed using thematic analysis. Data were organised into codes, and links between codes informed the development of themes. Analysis was conducted by two researchers independently and the final analysis was agreed through discussion. Member checking was undertaken.

Key findings: Four key themes emerged from the data: *interdisciplinary respect*; *patient and interdisciplinary expectations*; *path of least resistance*; and *wellbeing at work*. Paramedics reported a lack of respect from other professional groups. The general public and interdisciplinary colleagues have unrealistic expectations of the role of a paramedic. In order to deal with incivility, paramedics often reported taking the path of least resistance which impacts clinical decision making and potentially threatens best practice. Paramedics reported using coping strategies to support wellbeing at work.

Conclusion: The authors concluded that incivility from the general public and other health professionals can have a cumulative effect on paramedics, negatively impacting their mental wellbeing and clinical decision making. Expectations and lack of understanding about the scope of practice of a paramedic can lead to confusion, frustration and, often, confrontation from patients and other healthcare professionals.

Is the evidence rigorous and sufficiently reported?

Detailed questions from CASP

1. **Was the research design appropriate to address the aims of the research?**

   Consider:
   - *Whether the researcher has justified the research design.*

     The authors justified an interpretivist perspective 'to allow an in-depth exploration of incivility as experienced and understood by front-line paramedics'. Interpretivism is further justified based on aiming to gain knowledge of the world by understanding the meanings that humans attach to their actions and reactions. More broadly, the authors justify their use of qualitative research techniques 'to help us understand how people interpret and interact within their social environment'.

2. **Was the recruitment strategy appropriate to the aims of the research?**

   Consider:
   - *Whether the researcher has explained how the participants were selected.*

     The authors provide a clear description of the purposive sampling strategy used to select participants.
   - *Whether they explained why the participants they selected were the most appropriate to provide access to the type of knowledge sought by the study.*

     The participants selected appear to be broadly appropriate to meet the study's aims, although this was not explicitly justified. Purposive sampling was used to recruit paramedics through the Trust newsletter and Twitter feeds. The only inclusion criterion was that the participant must be a front-line paramedic. Although experience with incivility in the workplace was not a pre-specified inclusion criterion, this did not affect the recruitment strategy

since all participants stated that they experienced incivility on at least a weekly basis.
- *Whether there are any discussions around recruitment (for example, why some people chose not to take part).*

  There is no information provided regarding the number of potential participants who expressed interest in the study and the actual number recruited. It is unclear how many people chose not to take part and the reasoning behind this decision.

3. **Were the data collected in a way that addressed the research issue?**

   Consider:
   - *Whether the setting for data collection was justified.*
     The authors did not record the setting for data collection but outlined that interviews were conducted at the participants' convenience.
   - *Whether it is clear how data were collected (for example, focus group, semi-structured interview, etc.).*
     The collection of data by individual semi-structured interview has been made explicit. Interviews were conducted by a non-paramedic researcher to reduce bias.
   - *Whether the researcher has justified the methods chosen.*
     The authors justified that one-to-one semi-structured interviews were used 'to elicit discussion about experiences and their meanings'. This approach was chosen to give participants the opportunity to focus on issues most important to them in a confidential environment, avoiding the influence of a peer perspective.
   - *Whether the researcher has made the methods explicit. (For example, for interview method, is there an indication of how interviews were conducted, or did they use a topic guide?)*
     The authors provide the interview schedule used to guide interviews.
   - *Whether methods were modified during the study. If so, has the researcher explained how and why?*
     There is no indication that the methods were modified during this study.
   - *Whether the form of data is clear (for example, tape-recordings, video material, notes, etc.).*
     The authors have indicated that interviews were audio-recorded and transcribed for data analysis purposes.

Continued

◎ **PARAMEDICINE EXAMPLE—cont'd**

- *Whether the researcher has discussed saturation of data.*

    The authors indicated that recruitment, data collection and analysis occurred iteratively, and that these processes overlapped to allow for themes and codes to be saturated. The authors also state that despite the low numbers of participants, data saturation was achieved. However, it is unclear on what basis data saturation was deemed to have been achieved.

4. **Has the relationship between researcher and participants been adequately considered?**

    Consider:

    - *Whether the researcher critically examined their own role, potential bias and influence during:*
        - *Formulation of the research questions.*

            One of the authors appears to be a paramedic, but this has not been acknowledged in the formulation of the research question.

        - *Data collection, including sample recruitment and choice of location.*

            Interviews were undertaken by a non-paramedic researcher, and this was justified to reduce bias. However, the role, potential bias or influence of this researcher was not explicitly considered.

    - *How the researcher responded to events during the study and whether they considered the implications of any changes in the research design.*

        There were no events reported during the study that would have implications for changes in the research design.

5. **Have ethical issues been taken into consideration?**

    Consider:

    - *Whether there are sufficient details of how the research was explained to participants for the reader to assess whether ethical standards were maintained.*

        The authors provide an example of the call for participants that was circulated via internal newsletter and social media. This explicitly reveals that the research seeks to explore the incidence and impact of incivility in pre-hospital care. In addition, the authors indicate that paramedics who expressed interest in the study were given 7 days to consider the information sheet and decide whether to take part.

    - *Whether the researcher has discussed issues raised by the study (for example, issues around informed consent or confidentiality or how they have handled* the effects of the study on the participants during and after the study).

        Participants gave informed consent and were allocated numeric codes to ensure anonymisation. It is also foreseeable that being interviewed about incivility may affect some of the participants who have been adversely impacted. However, it is unclear how the researchers may have handled these effects.

    - *Whether approval has been sought from the ethics committee.*

        The authors have reported that ethics approval was obtained.

6. **Was the data analysis sufficiently rigorous?**

    Consider:

    - *Whether there is an in-depth description of the analysis process. Whether thematic analysis is used. If so, is it clear how the categories/themes were derived from the data?*

        The authors explain that thematic analysis was undertaken whereby data were organised into codes, and links between codes informed the development of themes. However, no detail or examples are provided about the coding or how codes were organised into themes.

    - *Whether the researcher explains how the data presented were selected from the original sample, to demonstrate the analysis process.*

        There is no explanation about how the data presented were selected from the original sample.

    - *Whether sufficient data are presented to support the findings. To what extent are contradictory data taken into account?*

        Several rich quotes are presented to support each of the four themes. The authors explored a range of strategies for coping with incivility and its impact.

    - *Whether the researcher critically examined their own role, potential bias and influence during analysis and selection of data for presentation.*

        There has been no critical examination of the researcher's role, potential for bias or influence during analysis, although they briefly make reference to the final analysis being guided by 'reflexive field notes' and selection of data for presentation.

7. **Is there a clear statement of findings?**

    Consider:

    - *Whether the findings are explicit. Whether there is adequate discussion of the evidence both for and against the researcher's arguments.*

The findings are explicitly described in terms of four themes. A range of impacts of incivility appear to have been considered and differences between incivility from patients and colleagues were noted.

- *Whether the researcher has discussed the credibility of their findings (for example, triangulation, respondent validation, more than one analyst).*

  The researchers have added to the credibility to their findings by using two analysts where agreement was reached through discussion, incorporating reflexive field notes in their analysis, and by undertaking member checking through discussion and reading of transcripts with participants who confirmed resonance with their experiences. It is unclear whether or not respondent validation of the final themes was undertaken.

- *Whether the findings are discussed in relation to the original research question.*

  The study's findings are discussed in relation to the research question and explore a range of experiences and impacts of incivility.

8. How valuable is the research?

Consider:

- *Whether the researcher discusses the contribution the study makes to existing knowledge or understanding. (For example, do they consider the findings in relation to current practice or policy, or relevant research-based literature?)*

  The researchers discuss the study findings within the context of the wider literature and consider both clinical and interprofessional implications.

- *Whether they identify new areas where research is necessary.*

  The researchers identify that further qualitative research is needed to explore experiences of incivility in relation to working with patients and their families, along with interprofessional and intraprofessional working to support a holistic approach to addressing incivility. They also recommend further research to explore potential intervention strategies to support front-line paramedics and indirectly suggest further research using a more diverse sample to improve the transferability of findings.

- *Whether the researchers have discussed whether or how the findings can be transferred to other populations or considered other ways the research may be used.*

  The authors acknowledge limitations in transferability of the study findings to other populations given that the participants were drawn from a single ambulance trust and were predominantly male. They also acknowledge that the sampling strategy may have resulted in a participant group that does not reflect the full range of experiences across the paramedic workforce.

What are the main findings?

Four themes were identified: *interdisciplinary respect*; *patient and interdisciplinary expectations*; *path of least resistance*; and *wellbeing at work*. Incivility from the general public and other health professionals can have a cumulative negative effect on paramedics' mental wellbeing and clinical decision making. Expectations and lack of understanding about the scope of practice of a paramedic can lead to confusion, frustration and, often, confrontation from patients and other healthcare professionals. Paramedics often reported taking the path of least resistance when confronted with incivility which impacts clinical decision making and potentially threatens best practice. Coping strategies were used by paramedics to support wellbeing at work.

How might we use this evidence to inform practice?

You now have a better appreciation of the cumulative effects of incivility on your staff and their subsequent clinical practice. This study has revealed the role of supervisors in proactively supporting paramedics. You decide to discuss key findings of this study with your team and to use this as a starting point to encourage open and transparent dialogue about incivility and how you can better support your team. This study also highlighted that a cultural shift towards strategies that actively support professional respect and understanding is likely to be needed. You therefore plan to discuss how you and your team can promote a clearer understanding of the role and skills of paramedics within the healthcare system.

◎ COMPLEMENTARY AND INTEGRATIVE MEDICINE EXAMPLE

Clinical scenario

You are a general practitioner (GP) working in a busy practice. Recently, several of your patients who have been diagnosed with dementia or their carers have asked you about using various types of complementary medicines (CM). You seek to understand the reasons behind why people with dementia consider using CM, and your role in this.

Clinical question

What motivates people living with dementia and their carers to consider using complementary medicine, and what is the role of the GP?

Search terms and databases used to find the evidence

Database: PubMed

Search terms: MeSH Major Topic: Dementia AND MeSH Major Topic: complementary therapies AND all fields: qualitative. Limited to last 5 years in order to be as up to date as possible.

The search yielded 38 results. Not all results were qualitative studies. Many examined the use of one CM modality alone—for example, tai chi. You choose one that has a broader scope—that is, it is not limited to one modality—and which has recruited people living in the community, rather than in residential aged care.

Article chosen

Steiner GZ, George ES, Metri NJ, et al. Use of complementary medicines and lifestyle approaches by people living with dementia: exploring experiences, motivations and attitudes. Int J Older People Nursing 2021;16:e12378. doi: 10.1111/opn.12378.

Structured abstract (adapted from the above)

Study design: A general qualitative study with individual interviews using a thematic (inductive) analysis approach.

Study question: The aim of this study was to explore the experiences, motivations and attitudes towards complementary medicine use by people living with dementia in an Australian setting.

Setting: Community-dwelling people living with dementia in Australia, and their caregivers.

Participants: The final sample ($N = 18$) included people living with dementia ($n = 4$), dyads involving a person living with dementia and their nominated third party ($n = 4$), current caregivers ($n = 7$) and former caregivers ($n = 3$). The mean age of participants with dementia was 72 years (SD = 11.2 years), 11 were male, and mean time since diagnosis was 4 years (SD = 3 years).

Data collection method: Sampling was purposive, and potential participants were recruited through social media and university webpages and consumer networks. In-depth semi-structured interviews were conducted by telephone between September and December 2016. Participants with dementia were encouraged to invite a third-party family member or friend if they felt they needed support during research participation. The interview schedule was grouped into the following four topic areas associated with three aims: (1) types of CM and/or lifestyle interventions used (aim 1); (2) reasons for use or non-use (aims 2 and 3); (3) the impact that CM or lifestyle intervention use has had on life (aims 2 and 3); and (4) conversations with doctors and health professionals about the use of CM and lifestyle interventions (aims 1 and 2). All interviews were recorded and transcribed verbatim by an independent transcription company.

Analysis: Transcripts underwent thematic analysis using an inductive approach with a six-phased method and constant comparison. This consisted of systematically identifying, comparing and coding themes within and between interviews. Emerging categories and associations among the codes led to the development of several themes and sub-themes. All transcripts were initially coded by one researcher, with independent coding of 44% of the transcripts among six members of the research team to achieve analytical rigour.

Key findings: Three overarching themes with multiple sub-themes were identified. (1) *CM knowledge and use:* people living with dementia and caregivers' understanding of CM, types of CM used and CM usage patterns. (2) *Self-determined reasons for use/non-use:* maintain or improve quality of life, hope, management of dementia symptoms, level of awareness, willingness and evidence, perceptions on efficacy and safety of CM, experiences of conventional medicine and holistic approach to wellness. (3) *External determinant of use:* information on CM, relationship influences on CM use and experiences with general practitioners and CM.

Conclusion: The authors concluded that complementary medicine use is widespread and is positively viewed by people living with dementia and their caregivers. Decisions regarding CM use were based on personal opinions. Findings have implications for conversations with health professionals regarding CM use in order to improve communication and health literacy, and to reduce the risk of adverse effects through polypharmacy.

Is the evidence rigorous and sufficiently reported?
Detailed questions from CASP

1. **Was the research design appropriate to address the aims of the research?**
   Consider:
   - *Whether the researcher has justified the research design (that is, type of qualitative research). (For example, have they discussed how they decided which method to use?)*
   No justification was provided for the use of a qualitative study design. However, given that the aim of the study was to gain an understanding of the experiences of, motivations for and attitudes towards complementary medicine use by people living with dementia, the research design is appropriate.

2. **Was the recruitment strategy appropriate to the aims of the research?**
   Consider:
   - *Whether the researcher has explained how the participants were selected.*
   The researchers stated that they used a purposive sampling strategy to recruit community-dwelling people living with dementia and their caregivers. Although the study was promoted online via social media and university webpages, and consumer networks, it is unclear how participants with dementia and their caregivers were specifically targeted. The researchers also state that efforts to balance users and non-users of complementary medicine were made by recruiting through a wide range of avenues and advertising, and that views from both users and non-users were of interest.
   - *Whether they explained why the participants they selected were the most appropriate to provide access to the type of knowledge sought by the study.*
   Eligibility criteria for study participants are not explicitly described. For example, it is unclear whether or not there were criteria around how participants were diagnosed with dementia (Table 1 in the article suggests the type of dementia may have been self-reported), the duration of their diagnosis or the extent of their symptoms. The protocol did specify that participants who were unable to engage with—or did not understand the purpose of—the study, according to the judgment of the research psychologist, would not be enrolled. There was also no direct rationale as to why caregivers were

interviewed, only that 'no prior research has explored intrinsic and external determinants of complementary medicine use/non-use in people with dementia and their caregivers'.
   - *Whether there are any discussions around recruitment (for example, why some people chose not to take part).*
   There is no discussion in the article regarding the number of potential participants who expressed interest in the study, the number who were eligible or reasons why some people chose not to take part. However, the researchers state that one person decided not to continue with the study due to their dementia symptoms.

3. **Were the data collected in a way that addressed the research issue?**
   Consider:
   - *Whether the setting for data collection was justified.*
   Participants were offered the choice of conducting their interview by videoconference or telephone interview. Although this is not explicitly justified, these settings are appropriate given their convenience, especially when recruiting participants from such a large geographical area (Australia).
   - *Whether it is clear how data were collected (for example, focus group, semi-structured interview, etc.).*
   The collection of data through in-depth semi-structured interviews was clearly described.
   - *Whether the researcher has justified the methods chosen.*
   The methods of data collection were not justified by the researchers, although the use of semi-structured interviews appears appropriate for the topic.
   - *Whether the researcher has made the methods explicit. (For example, for interview method, is there an indication of how interviews were conducted, or did they use a topic guide?)*
   The researchers outline that an interview schedule grouped into four topic areas according to the aims of the study was used. Although participants were posted interview questions to help them prepare for the interview, the schedule has not been provided to readers of the article.
   - *Whether methods were modified during the study. If so, has the researcher explained how and why?*
   The methods do not appear to have been modified during the study.

Continued

◎ COMPLEMENTARY AND INTEGRATIVE MEDICINE EXAMPLE—cont'd

- *Whether the form of data is clear (for example, tape-recordings, video material, notes, etc.).*

  All interviews were audio-recorded and transcribed verbatim by an independent transcription company. Quantitative demographic information was also collected.

- *Whether the researcher has discussed saturation of data.*

  Although the researchers state the sample size of 18 participants is considered sufficient for data saturation in exploratory work, there is no evidence that data collection and analysis occurred iteratively. It is also unclear how data saturation was defined, only that the researchers considered data saturation was achieved 'with many participants reporting similar experiences with CMs'.

4. **Has the relationship between researcher and participants been adequately considered?**

   Consider:

   - *Whether the researcher critically examined their own role, potential bias and influence during:*
     - *Formulation of the research questions.*

       The authors'/researchers' affiliations and qualifications suggest that they may have some deeper experience with dementia and psychology or neuroscience; however, this has not been acknowledged in the formulation of research questions.

     - *Data collection, including sample recruitment and choice of location.*

       It appears unlikely that the researchers had any connection with the participants, although this was not made explicit.

   - *How the researcher responded to events during the study and whether they considered the implications of any changes in the research design.*

     There were no events reported during the study that would have implications for changes in the research design.

5. **Have ethical issues been taken into consideration?**

   Consider:

   - *Whether there are sufficient details of how the research was explained to participants for the reader to assess whether ethical standards were maintained.*

     Informed consent was obtained from all participants and third-party proxies prior to each interview. Study materials were posted out to participants and receipt was confirmed by telephone. A rigorous process was used to determine that participants had sufficient cognitive capacity to provide informed consent, including the use of a psychologist for a research assistant, and an objective measure of cognition which was used to gauge the participant's ability to engage with the interview content. If participants were unable to provide the necessary information themselves, they were able to nominate a proxy.

   - *Whether the researcher has discussed issues raised by the study (for example, issues around informed consent or confidentiality or how they have handled the effects of the study on the participants during and after the study).*

     The authors indicate that all participants provided written informed consent. Participants were de-identified in the transcription of audio-recording. The authors did not report if any issues arose as a result of this study or how such issues may have been handled.

   - *Whether approval has been sought from the ethics committee.*

     Ethics approval was sought from Western Sydney University Human Research Ethics Committee.

6. **Was the data analysis sufficiently rigorous?**

   Consider:

   - *Whether there is an in-depth description of the analysis process. Whether thematic analysis is used. If so, is it clear how the categories/themes were derived from the data?*

     A description of the thematic analysis process using inductive coding and the method of constant comparison is provided. Although supporting quotes for each theme are provided, it is unclear how the themes and sub-themes were derived from the data.

   - *Whether the researcher explains how the data presented were selected from the original sample, to demonstrate the analysis process.*

     Although representative quotes to support each theme are provided, there is no explanation as to how these quotes were selected from the original sample.

   - *Whether sufficient data are presented to support the findings. To what extent are contradictory data taken into account?*

     Sufficient data are presented, and both positive and negative views of complementary medicine are presented.

- *Whether the researcher critically examined their own role, potential bias and influence during analysis and selection of data for presentation.*

  There was no critical examination of the researcher's role, potential bias or influence on the analysis or selection of data for presentation.

7. Is there a clear statement of findings?

Consider:

- *Whether the findings are explicit. Whether there is adequate discussion of the evidence both for and against the researcher's arguments.*

  There is a clear statement of findings and an adequate discussion of the evidence both for and against the researchers' arguments. For example, the researchers note that participants used complementary medicine to improve quality of life and cognition/mood, but also highlight that the placebo effect cannot be ruled out when using complementary medicine for chronic conditions.

- *Whether the researcher has discussed the credibility of their findings (for example, triangulation, respondent validation, more than one analyst).*

  Data were provided by people with dementia, dyads involving a person with dementia and their caregiver and current or former caregivers. The authors acknowledge that collecting information from caregivers can work as a strength when dyads involving the person with dementia are interviewed but that speaking solely with a caregiver can introduce reporting bias. Although independent coding of 44% of the transcripts was completed, there is no indication that more than one analyst was involved in the development of themes or sub-themes. In addition, there does not appear to have been any attempts at respondent validation.

- *Whether the findings are discussed in relation to the original research question.*

  The researchers discussed the findings in relation to experiences, motivations and attitudes towards complementary medicine use by people living with dementia in an Australian setting. This is consistent with the original research question.

8. How valuable is the research?

Consider:

- *Whether the researcher discusses the contribution the study makes to existing knowledge or understanding. (For example, do they consider the findings*

in relation to current practice or policy, or relevant research-based literature?)

The researchers consider the findings in relation to current evidence on information-seeking from healthcare providers on complementary medicine use, and explicitly present the new knowledge and implications for practice in a separate box: 'Summary Statement of Implications for Practice'.

- *Whether they identify new areas where research is necessary.*

  The researchers call for international population-based research to examine the prevalence and variety of complementary medicine use and perceptions of complementary medicine within this population group and their healthcare providers, especially nurse practitioners.

- *Whether the researchers have discussed whether or how the findings can be transferred to other populations or considered other ways the research may be used.*

  The findings will inform the development of standardised information on complementary medicine for people living with dementia, their caregivers and other healthcare providers. It will also provide direction for areas of focus for future international studies where evidence of efficacy and/or safety are lacking.

What are the main findings?

Findings highlight that CM use is widespread and positively viewed by people living with dementia and their caregivers. Three overarching themes emerged from the data: (1) *CM knowledge and use.* This relates to older people being likely to use natural products in order to manage and slow the progression of their dementia symptoms. (2) *Self-determined reasons for use or non-use.* This theme relates to motivations for using or not using CM (including maintaining or improving quality of life, a holistic approach to wellness and improving cognition and mood) and external determinants of use. (3) *External determinants of CM use.* These include media sources, dementia advocacy organisations, information discussed in scientific research, interaction with CM practitioners, pharmacists, GPs and nurses, as well as personal relationships.

Continued

⊚ COMPLEMENTARY AND INTEGRATIVE MEDICINE EXAMPLE—cont'd

How might we use this evidence to inform practice?
This article helps you to understand reasons motivating people with dementia to use complementary medicine. These findings indicate that GPs and other health practitioners should be educated on complementary medicine use in people living with dementia, as well as on potential contraindications with conventional treatments. You are now also aware that GPs and health practitioners can play an important role in initiating conversations about complementary medicine use and ensuring that adverse effects through polypharmacy are prevented.

⊚ PODIATRY EXAMPLE

Clinical scenario
You have been referred a patient living with rheumatoid arthritis (RA) for three years. They have never seen a podiatrist before and have been told to come and see you to help with footcare. At the first appointment, you discuss the role of the podiatrist and what can be offered, including the use of customised foot orthoses. The patient responds: 'I'm not sure what benefit they will be. I am taking prescribed medication to manage my pain. This will just be an additional thing to worry about and [may] become burdensome.' You acknowledge that medication will play a large role, but you suggest to them that you provide some information about the experience people with rheumatoid arthritis have had using orthoses to appease their concerns. As you only have anecdotal evidence from three patients who you have managed previously, a search of the literature and evidence base on this seems prudent.

Clinical question
What is the experience of using customised foot orthoses in people living with rheumatoid arthritis?

Search terms and databases used to find the evidence
Database: PubMED
Search terms: rheumatoid AND arthritis AND (feet OR foot) AND orthos* (orthosis and orthoses) AND Qualitative
  This search strategy retrieved nine articles. You choose a study that matches your question and focuses on the experiences of patients with rheumatoid arthritis before and after wearing foot orthoses for a period of 6 months.

Article chosen
Ramos-Petersen L, Nester CJ, Ortega-Avila AB, et al. A qualitative study exploring the experiences and perceptions of patients with rheumatoid arthritis before and after wearing foot orthoses for 6 months. Health Soc Care Community 2021 May;29(3):829–36. doi: 10.1111/hsc.13316. Epub 2021 Feb 9.

Structured abstract (adapted from the above)
Study design: A general qualitative study utilising thematic analysis.
Study question: The aim of this study was to explore the experiences of people with RA, before and after wearing foot orthoses for 6 months.
Setting: A podiatry department of a hospital in Granada, Spain.
Participants: Six adult participants (aged 32–75 years, all female) who had consented to participate in a randomised controlled trial comparing the effects of three different types of foot orthoses.
Data collection method: Semi-structured interviews employing open-ended questions were conducted by a podiatrist researcher with experience in rheumatoid arthritis and foot orthoses. Two interviews for each participant were conducted, one before the participant had been issued with their foot orthoses and a second interview 6 months after (September 2019 to March 2020). Interview questions were developed from a review of the literature on outcomes and measurement related to the use of foot orthoses. Field notes supplemented the interview data.
Analysis: A thematic analysis of the transcripts was conducted by one researcher and verified by another. Codes and themes were identified inductively using NVivo qualitative data analysis software (QSR International, Doncaster, Victoria, Australia). Once codes had been generated, themes and groups were developed iteratively. Codes from the initial interviews were generated first, followed by codes from the interviews conducted 6 months later. All codes were compared and themes were developed from the whole dataset.

Key findings: Three key themes emerged from the data: (1) improvement in physical activity; (2) footwear…a tricky situation; and (3) social implications of RA feet.

Conclusion: The authors concluded that although orthoses require time to adapt, wearing foot orthoses had a positive impact on comfort, pain and physical activity, and associated improved general wellness and quality of life. However, barriers to use and negative aspects of experiences related to complexities of finding suitable footwear.

Is the evidence rigorous and sufficiently reported?

Detailed questions from CASP

1. **Was the research design appropriate to address the aims of the research?**

   Consider:

   - *Whether the researcher has justified the research design (that is, type of qualitative research). (For example, have they discussed how they decided which method to use?)*

     The authors justify the use of qualitative research as it can 'add depth and richness to understanding the outcomes from quantitative studies, and it may provide information around factors that influence the attitudes of patients with RA towards orthoses'. However, the authors did not clearly state which qualitative research methodology (design) was used to inform the methods of the study.

2. **Was the recruitment strategy appropriate to the aims of the research?**

   Consider:

   - *Whether the researcher has explained how the participants were selected.*

     The authors explain that participants were recruited from those who had previously consented to participate in a randomised controlled trial comparing the effects of three different types of foot orthoses. However, the recruitment method for this trial was not adequately described, only that 'participants were recruited from the Hospital Virgen de las Nieves, Granada (Spain)'. Since the aim of the wider trial was to compare physical activity, general and foot health, and foot health experiences in people with RA when wearing three different types of foot orthoses, it is inferred that participants had been prescribed foot orthoses.

   - *Whether they explained why the participants they selected were the most appropriate to provide access to the type of knowledge sought by the study.*

     The authors clearly outline eligibility criteria. In addition to these criteria, however, participants also had to have consented to participate in a randomised controlled trial comparing the effects of three different types of foot orthoses. The authors do not explicitly explain why selected participants were the most appropriate for the study. It is inferred that these participants were deemed appropriate because they had been diagnosed with rheumatoid arthritis and had presumably been prescribed foot orthoses. It is also unclear why patients reliant on walking aids were excluded from the wider trial.

   - *Whether there are any discussions around recruitment (for example, why some people chose not to take part).*

     The authors state that four of the ten people who expressed interest by telephone and were sent a participant information sheet did not respond. However, the recruitment strategy for the wider trial is not described, although a separate publication of the trial protocol estimates a sample size of 45 (15 in each group). It is also unclear how many 'eligible' patients from the randomised controlled trial were initially contacted to take part in this qualitative study.

3. **Were the data collected in a way that addressed the research issue?**

   Consider:

   - *Whether the setting for data collection was justified.*

     The authors state that interviews were conducted face-to-face. Although it is inferred that these interviews were conducted 'in a clinical setting', the specifics of this are unclear and this decision was not justified.

   - *Whether it is clear how data were collected (for example, focus group, semi-structured interview, etc.).*

     Data were collected using semi-structured interviews performed face-to-face and recorded digitally. Demographic information was collected through a questionnaire completed prior to the start of the interview.

   - *Whether the researcher has justified the methods chosen.*

     The authors have justified the use of semi-structured interviews employing open-ended questions 'to elicit in-depth responses in a clinical setting'.

Continued

⊚ PODIATRY EXAMPLE—cont'd

- *Whether the researcher has made the methods explicit. (For example, for interview method, is there an indication of how interviews were conducted, or did they use a topic guide?)*

  The questions for the semi-structured topic guide were developed from a review of the literature on outcomes and measurement related to the use of foot orthoses. Questions for the first interview (prior to wearing orthoses) were provided and were based on a previous qualitative study. Specific questions for the second interview (after wearing orthoses for 6 months) are not provided, but the authors vaguely state the focus 'depended on their previous answer(s)'.

- *Whether methods were modified during the study. If so, has the researcher explained how and why?*

  There is no indication that the methods were modified during this study.

- *Whether the form of data is clear (for example, tape-recordings, video material, notes, etc.).*

  The researchers have indicated that data were collected as digital voice recordings which were transcribed and supplemented by field notes. Demographic information was also collected through a questionnaire.

- *Whether the researcher has discussed saturation of data.*

  Saturation of data was not described by the authors. This may not have occurred since only 12 interviews among six participants (all female) were conducted.

4. **Has the relationship between researcher and participants been adequately considered?**

   Consider:

   - *Whether the researcher critically examined their own role, potential bias and influence during:*
     - *Formulation of the research questions.*

       The authors identify that at least one of the researchers (who undertook data collection) was a podiatrist with experience of treating patients with RA and foot orthoses. The remaining authors' affiliations suggest that they may have some experience with podiatry; however, this has not been acknowledged in the formulation of the research question.

     - *Data collection, including sample recruitment and choice of location.*

Although participants were made aware that the researcher was a podiatrist, they do not specify who approached eligible patients for recruitment or how the location was chosen.

- *How the researcher responded to events during the study and whether they considered the implication of any changes in the research design*

  There were no events reported during the study that would have implications for changes in the research design.

5. **Have ethical issues been taken into consideration?**

   Consider:

   - *Whether there are sufficient details of how the research was explained to participants for the reader to assess whether ethical standards were maintained.*

     The authors have provided details regarding ethical permission to conduct the study. Although those who had expressed an interest were provided with a participant information sheet before the appointment 'to allow participants to consider their involvement in the study', it is unclear what study details were provided to the participants in the initial phone conversation and in the participant information sheet.

   - *Whether the researcher has discussed issues raised by the study (for example, issues around informed consent or confidentiality or how they have handled the effects of the study on the participants during and after the study).*

     The authors indicate that all participants had provided informed and written consent. Participants were de-identified in the reporting of results. The authors did not report if any issues arose as a result of this study or how such issues may have been handled.

   - *Whether approval has been sought from the ethics committee.*

     Ethics approval was obtained by the local committee and the study was registered with 'Clinicaltrials.gov'. The authors note that the study was carried out in full accordance with the Declaration of Helsinki.

6. **Was the data analysis sufficiently rigorous?**

   Consider:

   - *Whether there is an in-depth description of the analysis process. Whether thematic analysis is used. If so, is it clear how the categories/themes were derived from the data?*

The authors provide an in-depth description of the data analysis process. The authors outlined that one researcher undertook a line-by-line analysis, from which codes were developed. The same researcher developed themes and groups iteratively. Although 'the findings were scrutinised by a co-author', the relationship between the codes and themes is not depicted.

- *Whether the researcher explains how the data presented were selected from the original sample, to demonstrate the analysis process.*

No examples of the coding, theme generation or groupings were provided. Although specific quotes to support each theme are provided, there is no explanation as to how these quotes were selected from the original sample.

- *Whether sufficient data are presented to support the findings. To what extent are contradictory data taken into account?*

For each theme, several rich quotes are provided to support and illustrate. Quotes showing different perspectives about finding footwear to accommodate orthoses were provided. Other than this example, contradictory data do not appear to have been taken into account, although there may have been limited variation in the data given the small sample of six participants.

- *Whether the researcher critically examined their own role, potential bias and influence during analysis and selection of data for presentation.*

There is no examination of the role of the researchers with respect to influence on the analysis and presentation of data.

7. Is there a clear statement of findings?

Consider:

- *Whether the findings are explicit. Whether there is adequate discussion of the evidence both for and against the researcher's arguments.*

Findings are explicit and summarised into three key themes. Although the authors describe benefits and harms of foot orthoses for people with RA, there was limited exploration of evidence against the researcher's arguments. For example, all participants declared that their physical activity levels had improved after wearing the foot orthoses for 6 months. The authors do not appear to consider a possible alternative perspective that some participants may not experience an improvement in physical activity levels after wearing orthoses. This is possible given the wider physical impairments that people with RA often experience.

- *Whether the researcher has discussed the credibility of their findings (for example, triangulation, respondent validation, more than one analyst).*

Discussion regarding the credibility of the findings is limited. The authors state 'resulting themes were agreed by the researcher and co-author (LRP and GGN), to enhance the validity of the data'. However, only one viewpoint was obtained (that of patients) and there was no evidence of respondent validation. The inclusion of field notes to supplement the data could be considered as a means of strengthening the credibility of the authors' findings.

- *Whether the findings are discussed in relation to the original research question.*

The findings are related directly to the original research question and aims. However, findings related to the experience of people with RA before wearing foot orthoses are limited.

8. How valuable is the research?

Consider:

- *Whether the researcher discusses the contribution the study makes to existing knowledge or understanding. (For example, do they consider the findings in relation to current practice or policy, or relevant research-based literature?)*

The authors claim this study is the first qualitative research study that focuses on 'illuminating both the impact of, and attitudes towards, the use of foot orthoses for people with RA in their feet, and how that use has impacted on physical activity participation, general wellness and quality of life'. The authors discuss their findings in relation to previous research and, in particular, note that their findings agree with a previous meta-analysis supporting the benefits of foot orthoses on pain and disability and also with previous qualitative research highlighting footwear limitations as a potential barrier to wearing foot orthoses. The authors also discuss the implications for current practice in terms of managing patient expectations about the time taken to adapt to foot orthoses and about footwear complexities.

Continued

PODIATRY EXAMPLE—cont'd

- *Whether they identify new areas where research is necessary.*

  The authors suggest that future research in terms of advice that clinicians can provide to their patients is required.

- *Whether the researchers have discussed whether or how the findings can be transferred to other populations or considered other ways the research may be used.*

  The authors acknowledge that their findings may not apply to men, to a wider population of people with RA who are not already participants of a randomised controlled trial and to foot orthoses with differing levels of customisation.

What are the main findings?

Three key themes were identified: (1) *Improvement in physical activity.* This related to an improvement in pain, comfort, safety and physical activity after adapting to the orthoses which also led to improvements in social and mental wellbeing. (2) *Footwear … a tricky situation.* This related to issues around footwear choice with respect to cost, quality, availability and aesthetics both prior to using

orthoses and when having to accommodate orthoses. (3) *Social implications of RA feet.* This reflected unique adaptations made to social activity to accommodate their condition and negative feelings about how their feet influenced their decision to engage with others.

How might we use this evidence to inform practice?

This research highlighted both positive and negative aspects experienced by people with RA wearing foot orthoses, including the need to manage patient expectation as some participants in this study took a while to get used to the devices, but persevering had been shown to be beneficial. You decide to use these findings to help your patient balance the potential advantages and disadvantages of foot orthoses in order to make an informed decision. If your patient decides to consider wearing foot orthoses, you plan to manage their expectations by explaining that it will take some time to adapt and also to encourage them to persevere by describing the potential benefits for their physical, social and mental wellbeing. You also feel better prepared to understand and discuss your patient's concerns about footwear complexities.

PHARMACY EXAMPLE

Clinical scenario

You are a pharmacist and owner of a small pharmacy working in the community and want to provide a service that differentiates your pharmacy from the very large chain pharmacies in the area. In particular, you have been considering approaches to improve customer service and know that part of this is about building stronger relationships with customers. You decide to look into the factors that will help build these relationships, such as improving trust.

Clinical question

What factors build trust between customers (patients) and pharmacists in the community?

Search terms and databases used to find the evidence
Database: PubMed

Search terms: patient AND trust AND "community pharmacists" AND interview

Your search gives 21 results, a few of which are highly relevant. You obtain a copy of them to read. The following article is the first one you read and appraise.

Article chosen

Gregory PAM, Austin Z. Understanding the psychology of trust between patients and their community pharmacists. Can Pharm J (Ott) 2021 Feb 16;154(2):120–8.

Structured abstract (adapted from the above)

Study design: An exploratory qualitative research method was used.

Research question: To identify factors associated with public trust in community pharmacists and to explore opportunities to build trust.

Participants: 13 patients (eight female, aged 29–72 years, with between four and nine current prescriptions) from five different community pharmacies involved in the University of Toronto's experiential education program in Ontario, Canada.

Data collection: Semi-structured interviews were undertaken.

Analysis: Interview data were transcribed, coded and categorised using an inductive thematic coding method. Two researchers independently coded each transcript, and an agreed coding dictionary was then developed and refined. During a second round of coding, researchers consolidated themes independently and then met to obtain consensus on the final thematic analysis.

Key findings: Factors that diminished trust included the business context, lack of transparency about pharmacists' pay, lack of awareness about how pharmacists qualify and are regulated, and inconsistent past experiences with pharmacists. Factors that improved trust included accessibility, affability, acknowledgment and respect.

Conclusion: The authors concluded that factors that reduce trust seem to be somewhat outside the day-to-day control of individual pharmacists; however, factors that enhance trust are those that pharmacists may have greater control over.

Is the evidence rigorous and sufficiently reported?
Detailed questions from CASP

1. **Was the research design appropriate to address the aims of the research?**
   Consider:
   - *Whether the researcher has justified the research design.*
     This study did not use a specific qualitative research methodology, but indicated it was exploratory due to the nature of 'trust' as a psychological phenomenon which has had little research to date in the context of pharmacist–customer relationships. The authors argued this was to 'signpost' avenues of inquiry for future research. A qualitative design is well suited for understanding the nature of such concepts and can often be exploratory when little is known about a topic.

2. **Was the recruitment strategy appropriate to the aims of the research?**
   Consider:
   - *Whether the researcher has explained how the participants were selected.*
     The researchers used convenience sampling from pharmacies involved in the University of Toronto's experiential education program. Within that group, they then used purposive sampling to identify five community pharmacies, representing different geographical locations and business models (for example, chains, independent, grocery) in Ontario, Canada. Purposive sampling did not extend to other demographic factors. Managers were asked to make flyers with information about the study

available to customers in the location where prescriptions were collected. The flyer asked interested customers to contact a research assistant by email to learn more about the study. Inclusion and exclusion criteria (described below) further guided who would be selected, with 13 people participating in the study.
   - *Whether they explained why the participants they selected were the most appropriate to provide access to the type of knowledge sought by the study.*
     Researchers sought adults with sufficient verbal English-language skills who had a minimum of six conversations with any pharmacist about any topic related to health and/or medication in the last year. This was so that participants would have had sufficient interaction with a pharmacist to have some familiarity with them. They excluded those who were relatives or friends, pharmacists or other health professionals, who may potentially influence the patient's sense of trust in the profession, who had formally complained about a pharmacist or who were a current or retired healthcare professional or enrolled as a student of a health-related profession. The rationale for these exclusion criteria was not discussed.
   - *Whether there are any discussions around recruitment (for example, why some people chose not to take part).*
     Eleven community pharmacies were approached to participate in this research and six agreed. It is unclear why five pharmacies chose not to participate. Five of the six pharmacies were selected and one pharmacy was reserved as a back-up, although it is also unclear how the back-up pharmacy was selected. Of the 5 × 100 patient-oriented flyers distributed, 36 potential participants contacted the research associate for more information. Of these 36, 16 agreed to be interviewed but three subsequently withdrew. It is unclear why 20 potential participants who asked for more information chose not to participate or why three participants later withdrew.

3. **Were the data collected in a way that addressed the research issue?**
   Consider:
   - *Whether the setting for data collection was justified.*
     Interviews were scheduled by phone, Skype, FaceTime, Google-Hangouts or other technological

Continued

◎ PHARMACY EXAMPLE—cont'd

options convenient to the researcher and participant. No discussion about the effect of using technology platforms on interviews was discussed.

- *Whether it is clear how data were collected.*

  The collection of data using a semi-structured individual interview format held through a technology platform (as mentioned above) has been made explicit. Field notes were also kept.

- *Whether the researcher has justified the methods chosen.*

  The authors explained that use of a semi-structured protocol provided flexibility for individualising interviews, with the goal of 'eliciting individual stories and supporting individual participants in undertaking their own interpretation and meaning-making to enhance credibility of analysis'. The authors state that they kept field notes during interviews to aid data interpretation and the analysis.

- *Whether the researcher has made the methods explicit.*

  A semi-structured interview guide was used and is provided as supplemental material. This clearly outlines the topics discussed and the open questions.

- *Whether methods were modified during the study. If so, has the researcher explained how and why?*

  There is no mention that the research methods were changed during the study period.

- *Whether the form of data is clear.*

  Yes. It is clearly stated that interviews were audio-recorded or video-recorded and then transcribed and field notes kept.

- *Whether the researcher has discussed saturation of data.*

  The researchers indicate that interviews were undertaken to the point of thematic saturation. This was further defined as the point at which no additional new information was emerging from subsequent interviews.

4. **Has the relationship between researcher and participants been adequately considered?**

  Consider:

  - *Whether the researcher critically examined their own role, potential bias and influence during:*
    - *Formulation of the research questions.*

      Author ZA was responsible for development of the research question. The authors' affiliations and qualifications suggest they may have some

deeper experience in this topic, but there is no comment about this in the article other than 'the authors have no conflicts of interest to report'.

- *Data collection, including sample recruitment and choice of location.*

  The author responsible for data collection was identified, but there is no comment about their role, potential bias or influence on data collection within the article.

- *How the researcher responded to events during the study and whether they considered the implications of any changes in the research design.*

  No changes during the study are reported.

5. **Have ethical issues been taken into consideration?**

  Consider:

  - *Whether there are sufficient details of how the research was explained to participants for the reader to assess whether ethical standards were maintained.*

    The authors have stated that full informed consent from all study participants and ethics approval were provided. General information regarding the study remit and process was provided by email, and permission for informed consent was sought during a follow-up telephone or video call. If patients directed questions to their pharmacist, pharmacists were instructed to ask the patient to contact the research associate by email.

  - *Whether the researcher has discussed issues raised by the study.*

    There is no discussion about issues around informed consent or confidentiality in the article. Participant quotes were de-identified within the manuscript.

  - *Whether approval has been sought from the ethics committee.*

    Ethical approval was provided by the University of Toronto Research Ethics Board.

6. **Was the data analysis sufficiently rigorous?**

  Consider:

  - *Whether there is an in-depth description of the analysis process. Whether thematic analysis is used. If so, is it clear how the categories/themes were derived from the data?*

    Data was analysed using an inductive thematic coding method. Two researchers independently analysed the data and met to develop a consistent coding dictionary and then to obtain consensus on the final thematic analysis. The manuscript describes two broad categories and sub-themes within each category but it is unclear how these categories and sub-themes were derived from the coding.

- *Whether the researcher explains how the data presented were selected from the original sample to demonstrate the analysis process.*

There is no discussion about how the data presented were selected from the original sample.

- *Whether sufficient data are presented to support the findings. To what extent contradictory data are taken into account.*

Sufficient participant quotes are presented to support each sub-theme. Contradictory data in terms of the two broad categories labelled as 'trust-diminishing' and 'trust-enhancing' factors appear to have been taken into account.

- *Whether the researcher critically examined their own role, potential bias and influence during analysis and selection of data for presentation.*

The researchers do not appear to critically examine their role, potential bias or influence during analysis and selection of data for presentation.

7. Is there a clear statement of findings?

Consider:

- *Whether the findings are explicit. Whether there is adequate discussion of the evidence both for and against the researcher's arguments.*

Although the findings are explicit and compare and contrast factors that diminish public trust in pharmacists to those that enhance trust, these findings are not discussed within the context of previous literature in this field.

- *Whether the researcher has discussed the credibility of their findings.*

The authors identify strengths of this research as the independent double-coding of all transcripts to establish themes and the inductive analytical method used to refine and confirm themes. Field notes were also used to support data interpretation and analysis. Validation of data from participants does not appear to have been undertaken and only the perspectives of patients were explored.

- *Whether the findings are discussed in relation to the original research question.*

The findings are discussed in relation to the original research question to identify and characterise factors associated with public trust in community pharmacists.

8. How valuable is the research?

Consider:

- *Whether the researcher discusses the contribution the study makes to existing knowledge or understanding.*

The researchers identify factors that can diminish and enhance trust between patients and pharmacists and suggest that pharmacists may have greater control over trust-enhancing factors rather than trust-diminishing factors. However, these findings are not discussed in the context of existing knowledge in this field.

- *Whether they identify new areas where research is necessary.*

A combination of qualitative and quantitative research focused on understanding the nature and evolution of trust in pharmacy–patient relationships is suggested in order to better understand how to build trusting relationships between pharmacists and their patients.

- *Whether the researchers have discussed whether or how the findings can be transferred to other populations or considered other ways the research may be used.*

The researchers acknowledge that their findings will have limited transferability since the participants were not demographically representative of pharmacy users and due to the relatively small number of participants. However, they have framed this research as exploratory research that can be used as a starting point for further exploration of the issue of trust in pharmacists.

What were the main findings?

Four trust-diminishing factors related to structural features of the pharmacy profession were identified. These include the business context within which community pharmacy is practised, lack of transparency regarding pharmacists' remuneration, lack of awareness of how pharmacists become qualified and are regulated, and inconsistent previous experiences with pharmacists. Four trust-enhancing factors related to personal behaviours of pharmacists were identified. These include accessibility, affability, acknowledgment and respect.

Continued

PHARMACY EXAMPLE—cont'd

How might we use this evidence to inform practice?
This research identified four pharmacist-specific behaviours—accessibility, affability, acknowledgment and respect—that enhanced trustworthiness of both individual pharmacists and the pharmacy profession as a whole. You decide to make a concentrated effort to display these behaviours to your patients in order to build stronger relationships and improve trust and to provide education to your staff about the importance of these approaches. Specifically, you decide to establish an area where you can have private conversations with your patients and use this to harness opportunities to build individual relationships with them.

REFERENCES

1. Critical Appraisal Skills Program (CASP). 10 questions to help you make sense of qualitative research. Oxford: CASP; 2010. Online. Available www.casp-uk.net/wp-content/uploads/2011/11/CASP_Qualitative_Appraisal_Checklist_14oct10.pdf (accessed 2 February 2023).

2. Guyatt GH, Rennie D. Users' Guides to the Medical Literature. JAMA 1993;270(17):2096–7.

3. Giacomini M, Cook D, for the Evidence-Based Medicine Working Group. Users' guides to the medical literature, XXIII: qualitative research in health care. Are the results of the study valid? JAMA 2000;284:357–62.

Appraising and Interpreting Systematic Reviews

Matthew J Page, Sally Bennett, Karin Hannes,
Romi Haas and Denise O'Connor

LEARNING OBJECTIVES

After reading this chapter, you should be able to:
- Understand what systematic reviews are
- Understand how quantitative systematic reviews and qualitative systematic reviews differ
- Know where to look for systematic reviews

- Understand how systematic reviews are carried out
- Critically appraise a systematic review
- Interpret the results from systematic reviews
- Understand how systematic reviews can be used to inform practice

A systematic review is a method for systematically locating, appraising and synthesising research from primary studies and is an important means of condensing the research evidence from many primary studies. This chapter will describe systematic reviews of quantitative evidence and reviews of qualitative evidence, discuss the advantages and disadvantages of reviews, and briefly illustrate the use of systematic reviews for different types of clinical questions. The methods for carrying out systematic reviews will be described, and key factors that can introduce bias into reviews will be explained. Using worked examples, we will also demonstrate how to critically appraise or assess the quality of a systematic review and how it can be used to guide decision making in practice.

WHAT ARE SYSTEMATIC REVIEWS?

Due to the massive increase in the volume of health research over the last 50 years or so, it was recognised that some system of synthesising this information was essential. The health literature has a long tradition of using literature reviews to help readers grasp the breadth of a particular topic. These literature reviews typically provide a reasonably thorough description of a particular topic and refer to many articles that have been published in that particular area. Nearly all students are required to do at least one

literature review as part of their studies, so you probably know what literature reviews are all about.

In the last few decades, **systematic reviews** have been embraced as a comprehensive and trustworthy means of synthesising the literature.[1] Systematic reviews differ from literature reviews in that they are prepared using explicit and predefined methods that are designed to increase the transparency of review procedures.[2] This enables users to assess the risk of bias in the results and quality of the review. In contrast to literature reviews, systematic reviews:
- include a clearly defined review question
- incorporate a comprehensive search to identify *all* potentially relevant studies (or a clear rationale for the choice to work with a purposeful sample of papers such as in the context of reviews of qualitative evidence aiming to generate theory[3])
- screen and select retrieved studies for the review based on a predefined set of reproducible and uniformly applied eligibility criteria
- rigorously appraise the risk of bias (quantitative research) or assess the quality (qualitative research) within individual studies
- systematically synthesise the results of included studies.[4]

Systematic reviews may summarise the results from quantitative studies, qualitative studies, or a combination of quantitative and qualitative studies, depending on the clinical question and the methods used to conduct the review.[5,6] In a *quantitative review*, the results from two or more individual quantitative studies are typically summarised using a measure of effect, which enables each study's effect estimate to be statistically combined and compared in what is called a **meta-analysis**.[4] Meta-analyses generally provide a better way of determining an overall estimate of a clinical effect than looking at the results from individual studies. However, sometimes it is not possible to combine the results of individual studies in a meta-analysis because data in the included studies are reported incompletely, or the interventions or outcomes used in the different studies may be too diverse for it to be sensible to combine them. In this instance, the results from these studies should be synthesised using alternative synthesis and visual display methods (for example, Harvest plot).[7,8]

It may help you to think about these different types of reviews visually. As you can see in Figure 12.1, literature reviews make up the majority of reviews that are found in the overall health literature.[5] Systematic reviews can be considered a subset of literature reviews, and meta-analyses are a smaller set again. Note that the circle representing meta-analyses overlaps both systematic and literature

reviews. This is because not all meta-analyses are carried out systematically. For example, it is technically possible to undertake a meta-analysis of an idiosyncratically collected group of randomised controlled trials; however, this would not be considered a systematic review because a systematic search had not been undertaken. Sometimes the terms 'systematic review' and 'meta-analysis' are used interchangeably, but in this chapter (and many other sources) they are conceptualised as different entities. A systematic review is not necessarily able to, nor does it need to, incorporate a meta-analysis.

A *review of qualitative studies* (or *qualitative evidence synthesis*) brings together the findings from primary qualitative research studies in a systematic way.[9] Its aim is to establish greater understanding of phenomena, often of a sensitive or subtle nature, addressed in original research.[9] Findings from a qualitative evidence synthesis can be used to advance understanding or to advise professional practice or policy. There are several different approaches to qualitative evidence synthesis.[10–14] Some seek to develop more powerful and conceptually rich explanations. They position qualitative research findings within a larger, interpretive discourse. Examples of such approaches include

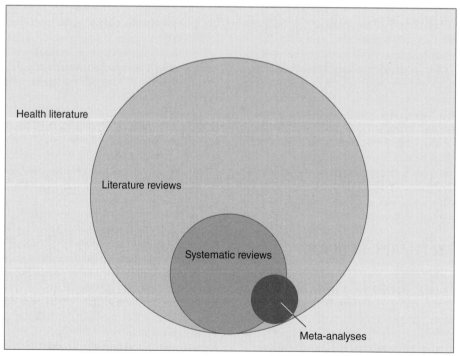

Fig 12.1 The relationships between the health literature, literature reviews, systematic reviews and meta-analyses.

Herbert R, Jamtvedt G, Hagen KB, et al. Practical evidence-based physiotherapy. 2nd ed. Edinburgh: Elsevier/ Churchill Livingstone; 2011.

meta-ethnography,[10] or critical interpretive synthesis.[11–14] Others are more appropriate for producing descriptive accounts of a particular reality or presenting a state of the art of existing evidence, including, for example, thematic synthesis,[12] the meta-aggregative approach to synthesis or mapping reviews. The latter may report on both quantitative and qualitative studies.

In a *mixed-methods review*, quantitative, qualitative or mixed-methods primary studies are combined and a mixed-method approach is used to synthesise and integrate the findings. Several types of mixed-method research syntheses have been developed: segregated, integrated and a contingent mixed-methods design.[15,16] More recently, the debate on what and how to mix has shifted in the direction of multimodality as a concept that explains how different types of evidence can be brought together.[17] It is beyond the scope of this book to explore this.

ADVANTAGES OF SYSTEMATIC REVIEWS

By combining the results of similar studies, a well-conducted systematic review can:
- improve the understanding of a phenomenon or situation
- assist in clarifying why results may vary between studies
- establish generalisability or transferability of the overall results
- guide decision making
- improve the dissemination of evidence from individual studies
- speed up the translation of research evidence into practice and policy
- set a research agenda (where a gap in knowledge becomes evident from the systematic review).

Systematic reviews are therefore important for health professionals and patients who want answers to clinical questions; for those developing policies and guidelines; and for researchers who are setting research agendas.[6] Although systematic reviews have many advantages in design, they may be done badly, which may mean they give the wrong answer. Critical appraisal is therefore very important when reading a systematic review before considering implementing any of the results into practice. We discuss how to critically appraise reviews later in this chapter.

SYSTEMATIC REVIEWS FOR DIFFERENT TYPES OF CLINICAL QUESTIONS

A systematic review is a methodology that can be used for many different study designs and research questions. The type of study designs that will be synthesised in a systematic review depends on the review's research questions.[6] Systematic reviews are at the top of the hierarchy of

evidence for any question type, as we saw in Chapter 2. For example, a well-conducted *systematic review of randomised controlled trials* is usually the best study design for assessing the effectiveness of an intervention, because it identifies and examines all the evidence about the intervention from randomised controlled trials (providing these are rigorous themselves) that meet predetermined inclusion criteria.[18] This type of systematic review is by far the most common. However, systematic reviews can also address other types of questions, such as those about *diagnosis* and *prognosis*.

Systematic reviews that focus on questions of prognosis or prediction best undertake a *synthesis of cohort studies*. Consider the following example in which a systematic review of cohort studies of patients with non-specific low back pain was conducted with the aim of identifying whether recovery expectations predict disability outcomes.[19] The authors searched MEDLINE, EMBASE, CINAHL and PsycINFO, as well as reference lists and personal files to locate relevant studies. They then assessed the risk of bias of the 60 studies they had selected for inclusion. Although the review found individual recovery expectations are probably strongly associated with future work participation at 12 months follow-up, the association of recovery expectations with other outcomes (including functional limitations and pain intensity) was less certain.

Systematic reviews of diagnostic test studies are carried out to determine estimates of test performance and to consider variation between studies. This type of systematic review uses methods to assess study quality and to combine results different from those used for systematic reviews of randomised controlled trials.[20] An example of this type of review is one that used meta-analytic procedures in a review of the accuracy of chest ultrasonography versus X-ray for the diagnosis of pneumothorax (collapsed lung) in trauma patients in the emergency department.[21] Thirteen studies were included in the review, with a subset of these included in a meta-analysis. The results found that chest ultrasonography had a sensitivity of 0.91 and specificity of 0.99, whereas supine chest X-ray had a sensitivity and specificity of 0.47 and 1.00, respectively. (Refer to Chapter 6 as a reminder of how to interpret sensitivity and specificity.) It was concluded that trauma protocols and algorithms in future medical training programs could incorporate chest ultrasonography for the diagnosis of traumatic pneumothorax.

Systematic reviews of qualitative studies allow us to have a more comprehensive understanding, for example, of a phenomenon of interest (for example, women's conceptualisation of what good antenatal care looks like). In addition, these reviews help us to identify associations between the broader environment within which people live and the interventions that are implemented; the values and attitudes towards, and experiences of, health conditions and interventions by those who implement or receive them; and the complexity of interventions and implementation. They provide important insights into the impact of such interventions on different sub-groups of people and the influence of individual and contextual characteristics within different contexts.[22]

Qualitative evidence syntheses are increasingly recognised, both on their own and as a supplement to quantitative systematic reviews. An example of this type of review is one that synthesised 21 qualitative studies exploring patient and public understanding of over-testing (the use of diagnostic tests and screening which lack clear benefits) and overdiagnosis (medically indicated diagnoses that can cause a patient more harm than good).[23] Themes identified that people had difficulty comprehending these concepts but had a willingness to be better informed about and engaged regarding it.

As noted earlier, methods for combining results from both quantitative and qualitative studies within a single review are generally referred to as *mixed-methods reviews*. Several handbooks and documents have been developed to support review authors in conducting these syntheses.[16,24] Examples of mixed-method reviews are now readily available in the Cochrane Library. One example is a systematic review that analysed 33 randomised controlled trials evaluating the effects of school-based interventions to improve self-management of asthma among children, along with 33 studies with qualitative data exploring the intervention features that were aligned with successful implementation.[25] The authors found that the interventions probably reduce hospital admission and may slightly reduce emergency department attendance. The qualitative synthesis revealed the importance of interventions being theory-driven, engaging of parents, and being run outside of children's free time. The potential benefits of mixed methods in this review were that the qualitative data provided further understanding of the quantitative results, and suggested how interventions may be implemented more successfully in future. A successful integration of different types of evidence at a review level improves understanding of complex phenomena and provides a more holistic answer. The criteria by which such reviews need to be assessed partly overlap with those used for other types of review. However, specific criteria on the 'mixing component' are usually added.[26,27] These could, for example, relate to the different methods used to analyse the causal chain presented in an effectiveness review, how they may intersect and whether there is any use of program theory to support the conclusions and reach implications.[28]

LOCATING SYSTEMATIC REVIEWS

It has been mentioned several times in this book that a substantial difficulty in efficiently locating research evidence is the overwhelming quantity of information that is available and the diverse range of journals in which information is published. Unfortunately, systematic reviews are not immune to this problem. As you saw in Chapter 3, the premier source for systematic reviews of studies answering questions about intervention effectiveness is the Cochrane Database of Systematic Reviews. These are reviews coordinated by Cochrane (https://www.cochrane.org) groups, which are editorial teams which support the preparation and maintenance of the reviews, as well as apply rigorous quality standards. The Cochrane Library also now contains some diagnostic accuracy reviews, prognosis reviews, qualitative evidence syntheses and mixed-methods reviews.

Chapter 3 provided the details of other resources that can be used to locate systematic reviews. These include specialist evidence databases (such as Epistemonikos,[29] the TRIP database and PDQ-Evidence), discipline-specific databases (such as PEDro) and the large biomedical databases such as CINAHL and PubMed. (The latter contains a search strategy specifically for locating systematic reviews on the PubMed Clinical Queries screen.) The PROSPERO register is a valuable source for identifying systematic reviews that are underway.[30] When searching for systematic reviews indexed in these resources, the phrase 'systematic review' does not necessarily distinguish well between quantitative and qualitative reviews—or even literature reviews—so you must search and screen results carefully.

HOW ARE SYSTEMATIC REVIEWS CONDUCTED?

The time required to undertake a systematic review varies considerably. It has been estimated that, on average, it can take approximately one year from registration of a review to submission of the completed review for publication.[31] However, the time required will be less for topics in which very little research exists, compared with topics where there is a huge amount of research to find and sort through. Furthermore, there have recently been a few examples where the time to complete a review was as little as two weeks.[32] Such reviews were done by a small team of very experienced systematic reviewers with complementary skills, protected time to work on the review, and who used automation tools to speed up review tasks. Since it is easier to learn how to read, appraise and interpret a systematic review if you understand what is involved in performing one, the methods used for undertaking reviews will also be described in this chapter.

QUANTITATIVE SYSTEMATIC REVIEWS

Whatever the focus of the systematic review question, the overall methods are similar:

1. Define the research question and plan the methods for undertaking the review.
2. Determine the eligibility criteria for studies to be included.
3. Search for potentially eligible studies.
4. Apply eligibility criteria to select studies.
5. Assess the risk of bias in the included studies.
6. Extract data from the included studies.
7. Synthesise the data.
8. Interpret and report the results.
9. Update the review at an appropriate time point in the future.

Define the research question and plan the methods for undertaking the review

As with any research study, when conducting a systematic review the first place to start is with planning the overall project. Planning also ensures that all aspects important to the scientific rigour of a review are undertaken to reduce the risk of bias. Each stage of the review needs to be thoroughly understood prior to moving on to plan the next stage.

The question needs to be clearly focused, as too broad a question will not produce a useful review. The question should also make sense clinically. Involving key stakeholders (both health professionals and patients) may be helpful, as this will ensure that relevant areas of concern, such as the types of interventions or outcomes, are appropriately considered.[33]

Decisions also need to be made about the methods used for searching, screening, appraising and synthesising. They should be made before commencing the review itself and ideally should be written up as a protocol,[34] as this will help to make the whole process systematic and more transparent for all involved. To reduce the duplication of reviews, authors should prospectively register the protocol for the review—for example, in PROSPERO, the International Prospective Register of Systematic Reviews.[35]

Determine the eligibility criteria for studies to be included

The use of explicit, predefined criteria for including and excluding studies (eligibility criteria) is an important feature of systematic reviews. The eligibility criteria to be defined for, and applied in, a systematic review will depend on several factors, such as the type of review question (for example, whether the review is about effects of interventions, or about diagnostic test accuracy or patient experiences) and the population of interest.

Traditionally, eligibility criteria for systematic reviews of the effects of interventions have focused on defining *types of participants* (that is, people and populations), *types of interventions* (and, where relevant, *comparisons*) and *types of studies* (that is, the study designs most suitable for answering the review question). Although systematic reviews of the effects of interventions also typically pre-specify *types of outcomes* (the outcome measures that are important to answer the review question), these usually are not used to include or exclude studies but rather to guide which results from the included studies will be extracted. Generally, systematic reviews of the effects of interventions primarily focus on randomised controlled trials or quasi-randomised controlled trials. However, there are many reviews that include both randomised and non-randomised studies, or which only include non-randomised studies (because the review question of interest cannot be answered by randomised trials). While these reviews can provide a comprehensive overall picture of the available research, they require the reader to be particularly careful when interpreting the conclusions and to consider the study types (and their associated strengths/weaknesses) that may have been used to contribute to the conclusion of the review.

Search for potentially eligible studies

The search methodology needs to be developed prior to commencing the review and be clearly explained and reproducible. Generally, for a systematic review evaluating the effects of an intervention, the 'participant' and 'intervention' components of the review question, as well as the study design(s), should be considered when developing the search strategy (that is, it will inform the list of terms entered into the databases and other resources). A wide variety of synonyms for these key components of the search should be incorporated, using free text terms and appropriate controlled vocabulary (for example, MeSH, Emtree).[36] The search strategy should not be limited by publication date, publication format or language unless there is a good reason for doing so (such as an intervention only being available after a certain point in time).

Searching should occur across multiple health-related bibliographic databases (for example, MEDLINE, Embase), as search strategies that are limited to one database do not identify all of the relevant studies.[37] Attempts can also be made to obtain unpublished studies (including masters and doctoral research and conference proceedings) by searching the CENTRAL database in the Cochrane Library, grey literature databases and trials registers (for example, ClinicalTrials.gov). Ideally, the review authors should also contact authors in the field in an attempt to locate other studies that have not already been identified, identify ongoing or planned studies in the area, and to ask about and obtain written copies of unpublished studies.[38] The reason for doing this is to limit a problem called '**publication bias**', which can occur due to study authors being more likely to submit studies with statistically significant results that are favourable to the experimental intervention for publication, thus leading to the suppression of studies with 'negative' results.[39] Citation tracking, or use of the references from the studies found, may also help the reviewer to locate further studies on the topic and increase the comprehensiveness of the search.

As an illustration of how important it is that review authors use a comprehensive search strategy, one study found that across 58 systematic reviews, 20% of eligible studies were missed by searching only MEDLINE, but this reduced to 2% when MEDLINE, Embase, Web of Science and Google Scholar were searched.[37] Another study found that while searching for and including unpublished studies may not necessarily change meta-analysis summary estimates, doing so often leads to an increase in the precision of the summary estimates.[40] For qualitative studies, indexing in biomedical and health-related databases has considerably improved, with an analysis finding that 94% of the included studies in qualitative reviews were retrieved from nine major databases. The remaining studies need to be located using several other databases and alternative search strategies such as handsearching and consulting grey literature.[41]

Apply eligibility criteria to select studies

Once the search is completed and potentially relevant studies have been identified, the next task is to decide which of the studies should be included in the systematic review. Not all articles that are located during the search will be directly relevant to the review question. Eligibility criteria are established to guide the selection of studies to be included in the review. The criteria specify the studies, participants, interventions and outcomes that are to be included. Ideally, the selection process should then be carried out by two or more authors independently to minimise bias. Titles and abstracts are screened first for potential relevance and eligibility. At this point, some citations will be excluded as it will be clear from the title and abstract that they do not meet the review eligibility criteria. The full text of citations that appear eligible or for which eligibility is unclear due to insufficient information in the title and abstract is then retrieved so that a more detailed evaluation can be done. A final evaluation of the full-text articles is conducted and a decision is made whether to include or exclude the studies. A flow diagram summarising the study selection processes, showing the number of records screened and excluded at

each step (along with reasons for exclusion), should also be appended to the review.[2]

Assess the risk of bias in the included studies

The next step is to assess if the studies being accepted into the systematic review could be biased. This is appropriately called a 'risk of bias assessment'. Including studies with a high risk of bias can serve to magnify the impact of that bias, and thus may raise doubts about the validity of the systematic review's results and conclusions.[42] Where such studies are included in the review, it is important that the risk of bias is clearly communicated to the reader. To guard against errors and increase the reliability of the risk of bias assessment, it is recommended that more than one person independently assess the risk of bias in the results of the included studies.[42] The potential for bias in individual studies can be determined in several ways, such as using the approach to appraising randomised controlled trials that was explained in Chapter 4 of this book. Systematic reviews in the Cochrane Database of Systematic Reviews use a 'risk of bias' tool, which includes multiple key domains as set out in Table 12.1. Implementation of this tool requires two steps:

1. Extract information from the original study report about each criterion to describe what was reported to have happened in the study (see the 'Issues addressed' column in Table 12.1).
2. Make a judgment about the likely risk of bias in relation to each criterion (rated as 'low risk' of bias, 'high risk' of bias, or 'some concerns').

Extract data from the included studies

Various types of information about each included study need to be collected so that the findings can be interpreted appropriately. Generally, data collected from quantitative research studies include characteristics of the study (such as country in which it was set, and the funding source), characteristics of the study design (such as randomised or non-randomised study), characteristics of the participants (such as age and gender), characteristics of the interventions (such as how they were delivered, by whom and for how long) and the results (such as summary statistics and effect estimates).[45] Standardised data collection forms are typically used, so that the data are collected consistently. Having more than one author independently extract data from reports of included studies can minimise errors in the data presented in the review.[46]

Synthesise the data

Before we explain what review authors do at this stage of the process, you first need to understand the principles of meta-analysis in more detail. As mentioned at the beginning of

TABLE 12.1 **Domains of bias in the initial (RoB 1) and revised (RoB 2) Cochrane risk of bias tool for randomised controlled trials**

Domain in RoB 1	Domain in RoB 2	Issues addressed
Random sequence generation (selection bias) Allocation concealment (selection bias)	Bias arising from the randomisation process	Whether the method used to generate the allocation sequence was random, and whether the allocation sequence was concealed using a method that prevented intervention allocations from being foreseen in advance of, or during, enrolment.
Blinding of participants and personnel (performance bias)	Bias due to deviations from intended interventions	Whether study investigators used methods to blind study participants and personnel from knowledge of which intervention a participant received, and if not, whether deviations from the intended intervention (e.g. use of co-interventions, lack of adherence to interventions) arose and were unbalanced between groups.
Incomplete outcome data (attrition bias)	Bias due to missing outcome data	Whether outcome data were missing for some participants—for example, due to dropout and loss to follow-up—and if so, whether the amount and reasons for missing outcome data differed between groups.
Blinding of outcome assessors (detection bias)	Bias in measurement of the outcome	Whether any methods were used to blind outcome assessors from knowledge of which intervention a participant received, and if not, whether assessment of the outcome was likely to have been influenced by knowledge of the intervention received.
Selective reporting (reporting bias)	Bias in selection of the reported result	Whether trialists reported only a subset of results that were generated, based on the statistical significance, magnitude or direction of effect.

RoB 1: Based on Higgins JPT, Altman DG, Gotzsche PC, et al. The Cochrane Collaboration's tool for assessing risk of bias in randomised trials. BMJ 2011;343:d5928. RoB 2: Based on Sterne JAC, Savovic J, Page MJ, et al. RoB 2: a revised tool for assessing risk of bias in randomised trials. BMJ 2019;366:l4898.

this chapter, a meta-analysis combines the data obtained from all studies answering the same clinical question included in a systematic review and produces an overall summary effect. The rationale behind a meta-analysis is that combining the samples of individual studies means the overall sample size is increased. This improves the power of the analysis and therefore the precision of the estimate of the summary effect of the intervention.[4]

When review authors plan a systematic review, the process by which they will conduct the meta-analysis should be clearly outlined and include the following steps:[47]

1. Clearly match the analysis strategy to the goals of the review.
2. Decide what types of study designs should be included in the meta-analysis.
3. Set the criteria used to decide whether to undertake a meta-analysis (or not to—see below!).
4. Identify what types of outcome data are likely to be found in the studies and outline how each will be managed.
5. Identify what effects measures (for example, risk ratio, mean difference) will be used.

6. Decide the meta-analysis method (for example, inverse-variance) and model (for example, random-effects or fixed-effect) that will be used.
7. Decide how to manage studies' clinical and methodological differences (this is called 'heterogeneity'—discussed below).
8. Decide how risk of bias in included studies will be incorporated in the meta-analysis.
9. Decide how missing data in the included studies will be managed.
10. Decide how publication and other reporting biases will be managed.

There are two stages to doing a meta-analysis. First, an intervention effect estimate and a measure of precision (for example, standard error or confidence interval) is calculated for each of the studies, using the same effect measure so that each study can be described in the same way. The effect measure used will depend on the type of outcome data found in the studies, with commonly used effect measures including odds ratios, risk ratios (also known as 'relative risks') and mean differences.[48] As we

TABLE 12.2   Examples of statistical measures of intervention effect that can be used in a meta-analysis

Type of outcome data	Measures of intervention effect
Dichotomous or binary (one of two categories)	Risk ratio (RR) (also called 'relative risk')
	Odds ratio (OR)
	Risk difference (RD)
	Number needed to treat (NNT)
Continuous (numerical)	Mean difference
	Standardised mean difference (SMD)
Ordinal (including measurement scales)	Proportional odds ratio
	Recalculated as binary data
Counts and rates (e.g. number of events)	Rate ratio
Time to event (survival data)	Hazard ratio

saw in Chapter 4 when learning how to interpret the results of randomised controlled trials, if the outcome is dichotomous then odds ratios or risk ratios may be used. For continuous outcomes, mean differences may be used. Table 12.2 lists some of the effect measures that can be used in a meta-analysis based on the outcome data type as outlined in the *Cochrane Handbook for Systematic Reviews of Interventions*.[47]

The second stage in a meta-analysis is calculating the *overall* intervention effect. This is generally a weighted average of the effect estimates from the individual studies. This process is described in more detail later in this chapter.

Not all systematic reviews can undertake a meta-analysis. The most important reason is excessive heterogeneity—when the studies (usually the interventions or the outcomes, but also participants and settings) are not similar enough for it to make sense for them to be combined. For example, in a systematic review of the effects of consumers and health providers working in partnership to promote person-centred health services, five trials were found but the results were not combined in a meta-analysis as the studies were heterogeneous in terms of the 'working in partnership' interventions delivered, what they were compared to, and which outcomes were used to measure effectiveness.[49] These differences mean that it was not correct to combine the results in a meta-analysis, and the review authors summarised the results descriptively by comparison and outcome (in text and tables) instead.

Interpret and report the results

The results of a systematic review are presented narratively in the text, while the results of a meta-analysis are also displayed visually using a forest plot. Forest plots are made up of tree plots (explained in Chapter 4 and in Figure 4.4) represented in one figure. They display both the information from the individual studies included in the review (such as the intervention effect estimate and the associated confidence interval) *and* an estimate of the overall effect. We will take a closer look at interpreting a forest plot towards the end of this chapter when we look at the results from a specific systematic review (see Figure 12.2). In some systematic reviews in which it may not be advisable to statistically combine data, forest plots may still be presented but without an overall estimate (summary statistic). Forest plots are useful, as they allow readers to visually assess the amount of variation among the studies that are included in the review.[50]

Conclusions that may be reached in systematic reviews include:

- The results from a review consistently show positive (or negative) effects of an intervention. In this case, the review authors might state that the results (that is, the evidence) are convincing.
- There are conflicting results from studies within the review. In this case, the authors might state that the evidence is inconclusive.
- Only a few studies (or sometimes none) that meet the eligibility criteria were found. In this case, authors might conclude that there is insufficient evidence about the effects of the intervention.

Remember not to confuse 'no evidence' (or 'no evidence of an effect') with 'evidence of no effect': it is not correct to say the results of the review show that an intervention has 'no effect' or is 'no different' from the control intervention when there is inconclusive evidence.[51]

Another feature of recent systematic reviews is the use of Grading of Recommendations, Assessment, Development and Evaluations (GRADE).[52] This is a method for summarising the overall certainty in the body of evidence (and the strength of recommendations for guidelines, as you will see in Chapter 13). GRADE encourages us to evaluate the body of evidence overall for risk of bias across studies, inconsistency of results (heterogeneity), indirectness, imprecision (having wide confidence intervals) and other factors such as reporting bias (if sufficient trials were included in the meta-analysis). The GRADE ratings of *high*, *moderate*, *low* or *very low* indicate how certain we can be in the effect estimates. For example, a rating of *high* certainty means we are very confident that the true effect lies close to that of the estimate of the effect. A rating of *very low* certainty means we have very little confidence in the effect estimate: the true effect is likely to be substantially different from the estimate of effect.[53] A 'Summary of Findings' table summarises the GRADE certainty of evidence and the magnitude of overall effect for each outcome, and provides detailed information about the reason for the certainty of evidence rating.[54] The systematic review[55] that we appraise later in this chapter has a 'Summary of Findings' table that you can see if you look at the full review in the Cochrane Library. A version of GRADE for assessing certainty in qualitative evidence syntheses—GRADE-CERQual—also exists.[56] The use of GRADE is discussed in more detail in Chapter 13.

Update the review at an appropriate time in the future

At some point after a systematic review is published, new studies may be published which might overturn the results and conclusions of the review. Therefore, review authors should periodically consider whether there is a need to update the review—that is, search for new studies meeting the inclusion criteria and incorporate the results of eligible studies into the review.[57] Some review teams might decide they only need to update their review every couple of years. On the other hand, some teams might conduct a 'living systematic review', which involves continuously updating the review on a regular basis (for example, every month) and incorporating new evidence as it becomes available. Living systematic reviews are particularly important when evidence on the topic emerges rapidly and the new evidence might change policy or practice decisions.[58]

CRITICAL APPRAISAL OF QUANTITATIVE SYSTEMATIC REVIEWS

Now that you understand what is involved in undertaking a systematic review of quantitative studies, let us look at how to critically appraise systematic reviews. As with other types of studies, not all systematic reviews are carried out using rigorous methods and, therefore, bias may be introduced into the results and conclusions of the review. A review of 300 systematic reviews indexed in databases in November 2020 found that reporting was suboptimal, and would be improved if widely agreed reporting standards were adhered to by authors and journals.[59] Just because the evidence that you have found which appears to answer your clinical question is a systematic review, this does not mean that you can automatically trust its results. It is important that you critically appraise systematic reviews and determine whether you can trust their results and conclusions.

Using the three-step critical appraisal process that we have used elsewhere in this book to appraise other types of studies, the three key elements to be considered when appraising a systematic review are: (1) the **validity or overall methodological soundness** of the review methods; (2) the **magnitude and precision of the intervention effect** (or the trustworthiness of the findings for qualitative evidence syntheses); and (3) the **applicability of the review findings** to your specific patient or patient population.

There are a number of checklists or tools that can be used to critically appraise systematic reviews, many of which are based on the early Overview of Quality Assessment Questionnaire[60] and the article on systematic reviews in the *Users' Guide to Evidence-Based Medicine*.[1] Four commonly used appraisal checklists are the CASP checklist for appraising reviews (https://casp-uk.net/); A MeaSurement Tool to Assess systematic Reviews (AMSTAR-2) tool;[61] the Risk Of Bias In Systematic Reviews (ROBIS) tool;[62] and the appraisal criteria suggested by Greenhalgh and Donald.[63] Box 12.1 lists key questions that you can ask when critically appraising a quantitative systematic review. These questions are from the AMSTAR-2.[61]

BOX 12.1 Key questions to ask when critically appraising a systematic review (based on AMSTAR [A MeaSurement Tool to Assess systematic Reviews] 2)

1. **Did the research questions and inclusion criteria for the review include the components of PICO?**
   For yes, it should include:
   a. Population
   b. Intervention
   c. Comparator group
   d. Outcome
   e. Time frame for follow-up (optional, recommended)
2. **Did the report of the review contain an explicit statement that the review methods were established prior to the conduct of the review and did the report justify any significant deviations from**
the protocol? *For partial yes, the authors should state that they had a written protocol or guide that included ALL the following:*
   a. Review question(s)
   b. A search strategy
   c. Inclusion/exclusion criteria
   d. A risk of bias assessment.
   For yes, the protocol should also be registered and should have specified:
   e. A meta-analysis/synthesis plan, if appropriate
   f. A plan for investigating causes of heterogeneity
   g. Justification for any deviations from the protocol.

Continued

BOX 12.1 Key questions to ask when critically appraising a systematic review (based on AMSTAR [A MeaSurement Tool to Assess systematic Reviews] 2)—cont'd

3. **Did the review authors explain their selection of the study designs for inclusion in the review?** *For yes, the review should satisfy ONE of the following:*
   a. Explanation for including only randomised trials
   b. OR explanation for including only non-randomised studies for interventions (NSRI)
   c. OR explanation for including both randomised controlled trials (RCT) and non-randomised studies for interventions.

4. **Did the review authors use a comprehensive literature search strategy?** *For partial yes, the authors should state ALL the following:*
   a. Searched at least two databases (relevant to research question)
   b. Provided key word and/or search strategy
   c. Justified publication restrictions (e.g. language).
   For yes, should also have ALL the following:
   d. Searched the reference lists/bibliographies of included studies
   e. Searched trial/study registries
   f. Included/consulted content experts in the field
   g. Where relevant, searched for grey literature
   h. Conducted search within 24 months of completion of the review.

5. **Did the review authors perform study selection in duplicate?** *For yes, either ONE of the following:*
   a. At least two reviewers independently agreed on selection of eligible studies and achieved consensus on which studies to include.
   b. OR two reviewers selected a sample of eligible studies and achieved good agreement (at least 80%), with the remainder selected by one reviewer.

6. **Did the review authors perform data extraction in duplicate?** *For yes, either ONE of the following:*
   a. At least two reviewers achieved consensus on which data to extract from included studies.
   b. OR two reviewers extracted data from a sample of eligible studies and achieved good agreement (at least 80%), with the remainder extracted by one reviewer.

7. **Did the review authors provide a list of excluded studies and justify the exclusions?** *For partial yes, the authors should have:*
   a. Provided a list of all potentially relevant studies that were read in full-text form but excluded from the review.
   For yes, the authors must also have:
   b. Justified the exclusion from the review of each potentially relevant study.

8. **Did the review authors describe the included studies in adequate detail?** *For partial yes, the authors should have ALL the following:*
   a. Described populations
   b. Described interventions
   c. Described comparators
   d. Described outcomes
   e. Described research designs.
   For yes, the authors should also have ALL the following:
   f. Described population in detail
   g. Described intervention in detail (including doses where relevant)
   h. Described comparator in detail (including doses where relevant)
   i. Described study's setting
   j. Time frame for follow-up.

9. **Did the review authors use a satisfactory technique for assessing the risk of bias (RoB) in individual studies that were included in the review? Relevant to RCTs** *For partial yes, the authors must have assessed RoB from:*
   a. Unconcealed allocation, and
   b. Lack of blinding of patients and assessors when assessing outcomes (unnecessary for objective outcomes such as all-cause mortality).
   For yes, the authors must also have assessed RoB from:
   c. Allocation sequence that was not truly random, and
   d. Selection of the reported result from among multiple measurements or analyses of a specified outcome.
   Relevant to NRSI *For partial yes, the authors must have assessed RoB:*
   e. From confounding, and
   f. From selection bias.
   For yes, the authors must also have assessed RoB:
   g. Methods used to ascertain exposures and outcomes, and
   h. Selection of the reported result from among multiple measurements or analyses of a specified outcome.

10. **Did the review authors report on the sources of funding for the studies included in the review?** *For yes:*
    a. Must have reported on the sources of funding for individual studies included in the review. *Note:* Reporting that the reviewers looked for this information, but it was not reported by study authors, also qualifies.

BOX 12.1   Key questions to ask when critically appraising a systematic review (based on AMSTAR [A MeaSurement Tool to Assess systematic Reviews] 2)—cont'd

11. **If meta-analysis was performed, did the review authors use appropriate methods for statistical combination of results? Relevant to RCTs** *For yes:*
    a. The authors justified combining the data in meta-analysis.
    b. AND they used an appropriate weighted technique to combine study results and adjusted for heterogeneity if present.
    c. AND they investigated the causes of any heterogeneity.
    Relevant to NRSI *For yes:*
    d. The authors justified combining the data in a meta-analysis.
    e. AND they used an appropriate weighted technique to combine study results, adjusting for heterogeneity if present.
    f. AND they statistically combined effect estimates from NRSI that were adjusted for confounding, rather than combining raw data, or justified combining raw data when adjusted effect estimates were not available.
    g. AND they reported separate summary estimates for RCTs and NRSI separately when both were included in the review.

12. **If meta-analysis was performed, did the review authors assess the potential impact of RoB in individual studies on the results of the meta-analysis or other evidence synthesis?** *For yes:*
    a. Included only low risk of bias RCTs
    b. OR, if the pooled estimate was based on RCTs and/or NRSI at variable RoB, the authors performed analyses to investigate possible impact of RoB on summary estimates of effect.

13. **Did the review authors account for ROB in individual studies when interpreting/discussing the results of the review?** *For yes:*
    a. Included only low risk of bias RCTs
    b. OR, if RCTs with moderate or high RoB, or NRSI were included, the review provided a discussion of the likely impact of RoB on the results.

14. **Did the review authors provide a satisfactory explanation for, and discussion of, any heterogeneity observed in the results of the review?** *For yes:*
    a. There was no significant heterogeneity in the results.
    b. OR if heterogeneity was present the authors performed an investigation of sources of any heterogeneity in the results and discussed the impact of this on the results of the review.

15. **If they performed quantitative synthesis, did the review authors carry out an adequate investigation of publication bias (small study bias) and discuss its likely impact on the results of the review?** *For yes:*
    a. Performed graphical or statistical tests for publication bias and discussed the likelihood and magnitude of impact of publication bias.

16. **Did the review authors report any potential sources of conflict of interest, including any funding they received for conducting the review?** *For yes:*
    a. The authors reported no competing interests.
    b. OR the authors described their funding sources and how they managed potential conflicts of interest.

Overall confidence in the results of the systematic review

The authors of AMSTAR 2 recommend that individual item ratings are not combined to create an overall score but that users instead consider the potential impact of inadequate ratings for included items.[44] They suggest the following items are the most critical domains affecting the validity of a review's findings, so rating the overall confidence in the results should reflect the extent to which there are concerns with one or more of these areas:

- Protocol registered before commencement of the review (item 2)
- Adequacy of the literature search (item 4)
- Justification for excluding individual studies (item 7)
- Risk of bias from individual studies being included in the review (item 9)
- Appropriateness of meta-analytical methods (item 11)
- Consideration of risk of bias when interpreting the results of the review (item 13)
- Assessment of presence and likely impact of publication bias (item 15).

High overall confidence in the results of the review is obtained when *no or one non-critical weakness* is identified and the systematic review provides an accurate and comprehensive summary of the results of the available studies that address the question of interest.

Moderate overall confidence is obtained when *more than one non-critical weakness* is identified and the systematic review may provide an accurate summary of the results of the available studies that were included in the

Continued

> **BOX 12.1   Key questions to ask when critically appraising a systematic review (based on AMSTAR [A MeaSurement Tool to Assess systematic Reviews] 2)—cont'd**
>
> review (*Note:* Multiple non-critical weaknesses may diminish confidence in the review and it may be appropriate to move the overall appraisal down from moderate to low confidence.)
> **Low overall confidence** is obtained when *one critical flaw with or without non-critical weaknesses* is identified. The review has a critical flaw and may not provide an accurate and comprehensive summary of the available studies that address the question of interest.
> **Critically low overall confidence** is judged when *more than one critical flaw with or without non-critical weaknesses* is identified. The review has more than one critical flaw and should not be relied on to provide an accurate and comprehensive summary of the available studies.
>
> Based on AMSTAR (A MeaSurement Tool to Assess systematic Reviews) 2 Rationale for selection of items https://amstar.ca/Amstar_Checklist.php Copyright © 2021 AMSTAR All Rights Reserved.

CRITICAL APPRAISAL OF SYSTEMATIC REVIEWS—A WORKED EXAMPLE

To help you further understand how to critically appraise and use systematic reviews to inform clinical decisions, we will consider an extended clinical scenario (with two parts), formulate relevant clinical questions, locate a systematic review of quantitative studies—and, later, a review of qualitative studies, that might address those questions and then critically appraise the reviews. The box describes the clinical scenario that we will use.

◎ **CLINICAL SCENARIO (PART 1)**

Clinical question and finding the evidence to answer the question

A multidisciplinary team in an outpatient stroke rehabilitation facility attached to a large metropolitan hospital wants to encourage healthy lifestyle behaviours—in particular, physical fitness—among people who have had a recent stroke, because of the potential benefits for minimising disability after discharge and reducing the risk of readmission. To help provide current evidence about the benefits of physical fitness training for people after stroke, the team decides to conduct a search of the literature. The team formed a clinical question.

Clinical question
For people who have had a stroke, does fitness training reduce disability and improve fitness compared to usual care?

Search terms and databases used to find the evidence
Database: Cochrane Database of Systematic Reviews
Search terms: ("stroke survivors" AND "physical fitness training")

Using these terms there was only one systematic review in the Cochrane Database that focused on physical fitness training,[55] so the team decide to start reading the full text of this review.

◎ **CLINICAL SCENARIO (PART 1) (CONTINUED)**

Structured abstract of chosen quantitative article
Citation: Saunders DH, Sanderson M, Hayes S, et al. Physical fitness training for stroke patients. Cochrane Database of Systematic Reviews 2020, Issue 3. Art. No.: CD003316. doi: 10.1002/14651858.CD003316.pub7.[55]
Objectives: The primary objective of this review was to ascertain if 'fitness training' post-stroke reduces death, death or dependence, and disability. The secondary objective was to determine its effect on adverse events, risk factors, physical fitness, mobility, physical function, health status and quality of life, mood and cognitive function. This was an updated review.
Search strategy: The authors searched nine databases, ongoing trials registers and a range of other sources with the latest search in July 2018.

Selection criteria: Included studies were randomised trials of adults with stroke living in the community that compared either cardiorespiratory training or resistance training, or both (mixed training), with usual care, no intervention, or a non-exercise intervention, and considered any of the outcomes of interest to the objectives of this review.

Data collection and analysis: Eligibility, data extraction and risk of bias assessment were completed by two review authors independently.

Main results: Seventy-five studies were included, which tested cardiorespiratory (32 studies), resistance (20 studies) or mixed training interventions (23 studies). Results found that death was not influenced by any intervention.

Disability scores were improved post-intervention by cardiorespiratory training, and mixed training, with insufficient data to determine the effects of resistance training. There were benefits from training on physical fitness, mobility and physical function (balance). Cardiorespiratory fitness (VO_2 peak) increased after cardiorespiratory training. There were no serious adverse events, and insufficient data meant effects on mood, quality of life and cognition could not be determined.

Authors' conclusions: The authors concluded that exercise is safe, and that there is evidence for cardiorespiratory and mixed training to improve fitness, balance, and the speed and capacity of walking, which may benefit stroke survivors living in the community.

◎ CLINICAL SCENARIO (PART 1) (CONTINUED)

Critical appraisal of chosen quantitative review
Using the questions that are outlined in Box 12.1, we will now step you through a critical appraisal of this systematic review.

A. Were the methods used in the review valid?
1. Did the research questions and inclusion criteria for the review include the components of Population, Intervention, Comparator and Outcome (PICO)?
Yes. While the review did not articulate review questions per se, it stated the aims of the review were 'to determine whether fitness training after stroke reduces death, death or dependence, and disability' and 'to determine the effects of training on adverse events, risk factors, physical fitness, mobility, physical function, health status and quality of life, mood, and cognitive function'. The PICO are:
a. *Population:* Adult stroke survivors considered suitable for fitness training by the studies' authors, irrespective of the time after stroke.
b. *Intervention(s) and comparator(s):* Physical fitness interventions involving a systematic, progressive increase in the intensity or resistance, frequency or duration of physical fitness training through a scheduled program and including at least one of the following: (i) cardiorespiratory training (aimed at improving the cardiorespiratory component of physical fitness—for example, treadmills, cycling, rowing, walking, stairs); (ii) resistance training (aimed at improving muscle strength and endurance or power output—for example, body weight exercises, use of elastic devices, free weights, machine weights); (iii) mixed

training (aimed at improving cardiorespiratory fitness and strength, power or muscular endurance—for example, a program comprising both cycling and weight training). The authors excluded studies that focused on standard rehabilitation techniques without a physical fitness training component; combined fitness training with assistive technologies; virtual reality approaches; and studies comparing upper and lower body training in the absence of a non-exercise control group. Comparators were usual care, no intervention or wait-list control, or sham intervention, attention control or adjunct intervention.
c. *Outcome(s):* The primary outcomes were death, death or dependence, and disability. Secondary outcomes included adverse effects, vascular risk factors, physical fitness, mobility, physical function, health-related quality of life, mood and cognitive function. The *time frame for follow-up* was at the end of the intervention period and at the end of the longest follow-up.

2. Did the report of the review contain an explicit statement that the review methods were established prior to the conduct of the review and did the report justify any significant deviations from the protocol?
Yes. The review refers to a previous version of the review and associated registered Cochrane protocol that outlined the aims, search strategy, selection criteria, and methods for risk of bias assessment, meta-analysis/synthesis and investigation of heterogeneity. The authors justified not conducting previously planned sub-group analyses as there were too few studies in the meta-analysis, too many other influential factors, and the scope and breadth of the review made these unmanageable.

Continued

◎ CLINICAL SCENARIO (PART 1) (CONTINUED)—cont'd

3. Did the review authors explain their selection of the study designs for inclusion in the review?

No. The review authors stated they only included randomised controlled trials but did not justify this decision.

4. Did the review authors use a comprehensive literature search strategy?

Yes. The review authors searched nine databases, ongoing trials registers, dissertation and theses repositories, grey literature (Google Scholar), and screened reference lists of included studies, conducted forward citation tracking of included studies and contacted researchers in the field to identify additional relevant studies. The search strategy for each database is included in the appendices. The authors stated that they included studies published in languages other than English when a translation could be arranged and did not report exclusion of any study on the basis of language in the table of excluded studies. The review was published within 24 months of the search being conducted.

5. Did the review authors perform study selection in duplicate?

Yes. Two review authors independently screened studies against the review's eligibility criteria and selected studies for inclusion. They resolved any disagreements through discussion or by consulting a third review author.

6. Did the review authors perform data extraction in duplicate?

No. Only one review author extracted data from the included studies and entered it into Review Manager 5 software. This was cross checked by a second review author. Independent extraction and checking of data from a sample of eligible studies was not performed.

7. Did the review authors provide a list of excluded studies and justify the exclusions?

Yes. The authors included a PRISMA flow chart summarising the screening and selection process, including exclusions, and provided a table of excluded studies with reasons.

8. Did the review authors describe the included studies in adequate detail?

Yes. The authors summarised the populations, interventions, comparators, outcomes and research designs of the 75 included studies in the main text of the review and also provided detail for each study in the table of included studies.

9. Did the review authors use a satisfactory technique for assessing the risk of bias in individual studies that were included in the review?

Yes. Two review authors independently assessed the risk of bias in included studies using the Cochrane Risk of Bias tool. The review authors made minor amendments to the tool and justified the reasons for their amendments. For example, given participant blinding is often impossible to achieve in behavioural interventions they considered studies to be at low risk of bias if the study authors described some attempt to disguise the true purpose of the comparisons being made (for example, describing a study as a comparison of two different interventions or a 'sham' intervention) and considered studies to be at high risk of bias if there was an imbalanced exposure such as would occur with no control intervention or wait-list control.

10. Did the review authors report on the sources of funding for the studies included in the review?

No. The authors did not report on the sources of funding for individual studies or an attempt to look for this information.

11. If meta-analysis was performed, did the review authors use appropriate methods for statistical combination of results?

Yes. The review authors conducted meta-analyses when the included studies were sufficiently similar (that is, similar participants, interventions, comparators and outcomes). The authors reported six main comparisons:

- cardiorespiratory training versus control for people with stroke at the end of intervention and at the end of follow-up (comparisons 1 and 2)
- resistance training versus control for people with stroke at the end of intervention and at the end of follow-up (comparisons 3 and 4)
- mixed training (that is, cardiorespiratory plus resistance training) versus control for people with stroke at the end of intervention and at the end of follow-up (comparisons 5 and 6).

They used random-effects models to calculate a summary intervention effect estimate and 95% confidence interval for each outcome (for example, death, dead or dependent, disability) where there were sufficient data to combine. They assessed heterogeneity using the I^2 statistic and interpreted values of I^2 exceeding 50% as indicating substantial heterogeneity. For the main comparison (cardiorespiratory training versus control) and the primary outcome (death) there was no heterogeneity.

12. If meta-analysis was performed, did the review authors assess the potential impact of risk of bias in individual studies on the results of the meta-analysis or other evidence synthesis?

Yes. The summary effect estimates for some outcomes in the review were based on randomised trials at variable risk of bias and the authors took this into account in their assessment of the certainty of the evidence using the GRADE approach. They also performed analyses to investigate the possible impact of risk of bias on the summary effect estimates, where relevant.

13. Did the review authors account for risk of bias in individual studies when interpreting/discussing the results of the review?

Yes. The risk of bias of studies contributing to outcomes was taken into account by the review authors in their assessment of the certainty of the evidence for the summary effect estimates using GRADE.

14. Did the review authors provide a satisfactory explanation for, and discussion of, any heterogeneity observed in the results of the review?

Yes. While the summary effect estimates for several outcomes in the review displayed little or no heterogeneity (for example, $I^2=0\%$ for the primary outcome death in the main comparison cardiorespiratory training versus control), the authors found substantial heterogeneity in the summary estimates of effect for other outcomes and attempted to investigate the sources of the heterogeneity with subsequent analysis. For example, the summary effect estimate for disability with cardiorespiratory training versus control had an I^2 value of 61%; however, when one included study with multiple risk of bias concerns was excluded in a sensitivity analysis, the heterogeneity disappeared and the beneficial effect of cardiorespiratory training remained.

15. If they performed quantitative synthesis, did the review authors carry out an adequate investigation of publication bias (small study bias) and discuss its likely impact on the results of the review?

Yes. The review authors prepared funnel plots of treatment effect versus study size and discussed the potential for publication bias where meta-analyses contained at least ten studies. For example, a funnel plot of data from 17 studies assessing walking endurance using the 6-minute walk test for cardiorespiratory training versus control shows no evidence of asymmetry or potential for publication bias.

16. Did the review authors report any potential sources of conflict of interest, including any funding they received for conducting the review?

No. One review author declared they co-authored one included study and another review author declared they receive royalties for a book about fitness training after stroke and led one included study. However, the review authors did not describe how they managed potential conflicts of interest (for example, by not making study eligibility decisions, extracting data or conducting risk of bias assessments for the relevant study).

Overall confidence in the results of the review

This review on physical fitness training for people following stroke had weaknesses in four domains (items 3, 6, 10, 16) but no critical flaws and so is judged as providing an accurate and comprehensive summary of the results of the available studies that address the question of interest.

B. What are the results of the review?

Before looking at the results of the systematic review about physical fitness training for people after stroke, some explanations are needed about the effect estimates that are presented. You can see that the authors were dealing mostly with continuous data for the various outcomes. When combining continuous data from different studies, review authors can use either mean differences (as done for the outcome about mobility) or standardised mean differences (as used for disability). Standardised mean differences (SMDs) are used in meta-analysis when the same outcome is measured in different studies, but different instruments are used to measure it.

For the few dichotomous outcomes considered in the review (for example, death), the review authors reported risk differences.

1. What are the overall results of the review?

Seventy-five trials were included in this systematic review. Results from meta-analysis of eight trials found that cardiorespiratory training improved disability scores at the end of the intervention (standardised mean difference [SMD] 0.52, 95% confidence interval [CI] 0.19 to 0.84, $P = 0.002$; moderate-certainty evidence) and increased cardiorespiratory fitness (VO_2 peak) (MD, 3.40 mL/kg/min, 95% CI 2.98 to 3.83, $P < 0.00001$; moderate-certainty evidence) compared with control. Death was not influenced by any intervention; risk differences were all 0.00 (low-certainty evidence).

Continued

◎ CLINICAL SCENARIO (PART 1) (CONTINUED)—cont'd

There are several important things to note from these results. First, we need to understand the size of the effects reported. One way to interpret the size of an SMD is to use Cohen's effect size guidelines.[51] Cohen suggested that 0.2 represents a small effect size, 0.5 a moderate effect size and 0.8 a large effect size. Using these guidelines, the SMD for 'disability' (0.52) would be considered a moderate effect size.

Second, you can see that the authors have undertaken an evaluation of the certainty of the evidence using the GRADE approach, which was discussed earlier in this chapter. The authors have judged the evidence for cardiorespiratory training's effects on disability as moderate certainty, which means 'we are moderately confident in the effect estimate: the true effect is likely to be close to the estimate of the effect, but there is a possibility that it is substantially different'.[54]

For death, however, the authors judged the certainty of the evidence as low, which means we could really only have limited confidence in the effect estimate because the true effect could be substantially different from the estimate of the effect.[54]

2. How precise are the results?

The precision of the effect size estimates that were reported for disability and cardiorespiratory fitness (VO_2 peak) are not too concerning. For instance, the lower bound of the confidence interval for disability (SMD of 0.19) indicates a small effect, whereas the upper bound of the confidence interval (SMD of 0.84) indicates that a large effect size could be possible; however, the conclusion that cardiorespiratory training is beneficial does not change.

Earlier in this chapter, we introduced the idea of forest plots as a way of visually representing the results from multiple studies within a systematic review. Let us look at the forest plot for disability from the physical fitness for stroke systematic review,[55] shown in Figure 12.2, in a bit more detail:

- We find that the forest plot is labelled to show that effect measures to the *left* of the vertical line favour the control and those to the *right* of the line favour the intervention (cardiorespiratory training).
- The top of each forest plot is labelled to tell you what the **comparisons** are. The forest plot that is included in the systematic review (and shown in Figure 12.2) is titled 'Cardiorespiratory training versus control—end of intervention'.
- The **outcome** of interest in this forest plot is 'Disability—combined disability scales'.

- Each forest plot consists of several **horizontal lines**, with each horizontal line representing one of the individual studies that is included in the review. The length of the horizontal line represents the precision of the result or the confidence interval of the result of the study. In the forest plot in Figure 12.2, the analysis involved eight studies. There is a **square** on each of the lines which represents the intervention effect estimate from each of the individual studies.
- In Figure 12.2 you can see that the authors have run a sub-group analysis; that is, they have separated the studies into those delivering training during usual care from those delivering training after usual care. The **diamond** at the bottom of each sub-group represents the pooled quantitative result from the meta-analysis of that sub-group.
- There is then an overall diamond at the bottom ('total'), which indicates the pooled quantitative result from the meta-analysis of disability overall. For now, we will just consider the interpretation of overall disability.
- At the bottom there is a line that tells you the *scale* for the intervention effect that you are measuring and at the top of the vertical line the type of effect. In this forest plot the type of effect used is the standardised mean difference.
- The **vertical line** in the middle of the plot is the 'line of no effect' where the treatment and the control have the same effect on disability. If the diamond, the standardised mean difference and its confidence interval are more than 0 (and therefore sit to the right of the vertical line), the interpretation is that the intervention (cardiorespiratory training) has resulted in better disability scores compared with control. Had the diamond been to the left of the vertical line, and the standardised mean difference and its confidence interval less than 0, it would have meant that those receiving control had better disability scores than those in the cardiorespiratory training group.
- Looking at the different columns, you can see that the first column on the left is a list of the authors of the various studies. The second and third column provides 'N' (number of participants) and mean (and standard deviations [SD]) for the intervention group for each study. The fourth and fifth columns then provide the number of participants and mean (and SD) for the control groups for each study.
- To the right of the vertical line you can see a column of weights for each study, which is the percentage weight given to each of the individual studies in the pooled meta-analysis. The weight used is a function of the sample size and its variance.

Review: Physical fitness training for stroke patients
Comparison: 1 Cardiorespiratory training versus control—end of intervention
Outcome: 5 Disability—combined disability scales

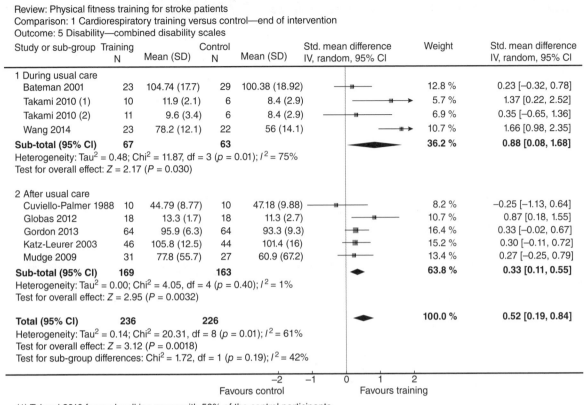

Study or sub-group	Training N	Mean (SD)	Control N	Mean (SD)	Std. mean difference IV, random, 95% CI	Weight	Std. mean difference IV, random, 95% CI
1 During usual care							
Bateman 2001	23	104.74 (17.7)	29	100.38 (18.92)		12.8 %	0.23 [−0.32, 0.78]
Takami 2010 (1)	10	11.9 (2.1)	6	8.4 (2.9)		5.7 %	1.37 [0.22, 2.52]
Takami 2010 (2)	11	9.6 (3.4)	6	8.4 (2.9)		6.9 %	0.35 [−0.65, 1.36]
Wang 2014	23	78.2 (12.1)	22	56 (14.1)		10.7 %	1.66 [0.98, 2.35]
Sub-total (95% CI)	**67**		**63**			**36.2 %**	**0.88 [0.08, 1.68]**

Heterogeneity: Tau^2 = 0.48; Chi^2 = 11.87, df = 3 (p = 0.01); I^2 = 75%
Test for overall effect: Z = 2.17 (P = 0.030)

2 After usual care							
Cuviello-Palmer 1988	10	44.79 (8.77)	10	47.18 (9.88)		8.2 %	−0.25 [−1.13, 0.64]
Globas 2012	18	13.3 (1.7)	18	11.3 (2.7)		10.7 %	0.87 [0.18, 1.55]
Gordon 2013	64	95.9 (6.3)	64	93.3 (9.3)		16.4 %	0.33 [−0.02, 0.67]
Katz-Leurer 2003	46	105.8 (12.5)	44	101.4 (16)		15.2 %	0.30 [−0.11, 0.72]
Mudge 2009	31	77.8 (55.7)	27	60.9 (67.2)		13.4 %	0.27 [−0.25, 0.79]
Sub-total (95% CI)	**169**		**163**			**63.8 %**	**0.33 [0.11, 0.55]**

Heterogeneity: Tau^2 = 0.00; Chi^2 = 4.05, df = 4 (p = 0.40); I^2 = 1%
Test for overall effect: Z = 2.95 (P = 0.0032)

Total (95% CI)	**236**		**226**			**100.0 %**	**0.52 [0.19, 0.84]**

Heterogeneity: Tau^2 = 0.14; Chi^2 = 20.31, df = 8 (p = 0.01); I^2 = 61%
Test for overall effect: Z = 3.12 (P = 0.0018)
Test for sub-group differences: Chi^2 = 1.72, df = 1 (p = 0.19); I^2 = 42%

```
         −2    −1    0    1    2
      Favours control   Favours training
```

(1) Takami 2010 forward-walking group with 50% of the control participants
(2) Takami 2010 backward-walking group with 50% of the control participants

Fig 12.2 Example of a forest plot: effect of cardiorespiratory training on disability.
Saunders DH, Sanderson M, Hayes S, et al. Physical fitness training for stroke patients. Cochrane Database Syst Rev 2020;(3):CD003316. doi: 10.1002/14651858.CD003316.pub7.

- Finally, in the column on the far right are the standardised mean differences with their confidence intervals for each study. The size of the square on each of the horizontal lines is proportional to the percentage of weight that is given to the study in the meta-analysis.
- If the horizontal line for a study crosses the vertical line, it means that the study found no significant difference between the two groups. In our example forest plot, all the studies except three (Takami et al. 2010 (1), Wang et al. 2014 and Globas et al. 2012) cross the vertical line. The study given the largest weight in the analysis is Gordon et al. 2013.
- The middle of the diamond is the summary treatment effect calculated in the meta-analysis. The **width of the diamond** is the precision of the result, generally the 95% confidence interval.[47] In both of the sub-group analyses shown in the forest plot, the intervention is

statistically significant, as can be seen by the associated diamonds not crossing the vertical line. Overall, the result is statistically significant and the diamond is clearly on the right of the vertical line. That is, the cardiorespiratory training interventions were more effective than control for improving disability scores in people after stroke.

C. How relevant are the results?
1. Were all important outcomes considered?
(From the points of view of individuals/patients, policy makers, healthcare professionals, family/carers and the wider community.)

For people who have had a stroke, many important outcomes were considered, with the primary outcomes being death, death or dependence, and disability. Other outcomes that would also be of interest to health

Continued

◎ **CLINICAL SCENARIO (PART 1) (CONTINUED)—cont'd**

professionals were physical fitness, mobility and physical function. Policy makers and managers would be interested in cost-effectiveness, which was not addressed in this review. The authors recommend that future studies should consider the effect on cognitive function and quality of life, and the long-term benefits of training.

2. Can the results be applied to my patient(s)?
If we go back to the clinical scenario raised at the beginning of this worked example, we see that the health professionals in the scenario are working in an outpatient stroke rehabilitation facility attached to a hospital and are particularly looking for evidence about physical fitness

training for people who have recently had a stroke. There should be enough similarity in the characteristics of the patients seen and those in the included studies that the results of the review are relevant. This systematic review of physical training interventions included 75 trials with 3,017 mostly ambulatory participants. However, participants' mean time since stroke had a wide range (8.8 days to 7.7 years), whereas the majority of people seen at the outpatient facility typically had a stroke recently. Given that there were benefits, despite the variation in time since stroke, it is reasonable that the results could be extrapolated from the review population to the patients being seen at the outpatient facility.

◎ **CLINICAL SCENARIO (PART 1) (CONTINUED)**

Resolution of clinical scenario: quantitative review
The question that was raised in the scenario was: *'For people who have had a stroke, does fitness training reduce disability and improve fitness compared to usual care?'* The results from this review provide important information that the therapists can discuss with their patients. It found physical fitness training probably has a moderate effect size for improving disability compared with usual care. However, because a range of different measures were used to measure disability, it would be helpful to look at the individual studies to understand this in more detail. Results also indicate that physical fitness training probably leads to better cardiovascular fitness compared with usual care, which the authors suggest may also reduce the risk of secondary events. Two other helpful conclusions the authors make are that regular training (3–5 days/week), tailored to be progressive in effort, may be more important than the dose of training (which varies

between studies). In addition, there was no evidence of serious adverse events with physical fitness training, which is important for both health professionals and patients to consider, although only a few studies specifically reported adverse events so this finding should be interpreted with caution. To use this information in practice with individuals, members of the multidisciplinary team would need to consider the individual's health status, fitness level and co-morbidities. They would need to have a conversation with each person about the likely benefits of fitness training and this conversation would also need to consider the context of their living situation, interest, motivation and preferences for engaging in fitness training, and other practical considerations. In our scenario, the team can use the evidence in this systematic review to work out how best to refine their service, given the resources available in their outpatient setting, including how best to provide this information to stroke survivors.

QUALITATIVE EVIDENCE SYNTHESES

We now look at qualitative evidence syntheses. We start by considering how these are undertaken, before we look at a specific example. The following steps (similar to the quantitative synthesis steps described earlier) are commonly followed, although not always applied chronologically in all synthesis approaches:

1. Define the review objective or question and, where possible, plan the methods for undertaking the review.

2. Determine the eligibility criteria for studies to be included.
3. Search for potentially eligible studies.
4. Apply eligibility criteria to select studies.
5. Assess the quality of the included studies.
6. Extract and analyse data from the included studies.
7. Synthesise the data.
8. Interpret and report the findings.
9. Update the review at an appropriate time in the future.

Define the review objective or question and, where possible, plan the methods for undertaking the review

The reviews start with a clear understanding of the purpose of the study, expressed as an objective or research question. The elements of the review are then planned, such as the search for individual studies, screening, assessment of quality and synthesis. Unlike quantitative reviews, the content of qualitative review protocols may be more subject to change. For example, in a review exploring the impact of arts-based methods on empowerment processes with vulnerable populations in the community,[64] the authors had to redefine their inclusion criteria, particularly on 'community-based research' and 'arts-based methods'. They moved the definition of communities away from its geographical character to a definition of communities that was centred around a common cause. They also changed their view on what were considered practical applications of arts-based methods by constantly renegotiating the meaning of arts-based methods, a label that was seldom used by the authors to describe their practice.[64]

Determine the eligibility criteria for studies to be included

The eligibility criteria for a qualitative evidence synthesis specify the topic or issue of interest, the types of studies to be included and information about the population of interest (perspectives) and the settings the authors are interested in. Authors of qualitative evidence syntheses are not necessarily studying interventions, or outcomes related to them. They might be interested in people's experiences of living with a particular disease or in challenging life circumstances. When interventions are the focus, though, the interest might be in the reasons for success or failure of an intervention, particularly in mixed-methods reviews. Qualitative evidence syntheses generally include all sorts of qualitative study designs: phenomenological studies, case studies, grounded theory designs and/or action research designs, although authors usually exclude opinion papers and editorials without a clear method. They may decide on a population of interest or a particular perspective they are interested in. For example, while people with a mental health condition might be the reviewers' target group, the experiences or opinions of family members and carers of such people might be of interest. A clear definition of the setting of interest is also important, given the fact that most qualitative studies are conducted 'in context'. For example, the introduction of a *doula* (a non-health-professional female to support young mothers) may be perceived quite differently by people in the West than by those in

African countries, where the active involvement of members of large, extended families is expected. Context relates to many factors, including geographical region, culture, type of care environment, and so on.

Search for potentially eligible studies

The search methods are similar to those of quantitative reviews, although they differ in the need to include terms for qualitative methods. Search filters that can be used to identify studies using qualitative methods in bibliographic databases are suggested in Chapter 3. While many authors of qualitative systematic reviews undertake an exhaustive search to retrieve all potentially relevant studies, a growing number of reviewers approach their pool of studies from a purposeful sample perspective,[3,65] using only a subset of the articles for further analysis, arguing that richness of ideas and concepts as well as variability in the perspectives invited is more important than representativeness.

Apply eligibility criteria to select studies

This step is also similar to the approach used in quantitative reviews, although review authors undertaking purposive sampling might report on the selection of studies based on, for example, a maximum variation strategy.[66]

Assess the quality of the included studies

In qualitative evidence synthesis, the focus is on 'assessing the quality' of the individual studies, rather than their 'risk of bias' (as in quantitative reviews). Various checklists and frameworks have been developed to assist. They include the CASP checklist for qualitative research, and the Qualitative Assessment and Review Instrument (QARI) tool (used in Chapters 10 and 11). The CASP checklist has a pragmatic focus on the different steps in the research project, and is relatively easy to use, while the QARI tool also addresses any influence of the researcher on the conclusions drawn. New quality appraisal instruments are currently being developed based on a systematic review of criteria used in different instruments to support quality assessment of primary research studies.[67] Sometimes it is appropriate to assign a judgment on individual findings in an included study, rather than rating the study quality only.[68] This allows the reviewer to decide which insights are valid enough to be considered for inclusion in the review. The following is an example of such judgments promoted by the Joanna Briggs Institute:

- *Unequivocal* evidence: if the evidence is beyond reasonable doubt and includes findings that are factual, directly reported/observed and not open to challenge.
- *Credible* evidence: if the evidence, while interpretative, is plausible in light of the data and theoretical framework.

- *Unsupported* evidence: in case the findings are not supported by the data and none of the other level descriptors apply.

Extract and analyse data from the included studies

The data to be extracted include setting, participant details, methodology and methods used, phenomena of interest, cultural and geographical information, and findings (such as the themes, metaphors or categories reported). In addition, review authors search for relevant ideas, concepts, metaphors and descriptors and use these as the basis for further synthesis.

Synthesise the data

There are several different approaches to synthesising data for qualitative evidence syntheses. One approach that has rapidly gained recognition is the *meta-aggregative approach to synthesis*.[69] This method takes an explicit integrative approach to synthesis, as opposed to the more commonly accepted interpretive approach. The meta-aggregative approach is designed to model the review process of performing systematic reviews that summarise the results of quantitative studies, while being sensitive to the nature of qualitative research and its traditions.[69]

In this chapter, we will focus on the meta-aggregative approach. It involves three steps: (1) assembling the findings of studies (variously reported as themes, metaphors or categories); (2) pooling them through further aggregation based on similarity in meaning; and (3) arriving at a set of synthesised statements presented as 'lines of action' for practice and policy. In extracting the themes (step 1) identified in the original studies, the reviewer takes into account the literal descriptions presented of original studies and maintains representativeness with the primary literature. Similarity of meaning on the level of categories (step 2) is contingent on the reviewer's familiarity with the included studies. After extracting the findings from each included study, the reviewer looks for commonality in the themes and metaphors across the studies. Similarity may be *conceptual* (where a theme or metaphor is identified across multiple papers) or *descriptive* (where the terminology associated with a theme or metaphor is consistent across studies). This process is similar to those used in primary qualitative research methods (such as constant comparative analysis and thematic analysis); however, in a primary qualitative research project, the result is a framework, matrix or conceptual model, while in a meta-aggregation it is declamatory statements or 'lines of action' (step 3).[70] An adapted version of the process of meta-aggregation[69] is illustrated in Figure 12.3.

Interpret and report the results

Supporting tools, such as the System for the Unified Management, Assessment and Review of Information

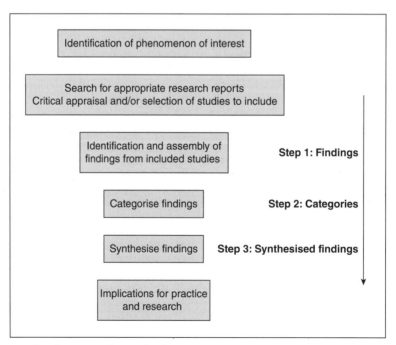

Fig 12.3 Process of meta-aggregative synthesis.
The Joanna Briggs Institute. Joanna Briggs Institute Reviewer's Manual. Adelaide: The Joanna Briggs Institute; 2008.

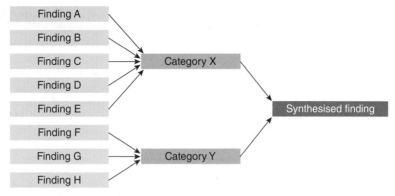

Fig 12.4 Meta-aggregative approach to analysis.
The Joanna Briggs Institute. Comprehensive Systematic Review Study Guide Module 4. Adelaide: The Joanna Briggs Institute; 2012.

(SUMARI) software and the QARI tool, have been developed to assist reviewers conducting a meta-aggregative approach. They document each step of the decision, and link synthesised statements to the findings retrieved from original studies.[71] Many other tools are available. The outcome of a meta-aggregation can be set out as a chart (see Figure 12.4), which is featured, for example, in a review on help-seeking behaviour of women after childbirth.[72]

The result may also be presented as a theoretical model, or a web of ideas, a narrative or a critique. In these cases, the graphical display is less linear than those of meta-aggregative analyses. A good example is seen in a qualitative evidence synthesis on people's resistance to taking medicine.[73]

Recently, two sets of guidelines have been developed to establish a transparent grading of the confidence of findings from qualitative evidence syntheses: CERQual (https://cerqual.org/)[74] and ConQual.[75] Confidence is broadly defined as the belief that a person can place in the results of these review findings. The CERQual framework is based on four components: (1) the methodological limitations of the qualitative studies contributing to a review finding; (2) the relevance to the review question of the studies contributing to a review finding; (3) the coherence of the review finding; and (4) the adequacy of data supporting a review finding. The ConQual framework was developed for meta-aggregative approaches and mirrors the GRADE system that was described earlier and is used in Cochrane's 'Summary of Findings' tables. It is based on two main concepts: 'dependability' and 'credibility'. Credibility evaluates whether there is a 'fit' between the authors' interpretation and the original source data. The concept of dependability is established if the research process is logical (that is, the methods are suitable to answer the research question and are in line with the chosen methodology), traceable and clearly documented.[76]

ASSESSING THE QUALITY OF QUALITATIVE EVIDENCE SYNTHESES

Here the focus is on assessing the overall quality of a qualitative evidence synthesis, rather than on 'assessing risk of bias' (as in quantitative reviews). There is still lack of general guidance for doing this. However, in the following example, the questions in Box 12.2 can be used as prompts to consider different aspects of the qualitative evidence synthesis (but should not be considered as standard criteria for appraisal).

BOX 12.2 Key questions to ask when critically appraising a systematic review using the CASP (Critical Appraisal Skills Programme) Checklist: Ten questions to help you make sense of a systematic review

1. Did the review address a clearly focused question?
2. Did the authors look for the right type of papers?
3. Do you think all the important, relevant studies were included?
4. Did the review's authors do enough to assess the quality of the included studies?
5. If the results of the review have been combined, was it reasonable to do so?
6. What are the overall results of the review?
7. How precise are the results?
8. Can the results be applied to the local population?
9. Were all important outcomes considered?
10. Are the benefits worth the harms and costs?

Critical Appraisal Skills Programme (CASP). 10 questions to help you make sense of systematic reviews. England: Public Health Resource Unit; 2013. Online. Available: www.casp-uk.net/casp-tools-checklists.

◎ CLINICAL SCENARIO (PART 2)

Finding qualitative evidence relevant to the scenario
Let us return to the clinical scenario outlined earlier in which an outpatient stroke rehabilitation team was looking for evidence from a systematic review about the effects of physical fitness training on disability and cardiorespiratory fitness. The team also wanted to better understand the views of people who have had a stroke about what factors help them to continue fitness training when they go home, and therefore decided to look for qualitative research (preferably a systematic review) on this topic. They search the PubMed database using the search terms 'stroke survivors' AND ('fitness training' OR exercise) AND (qualitative[tiab] OR themes[tiab]) and located a few relevant articles, including a systematic review about the barriers and facilitators to adhering to self-directed recovery exercises.[77]

◎ CLINICAL SCENARIO (PART 2) (CONTINUED)

Structured abstract of chosen qualitative article
Citation: Vadas D, Prest K, Turk A, et al. Understanding the facilitators and barriers of stroke survivors' adherence to recovery-oriented self-practice: a thematic synthesis. Disabil Rehabil 2021; Aug 30:1–12.[77]
Objectives: This study aimed to improve understanding of stroke survivors' adherence to recovery-oriented self-practice outside of clinical settings.
Selection criteria: After removal of duplicates, titles and abstracts were screened for relevance and the full text of studies remaining were then screened by one reviewer (with a second reviewer verifying 25%) using clear selection criteria. Studies needed to use a qualitative design with adult stroke survivors who were prescribed self-practice exercise programs targeting recovery of primary impairments or functional activities with findings pertaining to adherence.
Search strategy: Five databases were searched: MEDLINE, PsycInfo, CINAHL, Embase and ASSIA (Applied Social Sciences Index and Abstracts). Reference lists of included papers were reviewed, and three clinician peers were contacted.
Methodological quality: Quality assessment was undertaken using the CASP (Critical Appraisal Skills Programme) checklist for qualitative studies.
Data collection: Data for study aim, number and gender of participants, data collection and analysis methods, and main findings were extracted.
Data synthesis: Data were synthesised using thematic synthesis.
Results: Twelve papers ($n = 108$ post-stroke patients) were included. An overarching theme 'Tailoring and personalisation rather than standardisation' was informed by three analytical themes: 'The meaning of "self" in self-practice'; 'Identifying self-practice as a team effort'; and 'Self-practice that is grounded in one's reality'.
Conclusion: Clinicians are advised to tailor proposed exercise programs to stroke survivors' personal situations, preferences and needs to enhance adherence to self-practice.

◎ CLINICAL SCENARIO (PART 2) (CONTINUED)

Critical appraisal of chosen qualitative review
Using the questions that are outlined in Box 12.2 from the CASP Checklist, '10 questions to help you make sense of a systematic review', we will now step you through a critical appraisal of this systematic review. More detailed instructions on what to look for in an article for each criterion can be found on the CASP website (https://casp-uk.net/).

A. Are the results of the review valid?
1. Did the review address a clearly focused question?
Yes. Although the synthesis does not specify a review question as such, the aim of the synthesis is clear: 'to systematically collect, appraise and synthesise existing qualitative literature about the factors affecting stroke survivors' adherence to recovery-targeted prescribed self-practice'. The knowledge resulting from the qualitative

synthesis is meant to 'help support clinicians when recommending this type of activity to patients'. The inclusion criteria were specified as follows:

a. *The population studied:*

Post-stroke adult population. The duration of participants post-stroke is not specified but the practice was to be conducted outside of clinical settings.

b. *The intervention given:*

Exercise programs aiming at recovery of primary impairments or functional activities, with exercises to be practised at the stroke survivor's home or in another informal practice setting.

c. *The outcome considered:*

Factors affecting adherence to prescribed, recovery-oriented self-practice. These factors were described thematically and then interpreted to develop analytical themes which were used to produce recommendations for clinicians on increasing individuals' adherence to prescribed exercises.

2. Did the authors look for the right type of papers?

a. *Address the review's question?*

Yes. The studies selected appear to address the aim of this review.

b. *Have an appropriate study design?*

Yes. This study included all qualitative primary studies and qualitative parts of mixed-methods studies that could be separately extracted. This is appropriate for a qualitative evidence synthesis.

3. Do you think all the important, relevant studies were included?

It is difficult to judge if all the important, relevant studies were identified as the full search strategy for each database was not provided. In particular, the authors acknowledge the use of the 'qualitative' filter in the search strategy as a potential limitation. It is unclear whether a validated study design filter was used. In addition, two relevant papers identified using an updated search were not included because, according to the authors, they did not change the identified themes.

a. *Which bibliographic databases were used?*

The authors searched the following databases: MEDLINE, PsycInfo, CINAHL, Embase and ASSIA. These databases were chosen as they cover a range of disciplines and journals.

b. *Did the authors follow up from reference lists?*

Yes. The reference lists of the included studies were screened for more potential studies by two reviewers.

c. *Did the authors make personal contact with experts?*

Yes. Three clinician peers involved in research relating to rehabilitation were asked to forward suggestions

of articles that might be relevant. However, it is not known how these clinicians were chosen or whether, and on what basis, they were considered 'experts'.

d. *Did the authors search for unpublished as well as published studies?*

No. Studies that were not published in peer-reviewed journals were excluded. This may have introduced publication bias whereby studies with favourable findings are more likely to be published. In qualitative research, this may manifest as findings supporting preconceived notions of the researchers which were not specified in this review.

e. *Did the authors search for non-English language studies?*

No. The search is limited to studies published in or translated to English. This may introduce a culturally or geographically inspired bias in the set of selected studies, further evidenced by included studies that were conducted in countries where English is widely spoken (United States, Germany, United Kingdom, Singapore and Australia).

4. Did the review's authors do enough to assess quality of the included studies?

a. *Consider the rigour of the studies they have identified?*

In this review, the CASP checklist for qualitative studies was used to assess the quality of the included studies. This was conducted by one reviewer with a second reviewer independently assessing 2/12 studies. A transparent outline of how the studies score on each of the ten criteria is provided in the supplementary material. However, there appears to be some overlap in the interpretation between criteria 5 (data collection appropriate) and 6 (researcher/participant relationship), as two studies were rated 'can't tell' for criteria 5 because information about the researchers involved and their relationship with participants was lacking. In addition, the assessment of quality does not appear to be incorporated into the review findings. That is, the effect of the methodological limitations on the certainty or the strength of the findings does not appear to have been evaluated despite the authors' acknowledgment that 'one study failed to reflect many of the components of the CASP tool'.

5. If the results of the review have been combined, was it reasonable to do so?

a. *Were the results similar from study to study?*

Understanding the difference between studies is not a prerequisite for conducting a thematic synthesis. Outliers were not discussed, suggesting that the

Continued

◎ CLINICAL SCENARIO (PART 2) (CONTINUED)—cont'd

review was primarily focused on similarities between papers.

b. *Were the results of all the included studies clearly displayed?*

Yes. The main findings of all the included studies are summarised in a table and discussed further in the results section.

c. *Were the results of different studies similar?*

Similarities between studies seems to be the dominant focus in the analytical process. For example, the same influencing factor (for example, a caregiver or technology-based program) was portrayed as either a facilitator or a barrier to self-practice within different studies.

d. *Were the reasons for any variations in results discussed?*

Any search for alternative explanations was weak, with no mention of the review authors' sensitivity towards competing ideas. The review authors discuss how their findings compare to or differ from findings reported elsewhere; however, there is minimal discussion of potential disconfirming findings that challenge their synthesised findings.

B. What are the results?

1. What are the overall results of the review?

a. *Are you clear about the review's 'bottom line' results?*

Yes. The review's 'bottom line' results are clearly articulated using a model that emphasises the importance of tailoring rather than standardising self-practice programs and is underpinned by three analytical themes produced from the thematic synthesis.

b. *What are these results (numerically if appropriate)?*

An overarching theme was identified as 'Tailoring and personalisation rather than standardisation'. It was informed by the following three analytical themes: 'The meaning of "self" in self-practice'; 'Identifying self-practice as a team effort'; and 'Self-practice that is grounded in one's reality'.

c. *How were the results expressed (NNT, odds ratio, etc.)?*

The results are presented using themes rather than numerically, as is appropriate for a qualitative evidence synthesis.

2. How precise are the results?

Precision of results (which is very important for quantitative reviews) is not relevant to a qualitative evidence synthesis. Rather, we should evaluate the richness of the findings and ensure that the argumentation build-up (or systematic reasoning) is grounded in the study findings. The authors have provided the reader with a rich description of the factors affecting adherence to recovery-targeted prescribed self-practice in individuals after a stroke. Illustrative quotations, codes and descriptive themes are provided to justify the interpretation of the analytical themes and the overarching model. This allows users of the synthesis to evaluate the trustworthiness or believability of the findings.

C. Will the results help locally?

1. Can the results be applied to the local population?

It is difficult to judge whether the results can be directly applied to the local population as the patients and settings covered by the review are not described in sufficient detail. For example, participants' age, social situation, time since stroke and type or severity of impairment cannot be compared to the characteristics of the local population. However, the authors appear to justify the relevance to all post-stroke survivors by encouraging an individualised view of each participant whereby 'each factor that may affect a patient's adherence to self-practice should be judged as a facilitator or barrier for a specific patient in a specific context'.

2. Were all important outcomes considered?

Qualitative evidence syntheses are interested in the viewpoints, experiences and opinions, rather than health outcomes (which are important in quantitative reviews). Although this review only directly reports the perspective of individuals who had a stroke, it does consider the role of health professionals, caregivers, social and family support in doing self-practice through the lens of the stroke survivors. The broad 'outcome of interest' in this thematic synthesis is the factors affecting adherence to prescribed, recovery-oriented self-practice, and the review uses these factors to provide suggestions to health professionals about how to maximise adherence to self-practice.

3. Are the benefits worth the harms and costs?

Qualitative evidence syntheses are interested in understanding the reasons for human behaviour (for example, factors influencing adherence to self-practice) rather than weighing the potential benefits of an intervention (for example, self-practice) against the harms and costs.

◎ CLINICAL SCENARIO (PART 2) (CONTINUED)

Resolution of clinical scenario: qualitative review
The review concludes that it is important for health professionals who prescribe self-practice following stroke to identify and understand factors that patients experience as influencing their adherence. Factors relating to the individual, the team of prescribing therapists and carers, and practical factors (for example, cost, energy and time) were experienced as facilitators or barriers. Health professionals are advised to use this information to tailor self-practice programs to individuals' situations and preferences.

THE IMPORTANCE OF COMPLETE REPORTING IN SYSTEMATIC REVIEWS

Determining the quality of systematic reviews is influenced by how they are reported. Many reviews are poorly reported.[78] To help improve reporting, an increasing number of journals recommend, or insist, that authors follow a reporting guideline for quantitative systematic reviews, such as the Preferred Reporting Items for Systematic Reviews and Meta-Analyses (PRISMA) 2020 statement.[2] For qualitative systematic reviews, the Enhancing Transparency in Reporting the Synthesis of Qualitative Research (ENTREQ) statement has been developed to guide thorough reporting.[79] In addition to reporting guidelines, there are several design-specific guidelines, such as RAMESES (Realist And Meta-narrative Evidence Syntheses: Evolving Standards) for realist synthesis projects[80] and the Ch-IMP (Checklist to assess implementation) instrument that addresses process and implementation factors in reviews.[81] Increasingly, guidelines on how to translate review findings to a local context are being developed, among them the CONSENSYS instrument[82] and the TRANSFER framework.[83]

SUMMARY

- Systematic reviews differ from literature reviews because they are prepared using explicit, transparent and pre-specified methods to increase the reproducibility of the review and lower the risk of bias. They usually involve a comprehensive search of all potentially relevant articles; use explicit, reproducible and uniformly applied criteria in the selection of articles for the review; rigorously assess the risk of bias or quality of individual studies; and systematically synthesise the results of included studies.
- Systematic reviews synthesise the findings from different primary study designs dictated by the research question of interest.
- A well-conducted systematic review can hasten the translation of research into practice and policy. It can help to understand conflict (heterogeneity) between individual studies and establish generalisability of the overall findings. A review of qualitative studies can deepen the understanding of a phenomenon or situation and help clarify unexpected outcomes.
- Systematic reviews vary in quality, so you should know how to appraise them and to recognise the key features that introduce bias or flaws into these types of reviews. When examining whether the review used valid methods, key questions that need to be asked are whether the review:
  1. addressed a clearly focused question with clearly defined eligibility criteria;
  2. included high-quality, relevant studies;
  3. is unlikely to have missed important, relevant studies;
  4. included an assessment of the risk of bias or study quality of the included studies and incorporated this assessment into the review findings; and
  5. combined the results from studies and, if so, whether it is reasonable to do so?
- Other key questions that you need to ask when examining the results of a systematic review are: (1) What are the overall results? (2) How precise or grounded are the results? (3) Did the review consider all the important outcomes or evaluation measures? (4) Can the results be applied to your patients?
- Sensitivity for process and implementation factors and how to best adapt review evidence to the local context is important to consider to increase the uptake of a review's findings.

ACKNOWLEDGMENT

We acknowledge the help of Dr Sue Doyle in developing content for this chapter in the first and second editions of the book.

REFERENCES

1. Murad MH, Montori VM, Ioannidis JP, et al. How to read a systematic review and meta-analysis and apply the results to patient care: users' guides to the medical literature. JAMA 2014;312(2):171–9.

2. Page MJ, McKenzie JE, Bossuyt PM, et al. The PRISMA 2020 statement: an updated guideline for reporting systematic reviews. BMJ 2021;372:n71.

3. Benoot C, Hannes K, Bilsen J. The use of purposeful sampling in a qualitative evidence synthesis: a worked example on sexual adjustment to a cancer trajectory. BMC Med Res Methodol 2016;16:21.

4. McKenzie JE, Beller EM, Forbes AB. Introduction to systematic reviews and meta-analysis. Respirology 2016;21(4):626–37.

5. Gough D, Thomas J, Oliver S. Clarifying differences between reviews within evidence ecosystems. Syst Rev 2019;8(1):170.

6. Munn Z, Stern C, Aromataris E, et al. What kind of systematic review should I conduct? A proposed typology and guidance for systematic reviewers in the medical and health sciences. BMC Med Res Methodol 2018;18(1):5.

7. McKenzie JE, Brennan SE. Chapter 12: Synthesizing and presenting findings using other methods. In: Higgins JPT, Thomas J, Chandler J, et al., editors. Cochrane handbook for systematic reviews of interventions. The Cochrane Collaboration. Version 6.3 (updated February 2022); 2022. Available: www.training.cochrane.org/handbook.

8. Campbell M, McKenzie JE, Sowden A, et al. Synthesis without meta-analysis (SWiM) in systematic reviews: reporting guideline. BMJ 2020;368:l6890.

9. Flemming K, Noyes J. Qualitative evidence synthesis: where are we at? Int J Qual Methods 2021;20:1609406921993276.

10. Noblit GW, Hare RDR. Meta-ethnography: synthesizing qualitative studies. Newbury, CA: SAGE Publications; 1988.

11. Dixon-Woods M, Cavers D, Agarwal S, et al. Conducting a critical interpretive synthesis of the literature on access to healthcare by vulnerable groups. BMC Med Res Methodol 2006;6:35.

12. Thomas J, Harden A. Methods for the thematic synthesis of qualitative research in systematic reviews. BMC Med Res Methodol 2008;8:45.

13. Lockwood C, Munn Z, Porritt K. Qualitative research synthesis: methodological guidance for systematic reviewers utilizing meta-aggregation. Int J Evid Based Healthc 2015;13(3):179–87.

14. Hannes K, Lockwood C. Synthesising qualitative research: choosing the right approach. Chichester, UK: John Wiley & Sons; 2012.

15. Sandelowski M, Voils CI, Barroso J. Defining and designing mixed research synthesis studies. Res Sch 2006;13(1):29.

16. Heyvaert M, Hannes K, Onghena P. Using mixed methods research synthesis for literature reviews: the mixed methods research synthesis approach. Thousand Oaks, CA: SAGE Publications; 2016.

17. Hannes K. Artistically inspired systematic reviews. Campbell Collaboration; What Works Global Summit 2021: Evidence for Development, 18–27 October, Oslo; 2021.

18. Chandler J, Cumpston M, Thomas J, et al. Chapter I: Introduction. In: Higgins JPT, Thomas J, Chandler J, et al., editors. Cochrane handbook for systematic reviews of interventions. The Cochrane Collaboration. Version 6.3 (updated February 2022); 2022. Available: www.training.cochrane.org/handbook.

19. Hayden JA, Wilson MN, Riley RD, et al. Individual recovery expectations and prognosis of outcomes in non-specific low back pain: prognostic factor review. Cochrane Database Syst Rev 2019;2019(11):CD011284.

20. Salameh JP, Bossuyt PM, McGrath TA, et al. Preferred reporting items for systematic review and meta-analysis of diagnostic test accuracy studies (PRISMA-DTA): explanation, elaboration, and checklist. BMJ 2020;370:m2632.

21. Chan KK, Joo DA, McRae AD, et al. Chest ultrasonography versus supine chest radiography for diagnosis of pneumothorax in trauma patients in the emergency department. Cochrane Database Syst Rev 2020;7(7):CD013031.

22. Noyes J, Booth A, Cargo M, et al. Chapter 21: Qualitative evidence. In: Higgins JPT, Thomas J, Chandler J, et al., editors. Cochrane handbook for systematic reviews of interventions. The Cochrane Collaboration. Version 6.3 (updated February 2022); 2022. Available: www.training.cochrane.org/handbook.

23. Rozbroj T, Haas R, O'Connor D, et al. How do people understand overtesting and overdiagnosis? Systematic review and meta-synthesis of qualitative research. Soc Sci Med 2021;285:114255.

24. Stern C, Lizarondo L, Carrier J, et al. Methodological guidance for the conduct of mixed methods systematic reviews. JBI Evid Implement 2021;19(2):120–9.

25. Harris K, Kneale D, Lasserson TJ, et al. School-based self-management interventions for asthma in children and adolescents: a mixed methods systematic review. Cochrane Database Sys Rev 2019;1(1):CD011651.

26. Heyvaert M, Hannes K, Maes B, et al. Critical appraisal of mixed methods studies. J Mix Methods Res 2013;7(4):302–27.

27. Hong QN, Fàbregues S, Bartlett G, et al. The Mixed Methods Appraisal Tool (MMAT) version 2018 for information professionals and researchers. Education Inf 2018;34:285–91.

28. Jimenez E, Waddington H, Goel N, et al. Mixing and matching: using qualitative methods to improve quantitative impact evaluations (IEs) and systematic reviews (SRs) of development outcomes. J Dev Effect 2018;10(4):400–21.

29. Rada G, Pérez D, Araya-Quintanilla F, et al. Epistemonikos: a comprehensive database of systematic reviews for health decision-making. BMC Med Res Methodol 2020;20(1):286.

30. Page MJ, Shamseer L, Tricco AC. Registration of systematic reviews in PROSPERO: 30,000 records and counting. Syst Rev 2018;7(1):32.

31. Borah R, Brown AW, Capers PL, et al. Analysis of the time and workers needed to conduct systematic reviews of medical interventions using data from the PROSPERO registry. BMJ Open. 2017;7(2):e012545.

32. Clark J, Glasziou P, Del Mar C, et al. A full systematic review was completed in 2 weeks using automation tools: a case study. J Clin Epidemiol 2020;121:81–90.

33. Merner B, Lowe D, Walsh L, et al. Stakeholder involvement in systematic reviews: lessons from Cochrane's public health and health systems network. Am J Public Health 2021;111(7):1210–15.

34. Shamseer L, Moher D, Clarke M, et al. Preferred reporting items for systematic review and meta-analysis protocols (PRISMA-P) 2015: elaboration and explanation. BMJ 2015;350:g7647.

35. Stewart L, Moher D, Shekelle P. Why prospective registration of systematic reviews makes sense. Syst Rev 2012;1:7.

36. Lefebvre C, Glanville J, Briscoe S, et al. Chapter 4: Searching for and selecting studies. In: Higgins JPT, Thomas J, Chandler J, et al., editors. Cochrane handbook for systematic reviews of interventions. The Cochrane Collaboration. Version 6.3 (updated February 2022); 2022. Available: www.training.cochrane.org/handbook.

37. Bramer WM, Rethlefsen ML, Kleijnen J, et al. Optimal database combinations for literature searches in systematic reviews: a prospective exploratory study. Syst Rev 2017;6(1):245.

38. Isojarvi J, Wood H, Lefebvre C, et al. Challenges of identifying unpublished data from clinical trials: getting the best out of clinical trials registers and other novel sources. Res Synth Methods 2018;9(4):561–78.

39. Page MJ, Sterne JAC, Higgins JPT, et al. Investigating and dealing with publication bias and other reporting biases in meta-analyses of health research: a review. Res Synth Methods 2021;12(2):248–59.

40. Schmucker CM, Blümle A, Schell LK, et al. Systematic review finds that study data not published in full text articles have unclear impact on meta-analyses results in medical research. PLOS One 2017;12(4):e0176210.

41. Frandsen TF, Gildberg FA, Tingleff EB. Searching for qualitative health research required several databases and alternative search strategies: a study of coverage in bibliographic databases. J Clin Epidemiol 2019;114:118–24.

42. Boutron I, Page MJ, Higgins JPT, et al. Chapter 7: Considering bias and conflicts of interest among the included studies. In: Higgins JPT, Thomas J, Chandler J, et al., editors. Cochrane handbook for systematic reviews of interventions. The Cochrane Collaboration. Version 6.3 (updated February 2022); 2022. Available: www.training.cochrane.org/handbook.

43. Higgins JPT, Altman DG, Gøtzsche PC, et al. The Cochrane Collaboration's tool for assessing risk of bias in randomised trials. BMJ 2011;343:d5928.

44. Sterne JAC, Savović J, Page MJ, et al. RoB 2: a revised tool for assessing risk of bias in randomised trials. BMJ 2019; 366:l4898.

45. Li T, Higgins JPT, Deeks JJ. Chapter 5: Collecting data. In: Higgins JPT, Thomas J, Chandler J, et al., editors. Cochrane handbook for systematic reviews of interventions. The Cochrane Collaboration. Version 6.3 (updated February 2022); 2022. Available: www.training.cochrane.org/handbook.

46. Li T, Saldanha IJ, Jap J, et al. A randomized trial provided new evidence on the accuracy and efficiency of traditional vs. electronically annotated abstraction approaches in systematic reviews. J Clinical Epidemiol 2019;115:77–89.

47. Deeks JJ, Higgins JPT, Altman DG. Chapter 10: Analysing data and undertaking meta-analyses. In: Higgins JPT, Thomas J, Chandler J, et al., editors. Cochrane handbook for systematic reviews of interventions. The Cochrane Collaboration. Version 6.3 (updated February 2022); 2022. Available: www.training.cochrane.org/handbook.

48. Higgins JPT, Li T, Deeks JJ. Chapter 6: Choosing effect measures and computing estimates of effect. In: Higgins JPT, Thomas J, Chandler J, et al., editors. Cochrane handbook for systematic reviews of interventions. The Cochrane Collaboration. Version 6.3 (updated February 2022); 2022. Available: www.training.cochrane.org/handbook.

49. Lowe D, Ryan R, Schonfeld L, et al. Effects of consumers and health providers working in partnership on health services planning, delivery and evaluation. Cochrane Database Syst Rev 2021;9(9):CD013373.

50. Kossmeier M, Tran US, Voracek M. Charting the landscape of graphical displays for meta-analysis and systematic reviews: a comprehensive review, taxonomy, and feature analysis. BMC Med Res Methodol 2020;20(1):26.

51. Schünemann HJ, Vist GE, Higgins JPT, et al. Chapter 15: Interpreting results and drawing conclusions. In: Higgins JPT, Thomas J, Chandler J, et al., editors. Cochrane handbook for systematic reviews of interventions. The Cochrane Collaboration. Version 6.3 (updated February 2022); 2022. Available: www.training.cochrane.org/handbook.

52. Guyatt G, Oxman AD, Akl EA, et al. GRADE guidelines: 1. Introduction-GRADE evidence profiles and summary of findings tables. J Clin Epidemiol 2011;64(4):383–94.

53. Hultcrantz M, Rind D, Akl EA, et al. The GRADE Working Group clarifies the construct of certainty of evidence. J Clin Epidemiol 2017;87:4–13.

54. Schünemann HJ, Higgins JPT, Vist GE, et al. Chapter 14: Completing 'Summary of findings' tables and grading the certainty of the evidence. In: Higgins JPT, Thomas J, Chandler J, et al., editors. Cochrane handbook for systematic reviews of interventions. The Cochrane Collaboration. Version 6.3 (updated February 2022); 2022. Available: www.training.cochrane.org/handbook.

55. Saunders DH, Sanderson M, Hayes S, et al. Physical fitness training for stroke patients. Cochrane Database Syst Rev 2020;3(3):CD003316.

56. Lewin S, Booth A, Glenton C, et al. Applying GRADE-CERQual to qualitative evidence synthesis findings: introduction to the series. Implementat Sci 2018;13 (Suppl 1):2.

57. Garner P, Hopewell S, Chandler J, et al. When and how to update systematic reviews: consensus and checklist. BMJ 2016;354:i3507.

58. Elliott JH, Synnot A, Turner T, et al. Living systematic review: 1. Introduction—the why, what, when, and how. J Clin Epidemiol 2017;91:23–30.

59. Page MJ, Moher D, Fidler FM, et al. The REPRISE project: protocol for an evaluation of REProducibility and Replicability In Syntheses of Evidence. Syst Rev 2021;10(1):112.

60. Oxman AD, Guyatt GH. Validation of an index of the quality of review articles. J Clin Epidemiol 1991;44(11):1271–8.

61. Shea BJ, Reeves BC, Wells G, et al. AMSTAR 2: a critical appraisal tool for systematic reviews that include randomised or non-randomised studies of healthcare interventions, or both. BMJ 2017;358:j4008.

62. Whiting P, Savović J, Higgins JP, et al. ROBIS: a new tool to assess risk of bias in systematic reviews was developed. J Clin Epidemiol 2016;69:225–34.

63. Greenhalgh T, Donald A. Evidence-based health care workbook: for individual and group learning. London: BMJ Publishing Group; 1999.

64. Coemans S, Wang Q, Leysen J, et al. The use of arts-based methods in community-based research with vulnerable populations: protocol for a scoping review. Int J Educ Res 2015;71:33–9.

65. Ames H, Glenton C, Lewin S. Purposive sampling in a qualitative evidence synthesis: a worked example from a synthesis on parental perceptions of vaccination communication. BMC Med Res Methodol 2019;19(1):26.

66. Bengough T, von Elm E, Heyvaert M, et al. Factors that influence women's engagement with breastfeeding support: a qualitative evidence synthesis. Cochrane Database Syst Rev 2018;2018(9):CD013115.

67. Munthe-Kaas HM, Glenton C, Booth A, et al. Systematic mapping of existing tools to appraise methodological strengths and limitations of qualitative research: first stage in the development of the CAMELOT tool. BMC Med Res Methodol 2019;19(1):113.

68. Pearson A. Balancing the evidence: incorporating the synthesis of qualitative data into systematic reviews. JBI Reports 2004;2(2):45–64.

69. Aromataris E, Munn Z. JBI manual for evidence synthesis. Adelaide: Joanna Briggs Institute; 2020. Online. Available: https://synthesismanual.jbi.global.

70. Hannes K, Lockwood C. Pragmatism as the philosophical foundation for the Joanna Briggs meta-aggregative approach to qualitative evidence synthesis. J Adv Nurs 2011;67(7):1632–42.

71. SUMARI. User's Manual Version 5.0. System for the unified management, assessment and review of information. [computer program]. Adelaide: Joanna Briggs Institute.

72. Rouhi M, Stirling C, Ayton J, et al. Women's help-seeking behaviours within the first twelve months after childbirth: a systematic qualitative meta-aggregation review. Midwifery 2019;72:39–49.

73. Pound P, Britten N, Morgan M, et al. Resisting medicines: a synthesis of qualitative studies of medicine taking. Soc Sci Med 2005;61(1):133–55.

74. Lewin S, Glenton C, Munthe-Kaas H, et al. Using qualitative evidence in decision making for health and social interventions: an approach to assess confidence in findings from qualitative evidence syntheses (GRADE-CERQual). PLOS Med 2015;12(10):e1001895.

75. Munn Z, Porritt K, Lockwood C, et al. Establishing confidence in the output of qualitative research synthesis: the ConQual approach. BMC Med Res Methodol 2014;14:108.

76. Guba EG, Lincoln YS. Epistemological and methodological bases of naturalistic inquiry. ECTJ 1982;30(4):233–52.

77. Vadas D, Prest K, Turk A, et al. Understanding the facilitators and barriers of stroke survivors' adherence to recovery-oriented self-practice: a thematic synthesis. Disab Rehabil 2021;Aug 30:1–12.

78. Page MJ, Moher D. Evaluations of the uptake and impact of the Preferred Reporting Items for Systematic reviews and Meta-Analyses (PRISMA) Statement and extensions: a scoping review. Syst Rev 2017;6(1):263.

79. Tong A, Flemming K, McInnes E, et al. Enhancing transparency in reporting the synthesis of qualitative research: ENTREQ. BMC Med Res Methodol 2012;12:181.

80. Wong G, Greenhalgh T, Westhorp G, et al. Development of methodological guidance, publication standards and training materials for realist and meta-narrative reviews: the RAMESES (Realist And Meta-narrative Evidence Syntheses—Evolving Standards) project. Southampton, UK: NIHR Journals Library; 2014.

81. Cargo M, Stankov I, Thomas J, et al. Development, inter-rater reliability and feasibility of a checklist to assess implementation (Ch-IMP) in systematic reviews: the case of provider-based prevention and treatment programs targeting children and youth. BMC Med Res Methodol 2015;15:73.

82. Bengough T, Sommer I, Hannes K. CONSENSYS: a new instrument to support the development of context-sensitive implication sections in systematic reviews. Campbell Collaboration; What Works Global Summit 2021: Evidence for Development, 18–27 October, Oslo; 2021.

83. Munthe-Kaas H, Nøkleby H, Lewin S, et al. The TRANSFER Approach for assessing the transferability of systematic review findings. BMC Med Res Methodol 2020;20(1):11.

Clinical Practice Guidelines

Zachary Munn and Tammy Hoffmann

LEARNING OBJECTIVES

After reading this chapter, you should be able to:

- Describe what clinical practice guidelines are, their uses and their limitations
- Be aware of the major online resources for locating clinical practice guidelines
- Explain the major steps that are involved in the development of guidelines

- Appraise the quality of a clinical practice guideline to determine whether you should trust the recommendations that it contains
- Describe some of the issues related to using a clinical practice guideline

There are various forms of guidance that recommend how to manage clinical conditions. This guidance is developed in different ways and can range from consensus-based documents compiled by a group of individuals who are interested in the topic, to high-quality, evidence-based clinical practice guidelines that are informed by a systematic review of the research evidence and have undergone a transparent and rigorous development and review process. The latter is the type that we are interested in and what we focus on in this chapter. However, we will also discuss how to assess the quality of a clinical practice guideline, as it is likely that you will come across many types of guidelines in clinical practice.

In this chapter we will look at what clinical practice guidelines are, why they are used, where to search for guidelines, the steps involved in developing them and how to appraise their quality. We will also discuss some of the issues involved with using guidelines in clinical practice.

WHAT ARE CLINICAL GUIDELINES?

Clinical practice guidelines have been produced for many decades, with organised programs for guideline development introduced in some countries and clinical specialty societies from the 1980s and 1990s.[1] Guidelines are designed to help health professionals and their patients reach decisions about the most appropriate ways to investigate and manage presenting symptoms and specific conditions. In 2011 a report by the Institute of Medicine (IOM) in the United States proposed a standard definition that would reflect modern approaches to guideline development:[2]

Clinical practice guidelines are statements that include recommendations intended to optimize patient care that are informed by a systematic review of evidence and an assessment of the benefits and harms of alternative care options.[2]

According to this definition, a well-developed, trustworthy guideline contains rigorously compiled information *and* recommended actions to guide practice. It should be developed by a knowledgeable, multidisciplinary panel of experts and representatives from key stakeholder groups, and be based on a systematic review of existing evidence, using an explicit and transparent process that minimises bias. It should consider important sub-groups and patient preferences and values, clearly explain the relationship between alternative care options and health outcomes, and provide ratings of both the quality of the evidence and the strength of the recommendations. Finally, it should be revised when important new evidence becomes available.[2]

WHY USE GUIDELINES?

As we saw in Chapter 2, health professionals are continually exposed to an overwhelming amount of health research and there are thousands of new studies published each year. It is not possible for busy health professionals to keep abreast of this enormous volume of information, and the development of healthcare guidelines is one way in which information overload can be addressed. Guidelines are a useful tool for evidence-based practice as they help us to translate evidence into practice recommendations, which can then be applied to clinical situations.

Guidelines aim to help health professionals and patients make better decisions about health care. They aim to reduce unwarranted variations in practice across health professionals for the same condition and improve patient outcomes. The *development* of guidelines—the act of amassing and scrutinising the relevant research about a specific topic and making research accessible to health professionals and patients—is part of evidence-based practice at the organisational level. The subsequent *use* of guidelines in the clinical setting is more about evidence-based individual decision making, as well as the implementation of evidence into practice.

The number of clinical practice guidelines being produced has increased substantially over the last several years. A 2014 report from the National Health and Medical Research Council (NHMRC) of Australia notes that there were 1,046 guidelines produced by more than 130 Australian guideline developers between 2005 and 2013, with 648 of these produced in the most recent 5-year period studied.[3] International guideline-specific databases that are described later in this chapter contain many thousands of guidelines.

There is only a relatively small amount of research on the extent to which guidelines are used by health professionals. For example, the Australian Caretrack study assessed the extent to which a sample of adult Australians received appropriate care—defined as care in line with evidence-based or consensus-based guidelines—and found that people received appropriate care at only 57% of eligible healthcare encounters.[4] It has been estimated that only about 60% of care is in line with guideline recommendations.[5] How to improve the use of guidelines and increase the implementation of guideline recommendations in routine care is an expanding area of research, largely in the field of implementation science. (This refers to the scientific study of methods to promote the systematic uptake of clinical research findings into routine practice and is the focus of Chapter 16.)

The direct applicability to contemporary clinical practice is what makes a clinical guideline useful. As with other types of evidence, care should be taken to ensure that guidelines are of high quality, that the evidence they use is relevant for the setting and population where they will be used, and that they are implemented effectively. Guidelines will not address all the uncertainties of current clinical practice and are only one strategy that can help improve the quality of patient care.[6]

Guidelines: the benefits and challenges

High-quality guidelines differ from systematic reviews as they provide recommendations for care based on a combination of scientific research evidence, clinical expertise and patient values—whereas systematic reviews only provide implications for practice. They often provide an overview of the prevention, diagnosis and management of a condition or the use of an intervention, and so have a broader scope than systematic reviews, which tend to focus on a single clinical question. Potential benefits of guidelines include achieving better health outcomes, improving decisions about health care and saving time.[7,8]

However, guideline development is not easy and involves large amounts of time, money, expertise and effort. The development process can be lengthy and sometimes the evidence used in a guideline may not be the most current evidence by the time it is finally published. As such, we have seen the emergence of 'living guidelines', where guidelines are continuously updated as evidence changes.[9,10] For example, living stroke guidelines are produced by the Stroke Foundation in Australia[11] (informme.org.au/guidelines/living-guidelines-updates) and living guidelines on COVID-19 rehabilitation are produced and maintained by Cochrane Rehabilitation.

Many guidelines do not provide clear information about conflicts of interest within members of the guideline development group (for example, they may have financial or non-financial links with organisations or professions who have a vested interest in what the guidelines do and do not recommend) and how these were handled during the development process,[12] despite available guidance about how to do this.[13]

Duplication and overlap of guidelines is a problem. For many clinical conditions, there can be multiple guidelines—produced by different developers. This can make it confusing for health professionals, particularly when guidelines on the same clinical condition may have differing recommendations about the actions that should be provided. Sometimes this reflects a difference in the quality of production, with some guidelines undergoing more rigorous development processes than others. Differing recommendations may also arise because the guidelines have been developed for use in different settings, or with different population groups, or because of different views or approaches to valuing care outcomes.

When using a guideline, **the key word to remember is 'guide'**. Rigorously developed guidelines are the result of a comprehensive and systematic examination of the literature by a panel of experts with stakeholder input, including patients. This group considers how research findings should be applied in practice and aims to develop a useful, practical resource. However, guideline recommendations are *not* fixed protocols that must be followed. As with evidence-based practice in general, responsible and informed clinical judgment about the management of individual patients remains incredibly important. You should work together with your patient to develop an intervention plan that is tailored to their specific needs and circumstances, and is achievable, affordable and realistic. Guideline recommendations should be considered with appropriate consideration given to each patient's values, preferences and circumstances. This is a key component of shared decision making (see Chapter 14)—a process that allows the evidence about options, and their known potential benefits and harms, to be explicitly discussed with patients.[14] Unfortunately, most guidelines currently do little to enable shared decision making. For example, they may not clearly provide information about the benefits and harms of the options, or tools to facilitate conversations about these and collaborative decision making between health professionals and patients.[15,16] Recognition of the need for guidelines to incorporate tools, such as patient decision aids, that encourage this, and the development of methods for achieving it, are growing.[17–20] Box 13.1 contains examples from guidelines showing how this can be done.[21,22]

BOX 13.1   Examples and excerpts from clinical guidelines that (a) encourage shared decision making and provide links to tools and (b) encourage consideration of patient preferences.

a. Excerpt and example from a clinical guideline encouraging shared decision making and referring to decision support tools[21]

Management of acute bronchitis

As most cases of acute bronchitis are caused by a self-limiting viral illness, antibiotics are not indicated, as confirmed by a recent Cochrane review. Despite this, antibiotics are frequently inappropriately prescribed for acute bronchitis. Antibiotics are not indicated for acute bronchitis.

Many patients have an expectation of treatment with antibiotics. Effective communication with the patient about the role of antibiotics in acute bronchitis is essential. The discussion should address possible misconceptions about the effectiveness of antibiotic therapy and the expectation of an antibiotic prescription. Box 2.22 [in the guideline] provides a useful template for these discussions and outlines the approach to managing acute bronchitis with symptomatic therapy and patient education.

The Australian Commission on Safety and Quality in Health Care has created a patient decision aid to support discussions aimed at shared decision making and is available at https://www.safetyandquality.gov.au/our-work/partnering-consumers/shared-decision-making/decision-support-tools-specific-conditions.

b. Example of an excerpt from a clinical guideline that includes information about how patient preferences may influence the decision[22]

Guidance statements:

1. In patients with acute isolated distal DVT of the leg and (i) without severe symptoms or risk factors for extension (see text), we suggest serial imaging of the deep veins for 2 weeks over anticoagulation (weak recommendation, moderate-certainty evidence); or (ii) with severe symptoms or risk factors for extension (see text), we suggest anticoagulation over serial imaging of the deep veins (weak recommendation, low-certainty evidence).

2. In patients with acute isolated distal DVT of the leg who are treated with serial imaging, we (i) recommend no anticoagulation if the thrombus does not extend (strong recommendation, moderate-certainty evidence), (ii) suggest anticoagulation if the thrombus extends but remains confined to the distal veins (weak recommendation, very low-certainty evidence), and (iii) recommend anticoagulation if the thrombus extends into the proximal veins (strong recommendation, moderate-certainty evidence).

Remarks: Serial imaging refers to repeating ultrasound once weekly, or with worsening symptoms, for 2 weeks and anticoagulating only if distal thrombi propagate. Patients at high risk for bleeding are more likely to benefit from serial imaging. Evidence suggests uncertainty that anticoagulation is superior to no anticoagulation. Patients who place a high value on avoiding the inconvenience of repeat imaging and a low value on the inconvenience of treatment and on the potential for bleeding are likely to favour initial anticoagulation over serial imaging.

a. Excerpt from Therapeutic Guidelines Limited. Acute bronchitis, Respiratory tract infections other than pneumonia. In: Antibiotic Therapeutic Guidelines. Therapeutic Guidelines Ltd; [eTG March 2021 edition]. 2019. Online. Available: https://www.tg.org.au.
b. Excerpt from Stevens SM, Woller SC, Baumann Kreuziger L, et al. Executive summary. Antithrombotic therapy for VTE disease: second update of the CHEST Guideline and Expert Panel report. Chest 2021;160:2247–59.

Another potentially limiting factor about guidelines is that they generally tend to deal with single conditions in isolation. However, in practice, patients often present with a range of comorbid conditions. This can be problematic, because the studies used to develop guideline recommendations may specifically exclude people with comorbidities, resulting in conflicting recommendations within individual condition-specific guidelines. The additive effects of interventions recommended across multiple guidelines may also mean that a substantial, unfeasible, burdensome and potentially harmful combination of interventions would be involved. There has been increasing interest from the guideline development community in how to address multimorbidity in guidelines,[23] and a number of groups are working on this problem.[24]

HOW GUIDELINES FIT WITH OTHER EVIDENCE-BASED PRACTICE PRODUCTS

As well as clinical guidelines, there are other evidence-based practice products or aids that can help health professionals and patients to make decisions about care. Examples of these products include (some are only available with payment or membership of an organisation that provides access):

- 'Handbooks', of which there are many, and which differ from country to country. Some examples, primarily Australian ones, include:
  - *Therapeutic Guidelines* (www.tg.org.au)—covers over 2,500 topics of most relevance to medical practitioners.
  - *Asthma Management Handbook* (www.asthmahandbook.org.au).
- Decision support tools. (Sometimes these are available for both patients and health professionals.) More detail about patient decision aids is provided in Chapter 14.
- Clinical practice software that incorporates, or has links to, evidence-based guidelines.
- Educational modules and information packs that are sent out to health professionals by national and state health departments.

Guidelines can complement these other products when the information contained in them is aligned and consistent. Some of these products may contain guidelines, and sometimes the products may share the same evidence base as the relevant guidelines. However, there is not always consistency across products. Situations can arise where there are discrepancies in the recommendations made in various products. When discrepancies occur, you need to decide which resource to use. Later in this chapter, we discuss how to evaluate the quality of guidelines so that you can choose the highest-quality ones that will be of most use to your clinical situation.

WHERE AND HOW TO FIND GUIDELINES

It is probably clear to you by now that there are thousands of clinical guidelines across the health professions. The obvious question is: *Where and how should you look for guidelines relevant to your patient/clinical situation?* In general, there are two main electronic sources that can be used to locate clinical guidelines:

- large bibliographic databases (such as PubMed, Embase, CINAHL)
- guideline-specific databases (such as the Australian Clinical Practice Guidelines Portal, ECRI Guidelines Trust and the Guidelines International Network library).

Bibliographic databases

Although the large bibliographic databases do contain some clinical guidelines, the problem is that only a small proportion of guidelines are published in journals. Therefore, only a small proportion is indexed in the traditional databases. In addition, none of these databases appraise the quality of guidelines, and it may be difficult to access more than just the abstract from their sites. However, if you decide to search the large bibliographic databases to locate guidelines, here are a few tips:

- *PubMed:* you can select the limit 'practice guideline' under article types. Note that there is also the article type option of 'guideline'; however, this is a broader category and relates to the administration of healthcare activities, rather than clinical conditions.
- *MEDLINE (via Ovid):* you can select the limit 'practice guideline' in the publication types (practice guideline.pt). Methodological search strategies for locating methodologically sound guidelines in MEDLINE have been created[25] and are summarised in Table 13.1. Combine these methodological search strategies with your content terms (such as the keywords from your clinical question) when searching. It is important to note that although these filters exist, none of them appear perfect.[26]
- *CINAHL:* you can select the limit 'practice guidelines' under publication type.

Chapter 3 provides further details about these databases, as well as advice about how to use search strategies such as those shown in Table 13.1 when looking for evidence to answer a clinical question.

Guideline-specific databases

One of the best ways to find a clinical guideline can be by searching a guideline-specific database. Details of some of the major guideline-specific databases where guidelines can be found are provided in Box 13.2.

TABLE 13.1 **Search strategies (hedges) for locating practice guidelines in MEDLINE (via Ovid)**

Hedge	All classified guidelines	Methodologically sound guidelines
Best sensitivity	exp health services administration OR tu.xs. OR management.tw.	guideline:.tw. OR exp data collection OR recommend:. tw. guidelines.tw. OR practice guidelines.sh. OR recommend:.tw.
Best specificity	guideline:.tw.	guideline adherence.sh. OR physician's practice patterns. sh. practice guidelines.tw. OR practice guidelines.sh.
Best optimisation of sensitivity and specificity	guide:.tw. OR recommend:. tw. OR exp risk	exp "quality assurance (health care)" OR recommend:. tw. OR guideline adherence.sh.

colon (:) = truncation; exp = explosion; sh = subject heading; tu = therapeutic use; tw = textword; xs = exploded subheading.
From Wilczynski N, Haynes R, Lavis J, et al. Optimal search strategies for detecting health services research studies in MEDLINE. CMAJ 2004;171:1179–85.

BOX 13.2   Guideline-specific databases

ECRI Guidelines (https://guidelines.ecri.org/)
- Online repository of guidelines and is free to access.
- Includes profiles and snapshots of guidelines, along-side appraisals of guideline compliance with standards for trustworthy guidelines.

National Institute for Health and Care Excellence (NICE) (UK) (www.nice.org.uk/guidance)
- While some parts of the site are only available to people working within the NHS, most of the guidelines can be accessed by anyone and guidelines can be searched for by topic.
- An accreditation logo next to a guideline shows that the processes used by the guideline developers have been assessed as meeting NICE quality standards. However, as of late 2021, the accreditation program has been paused and its future scope has not been announced.

Guidelines International Network (G-I-N) (www.g-i-n.net)
- A global network with both organisational and individual members that aims to support collaboration on guideline development, adaptation and implementation.
- Has an International Guideline Library that contains more than 6,000 guidelines, evidence reports and related documents, developed or endorsed by G-I-N member organisations. Members who submit guidelines for listing on the database are asked to complete a standards reporting form to indicate whether specific standards (including a systematic review of the literature) have been met in the guideline development process, but completion of this form is voluntary.

- Anyone can access the library, but only network members can upload their guidelines.
- Also contains a registry of guidelines in development.

Turning Research Into Practice (TRIP) (www.tripdatabase.com)
- A search engine that searches multiple databases and sites for evidence. The search results are grouped according to the type of evidence (e.g. guideline). For guidelines, the search can be filtered further by choosing from Australia and New Zealand, Canada, the UK, the US or 'other'. See Chapter 3 for more detail about this database.

For some specialties and geographical regions, there are other smaller databases that collate guidelines. These include:
- **Physiotherapy** (PEDro—the Physiotherapy Evidence Database; www.pedro.org.au): contains evidence-based clinical guidelines of relevance to physiotherapy. Some guidelines are also of relevance to other health professions. PEDro is described in more detail in Chapter 3.
- **Canadian Medical Association Infobase—Clinical Practice Guidelines** (https://joulecma.ca/cpg/homepage): contains more than 1,200 guidelines developed or endorsed by an authoritative medical or health organisation in Canada.
- **Registered Nurses' Association of Ontario** (www.rnao.ca/bpg) contains about 50 guidelines relevant to nursing that are produced by this association and updated every 3 years.
- **Oncology** (www.nccn.org/index.asp): contains guidelines produced by the US National Comprehensive Cancer Network.

HOW ARE GUIDELINES DEVELOPED?

Clinical practice guideline development is a considered process that requires time and substantial resources along with intellectual investment. To meet standards from organisations such as the Guidelines International Network[27] and the NHMRC,[28] guidelines need to be based on the best available evidence, of high quality, suitable for their purpose and relevant for end users. An essential step in the development of appropriate guideline recommendations is determining the quality of the evidence on which recommendations are based.[29–37]

The steps involved in developing an *evidence-based* clinical guideline typically consist of:

1. Identifying the scope of a guideline—providing an outline of the aspects of care within the designated topic area that the guideline will cover.
2. Forming a guideline development group—usually made up of health professionals from a range of disciplines with expertise in the clinical area, representatives of patients and carers and people who have technical expertise in guideline development methods and in systematic literature reviewing.
3. Gaining agreement about the specific clinical questions or problems that will be addressed by the guideline and that will guide the types of evidence used and the search for evidence.
4. Searching systematically for evidence and appraising its quality.
5. Discussing and agreeing the implications of the evidence for clinical practice.
6. Formulating draft recommendations.
7. Obtaining external review and feedback on the guideline. Sometimes this may include a public consultation process.
8. Ongoing review and update of the guideline to ensure it remains based on the most current best available evidence—a time frame of 3 years is often used.

What gives rise to the variable quality of guidelines is that differences occur in this development process, typically in the following areas:

- the specific clinical questions that guide the search for evidence and the outcomes of interest
- the comprehensiveness of the search used to locate evidence
- the types and quality of the evidence reviewed
- the rigour of the processes used to assess/grade the evidence
- the mix of people reviewing the evidence
- the way in which conflicts of interest are identified and managed throughout the guideline development process

- decisions that are made about the desirability of different clinical outcomes
- assessments of the likelihood of harms and benefits of interventions and where the balance should fall
- the processes used to develop agreement on the final guideline recommendations
- the strength of guideline recommendations and the extent to which they are linked to evidence
- the process for obtaining review and feedback on the guideline and the modifications made to the guideline as a result.

Guides to guideline development have been published by a number of academic guideline developers and researchers and by international organisations, such as NICE, SIGN and the NHMRC, among others.[28,38,39] The GIN McMaster checklist also contains a comprehensive bibliography of resources available for each step of the guideline development process.[40] Specialist software applications for assisting in the development of clinical guidelines and systematic reviews have been developed to facilitate, streamline and support the systematic review and guideline development process.[41]

CAN I TRUST THE RECOMMENDATIONS IN A CLINICAL GUIDELINE?

With such a large number of clinical guidelines of varying quality available, you may be left wondering which guidelines you should, or should not, use in your clinical practice. You need to ask yourself the same question that we asked when appraising various study designs in earlier chapters of this book: '*Are the results of this study valid?*' When appraising clinical guidelines, the 'results' are the recommendations, so you are trying to determine whether you can trust the recommendations in a clinical guideline. As with the other types of evidence discussed in other chapters, it is important that you know how to appraise clinical guidelines and recognise the key features that discriminate high-quality guidelines (which can be used to guide practice) from low-quality clinical guidelines (which should only be used with caution and if no higher quality guidelines exist). High-quality guidelines can improve health care, but the adoption of low-quality guidelines can lead to the use of ineffective interventions, the inefficient use of scarce resources and, most importantly, possible harm to patients.[42,43] Unfortunately, studies of clinical practice guidelines have shown that there is substantial room for improvements to the quality, transparency and usability of guidelines.[44] In particular, studies have identified issues with the methods used for identifying, appraising and synthesising the evidence for guideline recommendations.[33,36,44–46]

The AGREE II instrument for appraising guidelines

The AGREE (Appraisal of Guidelines for Research and Evaluation) instrument is the most widely used and internationally accepted tool for assessing the quality of clinical practice guidelines. The original AGREE instrument[47] was developed in 2003 by an international group of guideline developers and researchers, the Appraisal of Guidelines Research and Evaluation (AGREE) collaboration.[48] The collaboration defined *quality of guidelines* as 'the confidence that the potential biases of guideline development have been addressed adequately and that the recommendations are both internally and externally valid, and are feasible for practice'.

The original instrument was revised and republished in 2009 as AGREE II.[49] Tutorials and training on its use can be found on the AGREE Research Trust website (www.agreetrust.org). The AGREE II tool appraises guidelines based on how they score on 23 items, which are grouped into six major domains, followed by two global rating overall assessment items. To increase reliability, it is recommended that each guideline is assessed by at least two people. Box 13.3 lists the domains and items of the AGREE II instrument. Each of the AGREE II items is rated on a 7-point scale (from 1 = strongly disagree

---

BOX 13.3 Domains and items contained in the AGREE II instrument

The AGREE II consists of 23 key items organised within six domains followed by two global rating items ('Overall Assessment'). Each domain captures a unique dimension of guideline quality.

Domain 1. Scope and purpose
1. The overall objective(s) of the guideline is (are) specifically described.
2. The health question(s) covered by the guideline is (are) specifically described.
3. The population (patients, public, etc.) to whom the guideline is meant to apply is specifically described.

Domain 2. Stakeholder involvement
4. The guideline development group includes individuals from all the relevant professional groups.
5. The views and preferences of the target population (patients, public, etc.) have been sought.
6. The target users of the guideline are clearly defined.

Domain 3. Rigour of development
7. Systematic methods were used to search for evidence.
8. The criteria for selecting the evidence are clearly described.
9. The strengths and limitations of the body of evidence are clearly described.
10. The methods for formulating the recommendations are clearly described.
11. The health benefits, side effects and risks have been considered in formulating the recommendations.
12. There is an explicit link between the recommendations and the supporting evidence.

13. The guideline has been externally reviewed by experts prior to its publication.
14. A procedure for updating the guideline is provided.

Domain 4. Clarity of presentation
15. The recommendations are specific and unambiguous.
16. The different options for management of the condition or health issue are clearly presented.
17. Key recommendations are easily identifiable.

Domain 5. Applicability
18. The guideline describes facilitators and barriers to its application.
19. The guideline provides advice and/or tools on how the recommendations can be put into practice.
20. The potential resource implications of applying the recommendations have been considered.
21. The guideline presents monitoring and/or auditing criteria.

Domain 6. Editorial independence
22. The views of the funding body have not influenced the content of the guideline.
23. Competing interests of guideline development group members have been recorded and addressed.

Overall guideline assessment
1. Rate the overall quality of this guideline (Scale of 1 to 7 with 1 being lowest possible quality and 7 being highest possible quality).
2. I would recommend this guideline for use (Options: Yes, Yes with modifications, No).

to 7 = strongly agree) regarding the extent to which the guideline meets the particular item.

A quality score can then be calculated for each of the six AGREE II domains. Domain scores are calculated by summing up all the scores of the individual items in a domain and by scaling the total as a percentage of the maximum possible score for that domain. The six domain scores are independent and should not be aggregated into a single quality score. AGREE II asks for the assessor to make two overall assessments of the guideline: (1) a judgment of the overall quality which takes into account the criteria considered in the assessment process; and (2) a statement about whether the assessor would recommend use of the guideline. A shorter item, AGREE II–Global Rating Scale Instrument (AGREE II–GRS Instrument) based on the AGREE II instrument, is also available on the website and, when time and resources are limited, may be used as an alternative appraisal tool.

Establishing the certainty of evidence and strength of recommendations

Determining the certainty of the evidence that underpins the recommendations within a clinical practice guideline is a key part of the guideline development process. Some guideline recommendations are based on higher certainty evidence, while others are based on lower certainty evidence, so it is important that users of guidelines are able to understand the certainty of the evidence that supports any particular recommendation.[50] Internationally, clinical practice guideline developers have in the past used a variety of systems to rate the certainty (sometimes called 'quality' or 'strength') of the evidence that underpins recommendations within the guideline and the strength of the recommendation that is being made.[51] The different systems were confusing for users as they used varying, and sometimes overlapping, combinations of letters and numbers to communicate the methodological quality of the underlying evidence and the strength of the recommendation.

Many groups around the world have now adopted the GRADE (Grading of Recommendations Assessment, Development and Evaluation) approach.[52–57] As you saw in Chapter 12, the GRADE approach forms the basis of the 'Summary of Findings' tables that now appear in many (particularly Cochrane) systematic reviews. GRADE is a structured and transparent approach to grading the certainty (sometimes called the 'quality of the evidence' or 'confidence in the estimates') of evidence and the strength of recommendations in health care, proposed by the GRADE Working Group in 2000.[29,58–60] GRADE provides a stepwise process to framing questions, selecting outcomes and rating their importance, evaluating the evidence, and considering evidence together with the values and preferences of patients and society to arrive at recommendations.[29,58–60] GRADE is used for systematic reviews and guidelines that evaluate alternative management interventions or strategies.[58,59] The working group that developed the GRADE system used the following definitions:

- **Certainty of evidence** indicates the extent to which one can be confident that an estimate of effect is adequate to support a particular recommendation.
- **Strength of a recommendation** indicates the extent to which one can be confident that adherence to the recommendation will do more good than harm.

The GRADE system takes several elements into account when judging the ***certainty of the evidence*** for each important outcome considered in the guideline, including: *study design* (for example, is the study a randomised controlled trial or a non-randomised study?); *risk of bias*; *inconsistency* (the similarity or variation of estimates of effects across studies); and *indirectness* (the extent to which the people, interventions and outcome measures used in the study are similar to those of interest); *imprecision* (the width of the confidence intervals around an effect estimate in relation to decision-making thresholds); and *publication bias* (and whether there is the potential for missing studies).

The ***certainty of evidence*** grading used by GRADE is:[54,55]

- **High**—further research is very unlikely to change our confidence in the estimate of effect.
- **Moderate**—further research is likely to have an important impact on our confidence in the estimate of effect and may change the estimate.
- **Low**—further research is very likely to have an important impact on our confidence in the estimate of effect and is likely to change the estimate.
- **Very low**—any estimate of effect is very uncertain.

Within the GRADE system, there are two levels of ***recommendation strength***:

- **Strong**—where there is considerable certainty that the benefits of intervention do, or do not, outweigh risks and burdens.
- **Weak** (may also be termed 'discretionary' or 'conditional')—where benefits, risks and burdens may be finely balanced; where there is considerable uncertainty about the magnitude of benefits and risks; or where fully informed patients may make different choices because of the different values they may attach to outcomes.

Alongside the establishment of the level of certainty in synthesised effect estimates, the GRADE working group has developed evidence-to-decision frameworks which can be used to guide a panel through the process of moving from the evidence to making a recommendation in a guideline.[61] The direction and strength of a recommendation is influenced by the balance of desirable and undesirable consequences; the priority of the problem; certainty of evidence; values and preferences of those affected; along with feasibility, equity implications, acceptability and resource use.[61]

The GRADE Working Group website (www.gradeworking group.org) has various resources for people wanting to learn more about the GRADE system, with a comprehensive list of published papers, presentations and aids to using the GRADE system.

CONSIDERATIONS FOR USING A GUIDELINE IN PRACTICE

- **Frame your clinical question of interest in a way that will help you to efficiently locate relevant information.** When searching for relevant guidelines, you should use the PICO method of formulating clinical questions, which was explained in Chapter 2.
- **Assess its applicability.** Once you have located and appraised a guideline and decided that it is valid, as with other types of evidence, you need to ask yourself: '*Is the guideline applicable to my patient/clinical scenario?*' Consider whether your patient is similar to the clinical population to which the guidelines apply. For example, your patient may have different risk factors to the clinical population who are the target group for the guidelines and, therefore, the guidelines cannot be applied to this patient.
- **Consider whether your healthcare setting is similar to the setting to which the guidelines apply.** This also involves considering organisational factors related to implementing a guideline, such as whether the appropriate resources are available and affordable (for example, specialised equipment or staff with the necessary skills).
- **Consider whether the values that are associated with a guideline (either explicitly or implicitly) match the values of your patient or your community.** As explained earlier in the chapter, application involves taking account of patient preferences as well as local circumstances. A clinical guideline is not a mandate for practice, but a 'guide'. Regardless of the strength of the evidence on which the guideline recommendations are made, it is the responsibility of the individual health professional to interpret their application for each particular situation. For example, while two patients may have the same risk for a particular health condition, we should not assume that they will react in the same way to a suggestion about interventions which are recommended in the guideline. As the two patients are likely to have different values, beliefs and preferences, and readiness to implement the intervention, one patient may wish to proceed with the intervention that the guideline recommends, whereas the other patient may decide not to.
- **Consider if additional tools may be useful.** Traditionally, guidelines were printed documents, sometimes with accompanying tools such as summaries, pathway maps or consumer versions. Information technology advances have enabled developers to produce guidelines differently (for example, some are moving to more dynamic, continuous updating so that changes occur not long after evidence changes) along with various guideline user tools.
- **Medico-legal implications.** It is beyond the scope of this book to discuss the medico-legal implications of guidelines in detail, as the situation and laws vary between countries. While guidelines can offer a standardised approach to clinical care for general situations, health professionals should interpret the guidelines within the context of an individual patient's circumstances. Because evidence-based clinical guidelines may be seen as providing normative standards for practice, departure from them may require some explanation. In clinical situations where there is a serious departure from evidence-based guidelines, this should be clearly documented in the patient's clinical records, along with the possible consequences of this, and that the benefits and harms of doing so have been thoroughly discussed with and understood by the patient, and the relevant clinical, or other (for example, patient choice), reasons for the departure provided.

DO CLINICAL GUIDELINES CHANGE PRACTICE AND IMPROVE CARE?

The use of clinical guidelines is not without some controversy. Extensive human and financial resources have been devoted to developing guidelines on a wide range of topics, but production and dissemination of a guideline alone has limited effect on uptake by health professionals.[62] It is clear that the effort and rigorous approach that goes into guideline development needs to be matched by a similar investment of time and resources into guideline implementation.

Implementing guideline recommendations often requires both a change in human behaviour and a change in the way systems work to deliver care, and this can be a difficult process. The process for implementing evidence into clinical practice, along with some of the barriers that may be encountered during the process and strategies for overcoming them, is discussed in Chapters 16 and 17. Unfortunately, there is a relative lack of high-quality research evidence on the impact of guideline implementation. There is some evidence that, when implemented, the use of guidelines can improve care processes and outcomes, but the effects are small and given the different delivery mechanisms and implementation strategies for these guidelines, difficult to measure.[63–67]

SUMMARY

- Clinical guidelines are systematically developed statements that are designed to help health professionals and their patients make decisions about patients' health care. Guidelines aim to reduce unwarranted variations in care, encourage best practice, and facilitate more informed and meaningful involvement of patients in making decisions about their health care.
- Clinical guidelines can be a useful tool for evidence-based practice. They translate evidence into actionable recommendations. They do not take the place of informed clinical judgment and patient choice in determining care but provide a summary of evidence and expert judgment about care that can be used to inform discussions with patients.
- A variety of online resources, such as guideline-specific databases, bibliographic databases, and the websites of disease-specific organisations and professional associations, can be used to locate guidelines.
- Guidelines are typically developed by a range of stakeholders, including clinical experts, researchers and patients. Ideally, the development of guidelines should follow a rigorous process. However, the quality of guidelines varies according to the processes that occurred during their development.
- Because guidelines vary in quality, you should know how to appraise clinical guidelines and recognise the key features that discriminate high-quality guidelines that can be used to guide practice from low-quality clinical guidelines that should be dismissed. The AGREE II instrument is a useful tool for appraising guidelines and helping you to determine if you can trust the recommendations that are in a clinical guideline.
- No matter how well clinical guidelines and their recommendations are linked to evidence, their interpretation and application should be guided by the health professional's clinical experience and judgment, and by the patient's preferences and values.

ACKNOWLEDGMENTS

The updated version of this chapter for this edition is based on Chapter 13 in the first, second and third editions of this book, which was co-authored by Dr Heather Buchan. Her valuable contribution to the content and structure of this chapter is gratefully acknowledged.

REFERENCES

1. Burgers JS, Grol R, Klazinga NS, et al. Towards evidence-based clinical practice: an international survey of 18 clinical guideline programs. Int J Qual Health Care 2003;15(1):31-45.
2. Institute of Medicine (US), Graham R, Mancher M, et al., editors. Clinical practice guidelines we can trust. Washington, DC: National Academies Press (US); 2011.
3. National Health and Medical Research Council. Annual report on Australian clinical practice guidelines. Canberra: National Health and Medical Research Council; 2014.
4. Runciman WB, Hunt TD, Hannaford NA, et al. CareTrack: assessing the appropriateness of health care delivery in Australia. Med J Aust 2012;197(2):100-5.
5. Braithwaite J, Glasziou P, Westbrook J. The three numbers you need to know about healthcare: the 60–30–10 Challenge. BMC Med 2020;18(1):102.
6. Feder G, Eccles M, Grol R, et al. Clinical guidelines: using clinical guidelines. BMJ 1999;318(7185):728-30.
7. Woolf SH, Grol R, Hutchinson A, et al. Potential benefits, limitations, and harms of clinical guidelines. BMJ 1999;318(7182):527-30.
8. Grimshaw J, Eccles M, Tetroe J. Implementing clinical guidelines: current evidence and future implications. J Cont Educ Health Prof 2004;24(Suppl 1):S31-S37.
9. Akl EA, Meerpohl JJ, Elliott J, et al. Living systematic reviews: 4. Living guideline recommendations. J Clin Epidemiol 2017;91:47-53.
10. Tendal B, Vogel JP, McDonald S, et al. Weekly updates of national living evidence-based guidelines: methods for the Australian living guidelines for care of people with COVID-19. J Clin Epidemiol 2021;131:11-21.
11. Hill K, English C, Campbell BCV, et al. Feasibility of national living guideline methods: The Australian Stroke Guidelines. J Clin Epidemiol. 2021;142:184-93.
12. Moynihan RN, Cooke GP, Doust JA, et al. Expanding disease definitions in guidelines and expert panel ties to industry: a cross-sectional study of common conditions in the United States. PLOS Med 2013;10(8):e1001500.
13. Schünemann HJ, Al-Ansary LA, Forland F, et al. Guidelines International Network: principles for disclosure of interests and management of conflicts in guidelines. Ann Intern Med 2015;163(7):548-53.
14. Hoffmann TC, Legare F, Simmons MB, et al. Shared decision making: what do clinicians need to know and why should they bother? Med J Aust 2014;201(1):35-9.
15. Scott IA, Guyatt GH. Suggestions for improving guideline utility and trustworthiness. Evid Based Med 2014;19(2):41-6.
16. McCormack JP, Loewen P. Adding 'value' to clinical practice guidelines. Can Fam Physician 2007;53(8):1326-7.
17. Elwyn G, Quinlan C, Mulley A, et al. Trustworthy guidelines–excellent; customized care tools–even better. BMC Med 2015;13(1):1-5.
18. Montori VM, Brito JP, Murad MH. The optimal practice of evidence-based medicine: incorporating patient preferences in practice guidelines. JAMA 2013;310(23):2503-4.

19. van der Weijden T, Boivin A, Burgers J, et al. Clinical practice guidelines and patient decision aids. An inevitable relationship. J Clin Epidemiol 2012;65(6):584–9.

20. van der Weijden T, Dreesens D, et al. Developing quality criteria for patient-directed knowledge tools related to clinical practice guidelines. A development and consensus study. Health Expect 2019;22(2):201–8.

21. Therapeutic Guidelines Limited. Acute bronchitis, Respiratory tract infections other than pneumonia. In: Antibiotic Therapeutic Guidelines. Therapeutic Guidelines Ltd (eTG March 2021 edition); 2019. Online. Available: https://www.tg.org.au/ (accessed 10 March 2022).

22. Stevens SM, Woller SC, Baumann Kreuziger L, et al. Executive summary. Antithrombotic therapy for VTE disease: second update of the CHEST Guideline and Expert Panel report. Chest 2021;160:2247–59.

23. Hoffmann T, Jansen J, Glasziou P. The importance and challenges of shared decision making in older people with multimorbidity. PLOS Med 2018;15(3):e1002530.

24. Goodman RA, Boyd C, Tinetti ME, et al. IOM and DHHS meeting on making clinical practice guidelines appropriate for patients with multiple chronic conditions. Ann Fam Med 2014;12(3):256–9.

25. Wilczynski NL, Haynes RB, Lavis JN, et al. Optimal search strategies for detecting health services research studies in MEDLINE. CMAJ 2004;171(10):1179–85.

26. Lunny C, Salzwedel DM, Liu T, et al. Validation of five search filters for retrieval of clinical practice guidelines produced low precision. J Clin Epidemiol 2020;117:109–16.

27. Qaseem A, Forland F, Macbeth F, et al. Guidelines International Network: toward international standards for clinical practice guidelines. Ann Intern Medicine 2012;156 (7):525–31.

28. National Health and Medical Research Council. Guidelines for guidelines handbook. National Health and Medical Research Council. Online. Available: https://www.nhmrc.gov.au/guidelinesforguidelines (accessed 10 March 2022).

29. Guyatt GH, Oxman AD, Vist GE, et al. GRADE: an emerging consensus on rating quality of evidence and strength of recommendations. BMJ 2008;336(7650):924–6.

30. Taylor-Phillips S, Stinton C, Ferrante di Ruffano L, et al. Association between use of systematic reviews and national policy recommendations on screening newborn babies for rare diseases: systematic review and meta-analysis. BMJ 2018;361:k1612.

31. Al-Ansary LA, Tricco AC, Adi Y, et al. A systematic review of recent clinical practice guidelines on the diagnosis, assessment and management of hypertension. PLOS One 2013;8(1):e53744.

32. Alonso-Coello P, Irfan A, Sola I, et al. The quality of clinical practice guidelines over the last two decades: a systematic review of guideline appraisal studies. Qual Saf Health Care 2010;19(6):e58.

33. Shaneyfelt TM, Mayo-Smith MF, Rothwangl J. Are guidelines following guidelines? The methodological quality of clinical practice guidelines in the peer-reviewed medical literature. JAMA 1999;281(20):1900–5.

34. Hoffmann-Esser W, Siering U, Neugebauer EA, et al. Guideline appraisal with AGREE II: systematic review of the current evidence on how users handle the 2 overall assessments. PLOS One 2017;12(3):e0174831.

35. Kung J, Miller RR, Mackowiak PA. Failure of clinical practice guidelines to meet institute of medicine standards: two more decades of little, if any, progress. Arch Intern Med 2012; 172(21):1628–33.

36. Grilli R, Magrini N, Penna A, et al. Practice guidelines developed by specialty societies: the need for a critical appraisal. Lancet 2000;355(9198):103–6.

37. Siering U, Eikermann M, Hausner E, et al. Appraisal tools for clinical practice guidelines: a systematic review. PLOS One 2013;8(12):e82915.

38. National Institute for Health and Care Excellence. Developing NICE guidelines: the manual: National Institute for Health and Care Excellence (NICE) (updated January 2022); 2014. Online. Available: www.nice.org.uk/process/pmg20 (accessed 11 March 2022).

39. Scottish Intercollegiate Guidelines Network (SIGN). A guideline developer's handbook. (SIGN publication no. 50). Edinburgh: SIGN; 2019. Online. Available: http://www.sign.ac.uk (accessed 11 March 2022).

40. Schünemann HJ, Wiercioch W, Etxeandia I, et al. Guidelines 2.0: systematic development of a comprehensive checklist for a successful guideline enterprise. CMAJ 2014;186(3): E123–E142.

41. Munn Z, Brandt L, Kuijpers T, et al. Are systematic review and guideline development tools useful? A Guidelines International Network survey of user preferences. JBI Evid Implement 2020;18(3):345–52.

42. Graham ID, Harrison MB. Evaluation and adaptation of clinical practice guidelines. Evid Based Nurs 2005;8(3): 68–72.

43. Shekelle PG, Kravitz RL, Beart J, et al. Are nonspecific practice guidelines potentially harmful? A randomized comparison of the effect of nonspecific versus specific guidelines on physician decision making. Health Serv Res 2000;34(7):1429.

44. Alonso-Coello P, Irfan A, Solà I, et al. The quality of clinical practice guidelines over the last two decades: a systematic review of guideline appraisal studies. Qual Saf Health Care 2010;19(6):e58.

45. Buchan HA, Currie KC, Lourey EJ, et al. Australian clinical practice guidelines: a national study. Med J Aust 2010; 192(9):490–4.

46. Van de Velde S, Heselmans A, Donceel P, et al. Rigour of development does not AGREE with recommendations in practice guidelines on the use of ice for acute ankle sprains. BMJ Qual Saf 2011;20(9):747–55.

47. Terrace L. Development and validation of an international appraisal instrument for assessing the quality of clinical practice guidelines: the AGREE project. Qual Saf Health Care 2003;12(1):18–23.

48. Makarski J, Brouwers MC. The AGREE Enterprise: a decade of advancing clinical practice guidelines. Implement Sci 2014;9(1):1–3.

49. Brouwers MC, Kho ME, Browman GP et al. AGREE II: advancing guideline development, reporting and evaluation in health care. CMAJ 2010;182(18):E839–E842.

50. Straus SE, Glasziou P, Richardson WS, et al. Evidence-based medicine E-book: how to practice and teach EBM. 5th ed. Elsevier Health Sciences; 2018.

51. Atkins D, Eccles M, Flottorp S, et al. Systems for grading the quality of evidence and the strength of recommendations I: critical appraisal of existing approaches The GRADE Working Group. BMC Health Serv Res 2004;4(1):1–7.

52. Guyatt GH, Oxman AD, Kunz R, et al. Going from evidence to recommendations. BMJ 2008;336(7652):1049–51.

53. Guyatt GH, Oxman AD, Kunz R, et al. Incorporating considerations of resources use into grading recommendations. BMJ 2008;336(7654):1170–3.

54. Guyatt GH, Oxman AD, Kunz R, et al. What is 'quality of evidence' and why is it important to clinicians? BMJ 2008; 336(7651):995–8.

55. Guyatt GH, Oxman AD, Vist GE, et al. GRADE: an emerging consensus on rating quality of evidence and strength of recommendations. BMJ 2008;336(7650):924–6.

56. Jaeschke R, Guyatt GH, Dellinger P, et al. Use of GRADE grid to reach decisions on clinical practice guidelines when consensus is elusive. BMJ 2008;337.

57. Schünemann HJ, Oxman AD, Brozek J, et al. GRADE: assessing the quality of evidence for diagnostic recommendations. Evid Based Med 2008;13(6):162–3.

58. Schünemann H, Brożek J, Guyatt G, et al., editors. Handbook for grading the quality of evidence and the strength of recommendations using GRADE approach. GRADE Working Group (updated October 2013); 2013. Online. Available: https://gdt.gradepro.org/app/handbook/handbook.html (accessed 11 March 2022).

59. Guyatt G, Oxman AD, Akl EA, et al. GRADE guidelines: 1. Introduction—GRADE evidence profiles and summary of findings tables. J Clin Epidemiol 2011;64(4):383–94.

60. Brozek JL, Akl EA, Alonso-Coello P, et al. Grading quality of evidence and strength of recommendations in clinical practice guidelines. Part 1 of 3. An overview of the GRADE approach and grading quality of evidence about interventions. Allergy 2009;64(5):669–77.

61. Alonso-Coello P, Schünemann HJ, Moberg J, et al. GRADE Evidence to Decision (EtD) frameworks: a systematic and transparent approach to making well informed healthcare choices. 1: Introduction. BMJ 2016;353:i2016.

62. Grimshaw J, Thomas R, MacLennan G, et al. Effectiveness and efficiency of guideline dissemination and implementation strategies. Health Technol Assess 2004;8(6):iii–iv,1–72.

63. Giguère A, Légaré F, Grimshaw J, et al. Printed educational materials: effects on professional practice and healthcare outcomes. Cochrane Database Syst Rev 2012;10(10): CD004398.

64. Kredo T, Bernhardsson S, Machingaidze S, et al. Guide to clinical practice guidelines: the current state of play. Int J Qual Health Care 2016;28(1):122–8.

65. Bighelli I, Ostuzzi G, Girlanda F et al. Implementation of treatment guidelines for specialist mental health care. Cochrane Database Syst Rev 2016;12(12):CD009780.

66. Agarwal S, Glenton C, Tamrat T, et al. Decision-support tools via mobile devices to improve quality of care in primary healthcare settings. Cochrane Database Syst Rev 2021;7(7):CD012944.

67. Giguère A, Zomahoun HT, Carmichael PH, et al. Printed educational materials: effects on professional practice and healthcare outcomes. Cochrane Database Syst Rev 2020;8 (8):CD004398.

Shared Decision Making

Tammy Hoffmann and Leigh Tooth

LEARNING OBJECTIVES

After reading this chapter, you should be able to:

- Understand what shared decision making is and describe its relationship with evidence-based practice
- Explain the importance of shared decision making and some of the challenges associated with it
- Explain the main steps in shared decision making and some of the strategies that can be used to facilitate it
- Explain key principles of effectively communicating statistical information to patients
- Describe the main considerations when deciding which communication format(s) to use with a patient

At the heart of the definition of evidence-based practice that was provided in Chapter 1 lies the involvement of patients and consideration of their values and preferences when decisions are being made regarding their health care. Patients often need to make decisions about aspects of their health care, such as whether to proceed with a particular intervention or test. Many patients and their families find it difficult to take an active part in healthcare decisions.[1] A health professional's ability to communicate effectively with patients and, often, also their family members is crucial to the successful engagement of patients in these decisions.[1] For these decisions to be fully informed and ones with which the patient is involved, patients need to know about the benefits, harms and risks, and uncertainties associated with the various options.[1] Even when a decision about intervention is not needed, there are often many other aspects of their health care that patients can benefit from being knowledgeable about. Many patients and their families have only a limited understanding about health and its determinants, and do not know where to find information that is clear, trustworthy and easy to understand.[1]

The main focus of this chapter, however, will be shared decision making (which is a type of communication and interaction with patients when a decision needs to be made)—including ways to facilitate it, challenges associated with it, how to assess it, and some of the skills involved in communicating statistical information to patients in an understandable and non-misleading manner. The aim of this chapter is to help you be aware of the importance of collaborating with patients as part of the decision-making process; of talking with your patients, where possible, about evidence relevant to the decision; and of being knowledgeable about the skills and resources that can assist you to do this successfully. However, this chapter will also briefly discuss some of the broader communication skills that health professionals need, as—despite its importance—specific training is often not provided in how to communicate effectively with patients.

PATIENT-CENTRED CARE

Many people do not think of communication as a particularly important or specialised skill for health professionals to have, and often health professionals do not give it the emphasis that it needs. Health professionals often think of communication as being secondary to their 'real' job of caring for patients. Yet, effective communication is central to a 'patient-centred' approach.

Patient-centred care (also referred to as *client-centred care* or *patient-centred practice*) is a broad umbrella term reflecting a particular approach to the health professional–patient relationship that implies communication, partnerships, respect, choice and empowerment, and a focus on the patient rather than their specific clinical condition.[2] This model of care sits between the 'paternalistic' and 'informed patient or independent choice' models of care.[3,4] In the traditional 'paternalistic' model of care, the health professional is in control, discloses information as and when suitable, and makes the decisions for the patient, who is expected to be passive, unquestioning and compliant. At the other end of the spectrum is the 'informed patient or independent choice' model, in which health professionals present the facts and leave the decision making solely up to the patient.[3] Central to patient-centred care is treating patients with dignity, responding quickly and effectively to their needs and concerns,[5] and providing them with enough information to enable them to make informed choices about their health care.[6] The last item is central to shared decision making; hence, shared decision making has been referred to as the pinnacle of patient-centred care.[7]

SHARED DECISION MAKING

Shared decision making is a consultation process where a health professional and patient jointly participate in making a health decision, having discussed the options, their benefits and harms, and considered the patient's values, preferences and circumstances.[8] Shared decision making can be viewed as a continuum,[9] along which the extent to which the patient or the health professional takes responsibility for the decision-making processes varies. At the extremes are health professional-led decisions and patient-led decisions, with many other possible approaches in between. The extent of involvement will vary between individuals, and between consultations, and according to the patient's preferences, the context in which the decision is occurring, and other circumstances.

While shared decision making is applicable to most situations, it is of most use, for example, where the evidence does not strongly support a single clearly superior option. This is the majority of clinical decisions! Here, it can help patients to understand the benefits, harms and trade-offs of the various options. It is also of particular value for *preference-sensitive decisions.* Preference-sensitive decisions are those where there is uncertainty as to which option is superior; where each option has different inherent benefits and harms; and, consequently, where the decision that is made is likely to be strongly guided by the patient's preferences and values.[10,11]

The connection between shared decision making and evidence-based practice

As you saw in Chapter 1, evidence-based practice should begin *and* end with the patient. After finding and appraising the evidence and integrating its inferences with their expertise, health professionals attempt to reach a decision, in conjunction with their patient, that reflects the patient's values and circumstances. Incorporating patient values, preferences and circumstances is probably the most difficult and poorly mapped step, but it has received the least amount of attention.[12] Shared decision making provides a mechanism for this to occur. As Figure 14.1 shows, shared decision making occurs at the intersection of patient-centred communication skills and evidence-based practice—all of which are necessary for optimal patient care.[13]

Shared decision making provides a process for explicitly bringing evidence into a consultation and discussing it with the patient. Through evidence-informed deliberations, patients construct informed preferences.[13] Without discussion, health professionals can only guess at a patient's preference. Authentic evidence-based practice cannot occur without shared decision making;[13] dictating to patients what they should do is not the intention of evidence-based practice. Shared decision making is also an important, but under-recognised, route by which evidence is incorporated into clinical practice.[8] Likewise, shared decision making is dependent on evidence-based practice as a number of its steps are inseparably linked to the evidence. For truly informed decisions to be possible, discussions with patients should incorporate the evidence. For example, the natural history of the condition, the possible options, the benefits and harms of each, and a quantification of these, must be informed by the best available research evidence.[13] Health professionals often have inaccurate expectations about the effect of health interventions and tend to overestimate the benefits and underestimate the harms.[14] As shared decision making requires health professionals to know the best available evidence about the benefits and harms of the options, it can be a mechanism by which they acquire this knowledge. This can be through the process of locating evidence as part of evidence-based practice or from synthesised evidence resources such as clinical guidelines, or even from patient decision aids.[15]

The importance, and benefits, of shared decision making

Many leading health organisations around the world now advocate shared decision making. Not only is it crucial to authentic evidence-based practice and an ethical imperative;[16] it also has other potential benefits. As it is a relatively

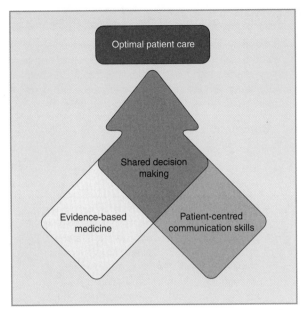

Fig 14.1 The interdependence of evidence-based practice and shared decision making and the need for both as part of optimal care
Hoffmann TC, Montori VM, Del Mar C. The connection between evidence-based medicine and shared decision making. JAMA 2014;312(13):1295–6.

new field, evidence about its effectiveness is still emerging. Most of the evidence to date comes from randomised trials of patient decision aids. (Decision aids are explained later in the chapter.) A Cochrane systematic review[17] of decision aids concluded that, compared with usual care, decision aids assist patients to have greater knowledge of the options, have more realistic expectations of possible benefits and harms, and make choices which better reflect their personal values and preferences, with no adverse effects on health outcomes or satisfaction. They also increase patient communication with health professionals, and participation in collaborative decision making, and reduce decisional conflict related to feeling uninformed.

Similar to health professionals, patients typically overestimate the benefits of interventions and underestimate their harms.[18] Shared decision making provides an opportunity for resolving this mismatch between expectations and the demonstrated benefits and harms of tests and treatments. As patients tend to choose more conservative options when fully informed about the benefits and harms,[17] shared decision making can reduce the inappropriate use of tests and treatments and has a role in reducing the problem of overdiagnosis and over-treatment.[19]

Steps in the process of shared decision making

Some of the things that shared decision making can mistakenly be perceived to be, but is *not*, are: (1) a single step to be added to a consultation; (2) the provision of patient education; (3) simply giving a patient a decision aid; and (4) a health professional presenting their recommendation to the patient and asking if they are okay with what is suggested. Remember that shared decision making is a *process*, and while it might additionally use patient education materials or decision support tools, it is not dependent on them. It involves establishing a partnership with the patient, a fundamental part of which is bidirectional communication, so just giving a decision aid to a patient does not mean that shared decision making has occurred. The exact nature and mode of shared decision making varies and needs to be tailored according to the patient, health professional and circumstances.[20] Typical elements of the shared decision making process that occur include: explaining the problem and the need for a decision; inviting the patient's engagement; explaining the options, and the benefits and harms of each; exploring the patient's preferences and values; clarifying understanding and answering questions; engaging in collaborative deliberation and consensus building; and making or explicitly deferring the decision.

There are various approaches that can be used to guide the process of shared decision making. Box 14.1 shows one way, with some questions that can be used to guide the process,[21] example comments for a particular clinical scenario and some general strategies.[22–24] Another approach breaks the decision-making part of the consultation into 'Team Talk' (helping patients to know that an issue, for which multiple options exist, needs to be discussed and a decision-making process started), 'Option Talk' (discussing the options and their benefits and harms), and 'Decision Talk' (helping patients to explore what matters to them, construct informed preferences and reach a decision).[25,26]

If a high quality and appropriate decision support tool is available for the decision under consideration, it can be incorporated into this process. The tool may be used before, during or after the consultation. For the scenario used in Box 14.1, the first page of an illustrative decision aid is shown in Figure 14.2. A summary of the process is illustrated in Figure 14.3. In 2021, a clinical guideline devoted to shared decision making was released by the UK's National Institute for Health and Care Excellence (NICE).[27] It contains information on how to engage patients in the process, resources and suggestions for organisational planning, training and healthcare delivery to assist with embedding shared decision making in an organisation's culture and practices.

BOX 14.1   An example of one approach to shared decision making

Clinical scenario: *You are a general practitioner and one of your patients today is Emma and her mother. Emma is a two-and-a-half-year-old who has had a cold for 3 days. Last night she became worse—she was restless and had a fever. Her mother was up with her for much of the night and Emma settled eventually with paracetamol. The only positive findings on clinical examination are a blocked nose and bulging red left ear drum. You diagnose acute otitis media. 'Okay,' you say. 'Emma has a middle ear infection.' Her mother asks, 'What can be done to help her?'*

Questions that health professionals can use to guide the process	Example phrases to illustrate each step, using a scenario of a child with middle ear infection	Comment
Before you start	*'Now that we've worked out what the problem is, there are some decisions to make about what to do next. I'd like to discuss the options (or choices) with you, and the pros and cons of each. Is that okay? We can then talk about how you feel about the options and if you have a preference for one or more, and any questions.'* *'Would you like to be involved in discussing with me and deciding together about what the best next step is for you/your child?'*	• Many patients may be unfamiliar with being invited to participate in the decision-making process, so you may wish to **explain the process briefly**. Outlining that they have some choices that you would like to go through with them before deciding together about the next step can provide reassurance to patients who may otherwise feel overwhelmed by the idea of participating in the decision, uncertain about being involved, or even abandoned. • Determine **the degree to which your patient wants to be involved in decision making**.
1. What will happen if we wait and watch?	*'In children, most middle ear infections get better by themselves, usually within a week. The best options to control pain and fever are paracetamol or ibuprofen.'*	• If it is clear what the problem is and that a decision about the next step needs to be made, this step involves describing the nature of the problem/condition. This should usually include providing information about the **natural history** of the condition—that is, what is likely to happen without any intervention ('watch and wait'). Quantitative information can be provided where possible, either at this step or in step 3. When this is not possible, descriptive information can be provided (e.g. *'Most people find that the symptoms go away by …'*). • Eliciting the patient's **expectations** about management of the condition (e.g. *'What have you heard or know about …?'*), including previously tested approaches and experiences, along with fears and concerns, is important and may occur here or later in the process.

BOX 14.1   An example of one approach to shared decision making—cont'd

Questions that health professionals can use to guide the process	Example phrases to illustrate each step, using a scenario of a child with middle ear infection	Comment
2. **What are the options?**	*'Waiting for it to get better by itself is one option. Another option is to take antibiotics. Do you want to discuss that option?'*	• This question triggers a discussion of the options and identification of those that the patient would like to hear more about. • For some decisions (such as in this example), the options may be familiar to patients and need little elaboration at this step. In others, a more detailed explanation about what each option is (and the practicalities of each, including options which are time-urgent) will be required.
3. **What are the benefits and harms of these options?**	*'We know from good research that of 100 children with middle ear infection who do **not** take antibiotics, 84 will feel better and have no pain after 2–3 days. Out of 100 children who **do** take antibiotics, 89 will feel better after about 3 days of taking them. So, about 5 more will get better a little faster. We can't know whether your child will be one of the 5 children who benefit, or not.'* [A graphical representation of these numbers can also be shown at this point, and again, as the harms information is discussed—see Figure 14.2.] *'There are some downsides to antibiotics, though. Out of 100 children who do take antibiotics, 27 will experience vomiting, diarrhoea or rash, compared to 20 who do **not** take them. That means about 7 children out of 100 will have side effects from antibiotics. But again, we can't know whether your child will have any of these problems. The other possible downside is antibiotic resistance—would you like to hear more about it?'*	• In addition to descriptively discussing the benefits and harms of each option, the **probability of each occurring or the likely size** of the benefit or harms, where this is known, should be provided. See the section 'Communicating numerical information to patients' later in this chapter for general principles about how to do this. • **Decision support tools**, if available, can be useful at this stage. Simple visual graphics can be particularly useful in helping to communicate the numbers. • The discussion about **harms** should extend beyond discussion about the risk of side effects and include other impacts that the option could have on the patient, such as cost, inconvenience and interference with daily roles (treatment burden) and reduced quality of life.

Continued

BOX 14.1   An example of one approach to shared decision making—cont'd

Questions that health professionals can use to guide the process	Example phrases to illustrate each step, using a scenario of a child with middle ear infection	Comment
4. **How do the benefits and harms weigh up for you?**	*'With all I've said, which option do you feel most comfortable with?'*	• This step includes eliciting the patient's preferences and working with them to clarify how each option may fit with their values, preferences, beliefs and goals. • Some decision aids include formal value clarification exercises and, if available, these can be used to supplement the conversation and/or enable the patient to reflect further on these issues following the consultation. • Clarifying the patient's understanding of what has been discussed so far, through the 'teach-back' method, can help to identify if any information needs to be repeated or explained in another way.
5. **Do you have enough information to make a choice?**	*'Is there anything more you wanted to know? Do you feel you have enough information to make a choice?'*	• This provides another opportunity to ask if the patient has additional questions and to determine the degree to which they understand the information you have provided to them. • The patient may feel ready to make a decision at this stage, or it may be jointly decided to defer the decision and to plan when it should be revisited. • The patient may wish to seek further information before deciding, to discuss the matter further with their family, and/or to take time to process and reflect on the information received.

Other general strategies
• Attend to the whole of the patient's problems and take account of their expectations, feelings and ideas.
• Tailor the amount and pace of information to each patient's needs and preferences.
• Value the patient's contributions—for example, the life experiences and values that they bring to the decision-making process.
• Provide clear, honest and unbiased information. Be well informed about the most current evidence.
• Be an active listener and provide a caring, respectful and empowering context in which the patient can be enabled to participate in decision making and feel comfortable asking questions.
• Do not assume that your patient will make the same decisions as you, just because the evidence has been provided to them in a manner that they can understand.

Adapted from Hoffmann T, Légaré F, Simmons M, et al. Shared decision making: what do clinicians need to know and why should they bother? Med J Aust 2014;201(9):513–14 © Copyright 2014. The Medical Journal of Australia—reproduced with permission. The Medical Journal of Australia does not accept responsibility for any errors in translation.

Middle ear infection: should my child take antibiotics?

- This decision aid is to help you and your doctor decide whether to use antibiotics when **your child** has a middle ear infection.
- This can help you to talk to, and make a **shared decision** with, your doctor about what is best for your child.

What causes middle ear infection?

- It can be caused by a viral or bacterial infection. It is hard for your doctor to tell which it is.
- It is also called 'acute otitis media'. 'Acute' means it is a short-term infection.

How long does the earache last?

- Symptoms (such as earache) usually get better in 2 to 7 days, without antibiotics.

What are the treatment **options?**

There are two options that you can discuss with your doctor:

1. Not taking antibiotics
This means letting the infection get better by itself.

2. Taking antibiotics

Symptoms, such as pain and fever, can be treated with over-the-counter medicines. They can be used with either option.

What are the likely **benefits and harms** of each option?

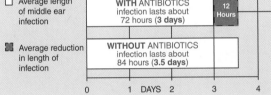

☐ Average length of middle ear infection

■ Average reduction in length of infection

WITH ANTIBIOTICS infection lasts about 72 hours (**3 days**) 12 Hours

WITHOUT ANTIBIOTICS infection lasts about 84 hours (**3.5 days**)

Children who take antibiotics have the earache for only about **12 hours less** than children who do not

These figures show what happens to children with middle ear infection who **do not** take antibiotics and those who **do**. Each circle is one child. We can't predict whether your child will be one of the children who is helped or harmed.

○ gets better by 2–3 days
● gets better by 2–3 days due to antibiotics
● not better by 2–3 days

○ has problems
● has problems due to antibiotics
● no problems

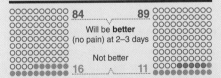

100 children who **don't** take antibiotics   100 children who **do** take antibiotics

84   89
Will be **better** (no pain) at 2–3 days
Not better
16   11

With antibiotics, **5 more children** will be better after 2–3 days.

After about **4 days** most children will be better anyway—without antibiotics.

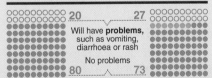

100 children who **don't** take antibiotics   100 children who **do** take antibiotics

20   27
Will have **problems,** such as vomiting, diarrhoea or rash
No problems
80   73

With antibiotics, 7 **more children** will have problems such as vomiting and diarrhoea. Other antibiotic harms are:

– the **cost** of buying them
– **remembering** to take them
– the risk of **antibiotic resistance**

Fig 14.2 Example of a section of a decision aid (for decisions about antibiotic use in middle ear infection), and also illustrating pictographs for communicating benefit and harm information
Reproduced with permission of Tammy Hoffmann, Chris Del Mar and Peter Coxeter of the Institute of Evidence-Based Healthcare, Bond University.

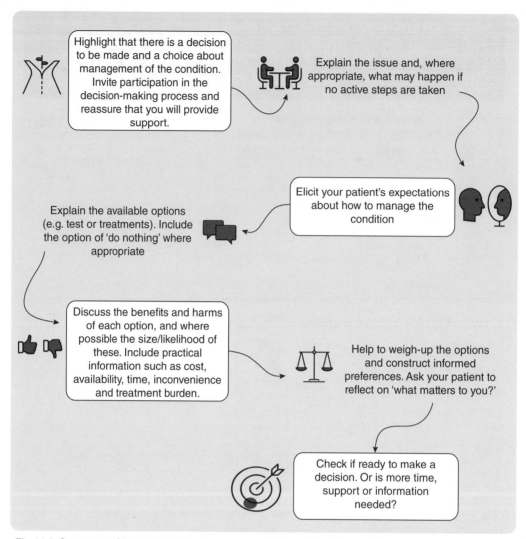

Fig 14.3 Summary of key elements in the process of shared decision making
Hoffmann T, Bakhit M, Michaleff Z. Shared decision making and physical therapy: what, when, how, and why? Brazil J Phys Ther 2022;26(1):100382.

Myths about shared decision making

There are a number of barriers and challenges to the widespread implementation of shared decision making.[28–32] Summaries of the main barriers, facilitators and strategies, at the level of the individual, organisation and system, to implementing shared decision making in practice can be found elsewhere.[33] While detailed discussion of these is beyond the scope of this chapter, it is pertinent that we list some of the barriers, as identified in a systematic review, as perceived by health professionals.[34] These are listed in Box 14.2, along with comments and, where possible, research findings about each perceived barrier.

Challenges in shared decision making

Some of the challenges that can be associated with shared decision making include:

- *Challenges related to the availability of evidence.* For some conditions there may not be sufficient, or any, evidence about the benefits and harms of the options, in which case the health professional needs to assist the patient to assess this uncertainty against the patient's values and preferences.[55]
- *Multi-morbidity.* Some patients, particularly older patients, have more than one chronic condition and this can complicate shared decision making as issues such as

BOX 14.2   Misconceptions about shared decision making and key research findings to refute them

Misconception	Research
The duration of the consultation will be lengthened.	
This concern is the most frequently reported barrier to shared decision making. Indeed, time constraint is the most frequently reported barrier to *any* clinical change.[35]	Systematic reviews indicate that there is no or minimal (for example, median 2.6 minutes) increase in consultation duration when shared decision making is implemented or decision aids are used.[17,36,37]
Patients will be unsupported when making healthcare decisions.	
There is a fear that shared decision making will make patients feel abandoned during difficult decisions.	This is a misinterpretation of the intent of shared decision making. The definition of shared decision making explicitly describes patients and their clinicians sharing the process of making a decision.[38] Shared decision making is not about insisting that every patient must make the decision (not all patients wish to); instead, it at least helps to ensure that patients are informed about their options and are offered the opportunity to participate in the decision making.
Not every patient wants to share in the decision-making process with their clinician.	
Critics of shared decision making argue that not every patient wants to be involved in making decisions with their clinician.	An Australian survey reported that over 90% of women preferred a shared role with their doctor in making decisions about screening and diagnostic tests.[39] A European survey of >8,000 people reported a high desire for shared health decision making (>70% of the sample).[40] A systematic review of 14 studies that examined the match between patient preferences about information and decision making with clinician–patient communication found that a substantial number of patients (26–95%; median 52%) were dissatisfied with the information given and would have preferred a more active role in decisions concerning their health, especially when they understood the expectations attached to this role.[41] A time trend in desired involvement in decision making has also been reported. Of the studies conducted in 2000 and later, 71% reported that the majority of respondents preferred a role in sharing decisions, compared to 50% of studies that were conducted before 2000.[42]
Most people are not able to participate in shared decision making.	
Critics of shared decision making question its complexity, believing that most people will not be able to manage it.	Shared decision making is comprised of a set of behaviours on the part of the clinician and the patient that can be learnt.[43,44] An increasing number of studies demonstrate successful shared decision making in clinical practice.[17,36,45]

Continued

BOX 14.2   Misconceptions about shared decision making and key research findings to refute them—cont'd

Misconception	Research
Shared decision making cannot be used with vulnerable people.	
Shared decision making requires a special set of skills that may be too complex for all patients to acquire and 'they may not ever be able to share decisions with their providers'.	Most surveys of patients regarding their willingness to engage in shared decision making systematically show that the most vulnerable people are those that are less willing to engage.[40] Therefore, we need to be careful not to increase health inequities by offering shared decision making solely to the most privileged patients. Individuals with low health literacy may want to be involved in health decisions but often lack the knowledge, skills and confidence to communicate with clinicians, navigate the health system and engage in shared decision making.[46] They receive less information, ask fewer questions and are less satisfied with healthcare provider communication.[47] More vulnerable patients may be less likely to engage in shared decision making because of lower self-efficacy—a modifiable factor to increase their willingness to do so.[48] Indeed, to decrease health inequities, more needs to be done to engage the most vulnerable patients to make informed decisions.[49,50] A recent systematic review found that decision aids did not reduce health inequalities; however, they resulted in better outcomes among socially disadvantaged populations.[51]
'I already do this.'	
Most clinicians feel they already successfully engage their patients in shared decision making—a belief that may arise from clinicians not really understanding what shared decision making is and how to do it.	A systematic review of 33 studies that assessed shared decision making with the OPTION (Observing Patient Involvement in Decision Making) scale found low levels of patient-involving behaviours (mean OPTION score of 23 +/− 14 on 0–100 scale, where higher scores indicate higher levels of patient involvement in decision making).[52] Lack of familiarity with shared decision making by health professionals has been found to be a frequent barrier to shared decision making.[34,45] Providing practical, interactive skills training and workshops (at entry-level education and in continuing professional development) can help to: dispel myths about it; improve clinicians' knowledge, along with risk communication skills and other shared decision making skills; identify differences between shared decision making and current practice; promote discussion and positive attitudes towards it (for example, 'We could do this better'). A free online course in shared decision making (four modules, takes about 2 hours to complete) has been developed to enable health professionals anywhere to undertake introductory training.[53] It is available at: https://www.safetyandquality.gov.au/our-work/partnering-consumers/shared-decision-making/risk-communication-module Versions tailored for various medical disciplines are available at: https://wintoncentre.maths.cam.ac.uk/resources/medicine/
Engaging patients in shared decision making will raise their anxiety level.	
Some clinicians are afraid that shared decision making will raise patients' anxiety levels as they become aware of the inherent uncertainty of evidence.	The Cochrane review of decision aids refutes this misconception, finding no effect on anxiety.[17] Anxiety should not be confused with decisional conflict, an intra-psychological construct that reflects the difficulty individuals can experience when comparing different options.[54]

polypharmacy and treatment burden need to be considered. Most guidelines and existing decision support tools do not consider multi-morbidity, and new approaches and tools for facilitating shared decision making among people with multi-morbidity are only just starting to emerge.[56]

- *Patients' involvement in shared decision making.* Shared decision making is not always possible—for example, in medical emergencies, or with patients who do not have the cognitive capacity to participate. Further, while desired by many, not every patient will desire or welcome shared decision making. As a health professional, you need to determine the role that each of your patients wishes to take in the management of their health. A simple question that you can ask to help establish this is: '*How do you feel about being involved in making decisions about your treatment?*'[57]

- *What if my patient chooses to do the 'wrong thing'?* Some health professionals, particularly those who are new to or unfamiliar with the principles of shared decision making, worry that once patients are fully informed about benefits, harms and risks, they may still decide not to undertake treatment for a health condition or to have a screening test because they are at low risk of developing future problems.[58] Health professionals can become frustrated if a patient makes a choice that the health professional perceives to be the 'wrong choice',[58] particularly if the patient is choosing a path that may result in harm or death.

Legal implications of shared decision making

Shared decision making is not the same as informed consent (such as when patients consent to a procedure), but the legal implications of shared decision making and associated requirements (such as documentation of it) are not yet clear. The inadequacies of the existing informed consent process are well documented.[59,60] In a significant legal case in 2015 in the United Kingdom, the Supreme Court ruled that the standard for what health professionals should inform patients about (in terms of benefits, harms and options) should be determined by what a 'reasonable patient' deems important.[60] This is a departure from the traditional approach in which a group of doctors determined what is important for patients to be told. As this 'reasonable patient' standard becomes more widely adopted, there is enormous opportunity (and incentive) for health professionals to embrace shared decision making and, in time, it is possible it may become the preferred standard for informed consent.[60] The importance of emphasising shared decision making as 'the way that health care decision making should occur' is reflected in an increasing number of official documents from healthcare organisations and governing bodies. For example, in November 2020 the UK's General Medical Council issued a guidance document that contains seven principles on decision making and consent.[61] The guidance clearly states: '*... the exchange of information between doctor and patient is essential to good decision making. Serious harm can result if patients are not listened to, or if they are not given the information they need—and time and support to understand it—so they can make informed decisions about their care.*' The Australian Commission of Safety and Quality in Healthcare has incorporated shared decision making into its National Safety and Quality Health Standards, which are the national accreditation standards.[62]

Tools to assess shared decision making

A number of scales have been developed to assess the involvement of patients and health professionals in shared decision making. These scales can also assist you by providing examples of competencies you can aim for in your own clinical practice. One of the most widely used tools to measure the extent to which shared decision making occurs in a consultation is the 12-item OPTION (Observing Patient Involvement in Decision Making; www.glynelwyn.com/) scale.[63,64] A five-item version of the OPTION scale also exists.[65] From the patient's perspective, questionnaires have been developed to assess their satisfaction with decision making,[66] degree of decisional conflict,[52] perceived involvement in care,[67] risk communication and confidence in decision making[57] and the extent of shared decision making.[68,69]

DECISION SUPPORT TOOLS

Various types of decision support tools exist, and most aim to help bring evidence into clinical decisions. A common type is a patient decision aid that is explicitly designed to facilitate shared decision making. Others provide information for some components of the process (for example, risk calculators, evidence summaries) or ways of initiating and/ or structuring conversations about health decisions. Examples of the latter include question prompt lists and communication frameworks such as Ask-Share-Know (https://askshareknow.com.au/ask-questions/overview/), BRAN (Benefits, Risks, Alternatives, do Nothing) (https://www.choosingwisely.co.uk/resources/shared-decision-making-resources/), and the Ottawa Personal Decision Guide (https://decisionaid.ohri.ca/decguide.html).

Patient decision aids

Decision aids are a communication tool that may assist patients who are facing decisions about the best way to manage their health. They contain information about the options, the benefits and harms of each option, and sometimes values clarification exercises (which aim to help patients think about what matters to them and what their preferences may be). They may be paper-based (such as a pamphlet), involve a video (often with accompanying printed information) or be based on the internet. Figure 14.2 shows an example of the first page of a two-page decision aid. The Australian Commission on Safety and Quality in Healthcare has produced a short video about decision aids and how to use them: https://www.safetyandquality.gov.au/our-work/shared-decision-making/shared-decision-making-symposium. One of the quality criteria for a patient decision aid is that it contains quantitative information;[70] hence, one of the skills that health professionals need is to be able to communicate that information well to patients. (See the next section of this chapter.)

Finding decision aids

Currently, the majority of decision aids that exist are on topics that are most appropriate for medical practitioners to discuss with their patients (for example, deciding between various treatments for cancer, or deciding whether to receive hormone replacement therapy). There are comparatively fewer decision aids that summarise the options and evidence for conditions that other health professionals, such as nurses and allied health professionals, discuss with patients. However, this is changing and new decision aids are continually being developed, so when you have a patient who needs to make a decision it is worth searching the internet to see if there is a relevant decision aid. Unfortunately, patient decision aids are scattered across various sites and there is not a single and comprehensive source of them, nor a reliable search strategy to locate them. Some of the resources to consider are:

- Ottawa Health Research Institute Inventory of decision aids—www.ohri.ca/decisionaid.
- In some countries, government agencies and health organisations contain collections of (usually) locally produced decision aids. Examples include: UK NICE (https://www.nice.org.uk/about/what-we-do/our-programmes/nice-guidance/nice-guidelines/shared-decision-making; you can filter by evidence type: patient decision aid); Med-Decs, an international database for support in medical choices (https://www.med-decs.org/en); and Harding Centre for Risk Literacy—aids here are called medical fact boxes (https://www.hardingcenter.de/en).
- MAGIC: https://magicevidence.org/magicapp/decision-aids/. Among the challenges of producing decision aids are the time it takes to do this and the need to keep them up to date as the evidence changes. A promising new initiative (although testing of the eventual output with patients is currently under way) enables the benefits and harms component of a decision aid to be produced automatically from evidence summaries (such as those in guidelines or systematic reviews).[71] As part of the MAGIC evidence ecosystem, and in conjunction with BMJ, rapid recommendation articles for various clinical questions have been published (https://www.bmj.com/rapid-recommendations) and decision aids that have been produced as part of this can be accessed.
- OPTION Grids are a brief decision aid. They mostly cover medical topics and require a subscription to be accessed: https://www.ebsco.com/health-care/products/my-health-decisions.

Using decision aids

If you are considering using a decision aid with a patient, you need to ensure that it is of good quality, reflects current evidence and is relevant to the decision that needs to be made and the setting that it will be used in. A set of criteria (from the International Patient Decision Aid Standards Collaboration—http://ipdas.ohri.ca/) has been developed for assessing the quality of decision aids,[72] although this set is currently being updated. As decision aids are added to the registry mentioned above, they are rated according to a shortened set of these criteria and the aid's score for each criterion is displayed.

Decision aids are a tool that can be used for facilitating shared decision making. However, there are many gaps in the research related to decision aids, such as how they affect communication between the health professional and the patient, factors that determine the successful use of decision aids in practice, and what types of decision aids work best with different types of patients. There are still many unknowns about the best way to select and incorporate evidence into patient decision aids,[73] and issues such as accounting for multimorbidity, which is the reality for many patients.[56] As mentioned earlier, use of a decision aid does not guarantee that shared decision making will occur. As decision aids currently do not exist for most of the decisions that occur in health care (and even when they do), it is incredibly important that health professionals are able to interpret and communicate numerical and statistical information, particularly about probabilities and risks, to patients in an appropriate way; hence, this is the focus of the next section of the chapter. This skill is often called *risk communication*, but as you will see, it involves more than just communicating risk.

Beyond the decision support tools described earlier, health professionals may wish to provide additional resources or health information to patients. The following resources may be of use:

- The Cochrane Consumer Network maintains a list of resources aimed at helping patients to use evidence when making decisions (https://consumers.cochrane.org/help-using-evidence).
- MedlinePlus (www.nlm.nih.gov/medlineplus)—a free service provided by the US National Library of Medicine that offers links to health information sites that meet pre-established quality criteria. It is designed to help provide high-quality health information to

patients and their families. Health professionals can also use this site to obtain quick access to images or videos to help when providing information.

- Choosing Wisely (www.choosingwisely.org.au; many countries have their own website with country-specific lists and resources)—a campaign that aims to help patients engage health professionals in conversations about health decisions, particularly about tests and treatments that may not be appropriate or necessary for them.

COMMUNICATING NUMERICAL INFORMATION TO PATIENTS

'Patients expect information about benefits and risks that is (as far as possible) accurate, unbiased, personally relevant to them and presented in a way that they can understand.'[74]

There are many examples of numerical information about health being presented in a non-transparent and/or incorrect manner by health professionals, public figures and journalists. (For good overviews, see Gigerenzer and colleagues[75] and Wegwarth and Gigerenzer.[76]) The impacts of incorrectly presented and/or misunderstood health statistics are many, including:

- incorrectly heightened or lowered appreciation of risk and the associated emotional reactions and health decisions that can occur
- impediments to shared decision making and informed consent procedures
- incorrect diagnosis,[75] overdiagnosis[77] or unnecessary medical procedures.[78]

There are often differences between how health professionals and patients understand probability and risk. Many health professionals have been trained to understand these as mathematical probabilities of an event happening within a whole population. Health professionals subsequently tend to view these statistics as objective and impersonal. Conversely, patients' views and understanding of these concepts are commonly influenced by their numeracy literacy; emotions; anxieties and concerns about the future; what they have seen and heard reported in media, online sources and social media; and the views and experiences of their social networks. As written cogently by Lautenbach:[79] 'An individual brings a lifetime of experience to how he or she perceives, interprets, understands, or even ignores these figures'. Indeed, patients often personalise risk and are less interested in what happens to 'populations'.[74] Information about risks can also be hard for patients to understand when they do not have medical knowledge or previous experience to compare the numbers against; for example, if the risk of an event is 20%, patients may not know whether this is relatively high or relatively low.[74]

There are different types of numerical and statistical information that health professionals need to understand[76] and communicate to patients. The next section describes frequently used statistics and how patients may misinterpret the meanings. Table 14.1 presents strategies that you can use to simplify how you present this information and ensure it is not misleading.

TABLE 14.1 **The problem of probabilities and risk, and how using natural frequencies can help when explaining this type of information**

The clinical scenario	Expressed as a probability	How probabilities may be incorrectly understood	Expressed as natural frequencies (event rates)
Patient needs to have a particular intervention but there is a 20% risk of a side effect	Single probability commonly expressed as 'There is a 20% chance that you will have a particular side effect if you follow the intervention'	That they will have the side effect 20% of the time	Of every 100 patients who have this intervention, 20 patients will experience this side effect

The clinical scenario	Expressed as a relative risk	How relative risks may be incorrectly understood	Expressed in natural frequencies as an absolute risk
By undergoing a particular screening test, the patient's risk of dying from a disease may be reduced	For example, 'By having a screening test, your risk of dying from the disease is reduced by 50%'	The large percentage may mislead the patient into thinking that the reduction in the risk of their own possible death is large	The patient's baseline risk of dying from the disease is 1 out of 1,000. By undergoing the screening test, this is reduced by half, or to 0.5 in 1000

Types of data that health professionals use and how to present them to patients

Probability

Probability refers to the chance of an event occurring. Values for probability lie between 0 and 1 and are often presented as a percentage. For example, a probability of 0.5 may be expressed as 50%. Probability can occur as a single probability or as a conditional probability. Consider the situation where a patient wants to know the likelihood of side effects that they might experience in relation to an intervention. An example of *single probability* is that there is a 20% chance that the patient will have a particular side effect if they receive a certain intervention. The problem with this concept is that how it should be interpreted may be confusing.[80] For example, a patient may interpret this as meaning that 20% of patients will have the side effect, or that all patients will have the side effect 20% of the time. The latter interpretation reflects the 'personal' as opposed to 'population' view that patients tend to have.[81] *Conditional probability* refers to the probability of an event, *given that another event has occurred*. An example of conditional probability is: if a person has a disease, the probability that a screening test will be positive for the disease is 90%.

Risk of disease or harm

Risk of disease (or *harm*) refers to the probability of developing the disease (or a harm) in a stated time period. As we saw in Chapter 4, risk is often presented as either absolute risk or relative risk. When referring to the risk of a disease or harm, these concepts can be interpreted as follows:

- *Absolute risk* refers to the incidence (or natural frequency) of the disease or event in the population.
- *Relative risk* is the ratio of two risks (or, as we saw in Chapter 4, the flip side of the concept of relative risk is relative benefit): the risk in the population exposed to some factor (for example, having received a particular intervention) divided by the risk of those not exposed. Relative risk gives an indication of the degree of risk.
  - If the relative risk is *equal to 1*, the risk in the exposed population is *the same* as in the unexposed population.
  - If the relative risk is *greater than 1*, the risk in the exposed population is *greater than* it is for those in the unexposed population.
  - If the relative risk is *less than 1*, the risk in the exposed population is *less than* it is for those in the unexposed population.

Box 14.3 provides an example of *relative* risk. Relative risk by itself should not be presented to patients as it tends to magnify risk perceptions and is not well understood.[82] The potential for relative risk to be misleading, to both patients and health professionals, was pointed out in Chapter 4.

Absolute risk: natural frequencies (incidence) versus probabilities (chance)

A recent review of presenting numerical information about the chance that an event will occur recommended that when the numerical information concerns the chance of a single event, then use of either of the following is suitable: natural frequencies (for example, 20 out of every 100 people every year) or probabilities or percentages (also called 'event rates'—for example, 20% of people with a certain condition will develop another condition).[70] When presenting natural frequencies or percentages, it is important to have a reference group to compare to, as this will help the patient to more accurately assess themselves against the reference group. For example, advising patients that every year, 5 in 100 people with hypertension will develop a certain condition. If time-based risk formats are used—for example, 'chance of a particular outcome at 5 years or 10 years'—it is important to use the same time frame for all outcomes.[83] Patients are also more likely to understand percentages out of 100, rather than 1,000 or 10,000. The use of 'one in X' formats should be avoided as these are difficult to understand and may lead to biased interpretations.[70]

The review by Bonner and colleagues of presenting numerical information about the chance that an event will occur also recommended that when the numerical information concerns the chance of two or more events occurring, the use of percentages is preferred over natural frequencies. For example, presenting that there is a 10% chance of side effects after taking drug A compared with a 15% chance with drug B.[70]

BOX 14.3 Example of relative risk

Incidence of a side effect among people exposed to medication $A = \dfrac{34}{1000} = 0.034$

Incidence of a side effect among people not exposed to medication $A = \dfrac{22}{1000} = 0.022$

$\text{Relative risk} = \dfrac{\text{Incidence in exposed}}{\text{Incidence in unexposed}} = \dfrac{0.034}{0.022} = 1.5$

Therefore, in people who have taken the medication, the risk of having the side effect is 1.5 times greater (or a relative risk increase of 50%) than in those people who have not taken the medication.

Absolute risk reductions (or increases) versus relative risk reductions (or increases)

A 2021 review of presenting numerical information about risk increase or decrease recommended that absolute risk reductions (or increases) be presented rather than relative risk reductions (or increases).[82] An example of how an absolute risk reduction (or increase) could be presented is 'after receiving treatment A, 5 out of 100 patients will develop condition B over the next year, compared to 8 out of 100 people developing condition B who do not receive the treatment'. In other words, 3 fewer people out of 100 will develop condition B over the next year if treatment A is received. Note that the simple number out of 100, the time frame and the comparison to baseline risk is conveyed in this message. This is also shown in Figure 14.2. Absolute risk reductions (or increases) are more intuitive and easier to grasp than relative risk reductions (or increases).[84]

As shown in the example in Box 14.3, while patients who take a medication may have a 50% higher risk of experiencing a side effect, in absolute terms, if a patient's initial risk was only 22 in 1,000 (or 2.2%), then taking the medication would increase this risk to only 34 in 1,000 people (or 3.4%). The importance of baseline risk was explained in Chapter 4. When explaining absolute risk reduction (or increase) to patients, the baseline or starting level of risk to the patient should also be presented to help the patient interpret the risks appropriately.[82,84] For example, a 1995 warning by the Committee on Safety in the United States stated that third-generation oral contraceptive drugs were associated with twice the risk compared with second-generation contraceptives. This warning was reported by the media, and it led to a dramatic reduction in the use of oral contraceptives and a subsequent increase in pregnancies and terminations. However, the media did not inform people that the baseline risk was extremely low, at 15 cases per year per 100,000 users, and that the increased risk was still extremely low, at 25 cases per year.[85,86]

Personalised risk estimates

In recent years there has been an increase in research into the effectiveness of personalised risk estimates. These are risk estimates that take into account characteristics of the patient—for example, their age, gender, body weight and level of physical activity. Reviews of their effectiveness have generally concluded that they are currently no better than more generalised risk estimates at aiding patient understanding and influencing behaviour change and often not trusted by patients or health professionals.[82,87,88]

Number needed to treat or number needed to harm

The concept of *number needed to treat* (or *number needed to harm*) was explained in Chapter 4 and we saw that it can be a clinically useful concept for health profession-als. However, it may lead to inaccurate perception of the treatment effect size, and studies have mostly found that it is a difficult concept for patients to understand, compared to absolute risk and should not be used to inform decision making.[82,89,90]

Table 14.1 provides two examples of the issues surrounding the presentation of probability and risk to patients and demonstrates the use of natural frequencies (for example, '8 out of 100').

Communicating uncertainty

'*The problem is not prognostic uncertainty, but how it is communicated.*'[91]

As we saw in Chapter 1, uncertainty is an inherent part of healthcare and of evidence-based practice. This includes uncertainty about the limitations, assumptions and generalisations that are inherent in the scientific process.[92] All data, whether prevalence estimates or absolute risk reductions, have some degree of imprecision. This uncertainty needs to be understood by health professionals and conveyed to patients as part of shared decision making. Health professionals need to be aware that patients often struggle to understand the probability of an event occurring, as well as the reliability and credibility of the numbers used to describe chance and probability. After all, as wisely stated by Bonner and colleagues, 'individuals experience only outcomes, not probabilities'.[70]

An increasing amount of research is investigating how to best communicate uncertainty to the general public as well as to patients in consultations, but more research is needed. Current recommendations are that in communicating information to the public, health professionals should be honest and transparent about knowledge limitations and, where possible, provide numerical messages about uncertainty (for example, a point estimate and range).[92] In addition, in consultations, health professionals should alert patients to the possibility of uncertainty (for example, 'The size of the likely benefit that we just discussed is only an estimate from research; you may experience a bigger or smaller amount of benefit than this'). Furthermore, they should try to gauge patients' perceptions about uncertainty and their tolerance for receiving this information, be flexible in how uncertainty is communicated, check patients' understanding of the information and provide hope and a sense of control where possible.[93] A good resource for information about strategies that health professionals can use is found in the article by Mendendorp.[93]

Factors for health professionals to consider when presenting numerical information to patients
Words versus numbers

So far in this chapter, we have focused on using numbers to present statistical information; however, words/verbal or qualitative descriptors can also be used. A meta-analysis of ten trials that compared the use of verbal and numerically presented information on consumers' comprehension of the frequency of adverse effects from medications found that the use of verbal descriptors (such as 'very common', 'common', 'uncommon', 'rare') led to an overestimation of the probability of adverse events.[94] It further found that consumers were more satisfied, more likely to take or continue taking the drugs, and less affected in their decisions when numerical presentations were used. Others have cautioned against using verbal descriptors such as 'low', 'high' and 'frequent' to quantify risk without clear explanation, as patients' and health professionals' perceptions of what such descriptors actually mean can vary dramatically.[95,96] For example, a patient may disregard being told they have a 'low' risk for a particular disease if a close friend has the disease.[79] It is recommended that where verbal descriptors are used, they be accompanied by natural frequencies or percentages.[79]

Framing

'Framing of information' refers to whether the information is presented in a positive or a negative manner. If information is positively framed, it is presented in terms of who will benefit or 'gain'. For example, out of 100 patients who have this treatment or test, 80 (or 80%) will benefit. If information is negatively framed, it is presented in terms of who will not benefit or 'lose' (or possibly be harmed). For example, out of 100 patients who have this treatment or test, 20 (or 20%) will experience an adverse side effect. In other words, positive (or gain) framing focuses on how to keep people healthy, and negative (or loss) framing focuses on identifying disease or disease risk.[97] The evidence about framing remains inconclusive. A Cochrane review concluded that, based on existing trials, the effect of framing on health behaviour was not consistent.[98] A meta-analytic review found positive (gain) framing was more effective than negative (loss) framing in promoting prevention behaviours (for example, skin cancer prevention, smoking cessation and physical activity), but not for other outcomes (such as patients' attitudes or intentions towards prevention, or behaviours towards disease detection).[99] Another meta-analysis also found no effect of framing on patients' attitudes or behaviour change intentions, but it did find an association between loss framing and patients engaging in cancer detection behaviours at least in the short term.[100] It is possible that the effects of framing are dependent upon the patient's underlying knowledge, beliefs and perceptions. Recommendations for the use of framing are that if it is used, it should be accompanied with pictorial or visual formats (see next section for more information), be unbiased and present patients with both the positive and the negative aspects of an intervention by using the same statistical denominator. For example, telling a patient that the risk of developing a disease is 3 in 100 people who have a certain treatment, and that the risk of not developing the disease is 97 in 100 people who have the treatment.[79,101] Gigerenzer and Edwards[81] describe an example of poor practice in an information brochure for patients about a particular screening test. In the brochure, health professionals presented information using relative risk statistics (to make the benefits appear large), while the harms of undertaking screening were presented using absolute risk statistics (which were smaller).

Using visual displays

Using visual displays such as graphs/charts, pictures, cartoons, symbols, tables and diagrams may assist patients to understand the information that you are presenting. Visual displays can be static, animated or interactive. The most well studied visual displays are pictographs (also called 'icon arrays') and graphs/charts, including bar charts. Pictographs and bar graphs have been found to have about equal efficacy in aiding comprehension, and these should be used with natural frequencies or event rates.[8] For example, a pictograph of a population of 1,000 people (represented by circles) which you can colour in to show how many will benefit (and conversely be harmed) by a particular intervention is one way of showing data in an absolute manner. Pictographs, such as in Figure 14.2, show how labels should indicate both benefit and harm where it is possible to quantify both. Far less research has been conducted on how to communicate information about prognosis than has been done on communicating intervention benefits and harms. A recent systematic review of visual methods for communicating prognostic information concluded that among the presentation evaluated (pictograph, bar graph, survival curve, tabular format), there was no clearly superior presentation.[102]

If no patient decision aid already exists, and you have the quantitative evidence and want to generate a visual display, an excellent resource is www.iconarray.com/. Graphs representing benefit and harm can also be prepared. Line graphs have been found to be better for showing trends over time, while bar graphs are better for showing comparisons between groups.[82] Figure 14.4 shows a hypothetical example of a graphical representation of the risk of experiencing a side effect from taking a particular medication. The vertical (y) axis shows the number of patients per 1,000 who experience this side effect. The horizontal (x) axis shows two groups. Group one is the general population (to represent baseline risk), and group two represents the patients who take the medication. The graph clearly shows the increased risk of experiencing the side effect for patients who take this particular medication, in

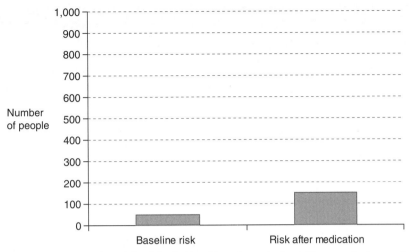

Fig 14.4 Graphical representation of the risk of side effects (harms) after taking a particular medication

comparison with the general population. Using this approach, graphs of benefit and harm can be presented side by side. However, if graphs of benefit and harm are presented side by side, the same y-axis should be used in both graphs to ensure consistency.[81]

As with all benefit–harm communication, it is important to:

- consider the suitability of the visual display for the intended user, including the necessary knowledge that they would require to understand it
- ensure that the main message in the visual display is simple and does not present confusing information
- check that the visual display itself contains the necessary information to ensure it is understood—for example, simple frequencies or percentages, evaluative labels and descriptions.[82,103] Consider time frames and cultural and social factors.

You should be aware that how patients perceive probabilities and risks can differ according to their age. A lifetime risk may not mean much to a young person, whereas a risk over the next 5 years may mean more to an older person.[74] There are also many social factors that can influence how patients interpret risk information. Patients can be influenced by the social context of the information—for example, the perceived relevance of it and the extent to which they trust the source. Health professionals need to understand that they are just one source of information about risk and may not be the source that patients trust the most.[104]

The nature of the risk also influences how patients may react. For example, patients may be more sensitive to high-consequence risks (such as being struck by lightning) than by the consequences of disease from smoking.[104] These

types of high-consequence, but rare, risks often evoke a strong emotional reaction and a disproportionately large popular media coverage. To help patients put risk numbers into perspective, it can be useful to compare risk numbers with other, more familiar risks—for example, dying of any cause in the next year.[105]

Less is more

Finally, health professionals should attempt to reduce the amount of numerical information they present to patients. Research has shown that limiting the amount to a few key points may result in higher comprehension, and therefore better and higher-quality decision making by patients.[106,107] Box 14.4 summarises the strategies that health professionals can use to ensure that numerical information is presented in the best possible way to facilitate understanding.

GENERAL PRINCIPLES REGARDING COMMUNICATION FORMAT

As shown in Figure 14.1, the skills that are needed for shared decision making are in addition to a health professional's general communication and relationship-building skills. Most health professionals receive training in these skills, even if only while doing their initial training; however, training in various communication formats rarely occurs. Using more than one format to provide the information can be a valuable way of increasing patients' retention of the information.[108] It is beyond the scope of this chapter to cover all the possible formats that can be used. We will briefly cover the formats of verbal and written

---

BOX 14.4   Tips for communicating numerical information to patients

- When there is uncertainty surrounding the benefits and harms of options (very often!), be open about this.
- Present natural frequencies (that is, plain numbers—e.g. '3 out of 100 people') where possible.
- When describing the risk of a single probability or event, clearly define the time scale and denominator and use simple frequency counts or percentages—e.g. 'In a 1-year period, 20 in 100 people who receive the intervention will have the side effect.'
- Use absolute risk (such as absolute risk reduction), rather than relative risks.
- Avoid using the number needed to treat or number needed to harm.
- Supplement explanation with visual aids such as icon arrays, pictographs or bar graphs, to aid in understanding where possible. Use evaluative labels to aid understanding.
- Use multiple formats—e.g. verbal and written descriptions—and, where possible, simple visual aids.
- Give information in terms of both positive (benefits) and negative (harms) outcomes.
- Use the same denominator when presenting positive and negative outcomes.
- Avoid using only qualitative risk descriptors—e.g. 'high', 'low', 'rare' and 'frequent'. If used, also present the quantitative information, such as in natural frequencies or percentages.
- Try to put the risk in perspective by presenting the comparative risk of other events.
- Less is more: avoid presenting too much information

---

information—these are the most common formats, and many of the principles that apply to them are also relevant to other formats (such as internet-based information).

Verbal information

General points that you should follow when providing patients with information verbally to improve the effectiveness of the information exchange[109] are listed in Box 14.5. One of the major limitations of this method is that people often forget what they have been told, with estimates that most people remember less than a quarter of what they have been told.[110] For this reason, using written materials including visual displays to supplement or reinforce information that has been presented verbally is recommended.[111]

Combination of verbal and written information

This combination has the potential to maximise a patient's knowledge. For example, a Cochrane review of providing written summaries or recordings (such as an audiotape) of consultations for people with cancer found that the majority of participants in the trials who received recordings or summaries used and valued them as a reminder of what was said during the consultation, demonstrated better recall of information and had greater satisfaction with the information received.[112]

BOX 14.5   Strategies for clearly and effectively providing information verbally to patients

- Sit down with the patient, maintain eye contact, remove any distractions and give the patient your full attention.
- Use effective communication skills such as active listening, gesturing, and responding to the patient's non-verbal cues to facilitate communication.
- Do not speak too quickly.
- Use clear and simple language. Avoid jargon where possible. Explain any medical terminology used.
- Where possible, use the same terms consistently throughout the discussion, rather than using a range of different terms that mean the same thing.
- Present the most important information first.
- Do not provide too much information at once. Present a few points and then pause to check that the patient understands.
- Observe for indicators that the patient may not have understood, such as a look of confusion or a long pause before responding to a question.
- Have the patient indicate their level of understanding. Having them repeat the main points of what you have said in their own words can often be more valuable than just asking, 'Do you understand?'

Written information

Regardless of the form (such as pamphlet, booklet, printed information sheet or online information), for written information to be useful to patients, it needs to be readable and understandable. Many written materials that health professionals use with patients are written and designed in a way that can make it difficult for patients to understand the content. One of the most common problems is that many materials are written at a reading level that is too high for the majority of the patients who receive them.[113,114] A fifth- to sixth-grade reading level (approximately a 10- to 11-year-old reading age in countries such as Australia) is recommended for written health information. There are various readability formulas that can be used to quickly and easily assess the readability of written information, including the SMOG[115] and the Flesch Reading Ease formula[116] (available in Microsoft Word). There are also online sources that provide readability checkers using different formulae—for example, https://readabilityformulas.com/ and https://www.textcompare.org/readability/.

Beyond readability, other features of written health education materials need to be given appropriate consideration to maximise the usefulness of the materials. They include features such as: the content (for example, is it evidence-based?); the language used (for example, what types of words are used, and how are sentences structured?); organisation of content (for example, are bulleted lists used where possible?); layout and typography (for example, appropriate font size); illustrations (for example, is each illustration appropriately labelled and explained in the text?); and incorporation of learning and motivation features (such as features that actively engage the reader). Further details of these features are readily available,[117] and there are a number of checklists that can be used to assess the quality of the written information that is used with patients.[117–119]

Choosing a communication format

Your choice of communication format will be influenced by a number of factors, including:

- *Patient's preference.* This may also be influenced by the patient's preferred learning style (for example, visual or auditory), cultural background, level of motivation, cultural background and primary language.
- *Patient's literacy level.* Health literacy is the degree to which individuals have the capacity to obtain, process and understand the basic information needed to make appropriate decisions about their health.[120] Poor or low health literacy has been associated with poorer health outcomes, lower uptake of preventive health behaviours, and lower quality of life.[121–123] You should be aware of your patient's literacy skills so that you can alter the educational

intervention accordingly.[124] There are a number of resources that provide strategies for how to do this (see, for example, the publication by Fischoff and colleagues).[125] Be aware that people with poor literacy often use a range of strategies to hide literacy problems[124] and are often reluctant to ask questions so as not to appear ignorant.[126] To have an indication of your patient's health literacy level, consider using a test that evaluates a patient's ability to understand medical terminology. Most are quick and straightforward to administer and score. Commonly used tests include: the Rapid Estimate of Adult Literacy in Medicine (REALM),[127] the Test of Functional Health Literacy in Adults (TOFHLA),[128] the Newest Vital Sign,[129] and Medical Achievement Reading Test (MART).[130] Recently, the use of a brief and simple screening tool to assess health literacy has been validated among patients with heart failure.[131] This tool consists of three items, each scored on a 5-point scale (with higher scores indicating lower literacy): (1) How often do you have someone help you read hospital materials? (2) How often do you have problems learning about your medical condition, because of difficulty reading hospital materials? and (3) How confident are you filling out forms by yourself? For more information, refer to government websites such as https://www.safetyandquality.gov.au/our-work/patient-and-consumer-centred-care/health-literacy or https://www.cdc.gov/healthliteracy/index.html.

- *Patient's cognitive ability and any impairments (for example, communication, hearing, visual, speech) they have that may affect their ability to communicate, understand or recall information or make decisions.* You need to consider how the presence of one or more of these impairments may result in the need for you to alter how you communicate with your patient and which communication tool(s) you choose to use. It is beyond the scope of this book to explain these strategies in detail. (For further information, refer to the patient education book by McKenna and Tooth.[6])
- *Educational resources/communication tools available to you.*
- *Time-related issues.* This includes the amount of time that is available for communicating with your patient, the timing of that communication, and (as discussed in the section on shared decision making) how quickly a decision needs to be made. Patients' needs vary at different times. For example, patients' informational needs during an initial consultation are different from their needs after a diagnosis or during follow-up consultations or treatment sessions. There may be various points in time (for example, after a diagnosis or when feeling acutely unwell) when patients are unable to process much information. You should be sensitive to when

this may be the case and adapt your communication with the patient accordingly. Providing only the most essential information may be sufficient initially. More detailed information can be provided to your patient at a later, more appropriate time.

One final comment

We have focused in this chapter on the crucial role and, indeed, responsibility that health professionals have in assisting patients to understand and use health information and authentically participate in decision making. At a broader level, we should also, at every opportunity, be helping the public in general to gain the skills and knowledge needed to be critical consumers of health information,

make informed decisions and understand issues such as how research knowledge is generated and presented. As a starting point, some highly recommended resources that have been written on these topics (and, wonderfully, are free to download as PDFs) include: *Testing Treatments* (www.testingtreatments.org), *Smart Health Choices* (https://www.ncbi.nlm.nih.gov/books/NBK63638/) and *Know Your Chances: Understanding Health Statistics* (https://www.ncbi.nlm.nih.gov/books/NBK115435/). Additionally, the book *Better Doctors, Better Patients, Better Decisions: Envisioning Health Care 2020*, by Gerd Gigerenzer and Muir Gray, is well worth reading (https://mitpress.mit.edu/9780262518529/better-doctors-better-patients-better-decisions).

SUMMARY

- Shared decision making is central to patient-centred care, and an integral component of evidence-based practice.
- In shared decision making, the patient and the health professional collaborate and jointly make decisions about the patient's health care.
- The steps involved in shared decision making include: communicating that a decision needs to be made; explaining the options and the benefits and harms (including the quantitative evidence) of each; eliciting, understanding and discussing the patient's experiences, expectations, preferences, values and circumstances; and incorporating the latter into the decision-making process.
- Shared decision making can assist patients to have a greater knowledge of their options, feel more informed, have more realistic expectations of possible benefits and harms, make choices that better reflect their personal values and preferences, improve patient–health professional communication and reduce decisional conflict.
- While shared decision making is desired by the majority of patients, it is not always possible. Sometimes

there can be challenges involved with achieving it, and myths that hinder health professionals from learning about and offering it.
- There are various types of decision support tools that can help to bring evidence into clinical decisions. A common tool is a patient decision aid, but simply giving a decision aid does not guarantee that shared decision making will occur, and shared decision making can occur in the absence of decision aids.
- It is important to communicate statistical information, such as risks and probabilities, to patients in a way that they will understand. A range of strategies—such as using natural frequencies, visual displays and absolute risks—can be used to aid patients' understanding.
- Adopt a flexible approach that uses more than one format where possible and assesses patients' comprehension of the content that is presented.
- When deciding which communication format/s to use with a patient, issues that need to be considered include the person's preference, health literacy, numeracy, and the suitability of the format/s for that person and their needs, abilities and clinical circumstances.

REFERENCES

1. Salzburg Global Seminar. The Salzburg statement on shared decision making. BMJ 2011;342:d1745.
2. Groves J. International Alliance of Patients' Organisations' perspectives on person-centred medicine. Int J Integr Care 2010;10(Suppl.):27–9.
3. Entwistle V, Watt I. Patient involvement in treatment decision-making: the case for a broader conceptual framework. Patient Educ Couns 2006;63:268–78.
4. Quill T, Brody H. Physician recommendations and patient autonomy: finding a balance between physician power and patient choice. Ann Intern Med 1996;125:763–9.

5. Coulter A. After Bristol: putting patients at the centre. BMJ 2002;324:648–51.

6. McKenna K, Tooth L, editors. Client education: a partnership approach for health practitioners. Sydney: University of New South Wales Press; 2006.

7. Barry MJ, Edgman-Levitan S. Shared decision making—the pinnacle of patient-centered care. N Engl J Med 2012;366(9):780–1.

8. Hoffmann TC, Légaré F, Simmons M, et al. Shared decision making: what do clinicians need to know and why should they bother? Med J Aust 2014;201:35–9.

9. Kon A. The shared decision making continuum. JAMA 2010;304:903–4.

10. Elwyn G, Edwards A, Kinnersley P, et al. Shared decision making and the concept of equipoise: the competences of involving patients in healthcare choices. Br J Gen Pr 2000;50:892–9.

11. Müller-Engelmann M, Donner-Banzhoff N, Keller H, et al. When decisions should be shared: a study of social norms in medical decision making using a factorial survey approach. Med Decis Mak 2013;33:37–47.

12. Straus S, Jones G. What has evidence-based medicine done for us? BMJ 2004;329:987–8.

13. Hoffmann TC, Montori V, Del Mar C. The connection between evidence-based medicine and shared decision making. JAMA 2014;312(13):1295–6.

14. Hoffmann TC, Del Mar C. Clinicians' expectations of the benefits and harms of treatments, screening, and tests: a systematic review. JAMA Intern Med 2017;177(3):407–19.

15. Hoffmann, TC, Jones, M, Glasziou P, et al. A brief shared decision-making intervention for acute respiratory infections on antibiotic dispensing rates in primary care: A cluster randomized trial. Ann Fam Med 2022;20(1):35–41.

16. Elwyn G, Tilburt J, Montori VM. The ethical imperative for shared decision-making. Eur J Pers Centred HealthCare 2013;1:129–31.

17. Stacey D, Légaré F, Lewis K, et al. Decision aids for people facing health treatment or screening decisions. Cochrane Database Syst Rev 2017;4(4):CD001431, pub5.

18. Hoffmann T, Del Mar C. Patients' expectations of the benefits and harms of treatments, screening, and tests. JAMA Int Med 2015;175(2):274–86.

19. Moynihan R, Doust J, Henry D. Preventing overdiagnosis: how to stop harming the healthy. BMJ 2012;344:e3502.

20. Hargraves IG, Montori VM, Brito JP, et al. Purposeful SDM: a problem-based approach to caring for patients with shared decision making. Patient Educ Couns 2019;102(10):1786–92.

21. Irwig L, Irwig J, Trevena L, et al. Smart health choices: making sense of health advice. London: Hammersmith Press; 2008.

22. Ford S, Schofield T, Hope T. What are the ingredients for a successful evidence-based patient choice consultation? A qualitative study. Soc Sci Med 2003;56:589–602.

23. Stewart A. Effective physician–patient communications and health outcomes: a review. CMAJ 1995;152:1423–33.

24. Elwyn G, Edwards A, Mowle S, et al. Measuring the involvement of patients in shared decision making. Patient Educ Couns 2001;43:5–22.

25. Elwyn G, Frosch D, Thomson R, et al. Shared decision making: a model for clinical practice. J Gen Intern Med 2012;27:1361–7.

26. Elwyn G, Durand MA, Song J, et al. A three-talk model for shared decision making: multistage consultation process. BMJ 2017;359:j4891.

27. Carmona C, Crutwell J, Burnham M, et al. Shared decision-making: summary of NICE guidance. BMJ 2021;373:n1430.

28. Légaré F, Witteman H. Shared decision making: examining key elements and barriers to adoption into routine clinical practice. Health Aff 2013;32:276–84.

29. Boland L, Graham ID, Légaré F, et al. Barriers and facilitators of pediatric shared decision-making: a systematic review. Implement Sci 2019;14(1):7.

30. Waddell A, Lennox A, Spassova G, et al. Barriers and facilitators to shared decision-making in hospitals from policy to practice: a systematic review. Implement Sci 2021;16(1):74.

31. Légaré F, Adekpedjou R, Stacey D, et al. Interventions for increasing the use of shared decision making by healthcare professionals. Cochrane Database Syst Rev 2018;7(7):CD006732, pub4.

32. Scholl I, LaRussa A, Hahlweg P, et al. Organizational- and system-level characteristics that influence implementation of shared decision-making and strategies to address them—a scoping review. Implement Sci 2018;13(1):40.

33. Hoffmann T, Bakhit M, Michaleff Z. Shared decision making and physical therapy: What, when, how, and why? Braz J Phys Ther 2022;26(1):100382.

34. Légaré F, Ratté S, Gravel K, et al. Barriers and facilitators to implementing shared decision-making in clinical practice: update of a systematic review of health professionals' perceptions. Patient Educ Couns 2008;73:526–35.

35. Cabana M, Rand C, Powe N, et al. Why don't physicians follow clinical practice guidelines? A framework for improvement. JAMA 1999;282:1458–65.

36. Légaré F, Turcotte S, Stacey D, et al. Patients' perceptions of sharing in decisions: a systematic review of interventions to enhance shared decision making in routine clinical practice. Patient 2012;5:1–19.

37. Dobler CC, Sanchez M, Gionfriddo MR, et al. Impact of decision aids used during clinical encounters on clinician outcomes and consultation length: a systematic review. BMJ Qual Saf 2019;28(6):499–510.

38. Charles C, Gafni A, Whelan T. Shared decision-making in the medical encounter: what does it mean? (or it takes at least two to tango). Soc Sci Med 1997;44:681–92.

39. Davey H, Barratt A, Davey E, et al. Medical tests: women's reported and preferred decision-making roles and preferences for information on benefits, side-effects and false results. Health Expect 2002;5:330–40.

40. Coulter A, Jenkinson C. European patients' views on the responsiveness of health systems and healthcare providers. Eur J Public Health 2005;15:355–60.

41. Kiesler D, Auerbach S. Optimal matches of patient preferences for information, decision-making and interpersonal behavior: evidence, models and interventions. Patient Educ Couns 2006;61:319–41.

42. Chewning B, Bylund CL, Shah B, et al. Patient preferences for shared decisions: a systematic review. Patient Educ Couns 2012;86:9–18.

43. Frosch DL, Légaré F, Fishbein M, et al. Adjuncts or adversaries to shared decision-making? Applying the integrative model of behaviour to the role and design of decision support interventions in healthcare interactions. Implement Sci 2009;4:73.

44. Hoffmann T, Bennett S, Tomsett C, et al. Brief training of student clinicians in shared decision making: a single-blind randomised controlled trial. J Gen Int Med 2014;29:844–9.

45. Joseph-Williams N, Lloyd A, Edwards A, et al. Implementing shared decision making in the NHS: lessons from the MAGIC programme BMJ 2017;357:j1744.

46. Smith S, Dixon A, Trevena L, et al. Exploring patient involvement in healthcare decision making across different education and functional health literacy groups. Soc Sci Med 2009;69:1805–12.

47. McCaffery KJ, Holmes-Rovner M, Smith SK, et al. Addressing health literacy in patient decision aids. BMC Med Inform Decis Mak 2013;13(Suppl. 2):S10.

48. Légaré F, St-Jacques S, Gagnon S, et al. Prenatal screening for Down syndrome: a survey of willingness in women and family physicians to engage in shared decision-making. Prenat Diagn 2011;31:319–26.

49. Muscat DM, Smith J, Mac O, et al. Addressing health literacy in patient decision aids: an update from the International Patient Decision Aid Standards. Med Decis Making. 2021; 41(7):848–69.

50. McCaffery K, Smith S, Wolf M. The challenge of shared decision making among patients with lower literacy: a framework for research and development. Med Decis Making 2010;30:35–44.

51. Yen RW, Smith J, Engel J, et al. A systematic review and meta-analysis of patient decision aids for socially disadvantaged populations: update from the International Patient Decision Aid Standards (IDPAS). Med Decis Making 2021;41(7): 870–96.

52. Couët N, Desroches S, Robitaille H, et al. Assessments of the extent to which health-care providers involve patients in decision making: a systematic review of studies using the OPTION instrument. Health Expect 2015;18(4):542–61.

53. Hoffmann TC, Del Mar C, Santhirapala R, et al. Teaching clinicians shared decision making and risk communication online: an evaluation study. BMJ Evid-Based Med 2021;26:253.

54. O'Connor A. Validation of a decisional conflict scale. Med Decis Making 1995;15:25–30.

55. O'Connor A, Légaré F, Stacey D. Risk communication in practice: the contribution of decision aids. BMJ 2003;327: 736–40.

56. Hoffmann T, Jansen J, Glasziou P. The importance and challenges of shared decision making in older people with multimorbidity. PLOS Med 2018;15(3):e1002530.

57. Edwards A, Elwyn G, Hood K, et al. The development of COMRADE: a patient-based outcome measure to evaluate the effectiveness of risk communication and treatment decision making in consultations. Patient Educ Couns 2003;50:311–22.

58. Bauman A, Fardy H, Harris P. Getting it right: why bother with patient centred care? Med J Aust 2003;179:253–6.

59. Krumholz H. Informed consent to promote patient-centered care. JAMA 2010;303(12):1190–1.

60. Spatz E, Krumholz H, Moulton B. The new era of informed consent: Getting to a reasonable-patient standard through shared decision making. JAMA 2016;315:2063–4.

61. The General Medical Council. Decision making and consent. Guidance on professional standards and ethics for doctors. Manchester: General Medical Council; 2020. Online. Available: https://www.gmc-uk.org/ethical-guidance/ethical-guidance-for-doctors/decision-making-and-consent (accessed 31 January 2022).

62. Australian Commission on Safety and Quality in Health Care. National Safety and Quality Health Service (NSQHS) Standards. Sydney: ACSQHC; 2019. Online. Available: https://www.safetyandquality.gov.au/standards/nsqhs-standards (accessed 31 January 2022).

63. Elwyn G, Edwards A, Wensing M. Shared decision making: developing the OPTION scale for measuring patient involvement. Qual Saf Health Care 2003;12:93–9.

64. Elwyn G, Hutchings H, Edwards A, et al. The OPTION scale: measuring the extent that health professionals involve patients in decision-making tasks. Health Expect 2005;8: 34–42.

65. Barr P, O'Malley A, Tsulukidze M, et al. The psychometric properties of Observer OPTION(5), an observer measure of shared decision making. Patient Educ Couns 2015;98(8): 970–6.

66. Holmes-Rovner M, Kroll J, Schmitt N, et al. Patient satisfaction with health care decisions: the satisfaction with decision scale. Med Decis Making 1996;16:58–64.

67. Lerman C, Brody D, Caputo G, et al. Patients' perceived involvement in care scale: relationship to attitudes about illness and medical care. J Gen Intern Med 1990;5:29–33.

68. Elwyn G, Barr P, Grande S, et al. Developing CollaboRATE: a fast and frugal patient-reported measure of shared decision making in clinical encounters. Patient Educ Couns 2013;93:102–7.

69. Kriston L, Scholl I, Hölzel L, et al. The 9-item Shared Decision Making Questionnaire (SDM-Q-9). Development and psychometric properties in a primary care sample. Patient Educ Couns 2010;80:94–9.

70. Bonner C, Trevena LJ, Gaissmaier W, et al. Current best practice for presenting probabilities in patient decision aids: fundamental principles. Med Decis Making 2021;41(7): 821–33.

71. Heen AF, Vandvik PO, Brandt L, et al. Decision aids linked to evidence summaries and clinical practice guidelines: results from user-testing in clinical encounters. BMC Med Inform Decis Mak 2021;21(1):202.

72. Elwyn G, O'Connor A, Stacey D, et al. International Patient Decision Aids Standards (IPDAS) Collaboration. Developing

a quality criteria framework for patient decision aids: online international Delphi consensus process. BMJ 2006;333:417.

73. Hoffmann TC, Bakhit M, Durand MA, et al. Basing information on comprehensive, critically appraised, and up-to-date syntheses of the scientific evidence: an update from the International Patient Decision Aid Standards. Med Decis Making 2021;41(7):755–67.

74. National Health and Medical Research Council of Australia. Making decisions about tests and treatments: principles for better communication between healthcare consumers and healthcare professionals. Canberra: Australian Government Printer; 2006.

75. Gigerenzer G, Gaissmaier W, Kurz-Milcke E, et al. Helping doctors and patients make sense of health statistics. Psychol Sci Public Interest 2007;8:53–96.

76. Wegwarth O, Gigerenzer G. The barrier to informed choice in cancer screening: statistical illiteracy in physicians and patients. Recent Results Cancer Res 2018;210:207–21.

77. Welch H, Schwartz L, Woloshin S. Over-diagnosed: making people sick in the pursuit of health. Boston: Beacon Press; 2012.

78. Malhotra A, Maughan D, Ansell J, et al. Choosing wisely in the UK: the Academy of Medical Royal Colleges' initiative to reduce the harms of too much medicine. BMJ 2015;350: h2308.

79. Lautenbach D, Christensen K, Sparks J, et al. Communicating genetic risk information for common disorders in the era of genomic medicine. Annu Rev Genomics Hum Genet 2013;14:491–513.

80. Gigerenzer G. Why do single event probabilities confuse patients? BMJ 2012;344:245.

81. Gigerenzer G, Edwards A. Simple tools for understanding risks: from innumeracy to insight. BMJ 2003;327:741–4.

82. Trevena LJ, Bonner C, Okan Y, et al. Current challenges when using numbers in patient decision aids: advanced concepts. Med Decis Making 2021;41(7):834–47.

83. Navar AM, Wang TY, Mi X, et al. Influence of cardiovascular risk communication tools and presentation formats on patient perceptions and preferences. JAMA Cardiol 2018;3(12):1192–9.

84. Zipkin D, Umscheid C, Keating N, et al. Evidence-based risk communication: a systematic review. Ann Intern Med 2014;161(4):270–80.

85. Berry D, Knapp P, Raynor T. Expressing medicine side effects: assessing the effectiveness of absolute risk, relative risk and number needed to harm and the provision of baseline risk information. Patient Educ Couns 2006;63: 89–96.

86. Edwards R, Cohen J. The recent saga of cardiovascular disease and safety of oral contraceptives. Hum Reprod Update 1999;5:565–620.

87. Scherer LD, Ubel PA, McClure J, et al. Belief in numbers: When and why women disbelieve tailored breast cancer risk statistics. Patient Educ Couns 2013;92(2):253–9.

88. Edwards AG, Naik G, Ahmed H, et al. Personalised risk communication for informed decision making about taking screening tests. Cochrane Database Syst Rev 2013;2013(2): CD001865, pub3.

89. Halvorsen P, Kristiansen I. Decisions on drug therapies by numbers needed to treat: a randomised trial. Arch Int Med 2005;165:1140–6.

90. Halvorsen PA, Selmer R, Kristiansen IS. Different ways to describe the benefits of risk-reducing treatments: a randomized trial. Ann Intern Med 2007;146(12):848–56.

91. Kirkebøen G. 'The median isn't the message': How to communicate the uncertainties of survival prognoses to cancer patients in a realistic and hopeful way. Eur J Cancer Care (Engl) 2019;28(4):e13056.

92. van der Bles AM, van der Linden S, Freeman ALJ, et al. The effects of communicating uncertainty on public trust in facts and numbers. Proc Natl Acad Sci USA. 2020;117(14): 7672–83.

93. Medendorp NM, Stiggelbout AM, Aalfs CM, et al. A scoping review of practice recommendations for clinicians' communication of uncertainty. Health Expect 2021; 24(4):1025–43.

94. Büchter R, Fechtelpeter D, Knelangen M, et al. Words or numbers? Communicating risk of adverse effects in written consumer health information: a systematic review and meta-analysis. BMC Med Inform Decis Mak 2014;14:76.

95. Epstein R, Alper B, Quill T. Communicating evidence for participatory decision making. JAMA 2004;291:2359–66.

96. Andreadis K, Chan E, Park M, et al. Imprecision and preferences in interpretation of verbal probabilities in health: a systematic review. J Gen Intern Med 2021; 36(12):3820–9.

97. Wilkes M, Srinivasan M, Coles G, et al. Discussing uncertainty and risk in primary care: recommendations of a multi-disciplinary panel regarding communication around prostate cancer screening. J Gen Intern Med 2013;28:1410–19.

98. Akl E, Oxman AD, Herrin J, et al. Framing of health information messages. Cochrane Database Syst Rev 2011;(12):CD006776.

99. Gallagher K, Updegraff J. Health message framing effects on attitudes, intentions, and behavior: a meta-analytic review. Ann Behav Med 2012;43:101–16.

100. Ainiwaer A, Zhang S, Ainiwaer X, et al. Effects of message framing on cancer prevention and detection behaviors, intentions, and attitudes: systematic review and meta-analysis. J Med Internet Res 2021;23(9):e27634.

101. Trevena L, Zikmund-Fisher B, Edwards A, et al. Presenting quantitative information about decision outcomes: a risk communication primer for patient decision aid developers. BMC Med Inform Decis Mak 2013;13(Suppl. 2):S7.

102. Abukmail E, Bakhit M, Del Mar C et al. Effect of different visual presentations on the comprehension of prognostic information: a systematic review. BMC Med Inform Decis Mak 2021;21(1):249.

103. Hallgren C, Mt-Isa S, Lieftucht A, et al. Literature review of visual representation of the results of benefit–risk assessments of medicinal products. Pharmacoepidemiol Drug Saf 2016;25(3):238–50.

104. Alaszewski A, Horlick-Jones T. How can doctors communicate information about risk more effectively? BMJ 2003;327:728–31.

105. Paling J. Strategies to help patients understand risks. BMJ 2003;327:745–8.

106. Peters E, Dieckmann N, Dixon A, et al. Less is more in presenting quality information to consumers. Med Care Res Rev 2007;64:169–90.

107. Zikmund-Fisher B, Fagerlin A, Ubel P. Improving understanding of adjuvant therapy options by using simpler risk graphics. Cancer 2008;113:3382–90.

108. McKenna K, Tooth L. Deciding the content and format of educational interventions. In: McKenna K, Tooth L, editors. Client education: a partnership approach for health practitioners. Sydney: University of New South Wales Press; 2006. pp. 128–58.

109. Tse S, Lloyd C, McKenna K. When clients are from diverse linguistic and cultural backgrounds. In: McKenna K, Tooth L, editors. Client education: a partnership approach for health practitioners. Sydney: University of New South Wales Press; 2006. pp. 307–26.

110. Boundouki G, Humphris G, Field A. Knowledge of oral cancer, distress and screening intentions: longer term effects of a patient information leaflet. Patient Educ Couns 2004;53:71–7.

111. Hill J. A practical guide to patient education and information giving. Baillières Clin Rheumatol 1997;11:109–27.

112. Pitkethly M, MacGillivray S, Ryan R. Recordings or summaries of consultations for people with cancer. Cochrane Database Syst Rev 2008;CD001539.

113. Griffin J, McKenna K, Tooth L. Discrepancy between older clients' ability to read and comprehend and the reading level of written educational materials used by occupational therapists. Am J Occup Ther 2006;60:70–80.

114. Hoffmann T, McKenna K. Analysis of stroke patients' and carers' reading ability and the content and design of written materials: recommendations for improving written stroke information. Patient Educ Couns 2006;60:286–93.

115. McLaughlin H. SMOG grading: a new readability formula. J Reading 1969;12:639–46.

116. Flesch R. A new readability yardstick. J Appl Psychol 1948;32:221–33.

117. Hoffmann T, Worrall L. Designing effective written health education materials: considerations for health professionals. Disabil Rehabil 2004;26:1166–73.

118. Helitzer D, Hollis C, Cotner J, et al. Health literacy demands of written health information materials: an assessment of cervical cancer prevention materials. Cancer Control 2009;16(1):70–8.

119. Paul C, Redman S, Sanson-Fisher R. The development of a checklist of content and design characteristics for printed health education materials. Health Promot J Aust 1997;7:153–9.

120. Institute of Medicine (IOM). Health literacy: a prescription to end confusion. Washington: IOM; 2004.

121. Kanejima Y, Shimogai T, Kitamura M, et al. Impact of health literacy in patients with cardiovascular diseases: a systematic review and meta-analysis. Patient Educ Couns 2021;S0738-3991(21)00767-9.

122. Lim ML, van Schooten KS, Radford KA, et al. Association between health literacy and physical activity in older people: a systematic review and meta-analysis. Health Promot Int 2021;36(5):1482–97.

123. Bostock S, Steptoe A. Association between low functional health literacy and mortality in older adults: longitudinal cohort study. BMJ 2012;344:e1602.

124. Weiss B, Coyne C, Michielutte R, et al. Communicating with patients who have limited literacy skills: report of the National Work Group on Literacy and Health. J Fam Pract 1998;46:168–75.

125. Fischoff B, Brewer N, Downs J. Communicating risks and benefits: an evidence-based user's guide. Silver Spring, MD: US Department of Health and Human Services, Food and Drug Administration; 2011. Online. Available: www.fda.gov/downloads/AboutFDA/ReportsManualsForms/Reports/UCM268069.pdf (accessed 28 January 2022).

126. Wilson F, McLemore R. Patient literacy levels: a consideration when designing patient education programs. Rehabil Nurs 1997;22:311–17.

127. Murphy P, Davis T, Long S, et al. REALM: a quick reading test for patients. J Reading 1993;37:124–30.

128. Parker R, Baker D, Williams M, et al. The Test of Functional Health Literacy in Adults: a new instrument for measuring patients' literacy skills. J Gen Intern Med 1995;10:537–41.

129. Shealy KM, Threatt TB. Utilization of the Newest Vital Sign (NVS) in practice in the United States. Health Commun 2016;31(6):679–87.

130. Hanson-Divers E. Developing a medical achievement reading test to evaluate patient literacy skills: a preliminary study. J Health Care Poor Underserved 1997;8:56–9.

131. Peterson P, Shetterly S, Clarke C, et al. Health literacy and outcomes among patients with heart failure. JAMA 2011;305:1695–701.

Clinical Reasoning and Evidence-Based Practice

Merrill Turpin and Joy Higgs

LEARNING OBJECTIVES

After reading this chapter, you should be able to:
- Understand different perspectives on the concept of 'evidence'
- Understand what is meant by the term 'clinical reasoning'
- Explain how clinical reasoning can be used to integrate information and knowledge from the different sources that are required for evidence-based practice
- Understand what is meant by the term 'critical reflection'

In this chapter we argue that clinical decision making is a process of professional judgment underpinned by a range of forms of evidence, rather than utilisation of prescriptions controlled by absolute and unequivocal evidence for all occasions. Evidence-based practice aims to improve outcomes for patients.[1] Patients, health professionals, funding bodies and policy makers all share in this aim. However, a range of issues make it problematic and undesirable to *uncritically* adopt an evidence-based practice approach, and the complexity of the problem becomes clearer when we question *how best* to achieve optimal health care.

Patient outcomes are dependent on a range of factors, such as:
- the uniqueness of the patient's circumstances and healthcare preferences
- the nature of the patient's health problem
- the types of services that are available to and accessible by the patient
- the fact that there are often treatment alternatives rather than just one treatment option
- the nature and quality of the interaction between the patient and the health professional
- the attitudes of the patient towards the services offered
- the patient's own conceptualisation of the health problem

- the ease with which any service recommendations made can be carried out by patients within the broader context of their lives.

This list illustrates the complexity of the issue of improving patient outcomes. If all of these factors interact together to affect the health outcomes for a particular patient, where should planned improvements focus? Will a change in one factor be sufficient to obtain the desired result, or do factors need to be considered in an integrated way? Health professionals face these kinds of questions on a daily basis, as well as the ever-present question, 'What *can* and *should* I do in this specific situation?'

Professional practice is complex and health professionals need to consider the range of factors that affect patient outcomes when planning and delivering services. They are required to make decisions about what services they can and should offer, given the particular needs of and circumstances surrounding each individual patient, as well as the broader organisational and societal context. Making these kinds of decisions requires complex thinking processes as the patient's 'problem' about which decisions have to be made is often poorly defined and the desired outcomes are often unclear.[2] These thinking processes are often referred to as *clinical or professional reasoning, decision making* or *professional judgment.*

Health professionals need to use their clinical reasoning to gather and interpret different types of information from a range of sources and combine it with their existing knowledge base to make judgments and decisions regarding complex situations under conditions of uncertainty. When health professionals make practice decisions, they have to be rational, pragmatic, ethical and patient-centred. They need to consider the likely effectiveness of their proposed actions and what their patients would accept and expect.

As you have seen throughout this book, evidence-based practice is a movement in health that aims to improve patient outcomes by supporting health professionals to incorporate research evidence into their practice. Evidence-based practice also recognises that research evidence alone is not sufficient for addressing the complex nature of professional practice and that health professionals must be able to integrate information from different sources in order to build their knowledge. Therefore, to practise in an evidence-based way, health professionals need to integrate research with their clinical experience, with their understanding of the preferences and circumstances of their patients, and with the demands and expectations of the practice context. The process by which health professionals integrate this information and add to their knowledge base requires clinical reasoning.

In this chapter, we explore the notion of evidence-based practice and the roles that information from different sources play in providing evidence for practice. We highlight how the concept of practice should be viewed as being embedded within particular contexts. We also explore the clinical reasoning processes that occur within practice and provide some brief suggestions for you to consider when critically reflecting on your own practice in terms of making it evidence-based.

THE EVIDENCE-BASED PRACTICE MOVEMENT'S CONCEPT OF EVIDENCE

The assumption underpinning the perceived need for an evidence-based practice is that basing practice on rigorously produced information or evidence (often referred to as *data*) will lead to enhanced patient outcomes. Given the complex range of factors that can affect patient outcomes, how can we be sure that basing our practices on such evidence will improve them, and what kinds of information and knowledge constitutes appropriate and sufficient evidence? These are important questions for health professionals to ask. The first question about whether basing practice on evidence leads to better patient outcomes has been examined widely in relation to specific interventions and specific outcomes and will not be addressed in this chapter.

The second key question pertains to what constitutes evidence. As we saw in Chapter 1, evidence-based practice across the health professions evolved from its medical counterpart, evidence-based medicine; consequently, many of the assumptions of medicine have been adopted in evidence-based practice. In the definition of evidence-based practice by Sackett and colleagues[3] that was examined in Chapter 1, the term 'current best evidence' was introduced. Predictably, clarifying the nature of 'best' evidence is a central concern of the evidence-based practice and evidence-based medicine movements. As the empirico-analytical paradigm is the dominant philosophy that underpins medicine, this also became the assumed perspective of the wider evidence-based practice movement.

The empirico-analytical paradigm is also known as the 'scientific paradigm' or the 'empiricist model of knowledge creation'. From the perspective of the empirico-analytical paradigm, the best form of evidence is that produced through rigorous scientific inquiry. According to Park and colleagues,[4] knowledge must be developed objectively using tightly controlled variables. When procedures are followed correctly, reliable and valid explanations and predictions are generated. Therefore, information and knowledge generated through research is the concept that is used by the evidence-based practice movement and is the approach taken throughout this text. Many people take this for granted, and the embedded nature of this assumption is highlighted by use of the clarifying term 'research-based practice' by some, rather than 'evidence-based practice'.

In some ways, the assumption that 'evidence equals research findings' has been problematic for the evidence-based practice movement and has contributed to a strong division between those who align themselves with it and those who oppose it. Critics of evidence-based practice argue that there are problems with the production, relevance and availability of research evidence, such as prioritising research that aligns with funding opportunities or deprioritising important research because it is difficult to measure,[5] and that it has limited capacity to address the problems of practice and enhance decision making in the context of complex practice and life situations.[6] Examples of criticisms include: that the research that is undertaken is often dependent on funding and, therefore, what is researched can be influenced by factors other than need and importance; that the research undertaken can reflect what is easier to measure more than what is important to understand or most important to professional practice; and that, often, research findings are not presented in forms that are easily accessible to health professionals.

These criticisms suggest that taking a balanced approach to the information that needs to inform practice (as the original definition of evidence-based practice proposed) is important. We now consider the concept of evidence and what might be valued as evidence from four different perspectives.

EVIDENCE OF WHAT?

What is evidence? The *Heinemann Australian Student's Dictionary* defines evidence as 'anything which provides a basis for belief'[7] and the *Macquarie Dictionary* defines it as 'grounds for belief'.[8] Therefore, *belief* requires substantiation of a position or argument or acceptance of its credibility. Using these definitions, evidence constitutes information or knowledge that supports some sort of belief, and an evidence-based practice would be a practice that is based on such information or knowledge. But whose beliefs are referred to? Is it an individual health professional's beliefs, the beliefs of a particular health profession, or the beliefs that underpin a particular health service or model of service delivery? Is it the beliefs of those receiving care from a particular service or of those funding or providing the service? Are the beliefs of the various stakeholders in health aligned and of equal value?

These questions highlight the argument that the types of information and knowledge seen as appropriate evidence for health practice can vary among different stakeholders. For example, if a service measures patient outcomes in terms of reducing (or eliminating) impairments, then it is information about the effectiveness of interventions in reducing impairments that will be valued most as evidence, regardless of the functional and practical implications and the matters of ethics, values and social justice related to using those interventions. However, people using health services might employ different criteria to measure outcomes. For example, they might value services that make an appreciable difference to their health experience, are accessible (physically and financially) and use interventions that are easy to implement within their own life contexts. Healthcare funding bodies might be most concerned with value-for-money and might seek information that substantiates the cost-effectiveness of interventions or services. That is, they might only look favourably on interventions and service provision models that have both evidence to support the effectiveness of an intervention in improving patient outcomes *and* an acceptable financial cost.

From the perspective of the empirico-analytical paradigm

As explained in an earlier section, the evidence-based practice movement has primarily taken its understanding of evidence from the *empirico-analytical paradigm* that underpins the assumptions of medicine. This paradigm aims to develop a knowledge base generated from a positivist perspective of 'reality' or 'how the world is', in which the world is taken to be observable (often with the assistance of technology) and information that is valued as knowledge is reliably generated and reproducible. In this perspective, to be dependable as evidence of reality (including how people's health responds to intervention), research data need to be as free of bias as possible when collected, the potential effects of the information collection process on the phenomena need to be minimised, and any changes observed must be able to be reliably attributed to the specific factors or variables under investigation.

To make the empirico-analytical concept of best evidence explicit, a number of hierarchies have been developed, based on the methodology used to generate research data. In Chapter 2, the authors explored in detail the hierarchies and levels of evidence for questions about intervention, diagnosis and prognosis. Developing levels of evidence was a strategy used to establish the degree to which research findings could be trusted as evidence. For example, the top two levels in the hierarchy for intervention effectiveness are randomised controlled trials and their systematic reviews. As we saw in Chapter 4, randomised trials (individual and systematically reviewed) generate knowledge that is considered to have a high degree of validity. By minimising potential bias and controlling for variables that might influence the outcome, the confidence that any observed change can be attributed to one factor is very high. Therefore, in the empirico-analytical paradigm, randomised controlled trials are the most trustworthy type of research-generated knowledge to use as evidence for the effectiveness of interventions. In general, from an empirico-analytical perspective, the most trusted research methods are quantitative, although rigorous qualitative research is being increasingly valued as a method to provide evidence for the utility of interventions and the experiences of groups of people or individuals.[9]

Understanding the origins of the evidence-based practice movement in the empirico-analytical paradigm helps to explain its assumption that 'evidence equals research findings'. As the imperative to identify 'current best evidence' remains a core value of evidence-based practice, determining ways to assess the quality of such research remains a central endeavour. Concern for the development and identification of critical-appraisal tools is an example.

While the empirico-analytical paradigm focuses on generating knowledge through the rigorous scientific methods with which research is often associated, other stakeholders might value other types of knowledge. The sections that follow explore some of the other types of information and knowledge that are valued to inform evidence-based practice.

From the perspective of technical rationality

Technical rationality is a second approach that addresses the type of information that could provide appropriate evidence for professional practice. This approach aims to improve patient outcomes by regulating practice to enhance quality through efficiency and cost-effectiveness. The major elements of this approach are problem solving and the rigorous use of scientific theory and technique. Whereas the empirico-analytical approach aims to facilitate quality by emphasising the trustworthiness of information, the aim of the technical rationality approach is to improve quality by enhancing the problem solving of health professionals. Therefore, a major difference between these two approaches is that the former centres on the *quality* of the information, whereas the latter targets the *use* of the information.

From a technical rationalist perspective, human reasoning and judgment is understood in health care as problem solving, which requires the framing and definition of a problem and the search for a solution within a defined problem space. From this approach, accuracy, efficiency and cost-effectiveness can be improved by providing tools that support the problem-solving process and minimise the likelihood of reasoning errors. As the technical rationalist approach values the rigorous use of the scientific method and technique, information that is generated using this method is incorporated into routines and procedures that aim to reduce and support the professional judgment required. The influence of technical rationality on health care is evident in the use of clinical pathways, protocols, decision trees and other tools that aim to systematise practice decisions. For example, the typical path to be taken by a health professional is clarified when a standard problem definition (often based on a medical diagnosis) can be used. Decision trees work in this way.

A major aim of using reasoning tools (based on knowledge generated using scientific methods) is to reduce reasoning errors and the potentially biasing effects that can arise from clinical opinions. For example, health professionals might rely on a narrow range of practices with which they are familiar or that are easily accessed, while being unaware of other potential courses of action. In contrast, clinical protocols and guidelines are generated from information from a broad range of sources. Examples include research evidence, broader trends in patient outcomes or statistics about adverse events, epidemiological trends in population health and the opinions and experiences of patients.

The technical rationalist approach shares a similar concept of evidence with the empirico-analytical approach in one important respect. Both approaches value information that is generated using rigorous scientific methods and consider this appropriate evidence for clinical practice. However, although they share a concern for quality and effectiveness, they often differ regarding cost-effectiveness. In the empirico-analytical approach it might be argued that an effective intervention is essential, regardless of the cost, whereas a technical rationalist approach values evidence regarding the reduction of both healthcare costs and the risk of adverse incidents occurring during service delivery.

What information helps health professionals to address the dilemmas of their practice?

A third approach to the matter of what constitutes evidence is to consider the question, 'What information helps professionals to address the specific and varied dilemmas and challenges of their practice?' While technical rationality aims to systematise practice, health professionals deal with the complexity of professional practice using judgment,[10] which relies on their clinical or *professional expertise*.

Socio-cultural theories of learning suggest that professional expertise is developed through interaction with communities of practice.[11,12] For health professionals, participation in practice leads to the development of identity as a member of a professional group, accumulation of experience and mastery of their practice area.[13]

The work of Dreyfus and Dreyfus[14] has been used widely to show that professional expertise develops with experience. They characterised into five stages the different ways that professionals think as they gain experience. These are: novice, advanced beginner, competent, proficient and expert. Essentially, these stages reflect a movement from a practice based on context-free information and generalised rules to a sophisticated and 'embodied' understanding of the specific context in which the practice occurs. The earlier stages focus on the application of generalised knowledge. In the later stages, with greater experience in the specific context, health professionals can recognise (often subtle) similarities between the current situation and previous ones and use their knowledge of previous outcomes to make judgments about what might be best in the current situation.

Professional expertise is difficult to quantify, because it is partly determined by understandings that are shared by members of the community of practice. In nursing, expertise has been associated with holistic practice, holistic knowledge, salience, knowing the patient, moral agency and skilled know-how.[15] In occupational therapy, Robertson and colleagues[16] linked expertise with the ability to engage in transformative critical reason, critical self-reflection and critical action. Carr and colleagues[17] investigated the use of observation of practice for developing clinical expertise in physiotherapy. It appears that members of a community of practice can recognise expertise, even though it involves unstated and embodied knowledge, skills and attributes that can be difficult to quantify.

As professionals have to make decisions about what action to take with patients in a specific organisational context, appropriate information could be conceptualised as including health professionals' memories of previous experiences and their specific outcomes. This is not to suggest that expert health professionals no longer use knowledge from research. Professional communities of practice have codes of ethics that usually include the need to maintain up-to-date knowledge of the field, and some professional bodies require members to undertake formal accreditation processes. Health professionals meet these requirements through a range of activities, including participating in conferences and workshops, reading professional journals, sharing this information and discussing cases and experiences with one another. All of these activities can increase professional knowledge through exposure to findings from systematic research and expand practice knowledge through experiential learning. Thus, using knowledge that is generated from research, practical experience and professional wisdom is important for health professionals when developing or undertaking an 'evidence-based' practice.

Considering evidence from the patient's perspective

A fourth perspective is brought into focus when we ask the question, 'What is going to make the biggest difference to my patient's life and health?' This question helps to turn our attention to the *patient's perspective*. Patients seek professional services because they need something that they cannot obtain in other ways. Professional services often come at substantial financial costs to patients (as well as other costs, such as time and effort). Attending to patients' predicaments, rights and preferences (see Sackett and colleagues'[3] definition of evidence-based medicine as presented in Chapter 1) requires a developed ability to understand people, both as individuals and as members of groups within the overall population. Examples of understanding preferences and rights include giving patients choices in relation to interventions (that is, considering their preferences) and understanding and advocating for the rights of marginalised people to participate in social roles such as work. Understanding 'predicaments' requires the ability to imagine patients within the context of their living situations and social roles (not just the service contexts in which they are seen). For example, a health professional might have to consider the need for support from a patient's carer or the logistics of whether a patient is able to follow an intervention recommendation when the patient returns to daily life, and their opportunities for social participation.

While patients expect health professionals to offer them services that will be effective, they also expect them to listen to their concerns and to validate their experiences of health. Increasingly, patients also acquire healthcare knowledge and information from sources such as the internet. Consequently, they are likely to expect health professionals to know about this information and help them to understand it, as well as to appraise its relevance and appropriateness for them. Patients might also expect shared decision making, 'evidence' of a health professional's interpersonal skills (for example, a professional's ability to listen to their concerns), 'value for money' and the accessibility (physical and temporal) of the services that are being offered. The importance of health professionals being able to communicate well with their patients was discussed in Chapter 14.

Evidence of what? A summary

In summary, asking the question 'Evidence of what?' emphasises that different stakeholders seek different types of information. People who work from an empirico-analytical paradigm are likely to seek information that is accepted as providing reliable and predictable representations of the world. Starting from this position, they are likely to value one kind of information (that is, research findings, especially quantitative research) over other types of information, as illustrated by the established hierarchies of evidence. People who work from a technical rationalist perspective are most likely to seek information that provides a combination of evidence of efficiency and cost-effectiveness and will aim to use this information to develop tools and strategies to standardise practice according to what is considered 'best practice'. Health professionals are most likely to value and seek information that provides evidence to support the decisions that they need to make about what they, as members of a specific health profession in a particular organisational context, should offer a certain patient, given their life circumstances. Finally, patients are most likely to value and seek information that provides evidence of services and health professionals that offer effective, accessible, and value-for-money interventions that they are likely to be able to incorporate into their daily lives.

All these different perspectives are important when considering what an evidence-based practice might look like for health professionals, because they highlight the complexity of professional practice. Health professionals are influenced by and need to consider in their practice the different types of knowledge and information or 'evidence' that different stakeholders might consider relevant and valid. Using information that can be 'trusted' is a key concern of evidence-based practice and will remain so as the movement explores a broader base upon which to make practice decisions. It also underpins the 'evidence' that the various stakeholders seek.

In this section, we explored some different types of information that can contribute to evidence-based practice. To come to well-reasoned decisions, health professionals need to integrate this complex range of information. The task of integrating these different types of information to make practice decisions can be difficult. To understand this process of integration, it is important to contextualise professional practice as requiring art, science and ethics. In the following section, we explore this process of integration.

INTEGRATING INFORMATION AND KNOWLEDGE: THE FORGOTTEN ART?

Evidence-based practice is currently conceptualised as a process that requires the integration of information from different sources. As discussed, much of the early attention of the evidence-based practice movement centred on specifying the nature of the evidence appropriate for health practice (mainly research evidence). Although it is well accepted that evidence-based practice uses different information sources such as research, clinical expertise, patient values and preferences, and the practice context, systematic investigation into how health professionals integrate this knowledge and information is more limited. Conceptualising evidence-based practice as a process of integration requires a focus on the activities of health professionals. This section of the chapter will explore the nature of professional practice.

Health professionals provide services to their patients. They think and act within specific contexts, which have been established to provide a particular type of service, and they remain accountable to their patients, employers and funding bodies. Health professionals also belong to certain professional groups or communities of practice. Therefore, professional practice needs to be understood within its social, organisational and professional contexts.

Professional practice is complex. It requires interaction between professionals and patients and among professionals from different disciplines, as well as ethical and professional behaviour. Health professionals need to be able to think critically, use professional judgment and practise wisdom when working with a range of patients. Professional practice is not just a problem-solving exercise (as technical rationalists might argue), although it requires problem solving. It is not just a process of applying theories and research-generated knowledge to practice (as an empirico-analytical approach emphasises), although these are vital in guiding practice. It includes the fulfilment of role expectations, professional judgment, ethical conduct and the delivery of patient-centred services. Professional practice requires systematic thinking, social and contextual understanding, deep listening, good communication, and the ability to deal creatively and ethically with uncertainty.

Health professionals need to use their judgment to make decisions about the best course of action to take under conditions of uncertainty. Part of the complexity is having to deal with different and often competing understandings from a variety of data and knowledge sources, and considering the individual nature of patient circumstances, needs and preferences. Professional practice is an ethical endeavour tailored to the individual patient and requires the credible use of theory and research, good judgment and problem solving, and the ability to implement protocols and procedures. Integrating information from research, clinical expertise, patient values and preferences, and information from the practice context requires judgment and artistry as well as science and logic.

Strategies for combining science and art in practice are embedded in the way that health professionals think about their work. For example, in reference to occupational therapists, Turpin (2007) stated that 'when occupational therapists refer to the paired concepts of art and science, they express their moral dissatisfaction with being constrained by either. In isolation, art somehow seems too soft and unquantifiable and science too hard and unyielding' (p. 482).[18] While science is generally associated with rigour, reliability and predictability, artistry is associated with judgment and being able to deal with unpredictability. In Sackett's 1996 definition of evidence-based medicine,[3] artistry is evident in the reference to 'thoughtful identification and compassionate use' of information that pertains to a particular patient. While various health professions emphasise art and science to different degrees, they all appear to accept that a balance of art and science is required for a practice that is rigorous, relevant and responds to human need.

Professional practice can be characterised as reasoned action, as it requires both knowing and doing. The concept of 'art and science' highlight that health professionals need different types of knowledge to undertake such reasoned action. Three types of knowledge used in practice are:[19]

- **Propositional knowledge** (also known as 'theoretical knowledge') is an explicit and formal type of knowledge that is generated through research and scholarship and is associated with 'knowing that'. This type of knowledge is often thought of as 'scientific knowledge' and has been emphasised most in evidence-based practice.
- **Professional craft knowledge** refers to 'knowing how' to carry out the tasks of the profession. It is often associated with the idea of an 'art' of practice and includes the particular perspectives that characterise each profession.

Yet, this knowledge requires the rigour of review and reflection to justify the claim of being knowledge.

- **Personal knowledge** refers to an individual health professional's knowledge of themselves in relation to others. This type of knowledge is important for professional practice as the relationships that health professionals build with their patients are often central to that practice.

Health professionals need to know what and how things work in specific contexts (both the setting and those of the patient), and to consider how they might need to alter their practice in response to features of these contexts. A common example is the influence of resource availability (such as funding, space, time, staffing levels and equipment) on practice decisions.[20] Less tangible is the influence of organisational culture and principles. While an organisation's policies and related structures determine practice aspects such as the amount of time health professionals have available to spend with patients, the culture of the organisation will determine how information is shared and what is expected of health professionals in particular disciplines. This information will affect decision making.

The complexity of professional practice becomes evident if you consider that it requires the following abilities: (1) to obtain and use different types of information from a range of sources; (2) to meet the demands of specific practice environments; (3) to fulfil roles consistent with the perspectives of the professional communities of practice to which the health professional belongs; and (4) to consider the predicaments, preferences and values of individual patients. Thus, the creation of a practice that is evidence-based is equally complex. 'Evidence' and 'practice' are both important for understanding evidence-based practice.

We now turn our attention to an important aspect of practice—the study of clinical reasoning. Because investigation of the thinking of health professionals was initiated in the field of medicine, the term *clinical reasoning* is commonly used. However, as many of the settings within which various health professionals work are not considered clinical, the terms *professional reasoning* and *professional decision making* are also used.

APPROACHES TO CLINICAL REASONING

Higgs (p. 1)[21] defined clinical reasoning (or practice decision making) as:

a context-dependent way of thinking and decision making in professional practice to guide practice actions. It involves the construction of narratives to make sense of the multiple factors and interests pertaining to the current reasoning task. It occurs within a set of problem spaces informed by practitioners' unique frames of reference, workplace contexts and practice models, as well as by patients or patients' contexts.

It utilises core dimensions of practice knowledge, reasoning and meta-cognition and draws upon these capacities in others. Decision making within clinical reasoning occurs at micro-, macro- and meta-levels and may be individually or collaboratively conducted. It involves the meta-skills of critical conversation, knowledge generation, practice model authenticity, and reflexivity.

Earlier approaches to the study of clinical reasoning were influenced by investigations into artificial intelligence, and conceptualised clinical reasoning as a purely cognitive process. These emphasised the iterative process of obtaining cues or information about the clinical situation, forming hypotheses about possible explanations and courses of action, interpreting information in light of these hypotheses and testing them. This process of generating and testing hypotheses using cues is referred to as hypothetico-deductive reasoning. Beyond this approach, Higgs's definition[21] emphasises that clinical reasoning is a process that involves cognition, meta-cognition (that is, the process of reflective self-awareness) and interactive and narrative ways of thinking. The work of Higgs and Jones[22] categorises approaches to clinical reasoning as *cognitive* and *interactive*. The wide range of clinical reasoning approaches presented in Table 15.1 relates to the following factors:

1. **The inherently complex nature of clinical reasoning as a phenomenon.** Clinical reasoning models are essentially an interpretation or an approximation of a very complex set of thinking processes at both cognitive and meta-cognitive (reflective self-awareness) levels. These processes use both domain-specific and generic knowledge. They operate in conjunction with other abilities such as communication and interpersonal interaction and are framed by the health professional's individual values, interests and practice model.

2. **The multiple, multi-dimensional ways of reasoning that evolve with growing expertise.** Health professionals, both within and across various health professions, do not reason in the same way. The assumption that there is one way of representing clinical reasoning expertise or a single correct way to solve a problem has been challenged. The different ways that health professionals think as they gain expertise was explained earlier in this chapter.

3. **The embedding of clinical reasoning in decision–action cycles.** As discussed, professional practice inherently deals with actions. These decisions and actions then influence each other. Decision making is a dynamic, reciprocal process of making decisions and implementing an optimal course of action. These decision–action cycles form the basis for professional judgment.

TABLE 15.1   Summary of clinical reasoning approaches

Model	Description
Hypothetico-deductive reasoning[23]	The generation of hypotheses based on clinical data and knowledge and testing of these hypotheses through further inquiry. It is used by novices and in problematic situations by experts.
Pattern recognition[24]	Expert reasoning in non-problematic situations resembles pattern recognition or direct automatic retrieval of information from a well-structured knowledge base. Through the use of inductive reasoning, pattern recognition/interpretation is a process characterised by speed and efficiency.
Forward reasoning; backward reasoning[24]	Forward reasoning describes inductive reasoning in which data analysis results in hypothesis generation or diagnosis, utilising a sound knowledge base. Forward reasoning is more likely to occur in familiar cases with experienced health professionals, and backward reasoning with inexperienced health professionals or in atypical or difficult cases. Backward reasoning is the re-interpretation of data or the acquisition of new clarifying data invoked to test a hypothesis.
Knowledge reasoning integration[22]	Clinical reasoning requires domain-specific knowledge and an organised knowledge base. A stage theory which emphasises the parallel development of knowledge acquisition and clinical reasoning expertise has been proposed. Clinical reasoning involves the integration of knowledge, reasoning and meta-cognition.
Intuitive reasoning[25]	'Intuitive knowledge' is related to 'instance scripts' or past experience with specific cases which can be used unconsciously in inductive reasoning.
Multidisciplinary reasoning	Occurs when members of a multidisciplinary team work together to make clinical decisions for the patient—for example, at case conferences and in multidisciplinary clinics.
Conditional reasoning[26]	Used by health professionals to estimate a patient's response to intervention and the likely outcomes of management and to help patients consider possibilities and reconstruct their lives following injury or the onset of disease.
Narrative reasoning[26]	The use of stories regarding past or present patients to further understand and manage a clinical situation. Telling the story of patients' illness or injury to help them make sense of the illness experience.
Interactive reasoning[26]	Interactive reasoning occurs between health professional and patient to understand the patient's perspective.
Collaborative reasoning[24]	The shared decision making that ideally occurs between health professionals and their patients. The patient's opinions as well as information about the problem are actively sought and utilised.
Ethical reasoning[24]	Those less recognised but frequently made decisions regarding moral, political and economic dilemmas which health professionals regularly confront, such as deciding how long to continue an intervention for.
Teaching as reasoning	When health professionals consciously use advice, instruction and guidance for the purpose of promoting change in the patient's understanding, feelings and behaviour.

4. **The influence of contextual factors.** It is important to remember that, in practice, health professionals are required to make decisions about particular actions that are going to be taken with particular patients in specific practice settings. The influence of context on clinical decision making has been examined, and it was identified that the nature of the task (such as its difficulty, complexity and uncertainty), the characteristics of the decision maker (including frames of reference, individual capabilities and experience) and the external decision-making context (such as professional ethics, disciplinary norms and workplace policies) all influence the decision-making process.

5. **The nature of collaborative decision making.** As presented in Chapter 14, there is a growing trend, and indeed societal pressure, for patients and health professionals to adopt a collaborative approach to clinical reasoning which increases the patient's role and power in decision making. Shared decision making and being able to work together are important for creating and providing services that result in satisfactory outcomes for patients.

Pursuing clinical reasoning capability

Too often, clinical reasoning is simply thought of as a process of thinking or a set of decisions that need to be made. Instead, clinical reasoning needs to be recognised as a capability, or set of capabilities. Capability places emphasis on being able to perform well in both known and unknown contexts and on having the capacity to solve complex and more straightforward clinical problems. The three elements of capability are ability (current competence and perceived potential), self-efficacy (confidence in capacity to perform tasks) and values (particularly the way that actions in uncertain conditions are guided by values and the capacity to articulate them).

HOW DO I MAKE MY PRACTICE EVIDENCE-BASED?

In this chapter, we have presented professional practice as a complex and fluid process that is characterised by high levels of uncertainty that arise from the context-dependent nature of the tasks that are undertaken. Professional practice is difficult to describe precisely, as it involves fulfilling professional roles with specific patients within certain contexts. Each of these factors contributes a unique aspect to the phenomenon, leading to a complex range of variations to what might be considered 'standard practice'. Therefore, there is no easy answer to the question, 'How do I make my practice evidence-based?' However, a number of principles and tools can provide health professionals with strategies for working towards improved patient outcomes through a practice that is evidence-based. The principle of critically reflecting on your practice underpins the ideas we present here. 'Critical reflection' refers to the process of analysing, reconsidering and questioning your experiences within a broad context of issues. The following list provides some ideas that you may wish to use as your practice and professional development requires:

- Be systematic in the way you collect and use information and knowledge so that you can be sure that the information and knowledge you are using is trustworthy and relevant to the decisions you make.

- Use sound and logical reasoning as well as compassion and understanding when making decisions and be clear about the information and knowledge you are basing those decisions on.

- Have a good working knowledge of the current propositional knowledge that is relevant to your professional community of practice or profession and the type of practice in which you are engaged. Be aware of the limits of your propositional knowledge and plan how you will systematically expand this knowledge to better inform your practice. Plan how you will determine the relevance of this knowledge to your practice more generally and to individual patients more specifically. Remember that evidence from a range of research approaches forms a key component of the propositional knowledge relevant to your practice.

- Be aware of your current non-propositional knowledge. Remember that non-propositional knowledge includes your professional craft knowledge (for example, knowing *how* to do things) and your personal knowledge (for example, understanding your strengths, weaknesses, preferences and interests). Ask yourself questions like: How have I systematically tested my practice experiences and derived knowledge from these experiences? Can I communicate this knowledge with credibility to my colleagues and patients and use it as sound evidence to support my practice? Is there personal knowledge derived from my life experiences (for example, working with people from different cultures) that I can use in my practice? What are my values and beliefs? What have I learnt about communicating with people who speak different languages to me or who experience hardship, disability or illness/injury that I can use to enhance my practice? Planning to systematically enhance or expand this type of knowledge is an excellent way of drawing on your practice expertise and individualising the services that you provide to patients.

- Engage in empathic visioning and collaborative questioning with patients about their experiences, knowledge and values. Listen to your patients' stories and experiences and try to understand their experience of and perspective on the situation. Ask them what they think would make the biggest difference in their life. Practise problem solving and mutual decision making with your patients to expand your collaboration skills and improve your decision making.

- Be aware of the degree to which your actions are informed by the different sources of information and knowledge: research evidence; your own clinical expertise; the patients' values, preferences and circumstances; and an understanding of the practice context and how it shapes your practice (for example, what demands and expectations it places on you; and in what ways it constrains what you can and cannot do).

• Critically reflect on and practise articulating your reasoning and your professional practice model.

Much professional expertise becomes 'embodied' knowledge or practice wisdom. You might not be aware of the details of this knowledge or be able to articulate this knowledge. To utilise this knowledge effectively as evidence for practice, it is important to raise awareness of those aspects of professional and personal thinking and action that have become taken for granted. This includes an ability to critically evaluate the types of knowledge that are available

to health professionals, including the assumptions about knowledge that are unquestioned. By engaging in critical reflection, you can become more systematic in your collection and use of the knowledge upon which you base your practice. To conduct truly evidence-based practice, you need to be aware of the types of knowledge that you are using and how you are using them, and asking yourself whether this constitutes appropriate evidence for the particular questions and problems about which you seek to be informed. You also need to be aware of the cognitive and meta-cognitive processes that you are using to combine information from different sources within the context of your discipline and practice context.

SUMMARY

• The notion of 'evidence' varies with different stakeholders and conceptual approaches.

• Integrating knowledge and information from different sources to create an evidence-based practice requires clinical reasoning and both art and science.

• Health professionals need to use clinical reasoning to collect, interpret and combine different types of information and knowledge from a range of sources to make judgments and decisions in professional practice, particularly in complex and uncertain situations.

• Health professionals are responsible for their clinical decision making, and so they need to be confident of their ability to reason well based on sound evidence and they need to be critical of both the knowledge they use as well as their own reasoning processes.

• Clinical reasoning is a process that involves cognition and meta-cognition plus interactive and narrative ways of thinking.

• Integrating knowledge from research, clinical expertise, patient values and preferences, and knowledge from practice requires judgment and artistry as well as science and reasoning.

• 'Critical reflection' refers to the process of analysing, reconsidering and questioning your experiences within a broad context of issues. By engaging in critical reflection, you can become more systematic in your collection and use of the information upon which you base your practice and more aware of your decision-making processes.

REFERENCES

1. Craik J, Rappolt S. Theory of research utilisation enhancement: a model for occupational therapy. Can J Occup Ther 2003;70:266–75.

2. Robertson L, Griffiths S. Problem solving in occupational therapy. In Robertson L, editor. Clinical reasoning in occupational therapy: controversies in practice. Oxford: Blackwell; 2012. pp. 1–14.

3. Sackett D, Rosenberg W, Gray J, et al. Evidence based medicine: what it is and what it isn't: it's about integrating individual clinical expertise and the best external evidence. BMJ 1996;312:71–2.

4. Park YS, Konge L, Artino AR. The positivism paradigm of research. Academic Medicine 2020;95(5);690–4.

5. Small N. Knowledge, not evidence, should determine primary care practice. Clin Governance 2003;8:191–9.

6. Rycroft-Malone J, Seers K, Titchen A, et al. What counts as evidence in evidence-based practice? J Adv Nurs 2004;47:81–90.

7. Heinemann Australian Student's Dictionary. Melbourne: Reed Educational and Professional Publishing; 1992.

8. The Macquarie Concise Dictionary. 3rd ed. Sydney: Macquarie Library; 1998.

9. Pearson A. Balancing the evidence: incorporating the synthesis of qualitative data into systematic reviews. JBI Reports 2004;2:45–64.

10. Higgs J, Jensen GM. Clinical reasoning: challenges of interpretation and practice in the 21st century. In: Higgs J, Jensen GM, Loftus S, et al., editors. Clinical reasoning in the health professions. 4th ed. Edinburgh: Elsevier; 2018. pp. 3–11.

11. Lave J, Wenger E. Situated learning: legitimate peripheral participation. Cambridge: Cambridge University Press; 1991.

12. Wenger, E. A social theory of learning. In: Illeris K, editor. Contemporary theories of learning: learning theorists … in their own words. 2nd ed. London and New York: Routledge; 2018. pp. 219–28.

13. Walker R. Social and cultural perspectives on professional knowledge and expertise. In: Higgs J, Titchen A, editors. Practice knowledge and expertise in the health professions. Oxford: Butterworth–Heinemann; 2001. pp. 22–8.

14. Dreyfus H, Dreyfus S. Mind over machine. New York: Free Press; 1986.

15. McCormack B, Titchen A. Patient-centred practice: an emerging focus for nursing expertise. In: Higgs J, Titchen A, editors. Practice knowledge and expertise in the health professions. Oxford: Butterworth–Heinemann; 2001. pp. 96–101.

16. Robertson D, Warrender F, Barnard S. The critical occupational therapy practitioner: how to define expertise? Aust Occup Ther J 2015;62:68–71. doi: 10.1111/1440-1630.12157.

17. Carr M, Morris J, Kersten P. Developing clinical expertise in musculoskeletal physiotherapy; Using observed practice to create a valued practice-based collaborative learning cycle. Musculoskelet Sci Pract 2020;50:102278.

18. Turpin M. The issue is ... recovery of our phenomenological knowledge in occupational therapy. Am J Occup Ther 2007;61:481–5.

19. Higgs J, Titchen A. Framing professional practice: knowing and doing in context. In: Higgs J, Titchen A, editors. Professional practice in health, education and the creative arts. Oxford: Blackwell Science; 2001. pp. 3–15.

20. Copley J, Bennett S, Turpin M. Clinical reasoning, evidence, and practice with children. In: Rodger S, editor. Occupation centred practice for children: a practical guide for occupational therapists. West Sussex, UK: Wiley-Blackwell; 2010. pp. 320–38.

21. Higgs J. The complexity of clinical reasoning: exploring the dimensions of clinical reasoning expertise as a situated, lived phenomenon. CPEA, Occasional Paper 6. Collaborations in Practice and Education Advancement. Australia: The University of Sydney; 2007.

22. Higgs J, Jones M. Multiple spaces of choice, engagement and influence in clinical decision-making. In: Higgs J, Jensen GM, Loftus S, et al., editors. Clinical reasoning in the health professions. 4th ed. Edinburgh: Elsevier; 2019. pp. 33–43.

23. Mahootian F, Eastman TE. Complementary frameworks of scientific inquiry: hypothetico-deductive, hypothetico-inductive, and observational-inductive. World Futures 2009;65(1):61–75.

24. Khatami S, Macentee M, Lofus S. Clinical reasoning in dentistry. In: Higgs J, Jensen GM, Loftus S, et al., editors. Clinical reasoning in the health professions. 4th ed. Edinburgh: Elsevier; 2019. pp. 261–70.

25. Pelaccia T, Tardif J, Triby E, et al. An analysis of clinical reasoning through a recent and comprehensive approach: the dual-process theory. Medical educ online 2011; 16(1):5890.

26. Mattingly C, Fleming MH. Clinical reasoning: forms of inquiry in a therapeutic practice. Philadelphia: FA Davis; 1994.

Implementing Evidence and Closing Research–Practice Gaps

Denise O'Connor and Ian D Graham

LEARNING OBJECTIVES

After reading this chapter, you should be able to:

- Appreciate the different types of theories, frameworks and models that can be used to describe, guide and/or explain implementation
- Describe the process of implementation and de-implementation
- Explain what is meant by an evidence–practice gap and how to assess for evidence-based gaps
- Describe how to adapt or contextualise evidence to the local context

- Explain types of barriers and enablers that may need to change for implementation to occur, and methods used to identify these
- Describe how to select implementation strategies that are most likely to target barriers and enablers of change
- Describe how to evaluate implementation processes and outcomes
- Identify factors that can help sustain post-implementation practice change

Searching for and appraising research articles are key steps in the evidence-based practice process. While these are fundamental activities, on their own they do not influence processes of care, or patient or health system outcomes. Findings from quality research studies and clinical practice guidelines that have involved years of effort, many participants and often substantial cost should not remain unused in journals. To improve healthcare and patient and system outcomes, health professionals need to do more than read research evidence and know what best practice is. They need to use this research evidence to inform their clinical decision making. While often seen as the final step in the evidence-based practice process, implementing best practice should be the end goal guiding all steps in the process.

Implementation is a complex, but active, process that may involve individuals, teams, systems and organisations, and is about facilitating the adoption of innovations. 'De-implementation' refers to the abandonment of ineffective or low-value practices, which may even be harmful (see the global

Choosing Wisely movement: https://www.choosingwisely.org/). Translating evidence into practice requires careful forward planning.[1,2] While some planning usually does occur, the process is often ad hoc and unsystematic. There may be little consideration of potential problems and barriers, of how to tailor implementation strategies to identified barriers or how to sustain practice change. As a consequence, results may be disappointing or short-lived. To help increase the likelihood of success when implementing evidence, this chapter provides guidance for individuals and teams to use when planning for evidence implementation.

This chapter offers a brief overview of implementation theories, frameworks and models and then focuses on process models of change—in particular, the Knowledge to Action Cycle.[3] The chapter then goes on to review the process of implementation in detail. This involves identifying evidence–practice gaps and specifying 'who needs to do what differently' to reduce the gap; contextualising the evidence to the local context; assessing barriers and enablers of evidence uptake to be targeted; matching implementation strategies to identified barriers and enablers to bring about change and sustain implementation; then selecting methods to measure the effectiveness of the implementation process and the impact or outcomes of the implementation; and, finally, considering sustainability and relevant strategies.

IMPLEMENTATION TERMINOLOGY

A number of terms appear in the implementation literature. Different terms may mean the same thing in different countries. To help you navigate this terminology, definitions relevant to the chapter are provided in Box 16.1.

BOX 16.1 Definitions of implementation terminology

Implementation of evidence: A planned and active process of using published research in routine practice. For example, delivering an effective therapy from an evidence-based clinical practice guideline or systematic review to patients in a local setting.

Implementation research (or science): The scientific study of methods to promote the systematic uptake of clinical research findings and other evidence-based practices into routine practice, and improve the quality of health care (effectiveness, reliability, safety, appropriateness, equity, efficiency).[4] This type of research typically involves studying the process of behaviour change, barriers to change, and the effects of implementation strategies such as reminders and decision support tools.

Diffusion of innovations: The process of spreading new ideas, behaviours or routines across a population. The adoption of new ideas typically starts with a slow initial phase, followed by a period of acceleration as more people adopt the behaviours of the innovators, then a corresponding period of deceleration with adoption by the last few individuals.[5] Examples of health 'innovations' include the introduction of a new outcome measure, screening procedure or treatment.

Knowledge translation: A process of synthesising and exchanging knowledge between researchers and users (professionals, patients and policy makers). A primary aim is to accelerate the use of research by professionals, in order to improve health outcomes.[6] Multiple disciplines, such as health informatics, health education, and organisational, social and behavioural theorists, may be involved in the knowledge translation process, to help close evidence–practice gaps.

Evidence–practice gaps: Areas of practice where clinical routines or behaviour differ from evidence-based guideline recommendations or known best practice. Areas of practice where quality improvement is required. For example, patients may be referred for an unnecessary test procedure, while others may not be receiving an intervention of proven effectiveness that could improve their health.

Determinants of practice: Factors that are thought to influence the effect of an implementation strategy on practice, sometimes referred to as 'barriers', 'enablers', 'obstacles' or 'facilitators'.[7] Seven domains with multiple determinants have been agreed, following a systematic review and consensus process: guideline factors; individual health professional factors; patient factors; professional interactions; incentives and resources; capacity for organisational change; and social, political and legal factors.[8]

Practice behaviour: A routine performed by health professionals that can be observed. For example, the ordering of tests, use of assessments and outcome measures, clinical report writing and the delivery of interventions.

Implementation strategy (or intervention): A strategy designed to facilitate, promote or encourage the uptake of evidence into practice in order to improve healthcare delivery and patient outcomes. Implementation strategies may target individual health professionals (e.g. provision of audit and feedback), teams of health professionals (e.g. educational workshops), organisations (e.g. computerised decision support) or health systems (e.g. financial incentives). Strategies may be tailored to prospectively identified barriers to change, such as health professional knowledge and/or skill gaps, addressed through providing education and training.[7]

Fidelity: The extent to which delivery of an intervention adheres to the protocol or program model originally developed. Adherence to a prescribed (or core) set of practices at an adequate dose or intensity, and competence in delivery.[9,10] Measures of fidelity include adherence to the original program and core components, and dose of intervention delivered.[11]

Sustainability: The continued use of a program and core elements of a program by organisations over time (i.e. years) to achieve a desired health outcome after initial funding/supports have been withdrawn. Some modifications and adaptations are likely to be necessary if an innovation is to persist,[12] but not so many adaptations that program 'drift' occurs;[13] that is, the program deviates so much from the original program that effects can no longer be assured. A program or intervention is considered sustained if core elements are maintained and delivered at a sufficient level of fidelity or intensity to replicate the desired health outcomes.[9]

USING THEORY, THEORETICAL FRAMEWORKS AND MODELS TO INFORM THE PROCESS OF IMPLEMENTATION

The implementation of evidence is a complex process involving change in attitudes, systems and behaviour by individuals, teams and organisations. Theories, frameworks and models can help to plan, describe and explain these complex processes, including how and why implementation efforts succeed or fail. Theoretical approaches are used to describe and/or guide the process of implementation, to understand and/or explain what influences implementation outcomes or to evaluate implementation.[14] For example, using theoretical approaches we can anticipate potential barriers, such as resistance to changing a professional's role, and then target these known barriers in advance. We can investigate why one profession or organisation succeeded or had difficulty with change compared to another—for example, delivering an intervention or ceasing to use a procedure.

A **theory** is defined as a set of principles or statements that help structure observations and understanding, and explain phenomena.[14] A useful theory will explain how and why specific relationships lead to particular outcomes or events in a predictable way. Theories can help us predict who might change, who might be resistant to change, how change might be experienced and the stages of change that most people will move through. Many theories have been developed within traditional disciplines such as psychology and sociology and are relevant to understanding and/or explaining how change occurs (for example, Social Cognitive Theory,[15] Theory of Planned Behaviour[16] and Theory of Diffusion[17]). Other theories have been developed within implementation science itself (for example, Normalisation Process Theory[18,19] and Capability, Opportunity, Motivation and Behaviour [COM-B][20]). For a comprehensive description of theories relevant to understanding change and implementation processes, see Nilsen,[14] Michie and colleagues,[21] Davis and colleagues[22] and Grol and colleagues.[23] For reviews of planned action theories, cognitive psychology theories of change in provider behaviour, education theories, organisational theories and quality improvement theories, see Straus and colleagues.[24] Theories have been used in implementation to inform the development of survey instruments[25,26] and interview questions about barriers to evidence uptake,[27] and to match interventions to identified barriers.[28]

Theoretical frameworks are structures consisting of various categories (for example, domains or constructs), and in some cases the relations between them, that are presumed to account for a phenomenon—for example, health professionals' behaviour change.[14] Frameworks in implementation science are typically descriptive in nature and outline factors believed or found to influence implementation outcomes. Examples include the Theoretical Domains Framework,[27,29] Diffusion of Innovations in Service Organisations[30] and the Consolidated Framework for Implementation Research.[31] For a comprehensive list of theoretical frameworks relevant to implementation, see Nilsen,[14] Flottorp and colleagues[8] and Tabak and colleagues[32]

Models are closely related to theory. Models in implementation science are used to describe and/or guide the process of translating research into practice rather than to predict or explain which factors influence implementation outcomes.[14] They refer to deliberately engineering change that occurs in groups. They can be used by change agents to consider variables that may increase or decrease the likelihood of the occurrence of change. One example of a process model is French and colleagues' Systematic Approach using the Theoretical Domains Framework.[1] The steps comprising this model are: (1) identify the evidence–practice gap and specify the evidence-based behaviour(s) to be implemented; (2) identify which factors (barriers and enablers) need to be addressed using relevant theory and/or theoretical frameworks; (3) select and deliver intervention components most likely to overcome the barriers and enhance the enablers, informed by theory and evidence; and (4) identify and select methods to measure implementation outcomes. Another example is Graham and colleagues' Knowledge to Action (KTA) Cycle, a model developed by reviewing 31 planned action theories, models and frameworks to identify common concepts that authors have offered to explain how planned change occurs.[3] Note that given the lack of consensus about the definitions of models and frameworks in the literature, the KTA Cycle is sometimes also referred to as a framework. The KTA Cycle is comprised of two components: a knowledge creation component (the knowledge to be applied or implemented) and an action component comprised of seven action phases identified by the review (Figure 16.1).

The knowledge creation funnel in the schema conveys the idea that knowledge needs to be increasingly distilled before it is ready for application. *Knowledge inquiry* refers to first-generation knowledge (for example, broad-base primary studies or information). *Knowledge synthesis* refers to the distillation of knowledge that identifies what is known in a given area or field and what are the knowledge gaps (for example, scoping reviews, systematic reviews, realist reviews, meta-analysis, etc.). The term *knowledge products or tools* refers to even more refined knowledge that can be more easily incorporated into decision making (for example, practice guidelines, decision aids, algorithms). Typically, the evidence or research to be implemented is generated externally to the setting that is wishing to implement it; however, in some cases, the setting may need to

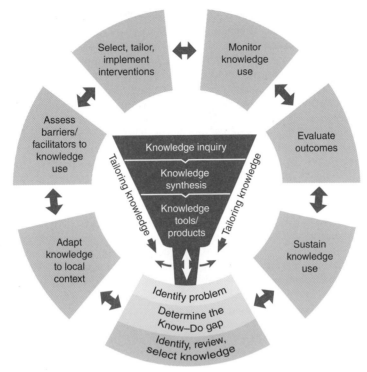

Fig 16.1 Knowledge to Action Cycle
Straus S, Tetroe J, Graham ID. Knowledge translation in healthcare: moving from evidence to practice.
2nd ed. Chichester, UK: Wiley Blackwell; 2013 (Figure 1.1.1, p. 10).

generate its own primary evidence, knowledge syntheses, or knowledge products or tools prior to or during the implementation process. Further, primary evidence, knowledge syntheses and knowledge products and tools can potentially inform each phase of the Action cycle.

The action component that is represented by the cycle is comprised of seven phases that can occur sequentially or simultaneously where any given phase may influence the next or subsequent phases. Each phase directs implementers to plan and collect local data to inform the phase. The interactive nature of implementation means that implementers may sometimes cycle back to earlier phases (for example, the need to continuously perform barriers assessments as implementation progresses). As shown in Figure 16.1, the action phases are: (1) determine the evidence–practice (or know–do) gap; (2) adapt or contextualise the evidence to be implemented to the local context; (3) assess barriers and enablers to adopting the evidence; (4) select and tailor implementation strategies to address the identified barriers; (5) monitor use of the evidence (adherence); (6) evaluate outcomes (impact) of using the evidence; and (7) sustain use of the evidence. While the phase of sustaining evidence use is positioned last in the cycle, sustainability considerations are to be incorporated into each action phase from the very beginning of the planned action process.

The KTA Cycle presents a holistic view of planned implementation by integrating the concepts of knowledge creation and application (or action). The KTA Cycle acknowledges that those who produce and use evidence are situated within a social system or systems that is responsive and adaptive, although not always in predictable ways. The KTA process is iterative, dynamic and complex. The boundaries between the knowledge creation and action components of the model are fluid and permeable. The research to implement may exist or may need to be produced. For example, a synthesis of best practice may exist, but a clinical protocol based on the synthesis needs to be produced to provide guidance on who needs to do what, with whom, how, under what conditions, and when. There are at least three ways to use the KTA model: (1) researchers generate the evidence to be implemented and push it to practice settings to implement; (2) practice settings decide what evidence–practice gaps they have and seek out relevant knowledge/evidence and pull it into their setting; or (3) researchers and implementers work together in an engagement approach to generate evidence and then implement it.

The KTA Cycle falls within the social constructivist paradigm which privileges social interaction and adaptation of evidence and takes local evidence and context into account. It is designed to be used by a broad range of prospective implementers (health system managers, clinicians, educators, researchers, etc.). As a process model that simply provides scaffolding to influence implementation planning, it also accommodates the use of other theories, frameworks and models that may be relevant and applied to guide or facilitate each phase of the cycle. An example of published uses of the KTA Cycle in one field (physical medicine and rehabilitation) has been reviewed by Moore and colleagues.[33]

Selecting theoretical approach(es) for an implementation project

As we have seen, there are numerous theories, frameworks and models that can be used to plan, describe and/or explain the process and outcomes of implementation. Selecting from among them can be challenging[34] and there is no right or wrong choice. Selecting one or more theoretical approaches should be guided by the 'goodness-of-fit' between the needs and aims of the implementation project and the characteristics of relevant theoretical approaches.[35] Lynch and colleagues[35] have proposed five questions that can be considered by health professionals when selecting theoretical approach(es). These are: (1) Who are you working with? (For example, individuals, groups or wider settings?) (2) When in the process are you going to use theory? (That is, are you planning, conducting or evaluating?) (3) Why are you applying a theory? (That is, what is your aim and what do you need to understand?) (4) How will you collect data? (For example, will you use routinely collected data or data informed by the theoretical approach?) (5) What resources are available (including the expertise of team in implementation projects)? More recently, the 'T-CaST' (implementation Theory Comparison and Selection Tool) has been developed. It is based on surveys and interviews with 37 implementation scientists across the United States, the United Kingdom and Canada and contains 16 items across four domains (usability, testability, applicability, acceptability).[36] The tool is available online (https://impsci.tracs.unc.edu/tcast/) and can guide the selection and transparent reporting of the rationale for theoretical approaches for implementation projects.

THE PROCESS OF IMPLEMENTATION IN DETAIL

This section of the chapter describes the implementation process in more detail using the phases of the KTA Cycle. However, before doing so, there are two important things to consider: *who to involve* in planning for implementation, and *what is to be implemented*.

Implementation as a team sport

There is growing appreciation that participatory approaches to implementation can be beneficial. The assumption is that implementation planning which is inclusive (by being interdisciplinary and including patients) is more likely to generate more relevant implementation plans by taking local context into consideration, attending to the implementation barriers of all diverse groups involved and selecting implementation strategies that are more context specific. In other words, engagement of eventual users of evidence in implementation planning and implementation can lead to more effective uptake and sustainability of evidence and this results in better implementation outcomes, be they patient or health system outcomes. An implementation working group should be formed to plan and execute an implementation initiative. This group should be diverse and inclusive of all the relevant stakeholders, including patients. Support for participatory implementation planning comes from the literature on user-centric design as well as on research coproduction.[37–39]

If you are looking for information on participatory approaches to implementation, a good place to start is Greenhalgh and colleagues' systematic review of patient engagement frameworks[40] and Jull and colleagues' review and synthesis of frameworks of knowledge user engagement in research.[41] Guidance on engaging and involving patients and informal caregivers can be found on the Canadian Strategy on Patient Oriented Research website (https://cihr-irsc.gc.ca/e/41204.html), the UK INVOLVE website (https://www.involve.org.uk/) and the US Patient-Centered Outcomes Research Institute website (https://www.pcori.org/).

What is to be implemented?

We want to emphasise that, with an evidence-informed approach to implementation, a critical step is ensuring that what is to be implemented actually deserves implementation. Implementing a practice that has not been sufficiently demonstrated to be effective or beneficial can contribute to squandering resources and potentially even doing harm. Hence, sometimes de-implementation is needed. There are always opportunity costs associated with implementation, so the benefits of implementation need to outweigh the harms and implementation costs. The resources that are put towards implementing a low-quality practice guideline might mean that a high-quality evidence-informed guideline with potential for greater impact is not implemented and patients are therefore denied best practice. For this reason, implementers need to have, or to have access to individuals with, strong critical appraisal skills in order to be able to identify high-quality evidence such as clinical practice guidelines and systematic reviews. (See earlier chapters of the book for guidance on how to search for and appraise evidence sources.) Judicious implementation is about ensuring there is always sufficient evidence to justify implementing or de-implementing practice. With few exceptions, practice should not be changed based on the results of a single clinical trial but, rather, on the accumulation of evidence via replication and synthesis.[42] Grimshaw and colleagues[43] have stated that the 'basic unit of knowledge translation should usually be up-to-date systematic reviews or other syntheses of research findings'.

The following breaks down the implementation process into the phases of the KTA Cycle and describes in greater detail the goals, considerations, required data and how it can be collected, and key decisions related to each phase.

Determine the evidence–practice gap

This phase can start with those in a practice setting raising concerns about a clinical issue. Conducting qualitative research on patients' and/or clinicians' perceptions, experiences or concerns about care can also be useful for identifying possible care gaps that will require more thorough investigation (see Chapter 10 on qualitative methods). Concerns might also be triggered by quality improvement reports. The literature is then reviewed for practice guidelines or knowledge syntheses about what is best practice for the identified problem. In some cases, the best available evidence may be primary studies such as randomised trials, but as already noted, changing practice based on the results of a single study should be done with care. Alternatively, this phase can start with those in the practice setting becoming aware of best practice (such as new evidence) that may have been recently reported in the literature and wondering about the extent to which current practice aligns with it ('identify the problem' on the KTA model;

Figure 16.1). In either case, the goal of this phase is to determine whether there is an evidence–practice gap by comparing current practice to best practice and deciding whether the gap needs to be closed or narrowed or no action is needed at this time.

The proposed best practice must be critically assessed to determine that it is, in fact, best practice based on the best available scientific evidence. For practice guidelines, we have found that having the implementation working group assess candidate practice guidelines using the AGREE II (Appraisal of Guidelines for Research and Evaluation Instrument II) or AGREE REX (Appraisal of Guidelines for Research and Evaluation Instrument – Recommendation Excellence) tool not only provides the group with their own evidence that the guideline they choose to implement deserves implementation (that is, the evidence is robust enough to justify implementation), but also builds group members' critical appraisal skills and positions them well to discuss the evidence with colleagues and the rationale for its selection.[44,45] Appraisal tools that can be used to assess the quality of systematic reviews include the AMSTAR 2 (A MeaSurement Tool to Assess systematic Reviews)[46] and ROBIS (Risk Of Bias In Systematic reviews).[47] For more detail on systematic review critical appraisal, please refer to Chapter 12.

The first phase in the KTA Cycle also involves specifying the behaviour(s) that need to be implemented to close the gap (that is, defining *who* needs to do *what differently, when, where* and *how*). This is informed by the guideline's recommendations or evidence syntheses that were selected for implementation and the behaviours that are 'audited' during a gap analysis. Examples of evidence–practice gaps and behaviours are presented in Box 16.2.

BOX 16.2   Examples of evidence–practice gaps

Only 17% of eligible stroke survivors (13/77) were receiving at least one targeted therapy session by an occupational therapist or physiotherapist to increase outdoor journeys.[48] An audit of 77 medical records across five stroke services highlighted 'underuse' of this evidence-based intervention, which was recommended in an Australian evidence-based stroke guideline.

Only one outdoor-related therapy session (median) was delivered per stroke survivor by occupational therapists and physiotherapists to increase outdoor journeys.[49] This audit of 311 medical records across 24 services again highlighted 'underuse' of an evidence-based intervention.

Only 26% of occupational therapists (67/253) reported using 'best practice' assessment for unilateral spatial neglect, and only 58% (147/253) reported providing any intervention for unilateral spatial neglect.[50] This national survey of 253 occupational therapists highlighted 'underuse' of

evidence-based practices, which were recommended in Canadian national stroke guidelines.

Only 9% of older inpatients admitted for surgery following hip fracture were identified as having a risk of falls, and only 8% had a documented referral to a community agency for follow-up regarding the prevention of falls.[28,51] This audit of 51 records at one site highlighted 'underuse' of evidence-based practices recommended in national clinical practice guidelines.

Only 42% of stroke inpatients were given a swallowing screen or assessment within 24 hours of admission and prior to being given oral food, drink or medications, and referred to a speech pathologist for full assessment after a failed swallow screen.[52] This audit of 1,062 medical records across 30 hospitals highlighted 'underuse' of evidence-based practices recommended in Australian national stroke guidelines.

Health professionals who seek funding for implementation projects, and postgraduate students who write research proposals, should demonstrate that a gap exists between evidence and practice. This gap can be quantified using data collection methods such as an audit of medical records or practice, or a survey.

An **audit** can be conducted of local medical records (for example, consecutive patient admissions over a 6-month period). Chart audits can determine how many people with a health condition received a particular test or evidence-informed clinical intervention. For example, we could determine the proportion of people with acute back pain for whom a plain X-ray had been ordered in a general practice over the previous 6 months. We could also count how frequently (or rarely) an intervention was used. In one study, the number of escorted outdoor sessions provided to stroke survivors by an occupational therapist or physiotherapist to help increase outdoor mobility was extracted from medical records.[48]

Baseline file audits of 77 consecutive referrals across five services in the previous year revealed that 57% of people with stroke had received at least one session targeting outdoor journeys, 35% had received two or more sessions and 17% had received six or more sessions. In the original randomised trial that evaluated this intervention,[53,54] a median of six sessions targeting outdoor journeys had been provided by therapists and this was considered the optimal 'dose' (or target) of the clinical intervention. Audits can also be conducted of practice behaviours, to help identify evidence–practice gaps. For example, by observing therapists we can obtain an accurate record of how often they ask target questions, screen patients, remember to offer or deliver an intervention, and so forth.

Surveys can also be used to explore current practice and clinicians' knowledge of or attitudes about best practice. If a large proportion of health professionals report rarely using an evidence-based test or treatment, this information can be used to demonstrate an evidence–practice gap. For example, surveys have been used to explore the practice of Australian chiropractors and physiotherapists, respectively, in managing acute low back pain and to assess concordance with an Australian evidence-based guideline.[55,56] The surveys incorporated vignettes of people who would typically present with acute low back pain, and respondents identified the investigations and interventions they would use for each scenario. In the survey of physiotherapists, 75% reported not ordering an X-ray, and 62% reported providing advice to stay active—both of which are consistent with the evidence-based guideline.[56]

Adapt or contextualise evidence to the context

Having identified appropriate evidence and established an evidence–practice gap, the implementation working group must review the specific best practice recommendations in detail to specify the exact practices/behaviours that need to be implemented to reduce the gap (that is, define *who* needs to do *what differently, when, where, how* and *with whom*). This level of detail is important, because anyone who is leading implementation efforts needs to be clear about what successful implementation looks like in order to bring about change. It is also necessary to consider if the practices/behaviours can be delivered as specified in the recommendations or whether some minor adaptations are required. For example, a recommendation may call for a nurse to conduct a cognitive assessment on admission, but if in the local setting, nursing resources would not enable another assessment to be conducted at admission, whereas a psychologist could, this could be an appropriate minor adaptation. Any adaptations to the best practice recommendations must be about customising the recommendations to the local context (that is, be relatively minor) and remain true to the evidence supporting the recommendation. Furthermore, specifying the change in a behaviour-specific manner will lead to more accurate assessment of the barriers and enablers to change. Barriers and enablers may vary for different behaviours. An example of a behaviour defined in behavioural terms is from the IRIS study,[57] in which the tailored implementation program aimed to increase the uptake of evidence-based guideline recommendations for the detection, diagnosis and management of people with dementia in Australian general practice.

- *What behaviour?* An assessment of cognitive function is undertaken in people with suspected cognitive impairment.
- *Who?* By general practitioners (GPs).
- *How?* Using the Mini Mental State Examination (a validated scale).
- *When, where, with whom?* Within the first three consultations from when a suspicion of cognitive impairment or dementia is first identified, conducted in the GP practice, with the patient.

Knowing what behaviours must be observed helps us identify factors that have to change for the evidence–practice gap to be closed.

Presseau and colleagues[58] have suggested a helpful mnemonic—'AACTT'—to specify the behaviour of interest: A—what is the Action/behaviour or practice to be implemented? A— who is the Actor or person to do the action? C—what is the Context in which the action is to be done? T—who is the Target for the action? And T—when is the action to be done (Time)? Typically, adaptations relate to the actors and context. The action, targets and timing, because they are often based on evidence, should only be adapted with great care. The adapted AACTT is the practice/behaviour that will now be implemented and the perceived barriers and enablers related to it then need to be assessed.

Assess barriers and enablers of use of the evidence

The next phase in the implementation process is to identify which factors need to be addressed (that is, the barriers to, and enablers of, change), informed by use of theory and/or a theoretical framework. As mentioned earlier, theory and/or theoretical frameworks can help us to understand how individuals, teams and organisations experience and think about behaviour change. This step can also prevent important factors being overlooked, such as unspoken beliefs or attitudes.

Barriers are factors or conditions that may prevent successful implementation of evidence (such as limited knowledge, skills or appropriate equipment). Conversely, enablers are factors that increase the likelihood of success (such as possessing relevant knowledge and skills). Barriers and enablers relate to what individuals know, think and feel (for example, knowledge, attitudes, emotions), and the environment in which they operate (for example, the social and environmental context). When barriers and enablers have been identified, a tailored implementation strategy can be developed (that is, a strategy to overcome the identified barriers and enhance the enablers).

Methods for identifying barriers and enablers to evidence uptake include a literature search for studies that have previously explored this problem, individual and group interviews, audits or observation of practice, and surveys. Sometimes more than one method is useful to enhance the validity of findings. The choice of method will be guided by time, finances, local circumstances, and the number of health professionals involved. Participant interviews, observation and surveys should include the health professionals and teams that will be the focus of the implementation initiative. The perspectives of patients, family members and managers can also be very informative.

Here are some examples of published studies that have used a theoretical approach to elicit barriers and enablers:[59,60]

- To inform the development and implementation of a similar intervention elsewhere, an evaluation was conducted of the implementation of an evidence-based upper limb stroke rehabilitation intervention (the 'Graded Repetitive Arm Supplementary Program', or GRASP) in Canada.[60] The researchers conducted semi-structured interviews with a purposive sample of 20 physiotherapists, occupational therapists and rehabilitation assistants involved in implementing GRASP across eight sites. One theory and two theoretical

frameworks were used to guide the interview schedule and data analysis:
- Normalisation Process Theory (NPT) was used to explore the processes involved in identifying, integrating and embedding GRASP in practice.
- The Conceptual Framework for Implementation Fidelity (CFIF)[61] was used to explore the coverage, content and dose when GRASP was used in practice, and to assess how it compared with the GRASP Guideline Manual (adherence).
- The Consolidated Framework for Implementation Research (CFIR)[31] was used during data analysis to identify emerging factors (that is, barriers and enablers) that influenced the implementation and use of GRASP.
- Therapists identified informal networks and the free online availability of GRASP as key factors that enabled them to know about the intervention and all reported positive opinions about the value of GRASP. At all sites, therapists identified individuals who advocated for the intervention; and in six of the eight sites, this person was the practice leader or senior therapist. Rehabilitation assistants were identified as instrumental in delivering GRASP in almost all sites, as they were responsible for organising the equipment and assisting patients to do the intervention. Almost all intervention components were adapted to some degree when GRASP was used in practice. Fidelity monitoring revealed that the dose of intervention provided was less than recommended, coverage was broader (that is, GRASP was provided to other populations) and program content was changed.

Other examples of barriers and enablers studies informed by theoretical approaches are published in a thematic series on the Theoretical Domains Framework (TDF) in the journal *Implementation Science* (see https://www.biomedcentral.com/collections/tdf). For example, Bussières and colleagues[62] used the TDF to identify the factors influencing uptake of diagnostic imaging guideline recommendations for back pain by chiropractors and identified patients' preferences for imaging as a barrier to change, among other factors, that would likely need to be addressed with an implementation strategy.

Select/tailor and deliver implementation strategies

The next phase in the implementation process is to select/tailor and deliver implementation strategies that are most likely to overcome the barriers and enhance the enablers to bring about and sustain evidence uptake. Implementation strategies (also known as implementation interventions) are strategies designed to facilitate, promote or encourage the uptake of evidence into practice to improve healthcare and patient outcomes (Box 16.1). The concept of tailoring strategies to optimise their impact makes intuitive sense and is supported by a systematic review by Baker and colleagues[7] which found that strategies tailored to prospectively identified barriers are more likely to improve health professional practice compared with no implementation intervention or to non-tailored strategies. However, the optimal method for tailoring strategies has not yet been established, and various approaches to tailoring have been reported in the literature.[63–69] These include theory-informed approaches such as that described by Moore and colleagues[63] who used the COM-B to identify health professional, patient and unit-level barriers to evidence uptake and map implementation strategies theorised to address the barriers in their MOVE ON (Mobilisation of Vulnerable Elders in Ontario) intervention. Another example is reported by Tavender and colleagues,[64] who used two theoretical frameworks (Theoretical Domains Framework and Diffusion of Innovations in Service Organizations) to identify factors influencing uptake of guidelines for managing mild brain injury in emergency departments and to guide the selection of implementation strategies and behaviour change techniques (the so-called active ingredients theorised to target the identified factors). Pragmatic or commonsense approaches to tailoring have also been described, including, for example, by Flottorp and Oxman[65] who report using an iterative process of identifying possible solutions to overcome barriers by drawing on the expertise of the implementation working group and conducting small group discussions and qualitative interviews with end users.

When selecting and tailoring implementation strategies it is important to consider the range of available options along with evidence of their effects, how the strategies are expected to bring about change, resources available to deliver the strategies and their acceptability to the target end users. Taking these factors into consideration during the design process will increase the likelihood of beneficial outcomes and minimise opportunity costs from investing in ineffective strategies. Several taxonomies that describe and organise implementation strategies for targeting different stakeholder groups (for example, healthcare providers, healthcare organisations, patients) at varying levels of granularity (for example, 'educational meetings'[70] versus 'action planning'[71]) are available.[71–76]

A useful starting point for locating evidence about the effects of implementation strategies is via systematic reviews prepared by authors from the Cochrane Effective Practice and Organisation of Care (EPOC) group and published in the Cochrane Library (https://www.cochranelibrary.com/). These reviews synthesise evidence from thousands of randomised and quasi-randomised studies of professional, organisational, financial and regulatory strategies using rigorous Cochrane review methodology.[43] Table 16.1 provides an overview of the effects of key implementation strategies summarised in Cochrane EPOC reviews. As can be seen, most strategies lead to modest changes in practice (typically, no greater than 10%). Larger changes can be expected if compliance with best practice at baseline is low. Health professionals and service managers who evaluate the outcomes of implementation efforts should not be surprised by changes of this magnitude. Additional searches for systematic reviews of implementation strategies targeting specific disciplines (for example, nurses[77]) or specific healthcare areas (for example, stroke rehabilitation[78]) may also be helpful. Other useful resources when designing implementation strategies include the Expert Recommendations for Implementing Change (ERIC), a list of 73 implementation strategies and definitions developed and refined through a literature review and modified Delphi process,[74,75] and the Behaviour Change Technique Taxonomy, which describes 93 discrete behaviour change techniques, considered the 'active ingredients' of interventions for changing behaviour.[71]

TABLE 16.1   Evidence of effects of key implementation strategies from Cochrane EPOC reviews

Intervention	Number of included studies in review	Effect size (median absolute improvement in desired practice)	Interquartile range
Printed educational materials[79]	84	+4.0%	+1.0% to +9.0%
Educational meetings[70]	215	+4.0%	+0.3% to +13.0%
Manually-generated paper reminders[80]	63	+8.5%	+2.5% to +20.6%
Audit and feedback[81]	140	+4.3%	+0.5 to +16.0%
Local opinion leaders[82]	24	+10.8%	+3.5 to +14.6%

Monitor the implementation process (adherence to the evidence) and evaluate outcomes (impact)

The primary aim of implementation is to change decision making and the behaviour of health professionals, teams and/or organisations; however, what is important, of course, is whether patient outcomes improve because of the practice change. Measures of health professional behaviour are most often used (88%) as outcomes in trials aimed at increasing the uptake of evidence, followed by patient measures (29%) and organisational measures (18%).[83]

The KTA Cycle distinguishes between monitoring knowledge use (monitoring adherence to the evidence, including knowledge, attitudes and intentions towards using the evidence) and evaluating outcomes produced by adhering to the evidence. To fully understand the impact of implementation it is often necessary to determine both the extent to which the evidence is being used, as well as the effect of the use of the evidence on patient outcomes, health professional outcomes or health system outcomes (as well as other relevant outcomes, including unintended outcomes). If only the impact of implementation is measured (for example, patient outcomes), it may be difficult to determine if the outcomes can be attributed to use of the evidence. If only adherence to the evidence is measured, it may be difficult to attribute broader impact to the adherence.

Adherence

To determine adherence to the evidence, the implementation working group should take each practice behaviour (*who? needs to do what? how? when? where? with whom?*) and develop indicators to measure whether the practice behaviour is occurring as intended. This is sometimes referred to as determining the fidelity with which the behaviour is being delivered.

There are several ways that adherence can be measured, each with its own advantages and disadvantages. Data on adherence can be self-reported or more objective. For example, questionnaires and surveys can be used to collect information on knowledge and attitudes about the evidence and self-reported adherence to it. Interviews are typically more labour-intensive to undertake than surveys, although both rely on self-report. Administrative databases and clinical databases can also be used to assess evidence adherence, but these rely on the accuracy of the data submitted to the databases. In determining how to monitor adherence, important considerations include: *How accurate will the data be? How easy will it be to collect the data? What are the costs associated with collecting the data? Will it be possible to use these methods after the implementation has been completed (that is, during the sustainability phase)?*

Outcomes/impacts

Many authors have described different ways to conceptualise implementation outcomes, often including indicators of adherence with impacts of adherence. Straus and colleagues have classified implementation outcomes at the patient level (the impact on patients of using the evidence), provider level (the impact on providers of using the evidence) and health system/society level (the impact on the health system of applying the evidence).[84]

Proctor and colleagues[85] defined implementation outcomes as the effects of deliberate, purposeful actions to implement new practices or services. In 2011, using a consensus process similar to Michie and colleagues,[20] Proctor and colleagues generated a taxonomy of eight conceptually different implementation outcomes: acceptability, adoption, appropriateness, costs, feasibility, fidelity, penetration and sustainability (see Box 16.3).[85]

Another framework that can be used to measure implementation outcomes is RE-AIM, with a focus on Reach, Effectiveness, Adoption, Implementation and Maintenance.[87,88] A similar, but smaller range of implementation outcomes was proposed by Chaudoir and colleagues (adoption, fidelity, implementation cost, penetration and sustainability) as part of a review.[89] Of the 62 implementation outcome measures identified during their searches, 39 contained items that measured adoption, five contained items that measured fidelity, but no studies measured implementation cost, penetration or sustainability.

An investigation of instruments for measuring implementation outcomes found few with respectable psychometric properties.[86] Of the 104 instruments appraised, 50 assessed *acceptability* of outcomes (the perception among stakeholders that a given intervention or service is agreeable or satisfactory) and 19 assessed *adoption* (the intention, initial decision or action to try or use an innovation or practice), but few other constructs were assessed. No *fidelity* instruments were identified during the review (the degree to which an intervention was implemented as intended). It was noted that implementation researchers do 'measure' fidelity, but tend to develop their own measure, which is specific to an intervention, typically psychometrically weak, and cannot be applied in other studies or contexts.[86]

Similar to what is suggested for measuring evidence adherence, the implementation working group should set out to determine what outcomes are of greatest interest and develop indicators for them. Strategies for collecting data on outcomes are similar to those that can be used to measure adherence and include using administrative databases and clinical databases (for example, to determine health status [morbidity or mortality], costs, wait times, length of stay), and questionnaires and interviews (for example, to

BOX 16.3 Proctor's taxonomy of implementation outcomes

Acceptability: Satisfaction with various aspects of an innovation such as content, complexity, comfort, delivery and credibility. Acceptability to patients or providers can be evaluated using a survey, semi-structured interview or local administrative data.

Adoption: Initial uptake, utilisation or intention to try an innovation. Adoption by individual providers and services can be evaluated through observation, a survey or semi-structured interview, or by using administrative data.

Appropriateness: Perceived fit of an innovation, including relevance, compatibility, suitability, usefulness and practicability. There is ambiguity and overlap in published instruments between the constructs of 'appropriateness' and 'acceptability', resulting in instruments measuring different constructs.[86] Appropriateness as perceived by patients, providers and organisations can be evaluated using a survey, semi-structured interview or focus group.

Feasibility: Actual fit or utility, suitability for everyday use and practicability. Feasibility as determined by providers and organisations can be evaluated using a survey or local administrative data.

Fidelity: Delivery of the innovation and adherence as intended, integrity and quality of program delivery. Fidelity has been widely evaluated, particularly in mental health, using observation, checklists and self-reporting.

Implementation cost: Cost of implementing an innovation, the resources and inputs involved, and benefits and effectiveness of the innovation. Cost to the provider and organisation is best evaluated using local data.

Penetration: Level of institutional spread and access by consumers. Penetration can be evaluated at the organisational level using audits and checklist.

Sustainability: Maintenance of an innovation, continuation, durability, incorporation, integration, institutionalisation, sustained use and routinisation. Sustainability can be evaluated over a longer period, typically years not months, at an organisational level using audits, semi-structured interviews, surveys and checklists.

Adapted from Proctor E, Silmere H, Raghavan R, et al. Outcomes for implementation research: conceptual distinctions, measurement challenges, and research agenda. Administration and Policy in Mental Health and Mental Health Services Research. 2011; 38(2):65–76.

determine health-related quality of life, or patients' experiences with care, or professionals' satisfaction with the new practice). It is also important for the working group to consider the feasibility of ongoing use of the measures, as being able to continue to measure outcomes can be a sustainability strategy. Evaluating outcomes over time can reveal when use of the evidence has stalled and more implementation or sustainability strategies are needed or when success should be celebrated and the continued use of resources planned.

Sustainability considerations

Sustainability has been defined as the continued use of programs and program components by organisations over several years to achieve desired health outcomes, as well as sustained use of an intervention by clients or patients.[9,90] Based on a literature review, Moore and colleagues[91] defined individual and organisational sustainability as the following, consisting of five key constructs: '(1) after a defined period of time, (2) the program, clinical intervention, and/or implementation strategies continue to be delivered and/or (3) individual behaviour change (i.e., clinician, patient) is maintained; (4) the program and individual behaviour change may evolve or adapt while (5) continuing to produce benefits for individuals/systems' (p. 5).

Sustainability is a key implementation outcome,[92] yet very little is known about how well or under what conditions clinical interventions are sustained. The limited literature suggests that adaptation, a good fit with the context, continued financial support, training, fidelity and leadership all contribute to sustainability.[9,90,92]

Adaptations and innovations are common to the content, design or delivery of a program, to make it 'fit' the local context. Elements may be added, substituted, reordered or removed, leading to program drift. For example, adaptations were made to an HIV risk-reduction video intervention to match presenter and participant ethnicity and gender, and patient outcomes were successfully retained despite adaptations.[12] The more that adaptations are allowed or encouraged when implementing an innovation, the more likely it is that the innovation will persist. However, there is a tension between adaptation and fidelity in implementation science. Organisations may continue a program but with limited fidelity to the original version and its core components. The type and extent of adaptation that can occur without compromising effectiveness and reducing fidelity requires careful monitoring.

Continued financial support is not synonymous with sustainability but seems to help. Availability of other resources, including volunteer services, can help sustain programs. Other influencing factors include the organisation's ability to mobilise appropriate resources, participation of the target population, the presence of a program network or community of practice, refinements and adaptations to program components and an internal need or 'pull' (versus an 'external push').[90] In a study that interviewed 90 hospital staff across ten sites, some of whom had successfully integrated new practices to reduce hospital admissions and some of whom had not, it was found that integration was successful when a small number of key staff devoted substantial effort to 'holding the innovation' in place for as long as a year while more permanent systems began to work and practice became more automated.[93] The key staff monitored the practice, made adjustments and adapted the innovation, which also helped to adjust staff attitudes.

Finally, some of the theories and theoretical frameworks mentioned earlier, such as the Normalisation Process Theory, include constructs related to sustainability. These theories can help researchers and service providers to think about long-term sustainability of a program earlier in the implementation process. For an overview of theoretical approaches that consider sustainability, see Nadalin Penno and colleagues.[94] Implementation of evidence is a crucial part of evidence-based practice and a way of closing evidence–practice gaps and this chapter introduced relevant theories, theoretical frameworks, and models, along with the key steps and strategies involved.

SUMMARY

- Implementation is a planned and active process of using published research in practice. Other terms for 'implementation' are 'knowledge translation' or 'knowledge mobilisation'. This process aims to help close evidence–practice gaps.
- The process of implementation involves a series of steps, starting with the need to demonstrate an evidence–practice gap, and specifying the behaviour(s) that need to be implemented. That is, defining *who* needs to do *what differently, when, where, how* and *with whom.*
- Barriers and enablers to implementation need to be identified early in the process, typically using interviews, observation and/or surveys. After this, a tailored implementation strategy can be developed.
- Common barriers to implementation include: knowledge, attitudes, skills, resources, social influences and systems. Barriers are unique to local teams and organisations, and time should be spent identifying local barriers.
- Implementation (or behaviour change) strategies include, but are not limited to, educational materials and meetings, reminders, audit and feedback, and local opinion leaders.
- Theory, theoretical frameworks and models can help us to understand how individuals, teams and organisations experience and think about behaviour change.
- Most implementation strategies lead to modest changes in practice (typically, no greater than 10%). Larger changes can be expected if adherence with best practice at baseline is low.
- Adherence measures that can be used to evaluate the success of implementation efforts include the level of adoption by individuals and teams, acceptability to patients and health professionals, fidelity and sustained use over time.
- Measures to assess impact of adherence include provider outcomes, patient outcomes, as well as health system outcomes.
- *Sustainability* refers to the continued use of a program, and program components by organisations over several years, to achieve desired health outcomes. Ideally, organisations should plan for sustainability beyond the period of initial funding.

ACKNOWLEDGMENTS

The updated version of this chapter for this edition is based on the chapter from previous editions of this book, which were co-authored by Annie McCluskey. Her valuable contribution to the content and structure of this chapter is gratefully acknowledged.

REFERENCES

1. French SD, Green SE, O'Connor DA, et al. Developing theory-informed behaviour change interventions to implement evidence into practice: a systematic approach using the theoretical domains framework. Implement Sci 2012; 7:38.

2. Grol R, Wensing M. Implementation of change in healthcare: a complex problem. In: Grol R, Wensing M, Eccles M, et al., editors. Improving patient care: the implementation of change in health care. 2nd ed. Chichester, UK: Wiley-Blackwell; 2013.

3. Graham ID, Logan J, Harrison MB, et al. Lost in knowledge translation: time for a map? J Contin Educ Health Prof 2006;26:13–24.

4. Eccles MP, Armstrong D, Baker R, et al. An implementation research agenda. Implement Sci 2009;4:18.

5. Greenhalgh T, Glenn R, Bate P, et al. Diffusion of innovations in health service organizations: a systematic literature review. Oxford, UK: Blackwell Publishing Ltd; 2005.

6. Davis D, Evans M, Jadad A, et al. The case for knowledge translation: shortening the journey from evidence to effect. BMJ 2003;327:33–5.

7. Baker R, Camosso-Stefinovic J, Gillies C, et al. Tailored interventions to address determinants of practice. Cochrane Database Syst Rev 2015;(4):CD005470. doi:10.1002/14651858. CD005470.pub3.

8. Flottorp SA, Oxman AD, Krause J, et al. A checklist for identifying determinants of practice: a systematic review and synthesis of frameworks and taxonomies of factors that prevent or enable improvements in health professional practice. Implement Sci 2013;8:35.

9. Stirman SW, Kimberly J, Cook N, et al. The sustainability of new programs and innovations: a review of the empirical literature and recommendations for future research. Implement Sci 2012;7:17.

10. Mowbray CT, Holter MC, Teague GB, et al. Fidelity criteria: development, measurement and validation. Am J Eval 2003;24(3):315–40.

11. Slaughter SE, Hill JN, Snelgrove-Clarke E. What is the extent and quality of documentation and reporting of fidelity to implementation strategies? A scoping review. Implement Sci 2015;10:129.

12. Stirman SW, Miller CJ, Toder K, et al. Development of a framework and coding system for modifications and adaptations of evidence-based interventions. Implement Sci 2013;8:65.

13. Chambers DA, Glasgow RE, Stange KC. The dynamic sustainability framework: addressing the paradox of sustainment and ongoing change. Implement Sci 2013;8:117.

14. Nilsen P. Making sense of implementation theories, models and frameworks. Implement Sci 2015;10:53.

15. Bandura A. Self-efficacy: toward a unifying theory of behaviour change. Psychol Rev 1977;84(2):191–215.

16. Ajzen I. The theory of planned behaviour. Organ Behav Hum Decis Process 1991;50:179–211.

17. Rogers EM. Diffusion of innovations. 5th ed. New York: Free Press; 2003.

18. Murray E, Treweek S, Pope C, et al. Normalisation process theory: a framework for developing, evaluating and implementing complex interventions. BMC Med 2010;8:63.

19. McEvoy R, Ballini L, Maltoni S, et al. A qualitative systematic review of studies using the Normalization Process Theory to research implementation processes. Implement Sci 2014;9:2.

20. Michie S, van Stralen MM, West R. The behaviour change wheel: a new method for characterizing and designing behaviour change interventions. Implement Sci 2011;6:42.

21. Michie S, West R, Campbell R, et al. ABC of Behaviour Change Theories. Bream, UK: Silverback Publishing; 2014.

22. Davis R, Campbell R, Hildon Z, et al. Theories of behaviour and behaviour change across the social and behavioural sciences: a scoping review. Health Psychol Rev 2015;9(3): 323–44.

23. Grol RP, Bosch MC, Hulscher ME, et al. Planning and studying improvement in patient care: the use of theoretical perspectives. Milbank Q 2007;85(1):93–138.

24. Straus S, Tetroe JM, Graham ID. Knowledge translation in healthcare. 2nd ed. Hoboken, NJ: Wiley; 2013.

25. Francis J, Eccles MP, Johnston M, et al. Constructing questionnaires based on the theory of planned behaviour: a manual for health services researchers. Newcastle upon Tyne, UK: Centre for Health Services Research, University of Newcastle upon Tyne; 2004.

26. Bowman J, Lannin NA, Cook C. Development and psychometric testing of the Clinician Readiness for Measuring Outcomes Scale (CReMOS). J Eval Clin Pract 2009;15(1):76–84.

27. Michie S, Johnston M, Abraham C, et al. Making psychological theory useful for implementing evidence based practice: a consensus approach. Qual and Safety in Health Care 2005;14:26–33.

28. Thomas S, Mackintosh S. Use of the TDF to develop an intervention to improve physical therapist management of the risk of falls after discharge. Phys Ther 2014;94(11): 1660–75.

29. Cane J, O'Connor D, Michie S. Validation of the theoretical domains framework for use in behaviour change and implementation research. Implement Sci 2012;7:37.

30. Greenhalgh T, Glenn R, Macfarlane F, et al. Diffusion of innovations in service organizations: systematic review and recommendations. Milbank Q 2004;82:581–629.

31. Damschroder LJ, Aron DC, Keith RE, et al. Fostering implementation of health services research findings into practice: a consolidated framework for advancing implementation science. Implement Sci 2009;4:50.

32. Tabak RG, Khoong EC, Chambers DA, et al. Bridging research and practice: models for dissemination and implementation research. Am J Prev Med 2012;43(3): 337–50.

33. Moore JL, Mbalilaki JA, Graham ID. Knowledge translation in physical medicine and rehabilitation: a citation analysis of the knowledge-to-action literature. Arch Phys Med Rehabil 2021;Feb 6:S0003-9993(21)00144-1.

34. Strifler L, Cardoso R, McGowan J, et al. Scoping review identifies significant number of knowledge translation theories, models, and frameworks with limited use. J Clin Epidemiol 2018;100:92–102.

35. Lynch EA, Mudge A, Knowles S, et al. 'There is nothing so practical as a good theory': a pragmatic guide for selecting theoretical approaches for implementation projects. BMC Health Serv Res 2018;18:857.

36. Birken SA, Rohweder CL, Powell BJ, et al. T-CaST: an implementation theory comparison and selection tool. Implementation Sci 2018;13:143.

37. Usability.gov. User-Centered Design Basics; 2022. Available: https://www.usability.gov/what-and-why/user-centered-design.html (accessed 19 August 2021).

38. Hoekstra F, Mrklas KJ, Khan M, et al. A review of reviews on principles, strategies, outcomes and impacts of research partnerships approaches: a first step in synthesising the research partnership literature. Health Res Policy Syst 2020;18(1):51.

39. Graham ID, Roycroft-Malone J, Kothari A, et al., editors. Research coproduction in healthcare. Chichester, UK: Wiley Blackwell; 2022.

40. Greenhalgh T, Hinton L, Finlay T, et al. Frameworks for supporting patient and public involvement in research: systematic review and co-design pilot. Health Expect 2019;22:785–801.

41. Jull JE, Davidson L, Dungan R et al. A review and synthesis of frameworks for engagement in health research to identify concepts of knowledge user engagement. BMC Med Res Methodol 2019;19:211.

42. Ioannidis JPA. Contradicted and initially stronger effects in highly cited clinical research. JAMA 2005;294(2):218–28.

43. Grimshaw JM, Eccles MP, Lavis JN, et al. Knowledge translation of research findings. Implement Sci 2012;7:50.

44. Brouwers MC, Kho ME, Browman GP, et al. AGREE II: advancing guideline development, reporting and evaluation in health care. J Clin Epidemiol 2010;63(12):1308–11.

45. Brouwers MC, Spithoff K, Kerkvliet K, et al. Development and validation of a tool to assess the quality of clinical practice guideline recommendations. JAMA Netw Open 2020;3(5):e205535.

46. Shea BJ, Reeves BC, Wells G, et al. AMSTAR 2: a critical appraisal tool for systematic reviews that include randomised or non-randomised studies of healthcare interventions, or both. BMJ 2017;358:j4008.

47. Whiting P, Savović J, Higgins JP, et al. A new tool to assess risk of bias in systematic reviews was developed. J Clin Epidemiol 2016;69:225–34.

48. McCluskey A, Middleton S. Feasibility of implementing an outdoor journey intervention to people with stroke: a feasibility study involving five community rehabilitation teams. Implement Sci 2010;5:59.

49. McCluskey A, Ada L, Kelly PJ, et al. Compliance with Australian stroke guideline recommendations for outdoor mobility and transport training by post-inpatient rehabilitation services: an observational cohort. BMC Health Serv Res 2015;15:296.

50. Menon-Nair A, Korner-Bitensky N, Ogourtsova T. Occupational therapists' identification, assessment and treatment of unilateral spatial neglect during stroke rehabilitation. Stroke 2007;38(9):2556–62.

51. Thomas S, Mackintosh S, Halbert J. Determining current physical therapy management of hip fracture in an acute care hospital and physical therapists' rationale for this management. Phys Ther 2011;91(10):1490–502.

52. Middleton S, Lydtin A, Comerford D, et al. From QASC to QASCIP: successful Australian translational scale-up and spread of a proven intervention in acute stroke using a prospective pre-test/post-test study design. BMJ Open 2016;6:e011568.

53. Logan P, Gladman J, Avery A, et al. Randomised controlled trial of an occupational therapy intervention to increase outdoor mobility after stroke. BMJ 2004;329:1372–7.

54. Logan P, Walker M, Gladman J. Description of an occupational therapy intervention aimed at improving outdoor mobility. Br J Occup Ther 2006;69:2–6.

55. Walker BF, French SD, Page MJ, et al. Management of people with acute low-back pain: a survey of Australian chiropractors. Chiropr Man Therap 2011;19:29.

56. Keating JL, McKenzie JE, O'Connor DA, et al. Providing services for acute low-back pain: a survey of Australian physiotherapists. Man Ther 2016;22:145–52.

57. McKenzie JE, French SD, O'Connor DA, et al. Evidence-based care of older people with suspected cognitive impairment in general practice: protocol for the IRIS cluster randomized trial. Implement Sci 2013;8:91.

58. Presseau J, McCleary N, Lorencatto F et al. Action, actor, context, target, time (AACTT): a framework for specifying behaviour. Implementation Sci 2019;14:102.

59. McCluskey A, Vratsistas-Curto A, Schurr K. Barriers and enablers to implementing multiple stroke guideline recommendations: a qualitative study. BMC Health Serv Res 2013;13:323.

60. Connell LA, McMahon NE, Harris JE, et al. A formative evaluation of the implementation of an upper limb stroke rehabilitation intervention in clinical practice: a qualitative interview study. Implement Sci 2014;9:90.

61. Carroll L, Patterson M, Wood S, et al. A conceptual framework for implementation fidelity. Implement Sci 2007;2:40.

62. Bussières AE, Patey AM, Francis JJ, et al. Identifying factors likely to influence compliance with diagnostic imaging guideline recommendations for spine disorders among chiropractors in North America: a focus group study using the Theoretical Domains Framework. Implementation Sci 2012;7:82. https://implementationscience.biomedcentral.com/articles/10.1186/1748-5908-7-82

63. Moore JE, Mascarenhas A, Marquez C, et al. Mapping barriers and intervention activities to behaviour change theory for Mobilization of Vulnerable Elders in Ontario (MOVE ON): a multi-site implementation intervention in acute care hospitals. Implement Sci 2014;9:160.

64. Tavender EJ, Bosch M, Gruen RL, et al. Developing a targeted, theory-informed implementation intervention using two theoretical frameworks to address health professional and organization factors: a case study to improve the management of mild traumatic brain injury in the emergency department. Implement Sci 2015;10:74.

65. Flottorp S, Oxman AD. Identifying barriers and tailoring interventions to improve the management of urinary tract infections and sore throat: a pragmatic study using qualitative methods. BMC Health Serv Res 2003;3:3.

66. Green SE, Bosch M, McKenzie JE, et al. Improving the care of people with traumatic brain injury through the Neurotrauma Evidence Translation (NET) program: protocol for a program of research. Implement Sci 2012;7:74.

67. Bosch M, McKenzie JE, Mortimer D, et al. Implementing evidence-based recommended practices for the management of patients with mild traumatic brain injuries in Australian emergency care departments: study protocol for a cluster randomised controlled trial. Trials 2014;15:281.

68. Riordan F, Racine E, Phillip ET, et al. Development of an intervention to facilitate implementation and uptake of diabetic retinopathy screening. Implementation Sci 2020;15:34.

69. Schmid AA, Andersen J, Kent T, et al. Using intervention mapping to develop and adapt a secondary stroke prevention program in Veterans Health Administration medical centers. Implementation Sci 2010;5:97.

70. Forsetlund L, O'Brien MA, Forsén L, et al. Continuing education meetings and workshops: effects on professional practice and healthcare outcomes. Cochrane Database of Syst Rev 2021;(9):CD003030.pub3.

71. Michie S, Wood CE, Johnston M, et al. Behaviour change techniques: the development and evaluation of a taxonomic method for reporting and describing behaviour change interventions (a suite of five studies involving consensus methods, randomised controlled trials and analysis of qualitative data). Health Technol Assess 2015;19(99).

72. Lokker C, McKibbon KA, Colquhoun H, et al. A scoping review of classification schemes of interventions to promote and integrate evidence into practice in healthcare. Implementation Sci 2015;10:27.

73. Effective Practice and Organisation of Care (EPOC). EPOC Taxonomy. The Cochrane Collaboration; 2015. Online. Available: https://epoc.cochrane.org/epoc-taxonomy (accessed 10 January 2022).

74. Powell BJ, McMillen JC, Proctor EK, et al. A compilation of strategies for implementing clinical innovations in health and mental health. Med Care Res Rev 2012;69(2):123–57.

75. Powell BJ, Waltz TJ, Chinman MJ, et al. A refined compilation of implementation strategies: results from the Expert Recommendations for Implementing Change (ERIC) project. Implementation Sci 2015;10:21.

76. Cochrane Consumers and Communication Group. Topic List. The Cochrane Collaboration; 2012. Online. Available: https://cccrg.cochrane.org/sites/cccrg.cochrane.org/files/public/uploads/Topics.pdf (accessed 1 April 2022).

77. Cassidy CE, Harrison MB, Godfrey C, et al. Use and effects of implementation strategies for practice guidelines in nursing: a systematic review. Implementation Sci 2021;16:102.

78. Cahill LS, Carey LM, Lannin NA, et al. Implementation interventions to promote the uptake of evidence-based practices in stroke rehabilitation. Cochrane Database Syst Rev 2020;(10):CD012575. doi:10.1002/14651858.CD012575.pub2.

79. Giguère A, Zomahoun HT, Carmichael P-H, et al. Printed educational materials: effects on professional practice and healthcare outcomes. Cochrane Database Syst Rev 2020;(8):CD004398. doi:10.1002/14651858.CD004398.pub4.

80. Pantoja T, Grimshaw JM, Colomer N, et al. Manually-generated reminders delivered on paper: effects on professional practice and patient outcomes. Cochrane Database Syst Rev 2019;(12):CD001174. doi:10.1002/14651858.CD001174.pub4.

81. Ivers N, Jamtvedt G, Flottorp S, et al. Audit and feedback: effects on professional practice and healthcare outcomes. Cochrane Database Syst Rev 2012;(6):CD000259. doi:10.1002/14651858.CD000259.pub3.

82. Flodgren G, O'Brien MA, Parmelli E, et al. Local opinion leaders: effects on professional practice and healthcare outcomes. Cochrane Database Syst Rev 2019;(6):CD000125. doi:10.1002/14651858.CD000125.pub5.

83. Hakkennes S, Green S. Measures for assessing practice change in medical practitioners. Implement Sci 2006;1:29.

84. Straus SE, Tetroe J, Graham ID, Zwarenstein M, et al. Monitoring use of knowledge and evaluating outcomes. CMAJ 2010;182(2):E94–E98.

85. Proctor E, Silmere H, Raghavan R, et al. Outcomes for implementation research: conceptual distinctions, measurement challenges, and research agenda. Adm Policy Ment Health 2011;38(2):65–76.

86. Lewis CC, Fischer S, Weiner BJ, et al. Outcomes for implementation science: an enhanced systematic review of instruments using evidence-based rating criteria. Implement Sci 2015;10:155.

87. Dzewaltowski D, Glasgow R, Klesges L, et al. RE-AIM: evidence-based standards and a web resource to improve translation of research into practice. Ann Behav Med 2004;28(2):75–80.

88. Gaglio B, Shoup JA, Glasgow RE. The RE-AIM framework: a systematic review of use over time. Am J Public Health 2013;103(6):e38–e46.

89. Chaudoir SR, Dugan AG, Barr CH. Measuring factors affecting implementation of health innovations: A systematic review of structural, organizational, provider, patient, and innovation level measures. Implement Sci 2013;8:22.

90. Scheirer MA, Dearing JW. An agenda for research on the sustainability of public health. Am J Public Health 2011;101(11):2059–67.

91. Moore JE, Mascarenhas A, Bain J, et al. Developing a comprehensive definition of sustainability. Implementation Sci 2017;12:110.

92. Proctor E, Luke D, Calhoun A, et al. Sustainability of evidence-based healthcare: research agenda, methodological advances and infrastructure support. Implement Sci 2015;10:88.

93. Brewster AL, Curry LA, Cherlin EJ, et al. Integrating new practices: a qualitative study of how hospital innovations become routine. Implement Sci 2015;10:168.

94. Nadalin Penno L, Davies B, Graham ID, et al. Identifying relevant concepts and factors for the sustainability of evidence-based practices within acute care contexts: a systematic review and theory analysis of selected sustainability frameworks. Implementation Sci 2019;14:108.

Embedding Evidence-Based Practice into Routine Clinical Care

Ian Scott, Chris Del Mar, Tammy Hoffmann and Sally Bennett

LEARNING OBJECTIVES

After reading this chapter, you should be able to:
- Understand that evidence-based practice occurs at micro, meso and macro levels of organisations
- Explain why organisations should promote evidence-based practice

- Describe the characteristics of organisations that integrate evidence-based practice
- Describe specific strategies that organisations might use to support evidence-based practice

---

Evidence-based practice can be conceptualised as operating at three organisational levels:
- *microsystems* of clinical departments, units, wards or clinical practices
- *mesosystems* such as hospitals and large group-practices
- *macrosystems* of health departments, general practice governing organisations, professional societies and clinical service networks.

Microsystems can be regarded as first-order units of practice in which health professionals, either as individuals or as tightly connected small groups, directly confront challenges in integrating evidence into the routine care of individual patients. This can occur at the bedside, clinic and community levels, and through regular interactions with nearby colleagues. Until this chapter, this book has focused primarily on the skills required to undertake evidence-based practice at this level and described the use of the five-step process for evidence-based practice.

Barriers to evidence-based practice at the microsystem level have been explored in many studies, across many settings and many professional groups, and in a range of countries.[1–5] There is remarkable consistency in the major barriers that have been identified, and some of these are summarised in Table 17.1.

But health professionals, as either individuals or small groups, do not work in a vacuum. They operate within the **mesosystems** of large organisations. These, in turn, are influenced by external forces that come from the **macrosystems** level of government and professional governance bodies that define healthcare policies, standards and norms of practice. All three levels are interdependent, and this is reflected in the evolution of our understanding of, and approach towards, translating evidence into practice over the last 20 years or so.[6]

The complexity and interrelatedness of these three levels was acknowledged in the previous chapter (Chapter 16), where we examined strategies that could be used to more consistently incorporate evidence into practice (either to accelerate the adoption of evidence-based practices or to discontinue interventions or assessment practices that are not supported by robust evidence). We overviewed strategies that can be used to narrow the gaps between current practice and practice based on the most rigorous evidence available, and also highlighted the influences and involvements of individuals, organisations and systems to achieve this aim.

Similarly, successfully using the steps of evidence-based practice in routine clinical work (as opposed to translating

TABLE 17.1 Commonly identified barriers to embedding evidence-based practice into routine clinical practice

Barrier	Description
Skills	A lack of skills in searching for, interpreting and applying research among health professionals means that they are insecure about changing practice from what they have read. There is also often too little support for doing so (including from senior colleagues with skills in evidence-based practice).
Time	In the chaos of everyday clinical practice, 'running behind', or dealing with urgent clinical situations, is common. The time pressure of administration and other responsibilities that health professionals have, coupled with the time taken for finding, let alone reading and appraising, the evidence, means that evidence-based practice is all too easily a casualty of being busy.
Attitudes	The traditional view of knowledge attainment (and thus, by extension, evidence-based practice) is that it is *separate* from clinical practice. That is, it is the responsibility of the individual health professional and, often, to be undertaken at the health professional's own expense and in their own time. These attitudes may be held by both health professionals and the organisations where they work.

specific research evidence into practice, as discussed in Chapter 16) is not solely a function of behaviour or responsibility of individual health professionals. It also requires enablers and reinforcers that operate throughout different levels of the systems of care in which health professionals work. There are enablers and reinforcers for each of the three major types of barriers to evidence-based practice listed in Table 17.1 (skills, time and attitudes). The primary focus of this chapter is the organisational settings (or systems of care) that determine the extent to which evidence-based practice becomes more (*much* more for some) an *everyday* part of the clinical work that is done at the level of individuals and small groups.

WHY IS A SYSTEMS APPROACH IMPORTANT?

A systems approach examines what can be done at the organisational level to foster evidence-based practice as a core component of organisational activity. What can we do to make evidence-based practice part of the mission statement or *modus operandi*, or even of the 'brand', of an organisation? How do we systematise the strategies for improving the translation of evidence into practice (which were discussed at the health professional level in Chapter 16) at the level of the organisation?

The premise is that if organisations endorse evidence-based practice as 'the way we do things around here', then their policies, procedures, infrastructure and governance are more likely to support evidence-based practice. This then makes it easier for the individuals within the organisation to practise this way. Organisations need structures, processes and cultures that can accommodate the complexity of implementing evidence-based practice in daily operations.

WHY SHOULD ORGANISATIONS *WANT* TO PROMOTE EVIDENCE-BASED PRACTICE?

1. To maintain their reputation and 'market share'

Organisations—not just the individual health professionals who work within them—are now held more accountable for ensuring that the care they provide is safe, effective and of high quality. It is no longer the sole responsibility of individual health professionals to provide good care: the organisation itself can now suffer loss of reputation, staff and revenue if it is not seen as proactively nurturing evidence-based practice. Moreover, organisations do not operate in isolation, but instead in a constantly changing environment of new healthcare and information technologies, novel multidisciplinary models of care and changing societal expectations. Evidence-based standards of care are increasingly being used in accreditation programs to assess whether healthcare organisations are providing optimal care;[7] simply having well-maintained physical infrastructure, or adequate staff-to-patient ratios, is insufficient. In Australia, hospitals and day hospitals must demonstrate they have systems in place aimed at ensuring compliance with national safety and quality health service standards.[8] Executive boards increasingly recognise that evidence-based practice may help prevent unsafe or inefficient practices as part of an organisational approach to improving the quality and safety of care.[9] All this necessitates clinical practice to be constantly informed (and re-informed) by good evidence if the organisation is to retain respect and authority within the community at large. Organisations also need to do this if they want to attract and retain health professionals who value working in an organisation where managers proactively facilitate the prerequisites for, and create a positive culture towards, evidence-based practice.[10]

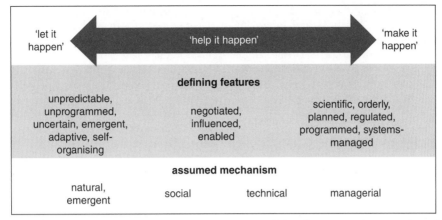

Fig 17.1 The spread of innovation in an organisation: its defining features and assumed mechanism
Adapted from Greenhalgh T, et al. Diffusion of innovations in service organizations: systematic review and recommendations. Milbank Q 2004;82:581–629, Fig 2.9. © 2004 Milbank Memorial Fund. Published by Black-well Publishing; reproduced with permission of John Wiley & Sons Inc.

2. To improve their delivery of care through innovation

Organisations that foster evidence-based practice are more likely to innovate, challenge orthodox practice and adopt new safety and quality initiatives that benefit patients. They are also more exciting and professionally satisfying to work in. A large-scale empirical study among the entire population of public hospital organisations that are part of the English National Health Service revealed a significant positive relationship between science- and practice-based innovation and clinical performance.[11] Data on measures of science and practice innovation, as well as patient mortality and satisfaction, were obtained for all 173 acute hospital trusts from sources such as published government records, databases, central authorities and the individual trusts. Regression models showed significant positive correlations (R^2 values between 0.19 and 0.44 after adjustment for other patient and organisational factors) between measures of science- and practice-based innovativeness and patient mortality and satisfaction. In a US study of Medicare beneficiaries in acute care hospitals, various clinical performance measures (mortality, complications, patient safety indicators and length of stay) were compared between institutions ($n = 424$) that have online access to an evidence-based knowledge source (UpToDate) and those that do not ($n = 3,091$).[12] Hospitals with access were associated with significantly better performance on risk-adjusted measures of patient safety ($p = 0.016$), complications ($p = 0.001$) and shorter length of stay (on average, 0.17 day, $p < 0.001$). An organisation's receptivity to, and readiness for, change are key determinants of how quickly and successfully new

innovations in practice are adopted.[13] This is illustrated in Figure 17.1. Importantly, theories around organisational change readiness and implementation emphasise that change is both a social and a technical innovation. That is, whether change occurs or not depends just as much on group psychology and mindsets, internal and external socio-political influences, peer opinions and cultural attitudes, as it does on implementing data systems or reconfiguring equipment and service resources.[14]

3. To increase their efficiency

In an era of limited resources but expanding demand for health care, organisations must learn to do more with less. This means they must discontinue—and disinvest from—clinical practices that consume resources but do not add value to patient care. Various ways of doing this have been proposed, including:

- eliminating waste—for example, avoiding duplication of tests as well as eliminating unnecessary tests, procedures and treatments that confer no health benefit.[15] It has been estimated that waste may account for as much as 30% of healthcare costs[16,17]
- minimising overdiagnosis and over-treatment of patients with medically benign conditions or physiological changes that do not impact on longevity or quality of life[18]
- reducing unwarranted variation in the use of diagnostic tests and treatments among health professionals and between communities[19]
- reforming medical liability laws to decrease the practice of defensive medicine.

Many of these approaches (for example, reducing over-use, avoiding preventable complications and improving inefficient processes) are under way in many organisations, in both private and public sectors.[20] Greater alignment of clinical practice with evidence-based practice could result in significant savings in healthcare expenditure[21] or, at the very least, in better-value care for the monies spent.

CULTURE AND CHARACTERISTICS OF ORGANISATIONS THAT INTEGRATE EVIDENCE-BASED PRACTICE

Introducing any innovation, including evidence-based practice, is challenging and occurs within a complex organisational context. The culture of an organisation influences attitudes towards the use of evidence-based practice and the change process itself.[22] An organisation's 'culture' refers to the norms and expectations about how work is performed in that organisation[23] or, more simply: 'how things are done around here'. An organisation's culture can affect staff attitudes, perceptions and behaviour.[22] Therefore, fostering a culture that is constructive and supportive of evidence-based practice is a key enabler of evidence-based practice. Some of the key characteristics of organisations that support the use of evidence-based practice are outlined below.

Active senior leadership commitment and support for evidence-based practice

Organisationally-driven evidence-based practice is more likely when senior leaders (such as clinical directors and managerial executives) promote change and foster a learning environment.[24,25] Leadership styles that positively influence the use of evidence-based practice have been described as transactional and/or transformative.[26] Transformative leadership supposes a strong attachment between the leader and their 'followers', such that the leader is then able to inspire and motivate others through role modelling and mentoring.[27] Role models are very powerful change agents in the behaviour of health professionals. If senior health professionals perform evidence-based practice as part of routine care themselves, this is an important influence on other staff. For this reason alone, organisations should expect competence in evidence-based practice in their senior staff when offering appointments and agreeing on role descriptions. Competency in this should be evaluated when undertaking professional performance reviews (perhaps based on documented evidence-based audits of clinical practice and 360° feedback from working colleagues). By spending their own time and effort on activities that directly support evidence-based continuous improvement and quality of care, senior leaders demonstrate the personal commitment and investment needed for sustained improvement.[25]

Transactional leadership makes use of rewards for meeting specific goals or performance criteria.[28] Examples of transactional leadership strategies that foster evidence-based practice include: performance appraisals for reviewing staff members' goals and learning needs *for evidence-based practice*; rostering time; providing remuneration; and organising physical resources (meeting rooms, audio-visual equipment, data systems, etc.) which encourage staff to undertake a myriad of activities that foster evidence-based practice.[29] Examples of these are journal clubs, practice reviews, bedside teaching, seminars and workshops, clinical audits and quality and safety improvement projects. Leaders may also create opportunities to communicate successes and failures, and reward those who have championed evidence-based practice. Examples of rewards include: academic or peer commendations, sponsorship of presentations at professional meetings, awarding credits for maintenance of professional standard programs or continuing professional development schemes,[27] and providing further training and leadership opportunities.[30]

Infrastructure of clinical informatics

For evidence-based practice to work, health professionals need ready access to three forms of data:

- evidence in response to specific clinical questions posed while doing routine clinical work
- guidelines and other forms of evidence guidance (for example, clinical decision support systems) that can inform commonly performed clinical decisions
- metrics of current practice for the purposes of conducting audits and identifying evidence–practice gaps—that is, the gaps between current practice (what we are doing) and best practice as defined by best available evidence (what we should be doing).

Access to evidence to answer specific questions

It is essential that organisations provide access to the relevant electronic literature databases for searching. This is normally provided through an organisation's library, although individuals, particularly medical professionals, can increasingly access reliable pre-processed syntheses of evidence online using proprietary software such as DynaMed, Up-to-Date and BMJ Best Practice. Observational studies suggest a positive association between increasing frequency of use of such online evidence retrieval systems and better patient care, along with fewer adverse events.[12] In the community or smaller organisations, library services and access to certain databases can be more of a problem. And without access to journal subscriptions through a library, it can be difficult to obtain full-text papers in some instances.

Health and medical librarians (now increasingly called 'clinical information specialists') are important in helping to seek out the evidence that is requested by health professionals. Information requests (in the form of clinical questions) received from health professionals are reformatted into 'answerable questions'; and evidence is then searched for, critically appraised (sometimes) and returned to the health professional who can then decide if and how to apply the evidence in the clinical setting from which the questions originated. In some organisations, health librarians also attend ward rounds and clinics, recording questions as they arise and then finding relevant evidence. Experiments featuring standardised literature searches and feedback of results to practising health professionals have changed practice for the better.[31] These services, in one form or another, exist in many organisations and target not only health professionals but also managers and policy makers.[32]

Several services have been tested over the years, some more successful than others. The ATTRACT service ran in Wales (UK)[33] and the database of questions asked has evolved into the TRIP database (www.tripdatabase.com), which was explained in Chapter 3. Question-answering services have been trialled in other countries, such as Australia and Canada.[34,35] However, these services come at a cost and although they are probably cost-effective in terms of cost savings resulting from better care, budgetary constraints probably act as a barrier to their wholesale introduction. They can also fail from poor demand, possibly because the culture of asking questions (itself an evidence-based practice skill, as discussed in Chapter 2) is underdeveloped in many organisations.

Access to clinical decision support systems

Such systems, especially if computerised, have great potential to assist evidence-based practice. If they are well designed and field-tested with health professional input,[36,37] they can significantly improve quality of care and patient outcomes.[38] The information devices that underpin clinical decision support systems are fast moving away from fixed desktop computers to portable and personal tablets and smartphones. This technology now allows instant availability of evidence search engines, evidence-based clinical guidelines, care pathways and clinical prediction rules. Research is starting to show benefits in terms of better and more-timely care.[39,40] Emerging evidence suggests that linking computerised decision support systems with electronic health records improves health professional performance and patient outcomes.[41] This technology places the individual health professional firmly in the driver's seat for accessing and applying evidence to patient care.

However, organisations must commit to resourcing and maintaining the physical devices (such as repairing and renewing them) and the quality of the content found on them (such as ensuring that evidence resources are valid and up-to-date), and ensuring a proficient skill level of those who use them (such as mandating ongoing health professional training and review of competency). It has been shown that when given access to online information sources, health professionals from different disciplines are able to find correct answers to at least half of their clinical questions.[42] In a cross-over controlled trial, health professionals using a locally designed web-based knowledge resource ('AskMayoExpert'), which was designed to provide quick, concise answers at the point of care to commonly asked questions, found answers with greater accuracy and confidence than when using other self-selected web-based resources.[43]

Access to databases for auditing current practice

In most healthcare facilities, data are collected routinely for non-clinical purposes (often financial reasons!). In hospitals, different clinical units centralise collection of discrete data that reflect the single focus of the clinical activity (for example, postoperative wound infections). In contrast, in community clinical settings, data are usually routinely collected only for individual patients. This presents challenges to getting aggregate data on outcomes. Aggregating data can also be complicated (for example, by ethical issues) by the use of electronic patient-held records which are used in some settings (www.digitalhealth.gov.au). In addition, community health settings usually deal with a far greater range of clinical problems (because there is less specialisation in community-based care). This means there are many more *categories* of care, with fewer *components* in each category. Both of these elements combine to mean that if data are needed to identify evidence–practice gaps, or to decide about the adoption of a change in practice based on new evidence, then the data may have to be collected as an independent effort, often as labour-intensive manual abstraction of data from paper medical records, rather than using data that is routinely collected for other purposes. However, the advent of electronic health records, already used in many primary care settings and increasingly in hospitals, has the potential for quicker extraction of de-identified clinical data relating to routine care of a wide range of conditions with reference to evidence-based standards as part of targeted quality improvement initiatives.[44,45]

Provision of training

Organisations must provide the necessary education and training to enable all health professionals to have skills in evidence-based practice. A systematic review of interactive teaching of evidence-based practice around clinical cases (that is, clinically integrated with everyday work) found that this style of teaching changes knowledge and skills much more effectively than didactic lectures or tutorials.[46] Focused teaching in evidence-based practice (and access to electronic searching facilities) has been shown to improve the quality of care and the number of evidence-based interventions used by health professionals.[47] When considering which educational format to use for learning about evidence-based practice, small-group interaction, role-play and simulation of real-world learning environments, mentorship and high educator-to-learner ratios have been found to be associated with more-effective learning.[48,49] In addition to the general evidence-based practice skills, health professionals also need to learn skills in decision making (that is, placing the evidence in perspective against the circumstances and needs of the patient)[50] and skills in communicating evidence to patients (which were described in Chapter 14).

Organisations need to maximise evidence-based practice learning opportunities. Some suggestions for ways of doing this are by:
- quarantining a little 'offline' time, away from clinical duties (perhaps weekly)

- expecting health professionals to attend courses/workshops to learn evidence-based practice skills[51]
- providing in-service training with face-to-face education at the bedside[52]
- delivering interactive educational resources such as online e-learning modules[53]
- supporting *evidence-based* journal clubs.

Evidence-based journal clubs (as opposed to the traditional, and more common, journal club which is typically *not* evidence-based) are especially important.[54] They focus on 'pull' strategies (see Chapter 2), in which health professionals bring along questions that have arisen during routine clinical work, search for the answers in the form of evidence and critically appraise the evidence. Such exercises require support from the organisation if they are to work well. Some examples of the support needed are outlined in Table 17.2.

TABLE 17.2 Organisational support required for running evidence-based journal clubs

Type of support	Details
Roster journal clubs	Minimise appointment conflicts so that as many members of the ward/team/practice as possible can attend. Enable 'pairing up' of more- and less-experienced appraisers for support and training. Periodically allow time for club members to prioritise topics/questions to be answered over the coming meetings (and advertise this 'schedule' in advance if possible).
Pragmatic resources	A (booked!) room. Data-projector, whiteboard or large flip-chart (so everyone can see). Online access to databases (such as PubMed). Sandwiches or other bring-your-own meal (to save time).
Organisation of the actual meeting	Ensure all members of the club get the chance to be involved in different roles. Consider all of the roles that are involved, such as: • managing the group process (e.g. who will lead the club process, each topic/article, etc.) • recording the discussion (e.g. writing on a whiteboard) • storing and disseminating the 'findings' of the meeting • doing 'homework' for any tasks (e.g. getting full-text articles) before the next meeting At the beginning of each meeting (or every alternate meeting), consider allowing time for discussion about 'what now?'. That is, discuss what to do with the topic/question just covered and, if needed, devise a plan to implement desired changes in practice.[45] Also consider scheduling a 'follow-up' session for each topic/question some time later (such as 6 months after the topic was initially discussed) to see what changes were made, how they are working, any refinements/further action needed, etc.
Share knowledge and experience	Librarians—if available—can provide enormous help with searching. Student health professionals should be included to experience the role modelling (and often can be great contributors, particularly if their evidence-based practice knowledge is fresh from a recent course/subject!).
Record notes	Provide a means for storing and disseminating the 'findings' of the club, so that others learn from the exercise and a sense of continuity is established, aided by a record of why clinical changes were considered desirable. Discuss ways to disseminate any practice-changing findings.

Using evidence-based practice to improve quality and safety

Evidence-based practice and the science of quality and safety improvement (QSI) complement each other. New evidence will drive new QSI initiatives. Conversely, QSI aspirations will need best available evidence. How you decide what changes to make takes you to the growing literature around evidence-based QSI interventions itself. One approach to QSI is predicated on the use of evidence, as shown in Figure 17.2.[55]

The focus of evidence-based practice is on 'doing the right things', whereas quality improvement focuses more on 'doing things right'. Combined, these processes help us to 'do the right things right'.[9] The implication is that those who work in quality-improvement teams need to consider the validity, applicability and value of the change being introduced,[56] and those who work from an evidence-based practice perspective need to look beyond the evidence to consider how behaviour change might be successfully implemented and sustained in the local context.[57] There is also a Cochrane group (The Cochrane Effective Practice

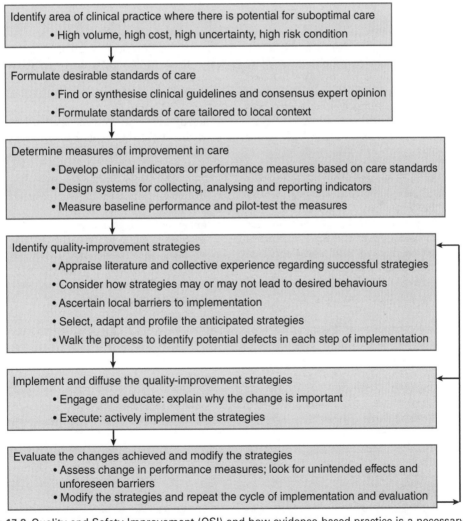

Fig 17.2 Quality and Safety Improvement (QSI) and how evidence-based practice is a necessary component

Scott I, Phelps G. Measurement for improvement: getting one to follow the other. Intern Med J 2009; 39:347–51, Fig 1.46. Reproduced with permission © 2009 Royal Australasian College of Physicians, John Wiley & Sons.

and Organisation of Care Group; epoc.cochrane.org) that reports on which QSI interventions are effective.

In recent times, several developments have consolidated the linking of evidence-based practice with QSI:

- **Clinical registries.** Registries that collect and analyse process and outcome data on large cohorts of patients from multiple hospitals and practices have grown in number in recent years[58] and provide an objective, audit-based window into real-world clinical practice and its possible shortcomings. Organisations that participate in such registries demonstrate evidence-based practice in action and are associated with higher quality care.[59] Registries can also generate new knowledge about effectiveness of care in unselected patients that may not be obvious in the results of randomised trials that seek to determine efficacy in highly selected populations.
- **Quality improvement collaborations.** Hospitals and other healthcare organisations can share data and experiences about care for specific patient populations and learn from each other about how to improve care and close evidence–practice gaps. Such collaborations can achieve substantial improvement in evidence-based care processes within relatively short time spans at relatively low cost.[60–62]
- **Health service accreditation.** This is increasingly looking not just at structures (such as buildings, staffing levels, physical infrastructure) but also at outcomes (quality of care). Accreditation teams now expect healthcare organisations to integrate an evidence-based quality improvement framework into their operations with proactive remediation of identified instances of suboptimal care. To date, particular attention has been given to the care of common presentations that are associated with high morbidity or high resource utilisation (such as stroke, heart attack, hip fracture and delirium), and for which prescriptive, evidence-based clinical care standards have been developed.[63]

Changing clinical processes

Finding better ways to do things, and putting them into practice, is dependent on the ability to change. The success and speed of adoption of evidence-based practice are related. Successful adoption of evidence-based practice in an organisation requires an organisational ethos and governance structure that are committed to the ongoing redesign of clinical care processes in response to new evidence about patient need and the effectiveness of interventions. Importantly, clinical process redesign, if it is to be successful and sustained, has to be driven and owned internally by the members of the organisation, not imposed or led by external consultants or agencies.[64] What should change is determined by evidence and data,[28,65] and the change itself needs to be supported by behavioural theory, concordant with professional values, able to be trialled and its effects directly observed, and able to be incorporated into work flows as a path of least resistance (that is, it needs to be easier to accept the change than resist it). Clinical redesign is made up of several stages:

- providing a platform for building evidence-based practice reliably into routine work, rather than layering it on top of existing work as an added demand[66]
- facilitating change by engaging health professionals in high-priority problem solving around concrete and meaningful issues and providing them with the training and information necessary to effect change[24,67]
- maintaining momentum for further change and improvement. Success motivates staff to go further with improvement to achieve more success.

Successful clinical process redesign relies on having all the enabling organisational characteristics that have already been discussed operating simultaneously within the one organisation. To illustrate this, several exemplars of large-scale clinical process redesign are described in Box 17.1.

BOX 17.1   Examples of large-scale clinical process redesign

Veterans Affairs healthcare system (United States)

The Veterans Affairs healthcare system in the United States underwent major transformation during the late 1990s and early 2000s.[68] This transformation included implementation of a systematic approach to measuring, managing and accounting for quality improvement. The focus was on high-priority conditions (such as diabetes and coronary artery disease), and emphasised health maintenance and management of care. Performance contracts held managers accountable for meeting improvement goals. An integrated and comprehensive electronic medical record system was instituted at all Veterans Affairs medical centres. This enabled performance data to be made public, and key stakeholders such as veterans' service organisations and politicians were targeted.

Payment policies for care delivery were aligned according to evidence of effectiveness. Health services, including ambulatory care, were integrated to achieve continuous and timely care. The widespread adoption of evidence-based practice was one of the central tenets of the new system of care.[69] Quality of care in the Veterans Affairs healthcare system substantially improved between 1997 and 2000, when the proportion of patients who received appropriate care was 90% or greater for nine of 17 quality-of-care indicators and exceeded 70% for 13 indicators. Compared against the Medicare fee-for-service program, the Veterans Affairs system performed significantly better on all 11 comparable quality indicators from 1997 to 1999, and in 2000 the Veterans Affairs system outperformed Medicare on 12 of 13 indicators.[70]

BOX 17.1   Examples of large-scale clinical process redesign—cont'd

Kaiser Permanente health maintenance organisation (United States)

A performance-improvement system was introduced in 2006, after variations in performance in quality, safety, service and efficiency in the organisation were recognised. This led to a strategy for continuous improvement systems: six 'building blocks' were identified to enable Kaiser Permanente to become a learning organisation: (1) real-time sharing of performance data; (2) training in problem-solving methods and adoption of evidence-based practice; (3) workforce engagement and informal knowledge sharing; (4) investing in leadership structures, beliefs and behaviours; (5) internal and external benchmarking; and (6) technical knowledge sharing. This required multiple complex strategies that combined top-down and bottom-up approaches.[71] Performance improvements were assessed in the 22 medical centres (in four of the eight regions) after implementation between January 2008 and September 2009. They achieved a 61% improvement in selected capabilities, and 84% of initial projects were successfully completed.[72] This was a cost saving—for each dollar invested, there was an estimated return of $2.36 surplus. Critical factors included: adequate dedicated time for performance improvement activities for staff, expert support, alignment of projects with regional and national strategic priorities, and a close working relationship between performance improvement staff and those who provide clinical care.

Intermountain Healthcare (United States)

Intermountain Healthcare is a conglomerate of hospitals and primary care organisations in Utah. A process management theory (W Edwards Deming's theory, which says that the best way to reduce costs is to improve quality) was applied after 1988 to its healthcare delivery.[73] Data systems and management structures were created to increase accountability, drive improvement and produce savings. All participants (patients, providers and systems), especially health professionals, were involved in planning, implementing, analysing and educating others in evidence-based practice, in assessing and refining guidelines, and in reassessing and continually modifying the care map. This redesign has been very successful. For example, a new delivery protocol helped to reduce rates of elective induced labour, unplanned Caesarean sections and admissions to newborn intensive care units. Implementation of this one protocol alone saves an estimated USD50 million every year.

Group Health Cooperative of Puget Sound (United States)

The Chronic Care Model was developed initially across a large health maintenance organisation as a way of improving the ambulatory care of patients with chronic disease—specifically, better disease control, higher patient satisfaction and better adherence to guidelines.[74] Redesign processes cluster in six areas: (1) healthcare organisation; (2) community resources; (3) self-management support; (4) delivery-system design; (5) evidence-based decision support; and (6) clinical information systems. The model stresses continuous relationships with the care team (which is very relevant to chronic care); individualising care according to patients' needs and values; providing care that anticipates patients' needs; providing services which are based on evidence; and cooperation among health professionals. Assessment of the model's processes shows that 51 organisations could effect 48 practice changes relating to evidence-based processes of care, and that in 75% of cases these changes were sustained for at least 12 months.[75] This assessment suggests that this redesign process has led to improved patient care and better health outcomes, although this assessment is only preliminary and cost-effectiveness work has not yet been undertaken.

South Australian Integrated Cardiovascular Clinical Network (Australia)

An integrated cardiac support network incorporating standardised risk stratification, point-of-care troponin testing, evidence-based cardiac care protocols and cardiologist-supported decision making was progressively implemented in non-metropolitan areas of South Australia from 2001 to 2008.[76] Hospital administrative data and statewide death records from 1 July 2001 to 30 June 2010 were used to evaluate outcomes for patients diagnosed with myocardial infarction in rural and metropolitan hospitals. Key components of the network were training clinicians in advanced life-support skills, cardiac monitor and defibrillator onsite, onsite electrocardiograph and remote interpretation capability, biochemical markers available at point of care, acute medications guided by agreed evidence-based protocols, timely access to invasive coronary procedures and cardiac rehabilitation service, and regular clinical follow-up, combined with clinical and technical quality assurance. Analysis of 29,623 independent contiguous episodes of myocardial infarction showed that, after adjustment for temporal improvement in myocardial infarction outcome, availability of immediate cardiac support was associated with a 22% reduction in 30-day mortality (odds ratio 0.78, 95% CI 0.65 to 0.93, $p = 0.007$). Evidence-based, cardiologist-supported remote risk stratification, management and facilitated access to tertiary hospital-based early invasive management were associated with an improvement in 30-day mortality for patients who initially presented to rural hospitals and were diagnosed with myocardial infarction.

Organisational policies that embrace evidence-based practice

An organisation's policies can influence the extent to which evidence-based practice is embraced within the organisation. Policy statements indicate an organisation's position or principles regardless of whether this organisation is at the level of government, a profession, a healthcare agency or a non-profit health organisation. Policies that support evidence-based practice (however specific this may be) are an essential means by which the organisation communicates a willingness to embrace a culture of evidence-based practice and helps to establish the norms and expectations about how things are to be done.[77]

Many organisations now incorporate the principle of evidence-based practice as part of their policies. In turn, this can influence governance structures, purchasing decisions and expectations for employees. Some organisations have position statements that are designed to be visionary in their support of evidence-based practice. However, other organisations go further and provide policies which inform governance structures that include expectations that employees will engage in evidence-based practice (for example, by meeting competency requirements or to support credentialling).[78] (This is not to be confused with evidence-based policy, which concerns the use of research evidence to inform policy development.) Tools have been developed for measuring the extent to which organisations embrace evidence-based practice according to the domains of vision, leadership, learning culture, the need for knowledge and the acquisition, sharing and use of knowledge.[79]

Most health professionals have an organisation (such as a college, association or academy) to support them in their professional development. Some have developed resources and methods of facilitating skill development related to evidence-based practice, especially upskilling in question asking, searching and critical appraisal. Maintenance of professional standards schemes also give increasing levels of credit points to audit and practice review activities that seek to align and remediate evidence–practice gaps.[80] Many health professional organisations also have specific policy statements about evidence-based practice in the form of position statements. A few extracts from position statements from different disciplines are provided in Box 17.2 as examples.

CONCLUSION

In this chapter, we have explained why promoting evidence-based practice is important to organisations and how they might go about it. Box 17.3 summarises the most pertinent strategies for supporting evidence-based practice. Ensuring that patients receive evidence-based health care requires healthcare organisations to be proactive in

---

BOX 17.2 Examples of position statements from different discipline-specific organisations

- **Physiotherapy** (The World Confederation for Physical Therapy):
  'The World Confederation for Physical Therapy (WCPT) believes that physical therapists have a responsibility to use evidence to inform practice and ensure that the management of patients, carers, and communities is based on the best available evidence.' www.wcpt.org/policy/ps-EBP
- **Nursing** (The Honor Society of Nursing, Sigma Theta Tau International):
  'As a leader in the development and dissemination of knowledge to improve nursing practice, the Honor Society of Nursing, Sigma Theta Tau International supports the development and implementation of evidence-based nursing (EBN). The society defines EBN as an integration of the best evidence available, nursing expertise, and the values and preferences of the individuals, families and communities who are served.' www.nursingsociety.org/connect-engage/about-stti/position-statements-and-resource-papers/evidence-based-nursing-position-statement

---

adopting evidence-based practice across the spectrum of their activities. This requires:

- active top leadership commitment and support
- managerial support
- a well-developed and user-friendly infrastructure of clinical informatics
- dedicated training of health professionals in the direct application of evidence to clinical care
- alignment of evidence-based practice with quality and safety improvement frameworks
- systematised clinical process redesign in response to new evidence-based clinical practices
- evidence-based health policy making at the level of senior executives.

Professional organisations also have a role in promoting evidence-based practice by developing resources and methods in question asking, searching and critical appraisal relevant to their members. While the key factor in advancing evidence-based practice will always remain the knowledge, skills and attitudes of the individual health professional, the existence of an organisational environment that recognises the value of, and encourages, evidence-based practice will add immeasurable value in accelerating and expanding the benefits of evidence-based practice to all who seek care within our healthcare organisations.

BOX 17.3   Organisational strategies for supporting evidence-based practice[81–84]

Active commitment and support from senior managers

- Direct and open endorsement of evidence-based learning and continuous quality improvement within mission statements and operations of boards, directorships and other sub-agencies of the organisation.
- Provide dedicated time, resources and remuneration for health professionals to practise evidence-based care:
  - Clinical decision support, evidence databases, other information technology infrastructure.
  - Resources (staff and physical resources such as meeting rooms) for conduct of evidence-based practice journal clubs, seminars and workshops.
  - Scheduling of 10% of normal working hours to be spent on evidence-based practice-related activities (journal clubs, clinical audits, quality and safety reviews, etc.).
- Recognise those who have championed evidence-based practice within the organisation and grant recognition awards.
- Sponsor presentations at professional meetings and/or attendance at professional development courses.

Use of evidence to inform care delivery

- Establish interdisciplinary panels for developing and updating evidence-based clinical standards (or guidelines or pathways) applicable to key areas of practice within the organisation.
- Develop easily accessible and searchable electronic repositories of evidence-based clinical standards (or guidelines or pathways) for use by health professionals and policy makers.
- Establish organisation-wide literature search services that staff can use to retrieve relevant and high-quality evidence to answer important clinical questions directly related to routine care.
- Sponsor clinician-led and organisation-wide restructuring of care processes and service delivery systems according to evidence of effectiveness in optimising care.
- Mandate that submissions for new clinical interventions or services include a rationale based on a systematic review of evidence of effectiveness compared with existing (or usual) care.

- Develop payment formulae that fully remunerate evidence-based practices while withholding payments for interventions for which robust evidence shows no benefit.
- Penalise providers financially for care that is consistently in violation of accepted evidence-based standards.
- Deploy performance appraisal and credentialling policies that restrict scope of practice of health professionals whose practice is consistently in violation of accepted evidence-based standards.
- Waive professional indemnity from litigation in cases where care resulting in serious patient harm was in clear violation of accepted evidence-based standards.
- Provide legal protection from defamation proceedings for whistleblowers who expose colleagues whose practice is consistently in violation of accepted evidence-based standards.

Alignment of evidence-based practice with quality and safety improvement

- Foster system-wide recognition that evidence-based practice and quality and safety improvement are symbiotic—they complement and reinforce one another.
- Establish evidence-based quality and safety teams at the level of clinical microsystems (group practices, hospital units or departments) that involve practising health professionals in identifying and remediating shortfalls in care.
- Provide the necessary resources for establishing quality and safety measurement and feedback systems for defined sets of key clinical indicators for commonly encountered conditions and procedures.
- Support the creation of clinical registries that collect and analyse process and outcome data on cohorts of patients which relate to key areas of practice within the organisation.
- Maintain an up-to-date inventory of evidence-based quality and safety improvement interventions relevant to key areas of practice within the organisation.
- Participate in evidence-based quality and safety improvement collaborations with other like-minded organisations.
- Seek organisational accreditation that recognises the integration of an evidence-based quality and safety improvement framework with all mainstream organisational activities.

Hess BJ, Weng W, Lynn LA, et al. Setting a fair performance standard for physicians' quality of patient care. J Gen Intern Med 2011;26(5):467–73; Oman K, Duran C, Fink R. Evidence-based policy and procedures: an algorithm for success. J Nurs Adm 2008;38:47–51; Wensing M, Wollersheim H, Grol R. Organisational interventions to implement improvements in patient care: a structured review of reviews. Implement Sci 2006;1:2; Lukas C, Engle R, Holmes S, et al. Strengthening organisations to implement evidence-based clinical practices. Health Care Manage Rev 2010;35:235–45; Powell B, McMillen J, Proctor E, et al. A compilation of strategies for implementing clinical innovations in health and mental health. Med Care Res Rev 2012;69:123–57; Correa VC, Lugo-Agudelo LH, Aguirre-Acevedo DC, et al. Individual, health system, and contextual barriers and facilitators for the implementation of clinical practice guidelines: a systematic metareview. Health Res Policy Syst 2020;18:74.

SUMMARY

- Evidence-based practice needs to be implemented into organisations at all levels: microsystems (such as the clinic/ward); mesosystems (such as hospitals or community practices); and macrosystems (such as health departments, professional societies and governing organisations). There is complexity at each level and interrelatedness of these levels.

- Evidence-based practice should be endorsed and actively supported at the organisational level. Organisations that foster a culture that is supportive of evidence-based practice often have some key characteristics, such as: (1) active senior leadership commitment and support for evidence-based practice; (2) appropriate clinical informatics infrastructure; (3) provision and support of learning relevant to evidence-based practice (including support of *evidence-based* journal clubs); (4) alignment of evidence-based practice with quality and safety improvement (that is, 'doing the right things right'); (5) the ability to change and redesign clinical processes on the basis of evidence and patient need; and (6) organisational policies that embrace evidence-based practice.

- Put simply, organisations need to provide the right culture and appropriate leadership, and set the policies that enable health professionals to have the skills, time and attitude to provide evidence-based practice. The benefits of doing this are immense: success means building reputation, improving morale and delivering better care more safely and efficiently.

REFERENCES

1. McColl A, Smith H, White P, et al. General practitioners' perceptions of the route to evidence based medicine: a questionnaire survey. BMJ 1998;316:361–5.
2. Burkiewicz J, Zgarrick D. Evidence-based practice by pharmacists: utilisation and barriers. Ann Pharmacother 2005;39:1214–19.
3. Bennett S, Tooth L, McKenna K, et al. Perceptions of evidence based practice: a survey of occupational therapists. Aust Occup Ther J 2003;50:13–22.
4. Al-Almaie S, Al-Baghli N. Barriers facing physicians practicing evidence-based medicine in Saudi Arabia. J Contin Educ Health Prof 2004;24:163–70.
5. Lai N, Teng C, Lee M. The place and barriers of evidence based practice: knowledge and perceptions of medical, nursing and allied health practitioners in Malaysia. BMC Res Notes 2010;3:279.
6. Scott I. The evolving science of translating research evidence into clinical practice. Evid Based Med 2007;12:4–7.
7. Office of Safety and Quality in Health Care WA. Clinical governance standards for Western Australian health services. Perth: WA Department of Health; 2005.
8. Australian Commission on Safety and Quality in Health Care. Assessment to the NSQHS Standards. ACSQHC; 2019. Online. Available: https://www.safetyandquality.gov.au/standards/nsqhs-standards/assessment-nsqhs-standards.
9. Glasziou P, Ogrinc G, Goodman S. Can evidence-based medicine and clinical quality improvement learn from each other? BMJ Qual Saf 2011;20:i13–i17.
10. Aitken LM, Hackwood B, Crouch S, et al. Creating an environment to implement and sustain evidence-based practice: a developmental process. Aust Crit Care 2011; 24:244–54.
11. Salge T, Vera O. Hospital innovativeness and organizational performance: evidence from English public acute care. Health Care Manage Rev 2009;34:54–67.
12. Bonis P, Pickens G, Rind D, et al. Association of a clinical knowledge support system with improved patient safety, reduced complications and shorter length of stay among Medicare beneficiaries in acute care hospitals in the United States. Int J Med Inform 2008;77:745–53.
13. Greenhalgh T, Robert G, Macfarlane F, et al. Diffusion of innovations in service organizations: systematic review and recommendations. Milbank Q 2004;82:581–629.
14. Srigley J, Corace K, Hargadon D, et al. Applying psychological frameworks of behavior change to improve healthcare worker hand hygiene: a systematic review. J Hosp Infect 2015;91:202–10.
15. American College of Physicians. How can our nation conserve and distribute health care resources effectively and efficiently? Policy paper. Philadelphia: American College of Physicians; 2011. Online. Available: https://www.acponline.org/system/files/documents/advocacy/current_policy_papers/assets/health_care_resources.pdf (accessed 12 January 2022).
16. Al-Khatib S, Hellkamp A, Curtis J, et al. Non-evidence-based ICD implantations in the United States. JAMA 2011;305:43–9.
17. Wennberg J, Fisher E, Skinner J. Geography and the debate over Medicare reform. Health Aff (Millwood) 2002;Suppl web exclusive:W96–W114.
18. Moynihan R, Doust J, Henry D. Preventing overdiagnosis: how to stop harming the healthy. BMJ 2012;344:e3502.
19. Australian Commission on Safety and Quality in Health Care. Australian Atlas of health variation. Sydney: ACSQHC; 2015.
20. Swensen S, Kaplan G, Meyer G, et al. Controlling healthcare costs by removing waste: what American doctors can do now. BMJ Qual Saf 2011;20:534–7.

21. Marshall M, Ovretveit J. Can we save money by improving quality? BMJ Qual Saf 2011;20:293–6.
22. Aarons G. Measuring provider attitudes toward evidence-based practice: consideration of organizational context and individual differences. Child Adolesc Psychiatr Clin N Am 2005;14:255–71.
23. Glisson C, James L. The cross-level effects of culture and climate in human service teams. J Organ Behav 2002;23:767–94.
24. Sirio C, Segel K, Keyser D, et al. Pittsburgh regional healthcare initiative: a systems approach for achieving perfect patient care. Health Aff (Millwood) 2003;22:157–65.
25. Lukas C, Holmes S, Cohen A, et al. Transformational change in health care systems: an organizational model. Health Care Manage Rev 2007;32:309–20.
26. Aarons G. Transformational and transactional leadership: association with attitudes toward evidence-based practice. Psychiatr Serv 2006;57:1162–9.
27. Bradley E, Webster T, Baker D, et al. Translating research into practice: speeding the adoption of innovative health care programs. Issue Brief (Commonw Fund) 2004;724:1–12.
28. Jung D. Transformational and transactional leadership and their effects on creativity in groups. Creat Res J 2001;13:185–95.
29. Ubbink DT, Vermeulen H, Knops AM, et al. Implementation of evidence-based practice: outside the box, throughout the hospital. Neth J Med 2011;69:87–94.
30. Caldwell E, Whitehead M, Fleming J, et al. Evidence-based practice in everyday clinical practice: strategies for change in a tertiary occupational therapy department. Aust Occup Ther J 2008;55:79–84.
31. Lucas B, Evans A, Reilly B, et al. The impact of evidence on physicians' inpatient treatment decisions. J Gen Intern Med 2004;19:402–9.
32. Davidoff F, Miglus J. Delivering clinical evidence where it's needed: building an information system worthy of the profession. JAMA 2011;305:1906–7.
33. Brassey J, Elwyn G, Price C, et al. Just in time information for clinicians: a questionnaire evaluation of the ATTRACT project. BMJ 2001;322:529–30.
34. Del Mar C, Silagy C, Glasziou P, et al. Feasibility of an evidence-based literature search service for general practitioners. Med J Aust 2001;175:134–7.
35. McGowan J, Hogg W, Campbell C, et al. Just-in-time information improved decision-making in primary care: a randomised controlled trial. PLOS ONE 2008;3:e3785.
36. Kawamoto K, Houlihan C, Balas E, et al. Improving clinical practice using clinical decision support systems: a systematic review of trials to identify features critical to success. BMJ 2005;330:765.
37. Roshanov P, Fernandes N, Wilczynski J, et al. Features of effective computerised clinical decision support systems: meta-regression of 162 randomised trials. BMJ 2013;346:f657.
38. Bright T, Wong A, Dhurjati R, et al. Effects of clinical decision support systems: a systematic review. Ann Intern Med 2012;157:29–43.
39. McCord G, Smucker W, Selius B, et al. Answering questions at the point of care: do residents practice EBM or manage information sources? Acad Med 2007;82:298–303.
40. Jones, DJ, Anton M, Gonzalez M, et al. Incorporating mobile phone technologies to expand evidence-based care. Cogn Behav Pract 2015;22(3):281–90.
41. Kruse CS, Ehbar N. Effects of computerized decision support systems on practitioner performance and patient outcomes: Systematic review. JMIR Med Inform 2020;8(8):e17283.
42. Westbrook J, Coiera E, Gosling A. Do online information retrieval systems help experienced health professionals answer clinical questions? J Am Med Inform Assoc 2005;12:315–21.
43. Cook DA, Enders F, Linderbaum JA, et al. Speed and accuracy of a point of care web-based knowledge resource for clinicians: a controlled crossover trial. Interact J Med Res 2014;3(1):e7.
44. Miller M, Strazdins E, Young S, et al. A retrospective single-site data-linkage study comparing manual to electronic data abstraction for routine post-operative nausea and vomiting audit. Int J Qual Health Care 2021;33(3):mzab116.
45. Gold J, Reyes-Gastelum D, Turner J, et al. A quality improvement study using fishbone analysis and an electronic medical records intervention to improve care for children with asthma. Am J Med Qual 2014;29:70–7.
46. Coomarasamy A, Khan K. What is the evidence that postgraduate teaching in evidence-based medicine changes anything? A systematic review. BMJ 2004;329:1017.
47. Straus S, Ball C, Balcombe N, et al. Teaching evidence-based medicine skills can change practice in a community hospital. J Gen Intern Med 2005;20:340–3.
48. Murad M, Montori V, Kunz R, et al. How to teach evidence-based medicine to teachers: reflections from a workshop experience. J Eval Clin Pract 2009;15:1205–7.
49. Menon A, Korner-Bitensky N, Kastner M, et al. Strategies for rehabilitation professionals to move evidence-based knowledge into practice: a systematic review. J Rehabil Med 2009;41:1024–32.
50. Slawson D, Shaughnessy A. Teaching evidence-based medicine: should we be teaching information management instead? Acad Med 2005;80:685–9.
51. Smith CA, Ganschow PS, Reilly BM, et al. Teaching residents evidence-based medicine skills: a controlled trial of effectiveness and assessment of durability. J Gen Intern Med. 2000;15(10):710–15.
52. Kitto S, Petrovic A, Gruen RL, et al. Evidence-based medicine training and implementation in surgery: the role of surgical cultures. J Eval Clin Pract 2011;17:819–26.
53. Kulier R, Coppus SFP, Zamora J, et al. The effectiveness of a clinically integrated e-learning course in evidence-based medicine: a cluster randomised controlled trial. BMC Med Educ 2009;9:21.
54. Glasziou P. ACP Journal Club. Applying evidence: what's the next action? Ann Intern Med 2009;150:JC1-2, JC1-3.

55. Scott I, Phelps G. Measurement for improvement: getting one to follow the other. Intern Med J 2009;39:347–51.

56. Scott I, Wakefield J. Deciding when quality and safety improvement interventions warrant widespread adoption. Med J Aust 2013;198:408–10.

57. Davies P, Walker A, Grimshaw J. A systematic review of the use of theory in the design of guideline dissemination and implementation strategies and interpretation of results of rigorous evaluations. Implement Sci 2010;5:14–19.

58. Evans S, Scott I, Johnson N, et al. Development of clinical-quality registries in Australia: the way forward. Med J Aust 2011;194:360–3.

59. LaBresh K. Quality of acute stroke care improvement framework for the Paul Coverdell National Acute Stroke Registry: facilitating policy and system change at the hospital level. Am J Prev Med 2006;31(Suppl. 2):S246–S250.

60. Scott I, Denaro C, Bennett C, et al.; for the Brisbane Cardiac Consortium Leadership Group. Achieving better in-hospital and post-hospital care of patients recently admitted with acute cardiac disease. Med J Aust 2004;180:S83–S88.

61. Scott I, Darwin I, Harvey K, et al. Multisite, quality-improvement collaboration to optimise cardiac care in Queensland public hospitals. Med J Aust 2004;180:392–7.

62. Wells S, Tamir O, Gray J, et al. Are quality improvement collaboratives effective? A systematic review. BMJ Qual Saf 2018;27(3):226–40.

63. Australian Commission on Safety and Quality in Health Care. Clinical Care Standards. ACSQHC; 2019. Online. Available: https://www.safetyandquality.gov.au/standards/clinical-care-standards.

64. Scott I, Coory M, Wills R, et al. Impact of hospital-wide clinical process redesign on clinical outcomes: a comparative study of internally versus externally led intervention. BMJ Qual Saf 2011;20:539–48.

65. Scott I, Guyatt G. Clinical practice guidelines: the need for greater transparency in formulating recommendations. Med J Aust 2011;195:29–33.

66. Bradley E, Holmboe E, Mattera J, et al. Data feedback efforts in quality improvement: lessons learned from US hospitals. Qual Saf Health Care 2004;13:26–31.

67. Beer M, Eisenstat R, Spector B. Why change programs don't produce change. Harv Bus Rev 1990;68:158–66.

68. Kizer K. The 'new VA': a national laboratory for health care quality management. Am J Med Qual 1999;14:3–20.

69. Demakis J, McQueen L, Kizer K, et al. Quality Enhancement Research Initiative (QUERI): a collaboration between research and clinical practice. Med Care 2000;38(Suppl. 1):I17–I25.

70. Jha A, Perlin J, Kizer K, et al. Effect of the transformation of the Veterans Affairs health care system on the quality of care. N Engl J Med 2003;348:2218–27.

71. Schilling L, Dearing J, Staley P, et al. Kaiser Permanente's performance improvement system, part 4: creating a learning organization. Jt Comm J Qual Patient Saf 2011;37:532–43.

72. Schilling L, Deas D, Jedlinsky M, et al. Kaiser Permanente's performance improvement system, part 2: developing a value framework. Jt Comm J Qual Patient Saf 2010;36:552–60.

73. James B, Savitz L. How Intermountain trimmed health care costs through robust quality improvement efforts. Health Aff (Millwood) 2011;30:1185–91.

74. Wagner E, Austin B, Davis C, et al. Improving chronic illness care: translating evidence into action. Health Aff (Millwood) 2001;20:64–78.

75. Coleman K, Austin B, Brach C, et al. Evidence on the Chronic Care Model in the new millennium. Health Aff (Millwood) 2009;28:75–85.

76. Tideman P, Tirimacco R, Senior D, et al. Impact of a regionalised clinical cardiac support network on mortality among rural patients with myocardial infarction. Med J Aust 2014;200:157–60.

77. Ubbink DT, Guyatt GH, Vermeulen H. Framework of policy recommendations for implementation of evidence-based practice: a systematic scoping review. BMJ Open 2013;3: e001881.

78. Oman K, Duran C, Fink R. Evidence-based policy and procedures: an algorithm for success. J Nurs Adm 2008;38:47–51.

79. French B, Thomas LH, Baker P, et al. What can management theories offer evidence-based practice? A comparative analysis of measurement tools for organizational context. Implement Sci 2009;4:28.

80. Hess BJ, Weng W, Lynn LA, et al. Setting a fair performance standard for physicians' quality of patient care. J Gen Intern Med 2011;26(5):467–73.

81. Wensing M, Wollersheim H, Grol R. Organisational interventions to implement improvements in patient care: a structured review of reviews. Implement Sci 2006;1:2.

82. Lukas C, Engle R, Holmes S, et al. Strengthening organisations to implement evidence-based clinical practices. Health Care Manage Rev 2010;35:235–45.

83. Powell B, McMillen J, Proctor E, et al. A compilation of strategies for implementing clinical innovations in health and mental health. Med Care Res Rev 2012;69:123–57.

84. Correa VC, Lugo-Agudelo LH, Aguirre-Acevedo DC, et al. Individual, health system, and contextual barriers and facilitators for the implementation of clinical practice guidelines: a systematic metareview. Health Res Policy Syst 2020;18:74.

INDEX

Page numbers followed by 'f' indicate figures, 't' indicate tables, and 'b' indicate boxes.